Anthr

Dedicated to our friend and teacher, Thomas McKeen (1953–1993),
to whom we owe the inspiration for this book.

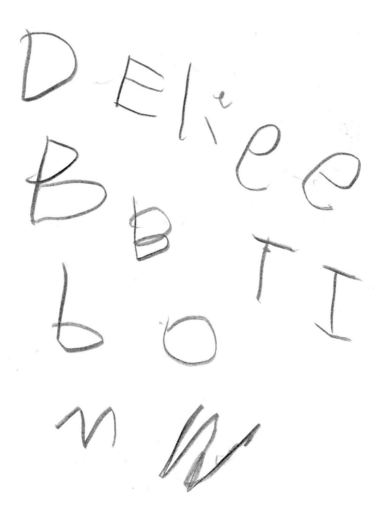

ANTHROPOSOPHIC NURSING PRACTICE

Foundations and Indications for Everyday Healthcare

ROLF HEINE, EDITOR

With contributions from Klaus Adams, Frances Bay, Gudrun Buchholz, Annegret Camps, Bernhard Deckers, Carola Edelmann, Sasha Gloor, Renate Hasselberg, Inge Heine, Rolf Heine, Christel Kaul, Monika Layer, Regula Markwalder, Heike Schaumann, Jana Schier, Ada van der Star, Christoph von Dach, Ursula von der Heide, Gabriele Weber, and Anna Wilde

With Forewords by Matthias Girke, and Michaela Glöckler

Introduction to the English Edition by Adam Blanning

In collaboration with Hanna Wäckerle, Karolin Steinke, and Ulrich Meyer

Portal Books | 2020

Published by Portal Books, an imprint of SteinerBooks / Anthroposophic Press, Inc.
402 Union Street #58, Hudson, New York 12534
www.steinerbooks.org

This book is a translation of *Anthroposophische Pflegepraxis – Grundlagen und Anregungen für alltägliches Handeln,* 4th corrected and expanded edition 2017, published by Salumed Verlag, Berlin, Germany, .

Translated from the German by Carol Brousseau.

ISBN: 978-1-938685-28-6

Important note: *Nursing care is in constant development. The information in this book has been compiled with care and in accordance with the current state of knowledge of the authors and the publisher but is subject to change as a result of new knowledge. Every user is required to handle the content on his or her own responsibility, as neither the authors nor the publisher can assume any liability. The publisher is grateful for feedback on any inaccuracies. Trade names and product names are used within the framework of the general freedom of the press, without regard to producer interests.*

Contents

Methodical-Didactical Foundations

Anthroposophy and Nursing

CHAPTER III   Frances Bay

The Anthropological Foundations of Nursing
Extended by Anthroposophy 31

CHAPTER IV   Renate Hasselberg • Rolf Heine

Illness and Destiny 58

CHAPTER V   Renate Hasselberg • Rolf Heine

Nursing as a Path of Development 78

CHAPTER VI   Rolf Heine

CHAPTER VII   Rolf Heine

CHAPTER XIV   Rolf Heine

Active Principles in External Applications
The Nature of External Applications—How They Differ from Other Medical and Nursing Interventions . 297

CHAPTER XVIII   Klaus Adams

CHAPTER XIX   Bernhard Deckers

CHAPTER XX   Jana Schier

CHAPTER XXI   Ada van der Star • Annegret Camps

CHAPTER XXII   Christel Kaul

CHAPTER XXIII   Heike Schaumann

CHAPTER XXV   Gudrun Buchhol

Introduction to the English Edition

This first English-language edition of *Anthroposophic Nursing Practice* shows not only the possibility, but already the practical experience of nursing care which is both holistic and optimistic in its orientation. That is a cause for celebration! Whole person paradigms and optimism are not so easy to find in our current medical environment, but to claim them as part of anthroposophic practice is no exaggeration. That is because the knowledge and perspectives gathered in this book have matured through the work of multiple generations of nurses, all striving to refine a truly integrative nursing practice.

The nursing care, gestures, and clinical tools described have roots in the generous tradition of nursing as a caring profession, and connect back to that deeper philosophy. For that reason, one might assume that anthroposophic nursing relies largely on a sentimental approach, on trying to balance the pressures of technology and limited time with kind stories and anecdotes. It does not—it goes much deeper. Anthroposophic nursing brings a true picture of the human being on the levels of body, soul, and spirit, and how they work together to create a whole. This is not about adding in an extra layer of kindness, it is about recognizing the fundamental one-sidedness of a medicine that continually places external material measures of care above a real cultivation of healing. We need this picture. It is very urgent, given the high burnout rates that are found across the nursing and medical professions, which on the one hand results from shifts towards greater patient loads, more time on electronic medical records, and hardly any time to actually be with patients, and at the same time states that the answer to this problem is for nurses to simply cultivate more self-care. More and more that feels like asking someone to swallow a large stone, made palatable by sprinkling a little sugar on top. The stone still sits in your stomach, and weighs on your heart. We do not need more saccharine sentiments, we need a fundamental reorientation. We need nursing that responds to the physical and spiritual needs of both patients and those who care for them at the foundation, not merely as an afterthought. That change can is possible.

Just as anthroposophic nursing does not rely on sentiment, it also does not rely on nostalgia. The natural substances, body treatments, compresses, poultices, and hot water bottles that are a core part of anthroposophic nursing do have a long history, one which might feel so far removed from the highly technical environment of most hospitals as to not even seem practical. But that too would be a misjudgment. That claim is easily disproved by simply receiving one of these nursing treatments, and then one very quickly realizes that they open a whole realm of clinical practices which actively nourish, calm, and soothe. When ill, they guide your body to an enhanced state of well-being, to a quieter, more regenerative state. They acknowledge the body's own intrinsic healing processes, and actively call on them. Once you have experienced a hot yarrow tea liver compress, you will no longer be tempted to dismiss the "simplicity" of these practices but will, instead, likely mourn our loss of knowledge about how deeply healing it is to be warmed, touched, calmed, and nurtured in this way. These nursing techniques are simple, safe, effective, and humane.

Now, the optimism. When we gain knowledge and tools to better meet the whole person, as a being of body, soul, and spirit, we cannot help but see the unique individual who stands inside all the symptoms and diagnoses. That is the true patient. The reality of that core spiritual kernel invites us to be a companion. It grants us eyes to see how illness can be a pathway for a fundamental change of being. From a strictly materialistic point of view, we might say that healing is just a "repair" that returns us to a previous level of functioning, a bit like swapping out a broken part in a car engine, but that addresses only the physical body, at best. In truth, we are different people on the other side of an illness. We are transformed in a way you may not be able to see on an x-ray. What was previously an unconscious part of our physiology has now been reclaimed because we have had to consciously meet an imbalance and work through it. A patient who has had a life-threatening illness may, once recovered, be told to "just go back to your old life," but that is hollow advice—life is different now. Even a child who has had flu and strong fever will take new step of immune maturation, of defining and claiming the boundaries of self, emerging on the other side of the illness a slightly different person. Indeed, when we accompany a dying patient, there are shifts in consciousness, burdens released, changes made, so that (and this is shared from personal experience) it is very possible to realize that even though a person's physical body has died the individual has healed in a profound way. There is always goodness that can come through care.

May we all find the seeds we need for future growth.

ADAM BLANNING, MD
PRESIDENT, ANTHROPOSOPHIC HEALTH ASSOCIATION (AHA)
JANUARY 2020

Preface

Twenty years have passed since the first publication of this book. That is a long time for a textbook! The hopes and fears that the authors associated with the first and second editions regarding developments in the European health care system have come true in the main areas. First, the fears: efforts to economize in hospitals, inpatient care for the elderly, and home nursing care has allowed the core task of the nursing profession, namely the relationship between people, to recede further into the background. Illness has long been a lucrative business—and nursing has become a branch of the economy in its own right. Economizing is nothing reprehensible, but when profit generation becomes a main motive of medicine and nursing care, when people profit primarily from the suffering and dependence of others, then a line has been crossed which also corrupts professional and ethical action. The excessive documentation that has resulted from the economization and legalization of the health care system, and quality assurance that acquires a questionable right to exist by collecting all kinds of indicators, are excesses of a system that serves itself more than the patient and the person in need of care.

This has an impact on the nursing profession, on professional action, on the motivation of newcomers to the profession and, of course, on the quality of care that patients, people in need of ongoing care and home residents experience in practice. For some years now, specialist literature has complained about the neglect of so-called soft skills in nursing practice. This refers to those areas in which social interactions, inner attitudes and ethical convictions shape the quality of care. The term 'soft skills' has an obvious analogy to computer software. Like software, these soft skills convey a quality that can be experienced directly by the 'user', while 'hardware' refers to aspects such as employee keys, employee qualifications and professional standards, which must be available but only become relevant through concrete human encounters. "I don't want to be operated on by either a badly trained surgeon or an ill-tempered one" is how the relationship between hard and soft qualities can be perfectly formulated from the patient's point of view. The term 'soft skills' thus refers to the phenomenon of a direct effect of people upon people. Particularly when treating people who have cognitive, mental or psychological impairments (perception disorders, delirium, dementia), the ability of nurses and doctors to communicate has an elementary influence on the patient's situation. This "rediscovery" is one of the particularly positive developments of the last decade. Especially in oncology and palliative medicine, yet also in the treatment of dementia, soft skills are once again considered to be standard principles of professional practice.

Anthroposophic nursing care goes beyond the communicative approach of soft skills. The nurse's valuing of the human body in anthroposophic nursing care, his or her attentiveness of touch, use of warmth, cold, air and light to promote healing processes, form a solid bridge between treatment of the body and treatment of the patient's soul and spirit. And this connection is needed more than ever today. For, although physical well-being, autonomy and youthfulness are central to our materialistic culture, our bodies actually receive little respect and appreciation, especially when they become old and ill. The nursing values that need to be rediscovered are those of respecting the debased human being, embracing illness as a part of existence, and allowing time for healing.

Anthroposophic nursing care has developed further in recent decades. Anthroposophic nursing practice is now substantiated by initial results of nursing research, especially in the field of external applications. In many areas, essential impulses from our anthroposophic work have been able to flow into general nursing care. External applications and embrocations are increasingly being integrated into the care provided at conventional facilities, especially palliative care. The conflict between 'conventional medicine' and 'complementary medicine' has long since ceased to be as ideological as it was in the previous century. How can anthroposophic nursing care contribute to this process of integration? To us, this question also seems existential for the future of anthroposophic nursing. With the new edition of this book we want to make a contribution to explaining the philosophical and anthroposophic-anthropological background of anthroposophic nursing care. Practical examples show how this type of nursing affects everyday life for patients and people in need of nursing care. The book's detailed descriptions of how to perform nursing applications are an important aid for those who want to learn anthroposophic nursing. A focal point of the book is the concept of nursing gestures, which relates inner attitudes and practical nursing activities to one another in detail, with numerous examples and overviews. Many new contributions in this edition have taken up the idea of nursing care gestures, illustrating how this concept has shaped the anthroposophic understanding of nursing in recent years.

It remains to say thanks to those who have made this book possible. They are first and foremost the patients and people whom we have been allowed to care for and who have taught us. We would also like to thank all our colleagues, friends and partners who accompanied the sometimes difficult birth of these texts with a critical and encouraging eye. The publication of this book would never have been possible within a year without the commitment of Salumed Verlag and its sure-eyed editors Hanna Wäckerle and Ulrich Meyer. Finally, we thank Matthias Girke from the bottom of our hearts for his faithful, encouraging commitment to the new edition of this nursing book.

ROLF HEINE
FILDERSTADT, JANUARY 2015

Foreword to the Fourth German Edition

It is with great pleasure that I look forward to the fourth edition of this important work on anthroposophic nursing care, which has already become necessary after just two years. This book presents the essential basics of professional nursing care for the ill, the elderly and children, looks at building relationships with patients, and discusses professional inner development in a transparent, comprehensible and practical way. The importance of this information seems to grow almost daily. The medical professions are currently subject to increasing fragmentation. Specialization is often accompanied by selective deprofessionalization of the profession as a whole: in the work of physicians, for example, increasingly complex interventional measures are required, for which comprehensive basic medical training no longer appears to be mandatory. Why should an intervening specialist deal with subjects such as psychiatry, psychosomatics or ophthalmology? Is it not enough—and therefore would it not also be cheaper—to offer specialized training in the respective process technique and avoid the "ballast" of a six-year course of study? The same applies to nursing care. Which tasks are inseparable from the nursing profession and which can be delegated? Some see even body care and the direct, everyday assistance that patients require as mere 'neighborly services', not professional activities. Many also think that preparing and administering medications can be delegated. The same applies to the other healing professions.

With this breakdown of the professions, their true nature and meaning are becoming increasingly "invisible," to the point where they might even disappear entirely from increasingly intervention-oriented hospitals. The result is detrimental to the decisive qualities needed by a kind of medicine that wishes to serve the patient, and it erodes the appreciation of the professions that are existentially connected with the art of healing.

Against this background, it is extremely important to reflect on the actual nature of the nursing profession, which this book edited by Rolf Heine does in detail. In every "external" activity live additional, "inner" dimensions, which are decisive for the action's effectiveness. Thus, it is not just "external" nursing care that affects the basic care of patients, it is the dynamic process of nursing that is reflected in the individual measures and their (if necessary, rhythmic) implementation. In addition, the nurse's mental and emotional accompaniment of the patient is of great importance: it is now well documented how important the soul is for healing and especially for wound healing. Patients who are depressed, agitated or tense have poorer wound healing.[1] Almost one hundred years ago Rudolf Steiner pointed out the importance of the soul for healing: "Contentment ... strengthens the etheric body in relation to its vital force [so] wounds heal more easily in a contented person."[2] The inner attitude of the nurse has a direct effect on the patient's inner world of soul and thus promotes the patient's vital forces in wound healing. Finally, therapeutic attitudes, the spiritual aims of healing, have essential significance: the measures taken have a stabilizing effect on patients when they follow a spiritual goal, an inner conviction and therapeutic intuition. The patient experiences a therapeutic will to heal that creates an outlook for the future, even hope, and has a positive effect on the course of the illness and possibly also on the prognosis. Different dimensions can thus be developed within nursing activities which are directly connected with healing and therapy. To delegate basic nursing care to a robot-supported "provision of services" would merely copy the mechanical aspect of nursing care measures and would not allow any dimensions of life, soul and spirit to enter in. The latter are certainly not "nice to have," they are significant, because they have a direct strengthening effect on healing processes, and they lead from mechanization to humanization in medicine. These qualities require ethical and spiritual development, as well as professional training, as is shown in this fundamental anthroposophic work. Training and developing one's own personality enables nurses to identify with the nursing profession, which is also indispensable in modern patient care, and it shows ways in which nursing measures and therapeutic applications can develop in a committed relationship with the patient that is supported by a therapeutic will. Many thanks are due to the editor, the authors, and of course the publisher for their commitment to human-oriented nursing care! May this fourth edition also find a large readership and may its many suggestions for anthroposophic nursing practice bear fruit. Especially patients will be grateful!

DR. MED. MATTHIAS GIRKE
MEDICAL SECTION OF THE SCHOOL OF SPIRITUAL SCIENCE AT THE GOETHEANUM /
HAVELHÖHE COMMUNITY HOSPITAL, MAY 2017

References

[1] Godbout, J.P.; Glaser R. Stress-induced immune dysregulation: implications for wound healing, infectious disease and cancer. *Journal of Neuroimmune Pharmacology* 2006; 4, pp. 427–427.
House, S.H. Psychological distress and its impact on wound healing. An integrative Review. *Journal of wound, ostomy, and continence nursing: official publication of The Wound, Ostomy and Continence Nurses Society* 2015; 42 (1), pp. 38–41.
[2] Steiner, R. Lecture of December 11, 1910, in *Paths and goals of the spiritual human being. Life questions in the light of spiritual science.* Rudolf Steiner Press, Forest Row UK 2015.

Foreword to the Third German Edition

The quality of nursing care determines how well cared for and in good hands a person can feel when he or she is in hospital due to an accident or acute illness—or how abandoned and helpless. Good outpatient nursing care enables many people in need of help and care to remain in their familiar home environment when their relatives are unable to cope with their care. Nursing care does not just accompany human life from birth to death, from cutting the umbilical cord to the last wash of the deceased. Nursing care is also a way of life, a cultural asset—it stands for human sympathy, "sisterliness" and "brotherliness"—for empathy and interest in what the other person needs. Perceptiveness, attentiveness and competent assistance belong just as much to the central values of this profession as universally human-oriented spirituality.

It is very much to be welcomed that this standard work on anthroposophic nursing practice is now being published in its third revised and significantly expanded edition—precisely because the academicization and economization of the nursing profession are continuing inexorably—often to the detriment of the quality of care in the everyday work environment. After all, this work is an essential contribution to a nursing culture that has developed and spread worldwide since its beginnings in 1921, in a small anthroposophic hospital in Arlesheim, Switzerland, founded by the Dutch physician Ita Wegman (1876–1943). The authors come from various clinics and institutions, which makes the spectrum of topics and specialties very varied, so that every nurse—no matter which field he or she is working in—is given valuable ideas as well as new techniques and possibilities for helping patients.

The authors wish to illuminate the general human and cultural dimensions of nursing, expanding it beyond what nursing is thought to be in a narrower sense. "Anthroposophy" means simply, translated into everyday language: "humanness." So, anthroposophic nursing is not bound to a specific 'anthroposophic' clinic, medical practice or institution for special needs. It can be used wherever the ideal of human-oriented and humanity-enhancing nursing care is sought. For this reason, the material presented here can also provide motivated laypeople, social workers, educators and a variety of other therapeutically oriented professions with inspiration for their daily work.

May this book contribute to a breakthrough of a consciously re-learned and practiced humanity in the nursing practice of our time, which is increasingly characterized by mechanization, rationalization and practical constraints. May it also contribute to forming and consolidating the identity of a profession that is decidedly an ideal for the future: for to voluntarily be a nurse to someone else, without asking for anything in return, is one of the basic Christian values, without whose consideration and cultivation the social problems of humanity cannot be solved—neither privately nor in society as a whole.

DR. MED. MICHAELA GLÖCKLER
MEDICAL SECTION AT THE GOETHEANUM, FEBRUARY 2015

Methodical–Didactical Foundations

CHAPTER I

How Do You Learn Anthroposophic Nursing? Learning Aid and Guide through this Textbook

ROLF HEINE

Anthroposophic nursing care is an extension of present-day professional nursing based on experience, tradition, and science. Anthroposophic nursing care has been practiced in hospitals, treatment centers, sanatoriums, institutions for the elderly, and in private homes for decades. Anthroposophic nursing care enables Anthroposophic Medicine to be applied to the everyday life of patients. In addition, it makes its own independent nursing contribution developed from anthroposophic spiritual science. Its theoretical and practical foundations are freely accessible. They can be learned firstly by working in anthroposophic institutions, secondly in advanced training courses, and thirdly in self-study. This textbook supports these three paths. It offers background knowledge for starting work in an anthroposophic nursing facility, orientation during the initial phase of familiarization, study material for basic and advanced training, as well as support and encouragement for independent study.

Each chapter is preceded by a brief summary and ends with suggested learning objectives for that chapter. One learning objective relates to fundamental practical skills, one to the relationship between patients and nurses, and one to the theoretical basis for the material presented. To achieve these or self-chosen learning goals, we suggest one of the three learning paths explained below.[1]

Learning path

Fundamental practical skills	Relationships	Knowledge
Learning path A	Learning path B	Learning path C

1. Working with the text

1.1 Read the chapter attentively.	**1.1** Read the chapter attentively.	**1.1** Read the chapter attentively.
1.2 Try to reproduce the content as accurately as possible from memory after each section.		**1.2** Mark the passages that explain the spiritual-scientific background or your learning objective.
1.3 Reread the passages that you cannot remember.		**1.3** Look up the cross-references in other chapters.
1.4 Try to clarify what you do not yet understand by reading the cross-references in the text, for example.		**1.4** Try to reproduce the content from memory.

2. "Warming up" to the topic

2.1 What do you find interesting in this chapter, what seems less important to you? What can you be enthusiastic about?	**2.1** What understanding of nursing care is the text based on?	**2.1** What makes sense to you, what do you find difficult to understand?
	2.2 Which inner attitudes do you find worth striving for?	
	2.3 Which inner attitudes do you not want to share in?	

3. Discussion

3.1 Compare the content of the chapter with your own experiences.	**3.1** Which positive and which negative experiences with patients shape your daily work?	**3.1** What prompts you to disagree?
3.2 Where have you had similar experiences? What must you contradict from your own experience? What can you add from your own experience?	**3.2** What do you find particularly stressful when encountering patients?	**3.2** How does the approach presented here differ from other concepts known to you?
	3.3 Ask colleagues to share their experiences with you.	

4.   Develop your own questions and set your own goals

4.1 What do you want to learn about the subject of the chapter? What skills do you want to acquire?	**4.1** Formulate your own learning objective or specify the proposed learning objective.	**4.1** Formulate your own learning objective or specify the proposed learning objective.
4.2 Formulate the learning objective differently for yourself. Maybe it needs to be narrowed down or expanded upon.	**4.2** What situations do you want to change?	**4.2** Which question moves you the most?
4.3 Determine your next learning steps in nursing practice. What do you want to practice?	**4.3** How do you want to act in these situations in the future?	**4.3** Write down this question.

5.   Practice

5.1 Practice the chosen exercise.	**5.1** Look for the described difficult situation in practice and try to look at it from the point of view that you have gained.	**5.1** Try to understand a matter that is of particular interest to you from the point of view presented.
5.2 How did the patient experience your nursing care?	**5.2** If you want to strengthen your mental powers, look for a suitable exercise. You can find suggestions for this in the chapter "Nursing as a Path of Development."	**5.2** Explain your discovery to a colleague.
5.3 How did you feel during the nursing procedure?	**5.3** Continue to actively seek out the situation that caused you problems.	**5.3** Which new questions arise?
5.4 What were you satisfied with, what were you dissatisfied with? Were your expectations fulfilled?		
5.5 What do you want to do better or differently next time?		
5.6 Repeat the selected exercise until you are satisfied with the result.		

Fundamental practical skills	Relationships	Knowledge
Learning path A	Learning path B	Learning path C

6. Deepening and expanding upon the material presented

6.1 Deepen what you have learned by reading the chapter again and taking note of additional or corrective suggestions.	**6.1** In the text, look for aspects that could give you an answer to your problem.	**6.1** Accept confidently your own objections or contrary arguments from third parties.
6.2 Share your experiences with colleagues.	**6.2** Observe how colleagues react in difficult situations.	**6.2** Ask yourself the written question again and again.
6.3 Ask colleagues to observe you providing nursing care.	**6.3** What impresses you about your colleague?	**6.3** Keep your question under constant review and follow up on any sugges- tions that you come across over time.
6.4 Search for complementary literature, attend continuing education courses.		

7. Acting creatively

7.1 Try to transfer your skills to new situations and cultivate them.	**7.1** Try to gain a fresh under- standing of the difficult situation and act freely.	**7.1** Examine whether the aspects gained make everyday nursing care easier to understand.

Example of working with the learning pathways

Learning path A (fundamental practical skills) below will show how the work with one chapter of the book can become fruitful. You can work with other chapters and self-chosen learning goals in the same way.

Chapter: "Variations in Whole-Body Washing"

Learning objective: You are confident in your ability to administer the three basic types of therapeutic washing.

Learning path A

1.1 Read the chapter attentively.
- Read the section on Variations in Whole-Body Washing once.

1.2   Try to reproduce the content as accurately as possible from memory after each section.

- Section 1: General aspects: In principle, washing can be done with four different objectives. We give preference to addressing the patient's physical body, life forces, mental state, or 'I', depending on the procedure.
- Proceed in the same way with the other sections.

1.3   Reread the passages that you cannot remember.

- The section on the "Invigorating wash" was difficult to remember. Read it again.

1.4   Try to clarify what you do not yet understand, for example by reading the cross-references in the text.

- You did not understand the following passage from the section on the "Invigorating wash": "The pressure exerted by the washing mitt or towel should not cause any tissue to be pushed forward (as with Rhythmical Einreibung)." [→ Chap. "Rhythmical Einreibung"] Look up the reference to Rhythmical Einreibung.

2.1   What do you find interesting in this chapter, what seems less important to you? What can you be enthusiastic about?

- You were especially interested in the statement that hand and foot baths can replace a whole-body wash for someone who is seriously ill.

3.1   Compare the content of the chapter with your own experiences.

- You compare your experiences with basal stimulation with the information in the chapter.

3.2   Where have you had similar experiences? What must you contradict from your own experience? What can you add from your own experience?

- Positive experiences with basal stimulation.

4.1   What do you wish to learn about the subject of the chapter? What skills do you wish to acquire?

- Washing according to principles known from Rhythmical Einreibung.

4.2   Formulate the learning objective differently for yourself. Maybe it needs to be narrowed down or expanded upon.

- "I'd like to learn to work with calm, rhythmic movements when washing a patient's whole body."
- "I'd like to gain experience in giving hand and foot baths to seriously ill patients."

4.3 Determine your next learning steps for nursing practice. What do you want to practice?
- I want to wash the patients entrusted to my care with calm, rhythmic movements on my next day of work. Give Mrs. T. a hand and foot bath as a substitute for the more strenuous whole-body wash.

5.1 Practice the chosen exercise.
- The next morning, you give Mrs. T. a hand and foot bath. Since she had been incontinent, you first clean her genital area.
- You then wash Mrs. M.'s back using calm circling movements.

5.2 How did the patient experience your nursing care?
- Mrs. T. was visibly less strained. After the wash, she fell asleep, relaxed.
- Mrs. M. noticed no difference to other washes, but she was satisfied with the treatment.

5.3 How did you feel during the nursing procedure?
- I experienced an almost meditative mood when giving the hand and foot bath.
- I was distracted by the fact that Mrs. M. wanted to tell me something.

5.4 What were you satisfied with, what were you dissatisfied with? Were your expectations fulfilled?
- I was satisfied by my work with Mrs. T.
- I was unhappy with the fact that I could not concentrate on my quiet movements with Mrs. M.

5.5 What do you want to do better or differently next time?
- Stay calm. Practice the rhythmic movement of the back wash on a colleague beforehand.

6.1 Deepen what you have learned by reading the chapter again and taking note of additional or corrective suggestions.
- You read the chapter again. As an additional aspect, you noticed the difference between washing towards the center of the body and towards the periphery.

6.2 Share your experiences with colleagues.
- They have no experience of their own with special types of washing. Some colleagues were familiar with other forms of therapeutic washing.

6.3   Ask colleagues to observe you providing nursing care.
- A colleague was happy to watch you give a hand and foot bath. She was impressed by the atmosphere created in the room. A fruitful conversation ensued.

6.4   Search for complementary literature, attend continuing education courses.
- You can obtain information about courses from *the North American Anthroposophic Nurses Association (www.anthroposophicnursing.org) or the International Council of Anthroposophic Nursing Associations (www. icana-ifan.org).*

7.1   Try to transfer your skills to new situations and cultivate them.
- After attending an advanced training course, you want to make this form of washing known to all your colleagues in an internal training course.

References

[1]   Cf. van Houten, C. *Awakening the will. Principles and processes in adult learning.* 2nd ed. Temple Lodge Publishing, 2000.

Anthroposophy and Nursing

CHAPTER II

Observation as a Method of Self-development
and a Therapeutic Element
in Care and Destiny

MONIKA LAYER

Perception and observation shape our image of the world. They are also the prerequisite for a differentiated understanding of the patient's situation in nursing care. This chapter presents exercises for training unbiased observation and prepares readers for nursing lessons. The relationship between perception and concept formation explains the epistemological background of anthroposophy.

→   Learning objectives, see end of chapter

1. Introduction

The first part of this chapter characterizes aspects of observation and offers a new understanding of the observation process and its relevance in nursing based on the epistemological principles explained in this context. It shows the personality-forming part of the observation process and explains its therapeutic effect on patients. The second part gives examples and exercises for observation training, which open up a focus on anthroposophically-oriented nursing training.

2. Starting out in nursing

What motivates people who decide to train to become a nurse? Interest in people, the desire to help, the desire to do something useful. This is how people starting out in their careers respond to questions about the reason for their choice of occupation. One could be inclined to put these statements into the drawer "helper syndrome," but this does not do justice to the prospective carers. Rather, these motivations express a basic humane attitude, perhaps also the desire to deal with questions about the meaning of life, illness, suffering and death and/or the search for real human encounters. It can be assumed that, in addition to existential questions and needs, young people also bring with them the necessary strength to cope with the goals they have set themselves.

In a nursing education these qualities and strengths should be preserved, promoted and substantiated by integrating and stressing personality-forming elements. In addition to the implementation of a socially-integrative educational philosophy, anthroposophically oriented education achieves this by teaching artistic subjects, by dealing with aspects of anthropology, and by a comprehensive training in observation. The points of view and methodologies presented here were developed at the "Freien Krankenpflegeschule an der Filderklinik" and are still being used there today in the design of nursing training.

3. Observation and maintenance

Although patient observation as a teaching subject has almost disappeared from curricula over the past twenty years, its real importance remains undiminished. The demand for accurate patient observation in nursing goes back historically to Florence Nightingale (1820–1919), who wrote:

> *"The most important practical lesson that can be given to nurses is to teach them what to observe–how to observe–what symptoms indicate improvement–what the reverse–which are of importance–which are of none–which are the evidence of neglect–and of what kind of neglect. All this is what ought to make part, and an essential part, of the training of every nurse."*[1]

Nightingale called for a systematic care based on observation and reflection. She thereby gave essential impulses for the development of the modern understanding of nursing as a calling.

As a consequence of the holistic and salutogenic orientation of nursing care, comprehensive observation that focuses on health is of great importance. Today, it is regarded as a means providing patient-oriented, professional care and is one of the first steps in the care process. The phenomena to be taken into account in observation are not only physical, but also the psychological and socio-cultural. The results are documented in the nursing anamnesis, then interpreted; results are incorporated into future planning, evaluated after implementation and possibly supplemented afterwards or already during the process. In all steps of the nursing process, attention, interest, and reflection are required, elements that are, in a comprehensive sense, part of observation.

3.1 Observation in care extended by anthroposophy

In nursing care extended by anthroposophy, observation is considered a core skill that must be intentionally developed. The physical, psychological, and socio-cultural dimensions are expanded to include the spiritual, and the results of the observations are integrated into the nursing process. The approach outlined here is based on the anthroposophical view of the human being and forms the basis for a more holistic approach to care. Learning and practicing careful observation is a type of training and can therefore play an important role in the process of individual self-development.

The following report, reproduced here in part, was written by a nursing student. In it, she describes questions and consequences that arose for her through the observation training in the context of her nursing training.

> *Can observation really be learned or is it a skill that is naturally available to everyone? What do I have to learn to acquire this ability? Is it useful or necessary to train my senses?*
>
> *These and other questions arose from practical tasks during the training at the nursing school. I had written a series of patient reports to practice observation. Subsequently, the question arose as to how I learn to observe. The following results became clear to me: My senses take in a great deal, but I can only grasp a little of it in my waking consciousness. In order to make myself aware of something, I need to be attentive and awake. In developing these two qualities, I see the actual possibility of learning to observe. It seems important to me that it is not about ... activities, but an inner attitude. This is already expressed in our everyday language. We say 'I see, I smell, I hear' but 'I am attentive, awake, interested.' Seeing, smelling, hearing are verbs; attentive, awake, and interested are adjectives. So, observation is not another activity I have to do, but I do what I do anyway, but with a changed basic attitude.*
>
> *In writing nursing reports, I experienced, like many of my classmates, that observing has clear effects on the one being observed. I was able to experience that the patients' behavior toward me changed when I observed them, without my changing my behavior toward them. That is why it has always been important to me that observations are not done in isolation. At the same time, it is important to pay attention to how the relationship between the other patients and the 'observed patient' changes.*
>
> *How can I learn to observe more precisely?*
>
> *Through my experiences with various patient descriptions I found that it was helpful if I directed my perceptions by asking questions. At the beginning of my observations a very general, indeterminate picture of the patient lived in me. I noticed it in the descriptions that were not very concrete. So I asked myself before the actual task began: What do I want to observe? What do I pay attention to the next time I meet the patient? At home I worked out the observations and tried to go through them again in response to these questions.*

Example

> *In one assignment, I dealt with the question of head and face. I talked a lot with the patient and looked at her face closely. At home I tried to describe it and suddenly noticed that I could see the eye, forehead, and nose area clearly in front of me and could describe it well. But there, where the mouth was, I found only an empty spot in my consciousness.*

This experience frightened me. I had the feeling that I had looked at the face closely. The jolt made me more alert, so that the next day I turned my attention to the lower part of the face. Thinking back on my observations, I also noticed that I could say a lot about certain things and nothing about others. In my opinion, this was due to the fact that certain features of the patient were particularly noticeable and that I am more attentive to certain areas. This means that I am more attentive to certain areas, which means I have a tendency to perceive selectively, i.e., only what I am interested in or what I have dealt with before. By working with my catalogue of questions, I was able to develop wakefulness, interest, and attention for aspects that I had not been aware of before.

Summary

In order to learn to observe more precisely and concretely it is:
- *important to reflect on your observations with temporal and spatial distance;*
- *very important to look at observations in regard to certain questions;*
- *essential to wake up to your own gaps in perception.*

The decisive factor for me was the practice of regularly carrying out the exercises. It was not necessary to spend much time with them; ten minutes of practice every day and I learned a lot.[2]

In her report, the author describes a number of issues that are essential in the context of patient observation:

1. the role of the sensory organs in the observation
2. the question of becoming aware of sensory impressions
3. the importance of attention
4. the relationship with the patient
5. the consistency of observation
6. the selective perception
7. the continuity of the observational process

In the following, these aspects will be illuminated from the perspective of anthroposophy. Prioritization of the areas addressed are made based on their relevance to nursing. Reference is made to literature for further reading. The order in which the aspects are dealt with varies. Since points two, three, and four form a thematic focus and are of greatest importance in this context, they are considered together last under the heading "Attention and Observation."

3.3 The function of the sense organs

Healthy sense organs are a prerequisite for observation. In anthroposophy, we exceed the number of senses described by general science and recognize twelve senses, each conveying different sensory qualities. Through them we experience our own body, our environment, and our fellow human beings in a very differentiated way. Anthroposophy understands perception mediated by the sense organs to have an objective character. Sensory experience within, and reality of life outside the individual are, therefore, the same in content but appear in different forms. Perception is not, as is the view of sensory physiology, changed by the various modifications it undergoes on the way from the object of perception to human consciousness (physical/chemical processes in the air, in the human organism etc.). Nor is it a personal construct of the individual. A detailed, systematic, and scientific explanation of the subject of perception can be found in Steiner's early writings, especially *The Philosophy of Freedom*,[3] *Truth and Knowledge*,[4] and *A Theory of Knowledge Implicit in Goethe's World Conception*.[5] In *The Philosophy of Freedom*, the activity of human perception is thoroughly examined and illuminated.

3.3.1 Outcomes from the observations

In the excerpted report above, the nursing student noted that observations are only meaningful if consequences are drawn from them, if actions result. These can be actions in the form of nursing interventions or in the form of correcting one's thoughts about things or people. If nursing interventions and corrections of ideas are carried out on the basis of observations—and not on the basis of speculations or assumptions—a relationship to reality is created.

What guides a person in his actions depends on many individual factors. The imprints of one's own personality, habits, preferences, experiences, ideals, traditions, societal rules and norms, role models, etc., all exert their influences. Ultimately, our actions are guided by our thoughts. Thoughts play a role in the formation of our motives, in the form of judgments or prejudices, of hypotheses or insights, of fantasies or reality-related ideas, and, last but not least, feelings. The awareness of the factors involved in the formation of motives depends on the degree of self-knowledge. The greater the inner work performed in this respect, the freer the individual becomes in working with past experiences or one's own conceptual framework.

How far this process of growing awareness has progressed and how much clarity a person gains about the way he or she forms motives has consequences for the person doing the work and of course plays a decisive role in their professional interactions. The degree of clarity about the motives and about the sphere from which they are formed will determine whether our actions are in accord with reality or not.

Steiner's *Philosophy of Freedom* deepens these brief remarks on ethics, developing an approach to ethical action which focuses on the individual who acts and dealing with the problem of freedom arising in this context.

3.3.2 Continuity in the observational process

At the end of her text, the nursing student suggests that the continuity and regularity of observation is a prerequisite for an in-depth observation process. This is because skills develop through repetition, i.e. practice. Our organization, whether physical, mental, or spiritual, requires repetition in order to incorporate something new. Without continuity, our efforts remain fruitless. In order to proceed developmentally in this area, clear motives, conscientiousness, and self-discipline are necessary. Anyone who has engaged in this process knows how strenuous it is. But all learning is based on practice. After some time, the first awkward beginnings become a skill that can then lead to healthy routine.

3.3.3 The selective perception

In the course of her observation exercises, the student nurse quoted above observes that she notices some things about the patient, and others she does not.
She sees a connection between the "selection" of observations and the prominence of certain phenomena in the patient and her own interests. The interest arises, in her view, out of questions that develop as a result of the engagement with certain things. Here "engagement with certain things" means the thoughtful examination of topics that precede the observation process or follow from it, based on experience. The form in which this examination takes place does not play a role in the development of interest or further-reaching questions, the only decisive factor is activity of thought. The question that is formed through thoughtful examination will depend on the concepts that one has dealt with.

In anthroposophically extended nursing, the conceptual framework is essentially that of the human being. In the human being, as a unity of body, soul, and spirit, corresponding physical, mental, and spiritual processes take place, which have to be taken into account in care. This book and the literature mentioned describe the image of the human being and point to consequences for nursing care. In forming questions, the individual is guided by the content of his or her mental work. In addition, past mental images, judgments, and prejudices influence the individual. It is therefore important to carry out exercises in self-observation in order to gain clarity about one's perspective. One's personal standpoint is quite justified as long as one has an open and yet critical attitude toward other points of view and as long as one continues to check and develop oneself. This is the only way to prevent one-sidedness and dogmatism, which are a hindrance to care that is humane and adequate for the whole human being.

3.3.4 Attentiveness and observation

The phenomenon of gaps in memory in connection with inattention is probably known to everyone. The following descriptions, derived from Rudolf Steiner's 1909 lectures on psychology, *A Psychology of Body, Soul, and Spirit*,[6] relate attention, as a special soul force, to the ability to remember. In addition, these descriptions contain aspects relevant to care that go far beyond attentiveness as a phenomenon of consciousness.

In the aforementioned lectures, Steiner pointed to two basic elements of human soul life, to reasoning, and to the experiences of love and hate. He describes how all feelings arise through a mixture of love, hate, and reasoning or judgment. The experiences of love and hate are connected with desire that arises from the inner soul life. Desire moves from the center of the soul to the periphery, to the gates of the senses.

> *"When you consider that the soul, as experience directly reveals, is really filled with the flood of desires, and you ask what it actually is that flows to the portals of the senses when the soul lets its own inner being surge there, you find it to be the desires themselves. This desire knocks at the gate; at this moment it actually comes in contact with the outer world, and while doing so it receives a seal imprint, as it were, from the other side . . . Just as the seal yields nothing out of itself but the crest, so the outer world furnishes nothing but the imprint. But something must oppose the seal if an imprint is to come about. You must therefore think of it so that in what opposes the sense experience an imprint has formed from without, and this we carry with us, this imprint come into being in our own soul life."[7]*

The transmission of the sense impression into the soul life takes place as an imprint. The medium in which the sense impression is imprinted is soul substance, the forces of love and hate that arise from desire. Steiner explained further how this relates to attention:

> *"That is what we take along, not the color or the tone itself, but what we have had in the way of experiences of love and hate, of desires. Is that altogether correct? Could there be something directly connected with a sense experience, something like a desire that must press outward? Well, if nothing of the sort existed you would not carry the sense experience with you in your subsequent soul life; no memory visualization would form. There is, indeed, a psychic phenomenon that offers direct proof that desire always makes contacts outward from the soul through the portals of the senses, whether the perceptions be those of color, smell, or hearing; that is the phenomenon of attention. A comparison between a sense impression during which we merely stare unseeing and one to which we give our attention shows us that in the former case the impression cannot be carried on in the soul life. You must respond from within through the power of attention, and the greater the attention, the more readily the soul retains the memory picture in the further course of life."[8]*

Steiner characterized attentiveness as a spiritual force that can be seen as part of the power of love or sympathy. It is soul substance into which the sensory impression is imprinted. "The greater the attention, the more readily the soul retains the memory picture." Therefore, if sense experiences (observations) take place without inner participation, these are dulled processes of consciousness that do not manifest themselves as a memory picture.

The next consideration will bring us even closer to an understanding of attention. The nursing student's report mentions the changing relationship between observer and patient. Is perhaps a reason for this the fact that the power of love in the form of attention was enacted by the observer, experienced by the patient, and led to a transformation of the relationship? According to Steiner, love is one of the forces that lead to real healing:

> "We have to instill love so that the act of love can be of help. All those healing acts that are more or less based on what can be called psychic healing processes have this character of transmitted love . . . it is love that we infuse the other person with as a balm. It must be attributed to love in the end, when we set simple psychological factors in motion, when we help another person to perhaps put his depressed mind in order." [9]

Love is the force that sets in motion healing processes in the soul. In the patient/nurse relationship, attentiveness, as a soul-spiritual phenomenon, can therefore become a factor in psychological healing. The extent to which the mental condition of patients suffers as a result of inattentiveness and carelessness on the part of their caregivers is well known from many accounts. In the experience of patients, "good care" is always characterized by carefulness and circumspection, not primarily by manual skill or adherence to hygienic guidelines. It is reasonable to say that patients experience a form of spiritual healing through the attention they receive through skillful, i.e., attentive and interested observation. This has an effect on their relationship with their caregivers. This aspect, which results from the form or process of observation, goes far beyond the interpretation of phenomena and is a clear contribution of care to the healing process.

4.   Observation and knowledge

Up to now, we have mainly dealt with soul processes in connection with observation; consideration of cognition and reality in relation to observation will follow. To this end, we will examine the elements of the activity of knowing and their interrelationships. The content follows from and references Steiner's writings *Truth and Knowledge, The Science of Knowing,* and *The Philosophy of Freedom,* which lay the scientific foundation for anthroposophy.

In cognition the human being becomes aware of the world in its regularities and co-herences. In her remarks on observation, Florence Nightingale suggested the elements that are essential for human cognition: perception, comprehension, and their being united in judgment or reasoning. Perception contains everything that is available to a human being as a sensory impression: color, smell, taste, etc. "The objects in space and in time approach us; we perceive a highly diversified outer world of manifold parts, and we experience a more or less richly developed inner world. The first form in which all this confronts us stands finished before us. We play no part in its coming about. Reality at first presents itself to our sensible and spiritual grasp as though springing from some beyond unknown to us. To begin with we can only let our gaze sweep across the manifoldness confronting us."[10]

> The world of perception, given without our active involvement is confronted with thinking, which penetrates it with the ordering mind.

If this did not happen, if our perceptions were not confronted with thinking, we would be perpetually faced with an incoherent aggregate of sentient objects: colors, sounds, pressure, warmth, taste and smell, as well as feelings of pleasure and displeasure. This aggregate is the content of pure perception without thought. It is met by thinking, which is ready to unfold its activity at the first opportunity. Thinking connects the elements of different observations, it links certain concepts to these elements and brings them into coherent relationship with one another. Through thinking, perception receives its ideational designation. It is placed in a context and thus becomes "understandable."

Perception in itself does not reveal anything about its meaning, and bringing a concept to bear on it is necessary for understanding. Imagine the following situation, for example: At night, as you walk down a dark alley, you notice a movement. As long as you cannot classify this perception through your thinking, you will not know what it is and you may be frightened. As soon as the concept "cat" is added to the perception, you recognize the situation and put the perception into context. Here, a judgment (in the epistemological sense) is formed. Thinking is the unobserved element of our mental life. We use it constantly in the formation of judgments but know little about it. Thinking is always ready to create connections by forming concepts.

However, before one learns more about the nature of concepts, one has to deal with thinking. Steiner wrote: "As long as philosophy goes on assuming all sorts of principles, such as atoms, motion, matter, will, the unconscious, it will be floating in the air. Only when the philosopher regards the absolute last as his first can he reach his goal. This absolutely last or latest thing that world development has arrived at is thinking."[11]

Thus thinking becomes the pivot point for all human understanding. Steiner consistently advocated that philosophy be free of all presuppositions by drawing attention to the instrument through which an understanding or recognition of the world is possible in the first place. This thinking must be observed and understood if the claim of unconditionality in philosophy is to be fulfilled. The scientist too must become conscious of thinking in order to know how and by what means one's scientific activity and research is possible. Only when this has been achieved can one speak of an immanently critical approach to science.

4.2 Thinking

For the human being, thinking belongs to the world of inner experience. We can observe this inner experience as just as we do the outer world, and thus make thinking an object of perception. In the experience of thinking, however, there is something completely different from the experience of the sense world.

> *"I can twist and turn the matter however I want: if I remain with what the senses provide, I find no connection between the facts. With thinking this is not the case. If, for example, I grasp the thought "cause," this leads me by its own content to that of "effect." I need only hold onto the thoughts in the form in which they appear in direct experience and they manifest already as lawful characterizations. What, for the rest of experience, must first be brought from somewhere else—if it is applicable to experience at all—namely, lawful interconnection, is already present in thinking in its very first appearance. With the rest of experience the whole thing does not already express itself in what appears as manifestation to my consciousness; with thinking, the whole thing arises without reservation in what is given me. With the rest of experience I must penetrate the shell in order to arrive at the kernel; with thinking, shell and kernel are one undivided unity. It is only due to a general human limitation that thinking appears to us at first as entirely analogous to the rest of experience. With thinking we merely have to overcome our own limitation. With the rest of experience we must solve a difficulty lying in the thing itself."*[12]

The "objects" of thought, the concepts, are of an ideal (non-sensual) nature, are determined by themselves and nothing else, and thus have an objective character. They originate in the realm of ideas and represent this realm in the consciousness of human beings. This means that human beings do not "create" the concepts themselves, but they do cause them to appear in consciousness through the activity of thinking. Thus, they exist independent of thinking. Concepts are valid, independent of time and space, and can be conceived by any thinking person at any time.

The facts presented here result from the observation of thought. Every human being is able to carry out these observations in their own consciousness and thus test the truth of these statements.

With the observation of thought, we live within spiritual experience. Through the observation of thinking, by means of thinking, the reality of the spiritual world becomes tangible for everyday consciousness.

A further observation of thinking shows that thinking does not occur by itself. The human being, as an individual, must carry out the activity of thinking in fullness; nothing is passively "delivered," as is the case with perception. The human being is self-determined only in the activity of thought; nothing foreign, nothing from outside the individual interferes with it.

With the activity of thinking, therefore, we have the possibility of experiencing our individuality, our 'I'. This thinking has two aspects:

- It is personal, because the 'I' performs the thinking activity—individual activity.
- It is universal, because through thinking the universally true world of ideas appears in the form of concepts in human consciousness—universal content.

Thinking itself follows certain laws (for example, the laws of logic) and is therefore also universal in form. Now that thinking has been characterized and its significance for the act of knowing has been described, we will further explore the act of cognition.

4.3 Forming judgments

"In all cognitive treatment of reality the process is as follows. We approach the concrete perception. It stands before us as a riddle. Within us the urge makes itself felt to investigate the actual what, the essential being, of the perception, which this perception itself does not express. This urge is nothing other than a concept working its way up out of the darkness of our consciousness. We then hold fast to this concept while sense perception goes along parallel with this thought-process. The mute perception suddenly speaks a language comprehensible to us; we recognize that the concept we have grasped is what we sought as the essential being of the perception. What has taken place here is a judgment."[13]

Only in judgment, in the synthesis of percept and concept, does the full reality of a thing exist.

In order to reach this full reality, two acts of thought are necessary: the first is finding the concept; the second is connecting the concept with the perception. In the cognitive judgment, there is no longer a pure concept, but a mental picture. Mental pictures are concepts related to perceptions and thus no longer "pure," since they are no longer of a completely spiritual nature. For the experience of pure concepts, we find examples in the field of mathematics or logic. By being a knower, whether in everyday life or in science, humanity overcomes the dualism of the world of the senses, with the help of thinking. Only in overcoming this dualism of the world of the senses and the world of ideas can we experience the full reality of the world. In this sense, practicing science also means uniting what was previously separate, an activity that only the thinking human being can perform. Knowledge creates a reality that did not exist before in this form.

About cognition and its extension from the sense world to the spiritual realm, Steiner wrote:

> "It is evident from the whole bearing of this epistemology that the point of its deliberations is to gain an answer to the question, What is knowledge? In order to attain this goal we looked, to begin with, at the world of sense perception on the one hand, and at penetration of it with thought, on the other. And it is shown that in the interpenetration of both, the true reality of sense existence reveals itself. With this the question, What is the activity of knowing? is answered in principle. This answer becomes no different when the question is extended to the contemplation of the spiritual. Therefore, what is said in this book about the nature of knowledge is valid also for the activity of knowing the spiritual worlds, to which my later books refer."[14]

5. Observation and intuition

Observation alone does not give us a complete picture of things; thinking must be "added" in order to illuminate the relationships. What role does intuition play in this process?

> "In contrast with the content of perception, which is given to us from outside, the content of thought appears within. The form in which this first appears, we will call intuition. It is for thinking what observation is for the percept. Intuition and observation are the sources of our knowledge."[15]

Observation and intuition are processes by which the perceptions and concepts, respectively, become accessible to human consciousness. The perceptions are the contents of observation, the concepts the contents of intuition. Here, therefore, process or activity is distinguished from content, and it is appropriate for a clear understanding of the term "intuition" to make this distinction consistently. By intuition we therefore understand a process that is a conscious experience of a spiritual content through thinking. Patricia Benner's work introduced the term intuition to the field of professional nursing. She defines intuition as "understanding without reasoning."[16] Does it refer to activity or content? With this definition, a certain rational element was emphasized (understanding), but at the same time it was relativized and thus negated (without justification). Is a real "understanding without reasoning" even conceivable?

Through conceptual intuition and the act of judgment, it is precisely the relationships that become transparent and understandable. As soon as the connections are clear, reasons can be given, because the "reasons" are aspects of the contextual-conceptual connection. This is experienced through intuition, therefore there can be no understanding without reasons. This prompts the question, which must for now remain open, what does the "intuition" referred to by Benner refer to?

Patricia Benner presents the path from newcomer to expert in nursing care as a stepladder in the acquisition of competence, culminating in the capacity for intuition. "A nursing expert is characterized by the fact that she no longer relies on analytical thinking (rules, guidelines, principles) to act in a situation. Rather, as a nurse with a broad background of experience, she intuitively grasps a situation correctly and immediately tackles the essential problem without time-consuming considerations of different alternatives."[17]

This characterization of an intuitive process can only be understood as a description of a psychological, not a cognitive process, taking into account the above considerations. The situation is grasped during "intuition," at lightning speed, so that the individual elements and actions of this process are no longer decisively carried out and consciously remembered. This immediacy of judgment, acquired through long practice, distinguishes the experienced nurse from the newcomer, who still has to struggle with the formation of concepts and the gradual acquisition of relevant judgments. It remains unclear in Brenner's statement whether "intuitive" comprehension is actually a current realization or whether it is a transfer of previously formed mental images to the current situation. If the latter is the case, then there is no current cognitive judgment, but rather a judgment from a previous experience. This was acquired at some point in the past and is applied in a supposedly similar situation.

An intuition understood in the sense of anthroposophy is always a cognitive process and is therefore always current. Through thinking activity a concept is formed and in a second act of intuition a judgment. Intuition cannot therefore be spoken of as a memory. The activity necessary for intuition is comparable to what is needed to solve a tricky mathematical problem. In this respect, it is something completely different from memory, because memory usually appears in the consciousness somehow without much activity. The novelty and accuracy of a real intuition makes it possible to relate realistically to a situation, since one is present in the here and now and not somewhere in the past.

This gives a rough outline of the psychological and epistemological foundations for observation in nursing care based on anthroposophy. Now we will focus on the practical consequences for nursing training.

6. Observation training as a component of nursing training

One of the aims of the observation and thinking training expanded by anthroposophy is to impart experience and insights into the elements of the act of cognition: "perception," "concept," "thinking," and "forming a judgment." This serves as the basis for the development of scientific awareness and thus also an understanding of professional nursing care. As explained in the previous chapters, observation and thinking training also develop self- and social competences. Therefore, these elements are repeatedly taken up and deepened throughout the training.

An instructional principle of experience-based teaching is to start from observations and experiences in the learning process. The exercises described below are structured according to this principle and can be used variably in different teaching units.

6.1 Sense perception

Rudolf Steiner's teachings about the twelve senses form the basis for a sensitization of perception. In the lessons, the twelve areas of sense perception are worked out through experiments and observation exercises. This is particularly enriched by artistic activities such as painting, drawing, music, movement, and sculpting. These subjects offer important opportunities for students to work with sense experience. Bothmer gymnastics has also proved its worth, especially for the so-called lower senses (the senses of touch, life, self-motion, and balance).

Examples of exercises to aid in differentiating the twelve fields of perception (senses):
- SENSE OF TOUCH: Exercises in which you sense objects with different qualities of touch, such as stones, plants, sand, rubber, etc.
- SENSE OF SELF-MOTION: gymnastics, eurythmy, observations during the mobilization of a patient
- SENSE OF SMELL: smell objects with different scents
- SENSE OF TASTE: Exploring the qualities of taste
- SENSE OF SIGHT: drawing, painting, viewing and contemplation of art, especially paintings
- SENSE OF WARMTH: Fill three bowls with water: one warm, one cold, and one lukewarm. Place the left hand in the cold water and the right hand in the warm water for about one minute, then place both hands in the lukewarm water. The experiment leads to the conclusion that the sensation of heat is relative to one's own body temperature, since the lukewarm water is felt to be a different temperature by each hand.
- SENSE OF HEARING: experience of sound qualities of different materials, music
- SENSE OF LANGUAGE: different languages/foreign languages, eurythmy, speech formation exercises
- SENSE OF THOUGHT: Exercises for observing thought using philosophical writings or mathematical examples

Further opportunities to experience sensory qualities arise for the learners in practical nursing lessons, for example when practicing Whole-Body Washing or Rhythmic Einreibung.

This practical work with the senses, and the related discussions, open up a spectrum of possibilities for comprehensive observation. This serves, among other things, to make people aware of habits in a particular realm of experience, and to enable them to change these habits, for example, with the sense of sight. A differentiated capacity for observation is developed, as well as the ability to articulate the contents of observations.

6.2   Training of thinking

Thinking plays a decisive role in cognition and thus in personality development. The goal is to increase the activity of thinking and to acquire the ability to learn to observe one's own thinking. In this way, certain prejudices, cherished or fixed ideas, and other limitations of our thinking can be discovered and overcome. The method of studying the texts can vary. It is possible to proceed paragraph by paragraph or chapter by chapter, to assign reports, to have records of the individual lessons drawn up and discussed in detail in a plenary session and—last but not least—to structure texts into individual or group work. It is recommended in particular to consider hygienic aspects when making the schedule (e.g., no philosophy lessons after lunch). The level of difficulty should be adjusted according to the wishes and abilities of the students.

6.2.1 The seedling observation

This exercise is particularly useful for developing stamina and precision in the observation process. It extends over a period of two to three weeks. Each student receives several seeds, such as vetch seeds (a fast-growing plant), on a water-soaked cotton pad. The students are asked to look at the seedlings once a day and to record their observations alternately in writing or drawing. At the same time, they are asked to pay attention to what happens inside them during the observation process. Once a day a short exchange of five to ten minutes takes place on the state of the plants' germination. After three weeks the exercise is evaluated, and everyone brings in the young plant and their notes. Again and again, the students describe that continuous observation requires patience, perseverance, and consistency. Usually a loving relationship develops toward the seedling. Through the exercise, the students get to know themselves in terms of their own endurance and commitment to observation.

6.2.2 The sage branch

With the help of this exercise the selection process occurring in sense perception becomes conscious. Each student is given a small branch of sage with the task of observing and recording the observations. After about ten minutes of individual work, the observations are collected on the blackboard and ordered according to the different senses. This exercise involves touch, smell, taste and sight.

It is experienced that each sense impression reflects only a part of the whole and that visual perceptions outweigh the others. The more differentiated the observations involving several senses, the more multi-faceted the resulting picture becomes.

6.2.3 Describing and considering paintings

This exercise touches on questions of personal judgment and systematic observation. The students come together in groups of six to eight and are given the task of writing about a painting together, e.g., by Wassily Kandinsky or Franz Marc. Abstract or semi-abstract paintings are best suited for this exercise. The more dynamic a picture, the more difficult it is to describe. The selection depends on the desired degree of difficulty.

The task is to describe the picture as precisely as possible, as it is, without interpretation. In the case of abstract pictures, the situation repeatedly arises that comparisons are made: "The one on the top left looks like a red elephant." "No, I really think that's a watering can," etc. The instructor must guide the description carefully and be sensitive to the important moments in which perceptual content and personal interpretation are mixed. An increase in the degree of difficulty lies in the challenge to relate each new contribution directly to the previous one. The exercise takes about twenty minutes, followed by a thorough evaluation. Experience has shown that participants repeatedly encounter similar difficulties in distinguishing between the visual impression and its personal interpretation. Furthermore, it can often be seen that two different approaches are taken in the description: the systematic, more distanced one or one that is more spontaneous and experiential. The students recognize the greater amount of discipline required by the former. They often do not enjoy the first approach as much as they do the second, but they also notice that the results are much more precise when the systematic approach is used. This insight helps them to consciously approach observation in a disciplined way.

The painting descriptions should be done several days in a row with different pictures in different sized groups. In this way, confidence in the discernment of picture content and the ability to articulate one's own experience is achieved. Different approaches in the descriptions can be worked out, e.g. from detail to overall composition, from the center to the periphery, or a focus on specific elements such as colors, shapes, movement, etc. The evaluation can be modified by not doing it verbally, but by asking the students to record their strongest impressions of the exercise by drawing pictures (chalk, wax crayons).

6.2.4 A journey through the hand

This exercise can be used for nursing instruction in many areas and has a special place in observation training. You can work with it in the context of observation as described here, but also in connection with personal hygiene or external applications. It is carried out blindfolded, the only seeing person present is the instructor. For this exercise one needs a large area, unfurnished except for chairs.

After blindfolding, the students are asked to hold hands and form a circle. During this time the instructor places chairs in pairs opposite each other, irregularly distributed in the room. From this time on, there is no more talking, only the instructor explains the next steps. The participants are taken out of the circle one by one and led to a chair. Pairs of chairs are created that have no contact with each other for the time being. When all participants are seated, the journey through the hand begins.

One of the partners explores the hand of the other person by touching it, so that he or she can get a picture of this hand. The instructor is the "tour guide" and gives the appropriate instructions.

First of all, the overall shape of the hand is explored, the relationship of wrist-palm-fingers. On the palm you have to experience the different "hills and valleys," the muscular layer and the skin. After that turn to the back of the hand with the same task. Next, attention is given to differences in warmth of the different parts of the hand, then to their mobility. Finally, the hand is grasped as a whole and the participants try to form a detailed picture of this hand. The whole "journey" takes about fifteen minutes. This is enough time to get involved in the tactile experience and yet short enough to avoid fear or impatience. It should be noted that sufficient opportunity must be given to gather the experiences and that there are pauses between the various instructions. The instructions given for the individual steps should be such that they do not give suggestions about what will be perceived, and yet do provide a guide for the observations. An example: "Please turn your fingers now. How long are they, how thick? How are the muscles on the fingers distributed? How do the bones feel?" etc.

The couples then line up blindfolded in such a way that the person whose hand has been palpated is behind the person who did the palpation and extends his/her hand forward. After the person who palpated the hand forms a clear mental image of the hand, he/she takes off the blindfold and looks at the hand. Does the mental image correspond to reality? To which person does the hand belong? Now everyone takes off their blindfold, the partners see each other and a lively exchange about their experiences takes place.

Again the evaluation of the exercise takes place in the plenum circle. The next day the exercise is repeated with swapped roles and different partners. Eliminating the sense of sight brings with it a great loss of security. By listening, a completely new experience of space is conveyed. A greater inner strength is needed to face this new experience. One's trust in other people is challenged. The hands as an "instrument" are experienced and become conscious in a completely new way. The diversity of the possible perceptions is surprising. The sense and quality of touch becomes a conscious experience. The aspect of freedom in relation to touch is addressed and the benefit of objective human touch can be experienced. Students often report deep impressions they have gained in connection with this exercise and that they have been able to take with them many suggestions for care. The experiences with and in this exercise are as inexhaustible as the subject of observation in general. Since the exercise requires a lot of courage and trust in the instructor, it should only be carried out after careful preparation and after a phase of getting to know each other in the classroom. It is important that there be no obligation to participate!

6.3   Transfer to the daily nursing routine

All acquired knowledge and experiences in observation obviously need to be consolidated and deepened in everyday nursing care. For this reason, it makes sense for us to provide observation tasks for the practical training right at the beginning of the training, which are then evaluated in clinical lessons or in conversation.

In the course of the training, the practical tasks are oriented towards the nursing process. In this way, the observation or the collection of information is continued by articulating nursing priorities in order to determine nursing goals and measures. The content gained from the observation is thus placed in context and becomes relevant for the nursing activity.

7.   Final remarks

Anthroposophy understands the human being to be a spiritual being who develops according to his or her destiny during life on earth. From this basic assumption a correspondingly differentiated view of humanity and an understanding of illness can be derived. For the nursing staff, the task is to approach the patient in a free, unprejudiced manner with the aim of supporting and accompanying each one on their unique path of development. The patient is to be recognized and accepted "as they are." It is important to develop interest and attention as virtues and to maintain them continuously in the daily work. But where does a caregiver with high ideals find the strength for this task? How do you ensure that the strengths and qualities of the next generation of caregivers are maintained and promoted, so that the practice of the profession does not lead to burnout?

Experience has shown that a great deal of inner activity is necessary, which goes beyond coping with the daily work routine. This activity includes, above all, working on oneself, on one's own attitude towards the profession, one's colleagues, and the work environment. This is the only way to develop and strengthen one's soul powers in order to be able to set a counterweight to today's demands.

Learning and development do not stop after the training is complete, but rather become a lifelong process. However, there is a marked difference between individuals trusting that development will take place somehow and those who work on their own development. Such development can take different courses. For me, the unfolding or development of 'I'-forces is the most significant. One way to do this is through the intentional training of thinking, since this is a pure 'I'-activity. Through this training the 'I,' the spiritual human being, is "nourished" and strengthened. At the same time, a feeling for the 'I' of the other person and the desire to meet him/her is developed. True human encounters become possible and a new kind of understanding of each other begins to form.

The training of thinking has another quality: In thinking, the individual core of the human being communicates with the eternal of the world. An act of devotion to a spiritual object takes place in the highest state of self-activity. The freedom of the person remains untouched, since they are self-determined and no external influences are effective. This kind of connection with the spiritual world is an actual source of strength; it strengthens the 'I'-forces of the person.

Training in observation has its rightful place in modern nursing curricula. On the one hand, it allows for a scientific understanding of the profession in the students. On the other hand, it presents a personal training that may be of value in their future life. In this context, I see the task of a training institution as pointing out the various paths and possibilities so that each person can make his or her own choice.

The process of observation and its practice thus shows its effect on caregivers as well as patients. But no matter what individual significance the observation training may have for trainees and nurses, the patient will always benefit from the fruits of good observation. He feels recognized in the issues that matter to him and receives attention and care. This places nursing care in the circle of those who make a significant contribution to the healing process of the people entrusted to it.

Category	Example learning objectives	Recommended learning path
Skill	You practice the appropriate exercises for nursing training.	A
Your own learning objective		
Relationships	Awareness of the senses increases interest in the environment.	B
Your own learning objective		
Knowledge	You think through the relationship between percept and concept.	C
Your own learning objective		

References

1   Nightingale, F. *Notes on Nursing.* Appleton & Co., New York 1860.

2   Reinert, B. *Kann man Beobachten wirklich lernen oder ist es eine Fähigkeit, die jedem Menschen selbstverständlich zur Verfügung steht?* ("Can you really learn to watch or is it a skill that is naturally available to everyone?") Rundbrief Verband für Anthroposophische Pflege, Bad Liebenzell 1992.

3   Steiner, R. *The Philosophy of Freedom.* Rudolf Steiner Press, London 2011.

4   Steiner, R. *Truth and Knowledge.* Rudolf Steiner Press, London 2007.

5   Steiner, R. *The Science of Knowing: Outline of an Epistemology Implicit in the Goethean World View.* Mercury Press, New York 1988.

6   Steiner, R. *A Psychology of Body, Soul, and Spirit.* SteinerBooks, Great Barrington 1999.

7   ibid.

8   ibid.

9   ibid.

10 Steiner, R. *The Science of Knowing: Outline of an Epistemology Implicit in the Goethean World View.* Mercury Press, New York 1988.

11 Steiner, R. *The Philosophy of Freedom.* Rudolf Steiner Press, London 2011.

12 Steiner, R. *The Science of Knowing: Outline of an Epistemology Implicit in the Goethean World View.* Mercury Press, New York 1988.

13 ibid.

14 ibid.

15 Steiner, R. *The Philosophy of Freedom.* Rudolf Steiner Press, London 2011.

16 Benner, P. *From novice to expert.* Prentice Hall, New Jersey 2000.

17 Benner, P., Tanner Ch. Die Intution der Pflegekompetenz. *Pflege Zeitschrift* 1990; 43 (3).

CHAPTER III

The Anthropological Foundations
of Nursing Extended by Anthroposophy

FRANCES BAY

This chapter will explain the spiritual-scientific foundations of anthroposophic nursing and discuss the nursing profession in the light of modern nursing theory. It will show that anthroposophic nursing is not merely a theory, rather it endeavors to develop humaneness in the nursing profession by applying a comprehensive anthroposophic understanding of what it means to be human. This chapter will describe the physically imperceptible, subtle members of the human being in their relationship to nature and the cosmos and illustrate them with practical examples from everyday nursing care and medicine.

→   Learning objectives, see end of chapter

It is difficult to write about nursing because it is an activity that takes place in the meeting and actions of two people. Every nursing activity is shaped by the situation in which the encounter between the patient and the nurse takes place. Thus, it may not seem very fruitful to theorize about nursing care. One might be inclined to accuse nursing scientists of drifting away from actual nursing care and straying into other fields, such as psychology and sociology. Nevertheless, our era demands that we bring awareness into our actions, awareness that takes our nursing work beyond purely functional and mechanical activity to a therapeutic level. Therefore, the question is: how can I, as a nurse, shape my encounters and actions in such a way that they become therapeutic? We need to think about nursing to approach an answer to this question. This should not result in a finished theory and no nursing model should emerge from it. Rather, it is an effort to point out a way to developing more insight and awareness in nursing.

1.   What do nurses do?

Nursing takes us to a new therapeutic level.

If you ask nurses about their work, they will probably answer briefly: "I ~~nurse~~ *take care of* people." Or they might add a long list of actions: "washing and positioning patients; accompanying them to the toilet; helping them with their meals; putting on bandages; administering injections, enemas, and inhalations; measuring temperature, blood pressure, and pulse; providing them with medication; comforting patients and their relatives;

giving advice for home care; supporting doctors and therapists; organizing ward tasks," and, depending on where they work, much more besides.

Regarding this long list, the question arises as to which of these actions are so specifically "nursing" that they justify three years of training. Is cleaning a bedside cabinet a nursing task or should it be done by a cleaning service? Is drawing blood a nursing activity or the task of the doctor or laboratory assistant? Couldn't the families of patients provide basic care and food for them? The same applies to talks with patients. We have specialists for this today, too. Any nurse would be reluctant to consider their work to be something that everyone could do, but no one wants to. What, then, is the special task of nursing care? The answer to this question is certainly not to be found only in what nurses do. The type and extent of the nurse's repertoire of tasks is influenced by progress in medicine, the disappearance of some diseases, and the emergence of new ones, as well as social and political developments. Therefore, nursing cannot find its identity in the changing roles of "what." Rather, it must learn to attain awareness in "how" things are done. How do we handle patients when settling, washing or mobilizing them? Is our touch purely functional in nature? Or are there other, additional qualities to consider?

We can ask: "How do I touch a patient in such a way that he feels it to be pleasant and reassuring, experiencing a sense of security? What do I convey to a patient when giving an injection? What are the thoughts and intentions of the nurse when he or she administers a rhythmic oil application or applies a compress? What is the content of the conversation between the patient and the nurse?"

The answer to such questions must be different for each person, because only then can we speak of individual care. We must learn to ask the right questions based on our observation of the patient. Then we can find individual answers, through which our nursing care can become healing.

Nursing activities are performed either functionally, or in such a way that the specific nursing-healing intention behind them has an effect. A simple example will illustrate this:

> A patient is lying in bed with a high fever and is bathed in sweat. It is advisable to quickly lower the fever and prevent macerations of the skin caused by moisture. To achieve this, we administer a fever-reducing agent prescribed by the doctor, wash off the sweat, and cover the moist, naked patient with a light sheet to further reduce the fever by means of water evaporation.

These purely utilitarian considerations will very likely achieve our objective: the patient is soon dry, and the fever has been reduced. A healing nursing approach to dealing with this situation would be to try to look at it from the patient's perspective: what does it feel like to lie hot and sweaty in bed?

It is not only the patient's body that is affected by this stressful situation. The patient suffers from the heat, he is restless, he feels oppressed and uncomfortable in the moisture. How does our treatment feel to him? Are we considering his mental state while we are caring for him? If we consider these questions, we can also treat the patient as follows:

> The aim is not primarily to reduce fever, but to make the patient feel comfortable in his skin. This is done by washing him. The temperature of the water is not simply cold, it is selected to feel pleasantly cool to this patient. He is then dried off so that he does not lie wet in bed and suffer a chill. This is followed by lukewarm lemon or vinegar calf compresses, which alleviate the symptoms caused by fever, such as headaches and aching limbs, feverish dreams and tachycardia, without exposing the patient to cold.

> INSTRUCTIONS: Pour approximately 2 liters of cold (or lukewarm for high fevers) water into a bowl. Cut a lemon under water and squeeze out the juice or add fruit vinegar. Then soak two cotton cloths in it and wrap them quite moist around the patient's calves, starting from the foot, and add a woolen cloth on top. Then cover the patient well. Change the calf wraps approx. every 15 minutes or as soon as the compresses are warm and dry. Check the body temperature after one hour; if the fever has not dropped, apply the compresses for another hour.

> With this application, the patient can enjoy the familiar covering of his pajamas and the bedclothes. He does not feel as if he is at the mercy of his environment. The treatment is repeated several times as needed, so that on an emotional level the patient comes to feel that the attention associated with it is beneficial and healing.

In this way, nursing procedures are not only carried out from a functional point of view, they are also assessed according to their value for the patient's well-being. In this sense, there are no nursing problems, only patient problems that nurses adopt as their own within the framework of the nursing process.

> *"When caring for the sick the aim is [...] to bring the person into conditions which allow the greatest possible scope for natural healing."*
>
> Florence Nightingale (1820–1910)[1]

In addition to shaping our own nursing tasks, nursing is also a prerequisite for the work of physicians and therapists. Our presence and our support of the patient around the clock gives us an overview of almost all the patient's personal activities. Nurses become intermediaries between physicians, therapists, relatives and the patient. This task can be compared to the effect of water in nutrition: without water, ingested substances are not effective. Water alone does not cause growth, maintenance or healing. Without water, however, the ingested substances do not get to where they need to go.

In this way, nursing finds a special task in being like water: it makes everything that happens around the patient healing.

2.   Developments in nursing

In recent decades, nursing care has developed from a medical auxiliary profession into an independent discipline with clear professional tasks and competencies. This has long since become the self-concept and image of professional care, especially in English-speaking countries. The academization of the nursing profession, with its own nursing science, research and teaching, has contributed to this on the one hand. On the other hand, the nursing profession has shifted from hospitals to inpatient nursing care for the elderly and outpatient care at home, so that "physician-free" areas have been created in which the doctor's view of the need for care has given way to independent evaluation and terminology by nurses. The demographic development of recent years and coming decades leads us to expect a massive increase in the number of elderly and very old people, who will have increasing care requirements. Due to lower birth rates, significantly fewer young people will be available on the labor market, so that a significant shortage of skilled workers will jeopardize decent nursing care. This scenario has influenced socio-political debate of recent years and has shifted care as a social task into unprecedented public awareness. The increase in dementia, associated with questions of lifestyle and quality of life in old age, creates strong personal concern and influences the emotional basis for political and ethical discussion, such as concerning personal advance health care directives and assisted suicide.

In the tension between demographic and social development on the one hand and the economic parameters of the health care industry on the other, nursing science of recent decades has arrived at striking advances. Supply contracts with payers of inpatient care for the elderly, outpatient care, nursing care in hospitals and rehabilitation facilities are nowadays bound to quality requirements, such as the establishment of a nursing model or the alignment of processes with patients, residents and clients in terms of the four-stage care process of collecting information, formulating a target/problem/resources, implementation and evaluation. Nursing care must follow evidence-based standards. Proof of the underlying nursing model, the individual steps of the nursing process, the implementation of the measures and their evaluation are prescribed by law and are checked regularly.

Every nursing model, every step of the nursing process, all evidence and each evaluation of results is based on a view of the human being. Our views are deeply rooted in our thinking habits, they influence our system of values and even our feelings. For example, if you consider the heart to be a pump, then heart-love symbolism and words such as "heartfelt" and "good hearted" must be interpreted as purely linguistic conventions, and heart transplantations seem to be comparable to replacing a pump in a washing machine. If you consider the heart to be an organ of the "human middle," then physiological and psychological levels of meaning arise that connect and support each other. In what follows we shall develop a picture of the human being that can bring about profound transformations in our relationships with patients, our environment and the social conditions in which we find ourselves.

3. Our view of the human being

It is not enough to have a simple definition of our view of the human being as a basis for nursing care. Rather, our view must become a realistic one that is alive in us and contributes to all our observations of patients and nursing procedures.

Rudolf Steiner's descriptions have contributed a great deal to our view of the human being. We shall therefore look at two fundamental aspects of anthroposophic anthropology:

- The fourfold nature of the human being: the human relationship to the environment and to other human beings.
- The threefold nature of the human being: the human being as an entity of body (biological), soul (psychological), and spirit in health and illness.

3.1 The fourfold nature of the human being

The fourfold nature of things is not unfamiliar to us in many areas of life. For example, we know the four cardinal points north, south, east and west, and the four seasons spring, summer, autumn and winter. Already the people of antiquity distinguished between four natural realms: the mineral, plant, animal and human realms. They recognized the four elements earth, water, air and fire. These elements only lead a shadowy existence in our present-day consciousness as the three states of aggregation—solid, liquid, gaseous—and energy. According to Hippocrates (ca. 460–370 BC), four juices flow through the human body: blood, mucus, yellow bile and black bile. When they are properly combined in the organism there is health, while imbalances cause disease. In the soul, dominance of one of the juices determines a person's temperament. There were thought to be four types of bile: sanguine (lat. sanguis = blood), phlegmatic (gr. phlegma = mucus), choleric (gr. chole = bile) and melancholic (gr. melan chole = black bile). Balance and harmonization of the juices was thought to cause healing.

If we consider the human being as a whole, we recognize numerous connections to the fourfold view of antiquity. Rudolf Steiner (1861–1925) used his spiritual-scientific methods to explain this anew and expand upon it for our time.[2,3,4] To illustrate the fourfold nature of the human being as represented by Steiner, we shall consider a patient being admitting to the hospital.

3.1.1 The human 'I'

During our first meeting with a patient, we ask questions and conduct examinations as part of preparing our nurse's case history. This is the first step in the nursing process. It is directed at the person as an individual personality. We ask for his name and numerous biographical details, such as his age, marital status, social circumstances and the genesis of his illness. The conversation allows us to begin to get to know the individuality of the person in front of us. He possesses a unique past that is shaped by his personality and experiences. Now, here in the present, he has become a patient in his search for help and healing.

Much of what happens in the following days and weeks during his illness and his interaction with doctors, therapists and nursing staff will influence his future.

If we look at the patient's past and possible future together with him, we arrive at a formulation of goals. If we look at him exclusively in the present, we run the risk of seeing only the disease or the problems associated with it. This limited vision often leads to the "gall bladder-in-room-3 syndrome."

In our conversation, in our exchange of ideas with the patient, we learn something about his 'I'—his individuality. This gift of human beings to think about themselves and others distinguishes them from all other living beings. The ability to think enables us to recognize ourselves as an 'I'. 'I' is a term that each human being can only apply to himself—never to another person.

Our physical form is designed for thinking.

This is different with animals. When an animal falls ill, it usually instinctively seeks healing in nature, such as a cat that eats grass. While human beings can freely, out of their own responsibility, do something to improve their health, as well as cause and prolong illness, animals instinctively seek the environment that provides them with what they need for survival. When an animal is taken to a veterinarian, we know that it is impossible for the animal to link the present illness to something in its biography. This is why it does not develop by means of the illness. The illness does not lead to increased biographical maturity. This is why it is merciful to kill an animal that is suffering severe pain. The same cannot be said for human beings, due to their potential for continued development throughout their entire lives. Adequate pain therapy must of course be given.

The entire body of the human being is designed to support the gift of thinking. Consider the human form: human beings are the only living beings to have an upright stance. They stand on two legs and balance themselves in this unstable posture. In contrast, four-legged vertebrates have stable postures. They need to develop strong neck muscles to hold up their skulls against gravity. The strength of the skull of an animal is comparable to that of a limb and can take over its function (e.g., a dog that retrieves a newspaper, or a lion that catches and tears its prey with its jaws). Human beings, in contrast, have both hands free thanks to their upright posture. Their hands can become creative servants: for artistic or technical activities—or the healing of others. The human head is emancipated from its function as a limb. It is at rest: a basic prerequisite for thinking. The need for this is easy to understand if we try to concentrate while shaking our heads. We find that a head that is constantly in motion like a limb cannot serve thinking. Similarly, the limbs of animals, which are specialized in keeping them stable, are not designed for free and creative action.

Apart from the ability to think and act creatively, the individuality or 'I' of human beings is also characterized by its relationship to warmth. To stay healthy, people need a relatively constant body temperature of 37°C (98.6°F). Gross fluctuations in either direction lead to damage to the organism, and they are ultimately incompatible with life. Many animals are less dependent on maintaining a specific body temperature. The body temperature of a field mouse drops to just a few degrees above freezing during its long winter sleep, for instance. This reduces its life processes to a minimum.

Due to their constant body heat, it is possible for human beings to arrange their lives largely independently of outside temperatures. In addition, human beings are the only beings who can control and use fire. Blacksmithing, pottery making, cooking and baking are expressions of this ability, which enables human beings to build a culture.

Another special feature of human beings is their freedom of choice. Animals depend on the natural world in which they live. Human beings do not instinctively follow the circumstances of nature. They must freely decide what is right for them. This also applies to drives and instincts. Each person decides for themselves whether to follow their hunger or sex drive. This freedom also creates room for the possibility of error. This is the cause of many diseases.

Our name for the individuality of the human being and the human ability to be free is the same term that each person applies to themselves: 'I'. The power with which the 'I' has found its expression in the human form down to the physical level is referred to in anthroposophic anthropology as the *I-organization.*

3.1.2 The soul body or astral body

Let us return to our example of the intake interview. We want to know how the patient feels. Often a person becomes a patient because he suffers from pain. Now he is looking for help from the doctor, therapist or nurse. The ability to feel and suffer is something that humans have in common with animals: no one doubts that a dog is suffering pain when they hear the animal howl.

Feelings change the rhythm of breathing: we "hold our breath" with tension, we laugh and speak while exhaling, we "shout with anger" and "sigh with relief." These and many other expressions of sympathy and antipathy interrupt the normal rhythm of breathing. When feeling antipathy, the soul contracts, when feeling sympathy, it expands. Breathing behaves similarly: as we inhale, the air flows into our lungs via the alveoli and comes into direct contact with the blood that pulsates through our body. During exhalation, the air saturated with carbon dioxide flows outwards and spreads throughout the space around us. In addition, we recognize the dynamics of breathing wherever there is contraction and expansion or an interplay between inside and outside. This shows how much our feelings are related to the breathing process.

Our awareness of feelings resembles that of our dreams. Sometimes they remain unconscious like healthy breathing, but sometimes they are vivid and dynamic like breathing stimulated by emotions. Goethe expressed the properties of the breathing process in a poetic way.

> *In breathing there are two blessings:*
> *Drawing in air and exhaling it again;*
> *One constrains and the other refreshes;*
> *So wondrously our life is mixed.*
> *So, thank God when He presses you,*
> *And thank Him when He releases you again.*
>
> J. W. von Goethe (1749–1832), Talismans[5]

Human beings have breathing and sensation in common with animals. These activities are expressions of the soul. But unlike animals, human beings are not dependent on their feelings. Because of their 'I', human beings can transform feelings. They can act independently of their emotions. The human soul thus opens itself on the one hand to body-bound sensations such as hunger and thirst or lust and disinclination, and on the other hand —via thinking—to spiritual content and ideals such as freedom and love. The human soul organization (and the soul of an animal) is referred to as the soul or astral body in anthroposophic anthropology. The soul forms the bodily organization of the human being into a carrier for the mental/emotional element acting in all the respiratory organs, which is closely connected with the element of air.

3.1.3 The life body or etheric body

Let us return to our example. While taking the case history we discuss the patient's life processes. We ask about his sleeping and eating habits and the nature of his excretions. We often observe that it is not only pain that makes people aware that "something is wrong." In addition to pain, the person often notices that disturbances have occurred in normal body functioning.

People are not aware of their life processes when they are healthy. What their liver does, how their muscles work or what is happening in their heart remains hidden to them.

The body simply does "what it has to do." It is only during illness or old age, when our life processes start to languish, that we are amazed at the miracle of a healthy organism. If we were constantly and consciously involved in our life processes, we would become mentally and spiritually unfree. We can be grateful that our awareness of our life processes in health is comparable to deep sleep. Only in illness do we become conscious of this functioning. Sexuality is also part of our life processes and life organization. Like the plant and the animal, human beings are also living beings that can reproduce. But as thinking, I-endowed beings, they have the possibility to decide in freedom where and how they will settle into the world. Animals can move freely in their environment but are bound to certain environmental conditions and places by their genus-specific instincts. In this respect, plants are fixed entirely to the place where they grow, flower, bear fruit and die. Only their seeds are passively carried away by the wind or by animals, to germinate in suitable locations. Plants are completely bound to their life processes, animals to their instincts and sensations, but human beings can make free decisions because they can think.

Nevertheless, plants, animals and human beings have the following in common: their life processes take place in a watery element. No life is possible without water. Unwatered flowers wither, animals and human beings die of thirst.

The life organization of plants, animals and human beings is called the *life body* or *etheric body*. Life is not to be understood as resulting from physical/chemical processes, but as a force that causes the structure of the organism to follow the regular laws of the species. In human beings, the activity of the etheric body is also shaped by that of the soul body and the I-organization.

3.1.4 The physical body

The 'I', soul body and etheric body are not directly perceptible to our senses, but their activity can be observed in the physical body.

When we physically examine a patient in our admission interview, we are dealing with visible, palpable and measurable phenomena, that is, with the physical body. We measure pulse, blood pressure, temperature, respiratory rate, height and weight. We examine the patient's skin surface (texture, color, scars, wounds and sore areas). All these phenomena are visible to the eye, palpable to the hands or measurable in numbers. Physical laws rule here.

When a human being, animal or plant dies, the physical body disintegrates into its chemical components. It returns to the mineral world, to the earth. There is no life in the inorganic world.

The physical form of the human body, i.e., its anatomy, is therefore easiest to study by using corpses. There everything can be accessed by analytical examination methods.

The etheric can only be properly studied as real physiology in entities that are alive.

Psychology deals with matters of soul when it is understood in its proper sense as knowledge of the soul. Anthroposophy tries to explore the entire human being while recognizing the spirit within.

> *"Anthroposophy is a path of knowledge that wants to lead the spiritual in the human being to the spiritual in the universe."*
> Rudolf Steiner (1861–1925)[6]

If we try to form an idea of our patient in this fourfold way, we recognize the 'I' as the force that integrates the entire personality into a whole. We can say:

- I have a physical body, as do minerals, created from the element of earth.
- I live in the etheric, as do plants, through the element of water.
- I feel, as do animals, in my soul body. My inner life of soul is related to the element of air.
- But I alone, as an individual human being, possess the gift of thinking and free decision making in my self-designed biography. I am a master of the element of fire, which enables me to access all the realms of nature. I recognize my affiliation with the four elements through my 'I', where the spiritual within me reveals itself.

3.2   Body, soul, and spirit and threefold functioning in the human being

Let us consider the human being as a threefold entity consisting of body, soul and spirit. This requires a more flexible kind of thinking than was necessary for our understanding of the fourfold aspect. To understand the human threefold nature, let us first characterize the differences between threefold and fourfold elements in our everyday environment.

Fourfoldness is a familiar ordering principle that we find in many contexts. Everything that is expressed in fours confers direction, stability and security. How confusing would a map or compass be with only three cardinal points? How sure-footed and dexterous would a cat or a mountain goat be with only three legs?

It is difficult for us to find connections that are determined by a trinity in everyday life. We have little inclination to divide things into three.

We find the archetype of three in the trinity of Christianity: the Father, Son and Holy Spirit. This trinity, however, is difficult to understand in its true essence if we want to comprehend it as a single unity.

In other contexts, we encounter trinity as a balance between polarities or as a combination of them, i.e., in the unification of two opposite dualities: above and below, left and right, front and back meet in the middle. Cold and hot come together in warmth, day and night meet at dusk. The borders and transitions of these trinities are usually not obvious and are therefore rarely exactly defined. Where does "left" end and become "center," where does "right" begin? When is "hot" only "warm" and when does it become "cold"? Neither is the threefold nature of human beings to be understood as a division into three, and it, too, often has flowing transitions.

The movement of our thoughts when we grasp the nature of four and three is comparable to the rhythms of two dances. Four is like a gavotte or march, three is like a waltz. Gavottes and marches are danced in four-four time. The movements of the dancers are determined by fixed and orderly figures. The waltz, on the other hand, conveys an impression of lively and freely circling movement, as the dancing couple whirls about in three-quarter time. They seem to be borne along unrestricted by rhythm and melody. The type of thinking that understands the threefold nature of things is comparable to the flowing movements of a waltz. But first—as with dancing—the separate steps must be learned and practiced before the dance appears as a flowing whole. In this sense, we shall now describe the individual components of threefoldness, in the hope that the reader will be able to bring them inwardly back to life as a living whole.

Since ancient times, the human being has been regarded as a threefold being consisting of body, soul and spirit. Over the centuries, this view met with less and less understanding, research and application in Christianity. On the contrary, it was gradually suppressed, and certain spiritual qualities were attributed to the soul. The dualism of Descartes (1596–1650) in the 17th century paved the way for a further division of the human being. Descartes' postulate of the separation of bodily and mental processes has shaped philosophical thinking to this day. In medicine, this view reached its peak in the middle of the 19th century with the cell pathology of Rudolf Virchow (1821–1902). This forms the basis of today's materialistic medicine:

"I have dissected thousands of corpses but found no soul in any."[7]

This famous quote was meant as a polemic against the church, since Virchow was deeply opposed to its dogmas. It is also a statement that wants the scientific method to be deemed the only appropriate one: the human soul cannot be seen with the eyes. It is not palpable, weighable or measurable, and consequently it cannot exist.

"All life is tied to cells, and cells are not merely vessels of life, they are the living part itself."[8]

With this statement, Virchow created the basis for a purely materialistic, mechanistic medicine that does not just consider soul and spirit to be separate from the body, it denies that those levels exist.

Psychosomatic medicine and modern medical psychology are trying to overcome this separation. As special disciplines, however, they have by no means penetrated all areas of medicine, so that the separation of the physical from the soul generally still predominates. This new attempt to view the human being as a whole, consisting of body, soul and spirit, can also be found in the literature on nursing. However, it seems questionable whether it is possible to gain insight into the threefold nature of the human being, which has been destroyed for centuries, in a new way within the framework of nursing care theory without extending our view of the human being. Such an extension is enabled by Rudolf Steiner's spiritual science, which opens up an understanding of the human body, soul and spirit.

We want to develop an approach to the threefold nature of the human being by contemplating body, soul and spirit and the qualities to be found in them.

3.2.1 The body

The body of the human being is closest to our ordinary understanding and is thus the easiest to initially understand. When we consider the human being as an entity having a body, we are dealing with a living organism, with both a physical and an etheric body. Modern anatomy and physiology give us the possibility to get to know the human body on a large scale, e.g., as organs and organ systems, as well as examining it down to the smallest structures of tissues, cells and genes. New and exciting discoveries in the human body are possible all the time with the help of modern technology, which unfortunately often leads to exclusively technical and mechanistic healing methods.

In our era, in which fixation on the physical predominates, we find an intensive preoccupation with the physical care of our patients. Basic care, prophylaxis, the supply of food and the disposal of excretions are all too often done purely with a view to expedience. Washing the whole body, for example, is limited to the aspect of physical cleanliness. This purely functional way of providing care does not take the mental and spiritual aspects of the patient into account and does not allow for any thought of deliberately aiming for a therapeutic effect, especially in the simplest care procedures. If we provide basic care from the point of view of bringing healing to body, soul and spirit, we can revive these necessities each day afresh and make our care more humane [→ see chapter "Variations in Whole-Body Washing"].

3.2.2 The soul

In medicine, as already described, the human soul was declared non-existent by Virchow. The psychologist Sigmund Freud (1856–1939), the "father" of psychoanalysis (gr psyche = soul), was born in 1856, two years before Virchow published his "Cellular Pathology." Freud and his successors took on a task that medicine covered less and less. While medicine was increasingly concerned with the body due to its scientific method, psychoanalysts concerned themselves with the soul.

What exactly do psychoanalysts, psychiatrists and psychotherapists concern themselves with? Those who seek help from these experts do not come with abdominal pain, a broken leg or other clearly definable physical symptoms. The pain is not primarily physical: physical symptoms are at most one of the reasons for visiting a psychotherapist and they often represent a plethora of diffuse symptoms that are difficult to define and which did not lead to a diagnosis during a medical examination. People go to a psychotherapist when they are experiencing a life crisis, are no longer able to cope with their life and cannot find a way out of their difficult situation on their own. Such crises manifest differently in different people. Often this has to do with problems that affect the *emotional life* of a person. Uncontrollable feelings resulting from one or more events put someone into a state in which he no longer feels free. These feelings can result from his relationships with other people: problems with family, partners, colleagues or friends. But they can also be of a more inner nature. Then the person no longer reaches his own aspirations, his self-imposed goals are too high, and feelings of failure, omission and unworthiness arise.

The latter feelings are often connected with a person's thoughts. No matter how he turns his thoughts, the long-awaited insights and solutions do not appear. The situation seems hopeless and he can only experience his life of thoughts as prison and torture. The person feels that he is not free to control his thoughts.

Excited and uncontrollable feelings, as well as aimless and confusing thoughts, also lead to problems in the *life of will*. The person seems to be paralyzed by the situation in which he finds himself. He is incapable of acting correctly, weakened in his will and unfree. The patient often asks the psychotherapist, "What should I do?"

Pathologically, emotional problems manifest as depressive or manic states. Difficulties in imagining and thinking can culminate in hallucinations. This is the case, for example, with schizophrenia. Pathological phenomena in the life of will can manifest in such a way that the person changes his behavior and carries out actions that he would never do in a healthy state. The terms "sociopath" or "criminal psychopath" are often used for these patients. On the other hand, a person's will can be so weakened that he no longer has the courage to live. This leads to the "suicidal patient."

> Three soul qualities can be seen from these aspects of the "psyche" or soul: *thinking, feeling, and willing.* These qualities do not act separately from each other, their interaction forms the rich content of our life of soul.

It is not only soul qualities that are closely linked, however. Body and soul cannot be considered separately in ordinary life, either. This results in a task of caring for the emotional and mental aspect of a person. And this applies not only to those who are mentally ill, but to all people who have become patients because of illness. Here, nurses serve as mediators in a similar way to water, in that we make sure that everything around our patients has a healing effect on their body, and we also design their surroundings in such a way that this has a beneficial effect on their soul. Practically speaking, we think in this context of the order and aesthetics of a hospital room. What does the patient see from his perspective in bed? A pale wall? Or can he look out of the window, at a beautiful picture or at photographs of loved ones? How light or dark is the room? Does it smell fresh—or used and musty? Is it peacefully quiet? Or are we so busy with our nursing task that we cause unnecessary noise? With these and similar questions, we as nurses are already paying attention to many things that contribute to the mental well-being of our patients.

3.2.3 The spirit

How can we gain an understanding of the human spirit? Is there something in the human being that differs so much from the soul and the body that it is recognizable as spirit?

Let us start by looking at the term "spirit" as it is ordinarily used. We may first think of religion. Chaplains, pastors and priests are its representatives. They are supposed to help people reconnect with the higher, eternally divine through religion (Latin religere = reconnecting). By recognizing an all-powerful, all knowing, good God, human beings seek development and refinement of their own spirit. Irrespective of religion or creed, the human spirit can be seen in the fact that we strive as aspiring individualities for eternal goodness, for refinement of our own being and for moral action. In individuals, this is also expressed in the feeling of having a task in this life. Spiritual striving is often not as conscious as just described, rather it exists as motivation in the background and as a reason to exist in daily life.

It follows from this that the human spirit is constantly developing its body and soul as instruments of its striving on this earth. The human spirit differs from the body, which is fully formed after 21 years, then ages and dies. The human spirit is not bound to the body or everyday events in the same way that the soul is through thinking, feeling and willing. The spirit represents the freely developing core of the human being which, through its interaction with the soul and body, aspires to attain a connection with the divine.

As the evolving, supersensible part of the human being, the spirit cannot fall ill. Suffering that manifests in the body or soul can be considered either as an obstacle to the development of the spirit, or as physical and mental resistance that the spirit must overcome to evolve. In this way, diseases can be viewed in a new light: they do not necessarily represent unnecessary and pointless events in life that must be eliminated as quickly as possible. They are challenges for the human spirit to overcome. They are opportunities to progress in developing the spirit. The biographies of individual human beings give insight into the individual aspirations of human spirits during their life on earth. Thinking about biographies can be a great help in understanding the motives for development and it often allows us to understand the meaning of illness in a person's life, when we look back on it.

The care of the spirit requires much more than mere respect and support for patients who want to lead a religious life. For the period of time when someone is a patient, we nurses can be companions to a certain extent. We can help them during the difficult time of their illness and perhaps assist them in regaining sight of the goals and direction of their life, so that they can continue on their way with fresh energy.

3.2.4 A bridge between body and spirit—the soul

In summary, we note that the body is the visible, living, physical part of the human being. The spirit is the inner, aspiring core, which at the same time has a share in eternal truth and goodness. The soul as a supersensible member forms the bridge between inside and outside, between body and spirit.

Anthroposophic anthropology allows us to discover divisions of three in body, soul and spirit as well. The threefold aspect of the soul, which has already been mentioned as thinking, feeling and willing, will be shown as it relates to the body's three-fold nature below. This will be followed by a short summary of the threefold nature of the spirit that arises from three levels of higher knowledge.

3.2.5 The threefold aspect in body, soul and spirit

In his book *Riddles of the Soul*,[9] Steiner described the threefold nature of the soul after many years of spiritual research. Its three fundamental powers are:

- Thinking
- Feeling
- Willing

As the physical foundations for these three soul powers, Steiner differentiated between:

- Neurosensory activity
- Rhythmic activity
- Motor-metabolic activity

Regarding the spiritual side, he described the corresponding further development of the three soul qualities into higher cognitive abilities that are not bound to the body's sense organs. He called these abilities:

- Imagination
- Inspiration
- Intuition

These words are to be understood only in terms of the capacities described by Steiner and explained here. They are not meant to convey the usual meaning, which uses them as synonyms for irrational methods of cognition. In particular, the concept of Intuition is not to be confused with the idea of intuition in nursing developed by Benner.[10]

3.3 Soul qualities and their physiological counterparts

A close examination of the soul qualities thinking, feeling and willing creates an understanding of underlying physiological processes. The assumption that mental qualities and physiology are connected distinguishes anthroposophic anthropology from both medical physiology and conventional psychology.

3.3.1 Thinking—the neurosensory system

In thinking, we concern ourselves with receiving and processing sensory impressions. The abundance of perceptions allows us to have a rich content of thoughts. We can hardly imagine what could be thought of if we were not able to perceive through our senses, and our sources of perception are not exhausted with the five classical senses. In addition to touch, taste, smell, sight and hearing, we also have perceptions of our own body: our movements, our balance and our physical condition. Furthermore, we possess a sense of warmth that can be distinguished from the sense of touch even by the anatomy of its receptors. We are also able to perceive the individuality of other people, as well as the feelings and thoughts expressed through language [→ Chapter "From the Question of Meaning in Cancer to the Cultivation of the Senses"]. The abundance of sense impressions thus forms the basis for the usual content of our thinking. Thinking also enables us to attain knowledge of spiritual things by liberating ourselves from all that is bound to the senses. We will go into this in further detail in relation to the three stages of spiritual development.

All sense impressions reach our consciousness via our nervous system and then become soul content. Our nervous system is not the source of our thoughts, but merely their physical carrier. Thinking is a process of soul and spirit that cannot be found in the anatomy of the nervous system.

The functional unity that conveys perception and consciousness is what Steiner called the *neurosensory system.*

The neurosensory system has its center in the head area, but it penetrates the body with innumerable nerve pathways that extend into the sensory organs. The prevailing principles of this system are static stillness, coldness and degeneration. As already described regarding the human fourfold nature, the head is freed from any function of the limbs by the upright stature of the human being. The firm skull reinforces this immobilization and prevents injury and overheating. In addition, the cerebrospinal fluid protects the brain floating in it from violent movements and vibrations. Only minimal metabolic activity occurs in the brain, because it would otherwise cause movement and warmth. Furthermore, there are no muscles. Shortly after birth, our nerve substance is already fully developed, so that any metabolic activity necessary for regeneration is largely eliminated in this area. The low ability of nerve substance to regenerate is also reflected in the poor healing tendency of the tissue. This organ system therefore provides ideal anatomical and physiological conditions for thinking: stillness, coldness and a tendency to degenerate.

3.3.2 Feeling—the rhythmic system

In feeling, the soul interacts with the surrounding world. In thinking it is possible to recognize objective facts; these can be seen equally by anyone. Feeling adds our personal impressions. We either like or dislike what we have perceived. Our opinion in this sense is an expression of our feelings about something. The will that is revealed in our actions is also often characterized by sympathy or antipathy. The soul's relationship with the world is comparable to a swinging back and forth: the world comes to us and we react to it with feelings.

The physical basis for feeling is found in the rhythmic processes of our organism. In the *lungs*, for example, the breath swings between the inner and outer world: air is inhaled and exhaled. It reaches the innermost part of each cell via the blood and is then exhaled off again to the outer world. The human being is thus in constant contact with the world through the activity of the lungs and the circulation. This physiological process is like a reflection of our soul life, which connects with the world in feeling and then must find its way back to itself.

The heartbeat relates to the breathing rhythm at a ratio of 4:1. A change in the rhythm of one organ always causes a change in the rhythm of the other in healthy people. In their close interaction, the heart and lungs are regarded as the two central organ systems of the *rhythmic system*. Thus, the center of rhythmic activity is in the human chest area, but it extends over all rhythmical processes in the body.

The predominant principles in the rhythmic system are balance, mediation and harmony. The ribs appear as a protective shell in the anatomy of the bone structure of the chest area. However, this protection has breaks in it, so it is much more flexible than the firm skull that protects the brain.

Movements in the rhythmic element are not chaotic. They are subject to balancing and harmonizing regulation resulting from the alternation between movement and rest [→ Chapter "Rhythm"]. The body's warmth is also regulated rhythmically. The blood, as the main mediator of warmth flowing through the whole body, must balance both the warmth generated in the liver and the relative coolness of the brain. Peripheral circulation in the form of vasodilation and vasoconstriction mainly causes the core temperature of 37°C (98.6°F) to be maintained inside and outside the body in relation to temperature fluctuations. These and numerous other physiological and anatomical conditions enable the rhythmic system to provide the physical basis for feeling through the underlying principles of harmony, mediation and balance.

3.3.3 Will—the motor-metabolic system

In volition, the soul has an impulse to do something in the world. Activity arises when human beings want something; human will is expressed in deeds.

The physical basis for implementing impulses of will is mainly found in the activity of the muscles. It is through our limbs that we can express our will. Our will is not only expressed in conscious impulses, it is also found in the unconscious primordial will to live, which constantly pushes us towards life.

Will finds its physical equivalent in the upbuilding and regenerating activity of the metabolic system. The metabolic system expresses the will to live by processing the nourishment that serves to build up the body. The activity of the limbs places deeds into the world; likewise, metabolic activity places the body into the world, ever again afresh, and maintains it.

The body's metabolic and muscle activity, which is summarized as the *motor-metabolic system*, generates the body heat that is indispensable for all life processes. The soft elasticity and high regenerative capacity of the metabolic organs, as well as the long tubular bones and their flexible joints, provide the ideal anatomical basis for the principles of movement, warmth and upbuilding that prevail in this system. The center of this system is in the abdomen, but its activity extends over the entire body and is found wherever metabolic activity and movement manifest as expressions of will.

3.4   Further examples of threefoldness

The above description of bone structure relating to the threefold nature of body and soul is only one example of how soul qualities and vital functions can be found reflected in the construction of the physical body. The firm, closed skull is ideal for giving the brain coolness and stillness, which serves consciousness and thinking. Opposite to this are the long, strong tubular bones, whose muscles surrounding them generate warmth through motion and allow the person's will to express itself in deeds. The ribs are located in between. The upper fixed and lower movable ribs form a kind of metamorphosis between the skull and the tubular bones. They are easily moveable, but not voluntarily, and they resonate with the rhythmic breathing that gives us the possibility to express feelings.

FACE: Let us continue our observations and look at the threefold aspect of the human face: we notice how the firmly closed forehead, behind which the brain is hidden, behaves as a resting pole in comparison to the movable mandible, which serves as a power pole for chewing and thus for metabolic activity. Between the two is the nose, which is the respiratory organ serving the rhythmic system. Smells, as sensory sensations of the nose, are also closely related to feelings and emotional memories.

EYE: The eye can also be seen to have a threefold structure: first, the cool, barely perfused cornea facing the light; hidden in the skull we find the base of the eye muscles and the choroid, which are characterized by blood circulation and metabolic activity. This allows the eye muscles to move. In between lies the sensitive iris, which adapts its involuntary movements to light conditions and perceived objects. Its activity, like that of breathing, is an interplay between inside and outside: the pupil narrows and opens like a gate between the inside and outside world.

ARM: A threefold structure is also evident in our arms. Here we find the strong, muscular upper arm with a supporting bone and a ball joint, which allows movements in all directions. Opposite this is the delicate hand, which can serve as an organ of perception for sensory activity. The forearm in between is less muscular, and its mobility is reduced by the ulna and radius to a back-and-forth movement in two directions.

DAY: Different organ systems operate differently at different times. During the day, while we are awake, there is the most demand for the degrading activity of our neurosensory system: during perception and when processing these perceptions in our thinking. During the night, when daytime consciousness is reduced, our metabolic organs work in a regenerative and upbuilding way, so that we wake up refreshed the next morning. This rhythmic activity bridges the gap between the two systems' degrading and regenerative activities day and night.

Just as thinking, feeling and willing permeate each other in the soul, we find that the body's neurosensory activity, rhythmic activity and motor-metabolic activity interact inseparably with each other. A closer examination of this physical threefold nature in health and illness will illustrate this interaction.

4.   Functional threefolding in health and illness

Anthroposophic anthropology describes this division into neurosensory, rhythmic and motor-metabolic systems as *functional threefolding.* Such a concept first directs our attention to activities and processes before considering anatomical facts. This view forms a basis for our understanding of disease in Anthroposophic Medicine, which does not primarily focus on the pathology of the cell with its biochemistry, but rather recognizes disease dynamics in disturbed relationships between the three functional systems.

To illustrate the dynamics of functional threefolding and not misunderstand it as a tripartite division, we can imagine the three functional systems as a figure-eight [Fig. A, B, C]. In health, their relationship would correspond to Figure A.

Figure A shows neurosensory and motor-metabolic activity in equilibrium: both sides of the figure-eight are equal in size and have the same proportion to each other. The rhythmic system has its center in the middle, where the lines cross. If we trace this figure with our finger, we find that the movement of our hand is very rhythmic. The organism is therefore healthy when the two poles are in balance. The rhythmic activity can mediate and harmonize unhindered between the neurosensory and motor-metabolic systems.

The figure-eight helps us to understand illness, which manifests in two fundamentally different types.

4.1 Type I diseases—cold predominates

Figure B shows what happens when neurosensory activity predominates (Type I diseases). Stillness (immobility), cold and degradation predominate, the tendencies already described. They encroach on the area of the rhythmic and motor-metabolic systems. If we trace this figure with our finger, we immediately notice how the rhythm changes and appears to be inharmonious. The organism has become unbalanced.

"Cold," sclerotic diseases with symptoms of hardening and stiffness are typical of this imbalance. Most of the diseases of our current civilization, such as arteriosclerosis, diabetes mellitus, carcinomas and dementia, are not accompanied by fever. These diseases often cause hardening of the blood vessels or poorly vitalized deposits such as tumors and plaque. Hardening can occur in all organs and is particularly noticeable in the formation of stones, such as kidney or gallstones.

Other expressions of this type can be found where cold, inflexibility and degradation occur in a place where warmth, movement and structure normally dominate. Here we recognize countless diseases that are so widespread today. The task of the nurse is then to ensure warmth, whether through administering compresses and rhythmical oil applications or through emotional warmth. The patient must also be protected against excessive sensory stimuli during illness and convalescence. This applies to television, radio and other activities that mainly appeal to the senses. How we work with rhythm is of great importance: in nursing we should support everything rhythmic in the daily routine and in the patient's life.

4.2 Type II diseases—heat predominates

Any predominance of motor-metabolic activity leads to a displacement of neurosensory activity. Here, too, there is a disturbance in the harmonious course of rhythmic activity, which can be seen in the figure-eight for Type II diseases [Fig. C]. If we consider the dominant principles of warmth, movement and upbuilding in the motor-metabolic system, we can quickly identify the type of disease caused by an excess of these processes. The increase in heat induces all diseases associated with fever. This is not contradicted by the fact that fever often arises as a reaction to an infection caused by microorganisms. After all, not all people get infected when they are exposed to influenza or other infectious diseases. Although the microorganisms are present in everyone, only those who are already in a state of imbalance are susceptible and fall ill.

Nowadays, the really "hot" inflammatory diseases are not only rarer than in earlier times, when epidemics such as cholera or the plague affected entire populations, the course of the illness is also no longer as spectacular today. Since antibiotics and antipyretics which suppress such diseases are used very quickly in most cases, we have little opportunity to observe these diseases in their natural course. The administration of antibiotics is undoubtedly justified in life-threatening situations—but we seem to be using them too quickly nowadays. This often happens before it has been determined whether the pathogens are viruses or bacteria. Antibiotics are known to have no effect at all on viral infections.

> It seems as if people expect drugs to be prescribed for the slightest problems, and if this does not happen, they feel that the doctor is not taking them seriously.

In many cases, we have forgotten how to deal with fever. We fear clouding of consciousness, losing control or suffering hallucinations and fever spasms. However, we can understand such febrile illness as an attempt by the organism to restore inner balance. For nurses, the aim is not primarily to reduce the fever, but to become aware of the specific role of warmth. This also means to carefully handle cooling, as already described with calf compresses. Feverish patients should drink a lot of fluids. In such cases, the aim is to strengthen the organism's disturbed rhythm, to restore inner balance, also because high fever is taxing for the heart and circulation. To get through the fever, we who accompany the patient can offer courage and trust. An inflammatory disease that someone overcomes with supportive help rather than with antipyretic drugs can thus be experienced as strengthening and as an achievement of balance. Support of the patient's rhythmic processes induces healing from the middle and strengthens the person's inherent healing powers.

Example: Migraine

Some ailments show aspects of both types of displacement. Migraines are a vivid example of this. On the surface, the second type of disease prevails (the motor-metabolic system predominates). Elements of the first disease type represent a late attempt by the organism to restore balance.

Migraines typically manifest in a (throbbing) headache, sensitivity to light, and nausea to the point of vomiting. Vasodilation with hyperemia in the head area and reactive vasoconstriction are considered to be its physiological causes. Usually, painkillers are given that reduce the patient's consciousness until the attack has subsided. Or substances such as triptans are administered to block the inflammatory reaction in the blood vessels and to dilate constricted blood vessels. As a side effect of these therapies, the person may experience a slight general feeling of weakness and undirected dizziness, discomfort, tingling, a feeling of warmth or heat and mild nausea. Overdose and excessive intake can lead to a permanent headache.

A functional examination of migraines leads us to interpret the increase in blood circulation and the inflammation of the vessels in the brain as an expression of increased metabolic activity. This is the area in which the activity of the neurosensory system should prevail. In this sense, the nausea that occurs later can also be regarded as consciousness—i.e., neurosensory activity—"in the wrong place." Often, vomiting brings a certain degree of relief. The organism tries to regulate itself to restore balance.

The diagnosis of a metabolic process that has shifted to the neurosensory area provides the basis for causal therapy. The displaced metabolic activity must be returned to where it belongs—to the organs of the motor-metabolic system. This might be done by means of a mustard foot bath, which has a strong metabolically stimulating, warming effect [→ Chapter "Compresses"]. With such treatment applied to the legs we are choosing an application location that is opposite the head region. The head is freed up again for its activity of consciousness. Side effects do not occur with this therapy if there is no hypersensitivity to mustard powder. This therapy makes sense from a conventional physiological point of view: the mustard powder's local stimulation on the lower legs causes local vasodilation, which in turn draws the blood from the head to the feet.

5. Illness and biography

Functional threefolding enables us to understand the physical and psychological causes of disease as displaced "normal" processes. This results in a causal therapy that brings the existing imbalances back into a harmonious relationship. However, this does not at first explain why in similar stressful situations one person suffers from migraines, another from stomach ulcers, a third reacts with neurodermitis and still others find that it manifests as mental illness. To come closer to an answer to this question, we must direct our attention to what is spiritual in the patient. We must look at the person's individuality and at how this unfolds in time, in his or her biography.

5.1 Threefoldness in spiritual development

The human being develops physically, mentally, emotionally and spiritually from the moment of conception to death [→ Chapter "Illness and Destiny"]. If we integrate the eternal character of the spiritual into our contemplation, then the idea of development gains an expanded meaning. When we consider the possibility of the human spirit developing over several lifetimes, then illness, disability and the premature death of a loved one appear in a new light. Blows of fate of all kinds then do not have to be accepted as senseless coincidences. Illnesses, whatever their nature, appear as specific expressions of an evolving individuality.

For nurses, this consideration results in the role of a companion. Our task is not to influence the spiritual development of our patients, i.e., we should not actively intervene in their developing lives or determine their direction. By caring for and nursing the patient, though, we can make it easier for him to find goals, as well as new courage and strength to follow his further path. An illness is often a drastic event in a person's life. People diagnosed with a "heart attack," "stroke," or "cancer" usually must radically alter their lifestyles, perhaps change careers or give up their hobbies. It can be very terrifying to contemplate what the future may hold. Sincere conversation allows us to hear what comes from the patient. We should not intervene with immediate help and advice. Nevertheless, we can assist and support him in reformulating his life goals. We can help him to find the strength and courage that he needs in his quest to follow the inner voice of his spirit.

5.1.1 Accompanying support—an opportunity in nursing

In nursing, we often have the unique honor of gaining insight into difficult decision-making moments in the destiny of people—our patients—and we can accompany them throughout this difficult time.

Rudolf Steiner described in many of his works how human beings can consciously follow a path of development that leads to knowledge of the spirit.[11, 12, 13]

We attain knowledge of higher worlds by liberating our thinking from all sense-bound impressions, so that our spiritual eye is opened for what is purely spiritual. The decision to follow such a path must be taken by everyone alone and in freedom. Since we in the nursing profession have made it our task to care for and accompany people in illness and at moments of severity in their destinies, our own path of development can appear as an urgent task, even a duty. Nursing becomes richer when nurses act out of understanding for the soul and spiritual connections behind the sense-perceptible world. Such a path of development not only serves to improve the care of our patients, it also helps us as caregivers to deal better with the many difficult, painful and sad situations that we encounter in our professional and personal lives.

6. Three levels of knowledge

Steiner described three levels of knowledge of higher worlds that result from consequential spiritual development. These are:

- Imagination
- Inspiration
- Intuition

These three levels of knowledge are closely connected with the principles active in the soul.

Thinking, feeling and willing are not directly perceptible with our eyes, but can be experienced as inner processes. Imagination, Inspiration and Intuition are different. These levels of knowledge are largely foreign to our experience, so you can understand why the following description must overcome some difficulties and remain sketchy. If we nevertheless succeed in remaining open to the spiritual aspect, it can reveal itself to us.

6.1 Imagination

Steiner used the term Imagination to describe spiritual insights that are reflected as thinking in the soul and as the neurosensory system in the body. At this level of knowledge, we perceive the spiritual world in the form of images. In doing so, however, we remain only on the pictorial surface of the spiritual world, just as we do not yet experience the inner essence of things when we only perceive them with our sense of sight in the sense-perceptible world.

Please do not misunderstand: Steiner does not mean that we can look into the spiritual world with our ordinary eyes. The dynamics of Imagination, however, can best be compared to our sense of sight.

6.2 Inspiration

Spiritual metamorphosis of feeling, which is expressed in rhythmic activity on the physical level, leads to Inspiration as a supersensible cognitive organ. Through Inspiration, we penetrate deeper into the essence of what is spiritual. Here the spiritual world reveals itself to the person who has trained himself in this level of knowledge, not just as an outer image, but from within. An example from the physical world can make this more understandable:

> When we meet a human being, our first impression is an image of his or her outer form conveyed by our sense of sight. An image comparable to the optical impression is derived from imaginative perception. If we now hear the voice of the person, his image comes to life and is complemented by more intimate expressions through sound and inflection.

6.3 Intuition

Will, the soul power which has its physical basis in the motor-metabolic system, forms the basis for a further level of spiritual knowledge—Intuition. To describe what is characteristic of this stage of knowledge, let us first remember the example above. Imaginative perception seemed to be comparable to visual impressions, Inspiration to deeper acoustic experiences. Intuition can now be imagined as an active encounter, for example, when we shake hands with the person opposite us. In Intuition perception and action unite into a unity: we are no longer an observer in intuitive cognition, we have become one with the spiritual world.

The soul forms a bridge to the physical world via will activity and opens itself towards the spiritual in thinking.

We have recognized that neurosensory, rhythmic and motor-metabolic activity permeate each other in the body and interact in thinking, feeling and willing in the soul. Similarly, the stages of knowledge Imagination, Inspiration and Intuition to be developed in the spiritual world cannot be understood separately. In their entirety they open the door to the spiritual world.

7. Final remarks

Understanding the human being as a threefold and fourfold being provides a basis for nursing that is extended by anthroposophy.

The fourfold aspect shows how we are related to the world and nature, and it refers to our relationship to the four elements earth, water, air and fire. It shows how the human being, through the 'I' and the mastery of fire, represents the fourth realm of nature above minerals, plants and animals. In our fourfold nature we are in harmony with the earth, with the four cardinal points, the four seasons and with all other fourfold principles that belong to this earth. Our understanding of the fourfold nature of the human being can be a stimulus for nursing. *Florence Nightingale* already formulated it as follows:

> "The word 'nursing' as I understand it, has a far deeper meaning than is attributed to it in ordinary life, where people don't think that it is much more than the administration of medicines and compresses and other mere handwork. Rightly understood, however, nursing means the proper use and regulation of fresh air, light, warmth, cleanliness, tranquility, the right choice and the timely supply of food and drink, and all this with the greatest possible protection of the life forces of the one who is ill."[14]

The threefold aspect shows how we as beings of body, soul and spirit stand in a living relationship between the physical and the spiritual worlds, between heaven and earth. The number three represents a divine aspect, as in the archetype of the Father, Son and Holy Spirit of Christianity.

Nursing finds a special task in working with rhythm when it works with the threefold aspect. Rhythm can harmoniously connect polarities (hot and cold, sleeping and waking, spirit and body) to support our patients' recovery.

These anthropological considerations are clearly not suitable as a method for theoretical care models or excessive documentation schemes. This would be contrary to the aim of anthroposophy and would impair the vital relationship between patients and nurses. Instead, if we endeavor to work with the view of the human being described here, we will deepen our relationship with patients and, in our day-to-day nursing work, be able to give direction to the "how" of our actions.

The following chapters will explain the practical application of anthroposophic anthropology.

Category	Example learning objectives	Recommended learning path
Skill	You can conduct intake interviews from the perspective of the patient's fourfold nature.	A
Your own learning objective		
Relationships	You are extending your understanding of your profession with respect to the holistic, patient-centered task of nurses.	B
Your own learning objective		
Knowledge	You are familiar with the basic concepts of anthroposophic anthropology.	C
Your own learning objective		

References

1   Nightingale, F. *Notes on nursing.* Translated from the facsimile reproduction of the German translation of 1878, Leipzig. Published by Bundesausschuss der Unterrichtsschwestern und Pfleger, Stuttgart 1980.

2   Steiner, R. *Occult science: An outline.* Rudolf Steiner Press, London 2013.

3   Steiner, R. *Theosophy. An introduction to the supersensible knowledge of the world and the destination of man.* Rudolf Steiner Press, London 2005.

4   Steiner, R.; Wegman, I. *Extending practical medicine. Fundamental principles based on the science of the spirit.* Rudolf Steiner Press, London 2000.

5   Translated from: Goethe, J.W. von. *Werke.* Vol. 2, Talismane. Hamburg edition. Deutscher Taschenbuch Verlag, Munich 1998.

6   Steiner, R. *Anthroposophical leading thoughts. Anthroposophy as a path of knowledge. The Michael Mystery.* Rudolf Steiner Press, London 2007.

7   Virchow, R. Translated from: Vasold M. *Rudolf Virchow. Der grosse Arzt und Politiker.* Deutsche Verlags-Anstalt, Stuttgart 1991.

8   Ibid.

9   Steiner, R. *Riddles of the soul.* Mercury Press, Spring Valley 1996.

10 Benner, P. *From novice to expert.* Prentice Hall, New Jersey 2000.

11 Steiner, R. *Occult science: An outline.* Rudolf Steiner Press, London 2013.

12 Steiner, R. *Theosophy. An introduction to the supersensible knowledge of the world and the destination of man.* Rudolf Steiner Press, London 2005.

13 Steiner, R. *How to know higher worlds—a modern path of initiation.* Anthroposophic Press, Great Barrington 2002.

14 Nightingale, F. *Notes on nursing.*

CHAPTER IV
Illness and Destiny

RENATE HASSELBERG · ROLF HEINE

Serious illness has an impact on a patient's biography. Anthroposophic Medicine integrates this aspect into treatment. In doing so, it is decisive to work with the question of meaning to find the thread of continuity running through the patient's biography. This is only possible for nurses and therapists who understand their own basic biographical patterns. This chapter examines the relationships between patients and nurses as encounters of destiny.

→ Learning objectives, see end of chapter

1. Introduction

We have chosen the unusual form of a dialogue for this topic. It will enable us to talk about it more personally and will avoid giving the impression that we have all the answers to life's "ultimate" questions. We thought that a conversation would enable us to show how we are wrestling with these questions and indicate the aphoristic character of our presentation.

When someone falls ill, they are hampered in performing their everyday life tasks. The flow of life slows down, and the patient is thrown back on himself. Especially serious, life-threatening diseases call into question the person's previous life plan or confront him with the question of what gives his individual life meaning.

Even mild, everyday illnesses, such as a cold or an occasional headache, often raise the question of why such an unpleasant disorder has to be experienced now of all times, at such an inopportune time.

Anyone who seriously asks himself such a question usually already suspects an inner connection between the disease and the individual biographical situation in which he is currently standing.

In this article we want to present some aspects of the problem of disease as it occurs in the course of a human life. Such questioning only make sense if we start from the goal-orientation of individual biography. The meaning of human life can only be felt. In a healthy child it is there as a matter of course. The child's whole attitude towards life is based on the certainty of the meaningfulness of the world. Adults no longer have this basic sustaining reason for existence at their immediate disposal. For them, the meaning and goal of life must rather be sought, experienced and suffered individually.

Against this background, we would like to discuss the role of disease and crisis in human biography.

2. The question of meaning

2.1 What is a biography?

[Renate Nadja Hasselberg **NH** | Rolf Heine **RH**]

NH What exactly is a biography? First we can say: only human beings have biographies. Animals, plants, and minerals have no biography—at least not in the sense that they could shape their life's path purposefully or develop self-awareness. When I have observed a rabbit, then I do not have to observe countless other rabbits to know what a rabbit is as a species. All its possible manifestations can be found in this rabbit type. Knowledge of this rabbit is sufficient to understand the creature "rabbit." If I meet a person and already know his mother, grandfather, and aunt, then I still know very little about this person himself. I need to have an individual relationship with him, I need to perceive him individually to be able to say anything about him.

If we look at a biography from a temporal point of view, it seems at first as if it begins with birth and ends with death.

This undoubtedly applies to the person's biological existence. It begins—hidden from view—with conception. But where are the limits to the existence of the individuality? Science tells us nothing about this. The millennia-old knowledge of the immortality of the soul is shaken by doubts. The pre-existence of human individuality before the moment of conception—its unborn nature—has not been taken into consideration in Christian Western culture for centuries, with a few exceptions (e.g., Goethe, Novalis, Lessing). Only at the beginning of the last century did Rudolf Steiner again present the idea of the pre-existence and after-death existence of the human being as something that is indispensable for understanding individuality. According to Steiner, every human being passes through a long series of embodiments (incarnations). In the time between death and a new birth, the individuality exists in a spiritual world and prepares for its next incarnation.

The concept of biography seems considerably expanded when considered from the point of view of repeated earth lives. We can now look at the events of the current life with a question: what impulses from a previous life will have an effect on the present, and what consequences will our present action have for our after-death existence and subsequent incarnations?

RH This is difficult to understand for a person who initially experiences his biography as being limited to the time between birth and death. It is only during this period that we are aware of our existence.

What possibilities are there for a person who is unfamiliar with the idea of reincarnation to approach an understanding of it? What is the difference between the concept of reincarnation based on anthroposophy and similar, Eastern ideas, for example?

NH In his book *Theosophy,* Steiner described a train of thought that substantiates the necessity of repeated earth lives to gain a satisfactory understanding of the human being. He starts with the question: "Where did I get what's expressed in my biography?"[1]

He continues: "As a physical person I come from other physical people, for I have the same human form as the whole human species. It was therefore possible for me to acquire the characteristics of the genus within the genus by heredity. As a spiritual being I have my own form, just as I have my own biography. I can therefore have this form from no one else but myself. And since I did not enter the world with indefinite, but with specific soul qualities, because my life's path, as it is expressed in my biography, is determined by these qualities, then my work on myself cannot have begun at my birth. I must have been present as a spiritual being before my birth [...] I must [...] as a spiritual being be the repetition of a spiritual being, from whose biography my own can be explained [...] Just as therefore the physical human form is again and again a repetition, a re-embodiment of a being of the human genre, the spiritual being must be a re-embodiment of the same spiritual being. For as a spiritual being, each person is a separate species."[2]

"In one lifetime, the human spirit appears as a repetition of itself with the fruits of its previous experiences gained in previous lifetimes."[3]

In contrast to some Eastern concepts of reincarnation, it seems absurd for a human individuality to embody itself in an animal or plant existence. Over many incarnations it becomes possible for human beings to rise to ever higher moral levels of humanity. According to an anthroposophic understanding, the meaning of reincarnation does not lie in liberation from the "wheel of births," as the Eastern tradition says, but in becoming a co-creator of creation.

RH The idea of reincarnation is not just a theory. It must prove its fruitfulness by bringing clarity and understanding to the often incomprehensible situations in our lives. Are there typical moments in a biography where people encounter the idea of reincarnation?

NH It can happen, for example, that you encounter someone who believes in such "superstitious stuff" as reincarnation, yet who otherwise seems to be quite reasonable. You become curious and think: how is it that someone who stands so solidly and capably in life can harbor such ludicrous thoughts? You can then perhaps notice how this idea of reincarnation carries that person in a special way and makes him fit for life.

Another possibility is that a person gets enmeshed in a life crisis in such a way that nothing carries him that carried him before. Something is breaking open that had been concealed by habits, phrases and routine until now. Out of this nothingness, a quality can appear that causes him to feel and wonder about things completely differently.

Or someone falls very, very ill, gets cancer or AIDS, and now in the face of imminent death the question arises: how have I lived my life, is there life after death or is it all over?

It always needs an experience that wakes you up, an experience where you suddenly catch your breath and for a tenth of a second the world seems to be turned upside down.

RH In conversations with seriously ill people I have often experienced that they said: "Reincarnation, that is something very familiar to me. It confirms something that I've actually felt for a long time. It has always felt to me as if my existence would go on after death, as if I was not born as a blank slate and as if I were carrying something from a very old past into this lifetime."

How can such a notion become practical in life and sustainable in a crisis?

NH Whether what I believe, or what has become certain to me, will actually carry me through, I can only know when it is actually demanded of me. It is not put to the test when my pension is secure, the sun is shining, and I have fried potatoes on the table. At such a time you can think splendidly about your personal maxims. This changes the moment the last building block holding you up starts to crumble. Life security and trust in life can only prove themselves when I am really challenged, for example during a biographical crisis.

2.2 A biography can be looked at on different levels

RH We started by talking about the nature of biography and you described different ways of looking at the life span. By referring to the idea of reincarnation, you have in a way opened a path to look at biography.

A biography can be looked at on different levels. One speaks, for example, of the biography of the body. A child is different from an elderly person and undergoes different physical development than the elderly person. The soul also matures. Other topics and goals become dominant. Over the course of our life we change the way we stand in life, how we shape our lives, how we shape the world and perform our life's tasks. Perhaps we should talk a little more about our physical, mental and spiritual biographies.

NH When we look at the biography of the body, it is true that the growing child needs all his powers to build up his physicality. One of Rudolf Steiner's most important discoveries in this regard concerns the relationship between consciousness and building up the physical body. Steiner explained that the forces that build up the human body in childhood are the same forces that are later available to the adult for thinking. In the first seven years of life these forces are still fully integrated into building up the body, and only around the time of the appearance of the secondary teeth do they gradually become free for thinking activity.

With sexual maturity the development of the body reaches a further stage. The forces that differentiated the body to the point of sexual maturity now enable us to develop independent life in our soul. The adolescent begins to deal consciously with his feelings. Sympathies and antipathies are experienced and acted out in extremes.

Around the age of 21, the young person comes of age. He is in a position to face the world as a free personality due to the physical and mental maturity acquired up to then.[4]

Awareness only arises where degenerative processes come into play. We need up-building processes to grow and develop the body. The more our corporeality is pushed back, the more our mental powers can become free. Up to about the middle of the third decade of life upbuilding processes predominate, then up to about the age of 35 upbuilding and degeneration balance each other out, after which processes of degeneration gain the upper hand.

This gives the biography a promising outlook. Degeneration in the body is up-building in consciousness, aging as a process of bodily degeneration offers the possibility to develop consciousness [→ Chapter "Geriatric Care as Care for Human Beings"].

That is why our culture, which absolutizes youth, is actually mistaken. The quality that flows into the world almost plantlike in children and young people is something tremendously beautiful and graceful. But it seems tragic when it is merely carried over to a later age. The upbuilding processes in the body must be sacrificed if consciousness is to develop!

When a child is growing up, its developmental processes are vital. That is why one-sided and premature intellectual education is so devastating. It introduces degenerative processes and ageing tendencies too quickly that do not belong at all to this age. Conversely, it is just as problematic to simply carry growth processes into a time in life when degenerative processes should predominate. An adult who spends a lot of time trying to keep her body in the condition of a teenager can seem just as disconcerting as a precocious teenager. So, you see, it really takes both, upbuilding and degeneration, but each in its own time.

Also, concerning the soul one can say: a soul in a youthful body is different from a soul in an aging one. The youthful soul needs joy so that it does not shrivel up in old age.

In youth until the fourth seven-year cycle, the main question is: what does the world have to offer me? I have been released into my freedom and can experiment in the world. It is hoped that during this time a young person will be given the fullness and richness of life and will be able to gather a wide range of experiences with himself and the world without worrying. Before processes of consciousness begin to dominate in the soul, the world should have been there for it as much as possible. The soul should have eaten its fill at the tables of life.

In many biographies, this is precisely the prerequisite for later selflessness that is not paid for with emotional draining. I must have experienced something on my travels in order to change from a wanderer into a counselor. Such wealth of experience is like a huge treasure of gold, which is to be transformed later. This original gold treasure cannot remain like this. The experience has to be forged into life experience:

"No illness should be forsaken without its blessing being wrung from it."

Friedrich Rittelmeyer (1872–1938), theologian

2.3 What actually falls ill and what happens during illness?

RH What role do illnesses play in biographies?

NH You can ask first: What actually falls *ill?*

RH The whole person always falls ill. There is a symptom, it becomes an obstacle, the life forces are impaired, one cannot move one's body as one normally does. This is where the disease first becomes noticeable.

NH At first I experience myself as being hindered from carrying out my intentions. I am thrown back to myself . . .

RH . . . or to my dependency on others. At first the body falls ill. Can the soul also fall ill?

NH Yes; in neurosis, for example, the soul falls ill, and the disease may also appear as a physical symptom in the body. This is not the case with so-called mental illnesses. Here we say from an anthroposophic understanding that the body falls ill, and the symptom appears in the soul.

In the case of physical and psychosomatic illnesses it is primarily the soul that falls ill. The illness manifests in physical symptoms, because the person did not consciously intervene in the soul's process of falling ill in time or did not do so energetically enough. One can also say that a symptom is a sign that something was not properly grasped via a conscious act.

"Any illness can be called a mental illness."

Novalis (1772–1801)

RH Why can't the spirit fall ill?

NH We have an everyday self. In that self, we are what we think we are. The self-image with which we define ourselves in everyday life corresponds to this everyday self. Above that we have, or rather, are a higher self, which is usually hidden from everyday consciousness. This higher self is the most significant writer of the biography. It guides us on our way, gives us our intentions and leads us to the human encounters and relationships that are essential for us. Just as the higher self ensures that we have the life partner or profession that suits us, so does it also ensure that we get the diseases that we should get. The higher self is an entity that remains unharmed by the fact of the disease, it progresses from incarnation to incarnation. It leads, it starts something new, it shapes the biography. Steiner wrote: "The human being who reflects on himself soon comes to the realization that, in addition to the self summed up in his thoughts, feelings and fully conscious will impulses, he carries a second more powerful self within him. He becomes aware of how he subordinates himself to this second self as a higher power [...] A human being is not alone: in him lives something that can always provide proof: the human being can lift himself above himself to something which is already growing beyond him and which will grow from lifetime to lifetime."[5]

RH Why would my higher self get me into such difficulties?

NH Take it as a hypothesis that it is no coincidence when a disease strikes you. If we include the thought of reincarnation in our reflection, what happens is that in the life between death and a new birth we take stock of our finished life and grasp impulses for a new life on earth. The higher self now leads us according to these impulses to the possibilities to compensate for the deficits that we became aware of in our life between death and new birth.[6]

> *"Illnesses, especially protracted ones, [are] years of apprenticeship in the art of living and the education of our soul. One has to try to use them by making daily observations. Is not the life of an educated person a constant invitation to learn?"*
>
> Novalis (1772–1801)

We want to take a phenomenological view of being ill. What happens when a disease progresses and you get better? After surviving suffering, you feel on top of the world. In children who have undergone one of the typical childhood illnesses, one usually observes a physical, mental and spiritual maturation process. Illnesses develop the soul. It is precisely because external activities are held back by the disease that something can condense inside and manifest as a great force.

If you really endure pain, it can be a profound experience in which your trust in life has to prove itself. You experience that something flows towards you from a completely unknown side, and you feel how little you are really alone. This can also be the experience of an angel or Christ.

The problem is that we are so little inclined to see the disease as a gift, we just want it to go away. We don't accept the fact of being confined to our bed as a question: do you want to continue as before, or do you want to take stock of your situation?
That is why it is so important to accompany people who are ill, because very few people come up with the idea of asking themselves: what is the developmental nucleus of this disease?

RH This is the one form of illness that can lead to a kind of conscious self-knowledge and where we find that our further life's path develops differently than it would have without the illness, as if reaching a crossroads. These are fortunate cases that occur time and again, especially in cases of serious illness. Predominantly, however, the phenomena of illness are likely to occur in the following way: the flow of life is interrupted, you are confined to your sickbed, but you are not in a position to think about anything because, for example, the fever so dampens your consciousness or the pain binds it in such a way that it is quite impossible to grasp a sensible thought about something more significant, let alone think about the meaning of life. Nevertheless, the following occurs at the end of the disease: not only do you feel physically healthier than before, you also feel mentally more capable.

For example, a child will not have to consciously experience the question of the meaning of her life or her future in a childhood illness, even if she suffers pain and anxiety. There seems to be something in the illness that enables developmental processes to happen physically, which cannot happen at all in the soul, because they would overwhelm the person in her present state of consciousness.

> *"Don't think that the disease is an obstacle to development. It is only another way of moving forward. In health you must use all your strength yourself to progress. Illness is a vehicle: all you have to do is hold on and you will move forward, you have no idea how fast."*
>
> Albert Steffen (1884–1963)

2.4 Inviting people to become inquirers

NH How can we meet a person who comes to us for treatment in a way that enables him to become aware of the connection between his illness and his life?

RH In disease, a physical process initially enables further development by taking the place of a process of consciousness. This does not mean that questions should not be consciously addressed when they arise.

NH When someone falls ill they do not have the feeling that they wanted it or intentionally made it happen, or that it is an opportunity for development happening in the body which they have not succeeded in accomplishing in their soul. But perhaps they notice during the illness that something has manifested itself somatically because they were not able to grasp it consciously. The body now continues in the form of a symptom what the soul had missed. A whole series of diseases could be intercepted if the body did not need to do something at this point that the soul could have done consciously. Under no circumstances should we judge this morally. In fact, we do not initially know why the soul did not address the matter consciously. The higher self then sets a task in the body through which the soul is now able to develop the abilities that it needs for a higher health.

RH If this does not succeed, it can often be observed that, although an illness has initially been overcome physically, its underlying cause in the soul still continues to have a harmful effect on the body. Then disease follows disease, with varying symptoms.

> *"If you yourself are lacking, dear sick man, what can I prescribe for you other than yourself?"*
> Ernst von Feuchtersleben (1806–1849)

NH If the golden moment passes unused, if the disease stops the flow of life for a moment and then you are healthy again and just live on as before, how can the disease become a real experience and strength for your further life?

Whether illnesses are chronic or highly acute, much depends on the quality of the therapist's relationship with the patient in terms of whether the patient will succeed in establishing a cognitive relationship to his illness and to himself and thus to his biography. One has to learn to help people to become inquirers.

There can also be hurdles in a person's destiny, where the person only rails against his fate. As a companion, one feels that the illness and suffering which actually belong to this person are being treated by him only as a kind of "occupational accident." This is so disturbing because one experiences that an opportunity is being missed and wasted. The patient has the suffering and pain anyway, but if he would make something out of this pain that would give him prospects for his future, then his pain would feel different to him. That is why the missed opportunity is often so difficult for onlookers to bear.

In such cases, as a companion, nurse or doctor, you can only straighten it out in your thoughts, or feel in yourself what is right on behalf of the person. This is a centrally Christian principle. Otherwise it is easy to fall into the temptation to reject the person, because it is so incredibly difficult to empathize with their situation. Loving understanding of the patient's current inability to recognize a meaning in suffering is just as much a prerequisite for accompanying him as is the attempt to awaken a sense of meaning.

RH So far we have looked at illnesses in terms of being the consequence of an unsolved problem of the soul and spirit. But now we can't just look at karma as affecting people from the past. It is also quite conceivable that a disease is not the result of such an unsolved problem, but is giving the patient an opportunity to develop capacities that will only come to fruition in the future.[7]

The knowledge that a disease has not only a "why" but also a "what for" makes it easier to deal with the patient. With this knowledge, the nurse stays open for the future. Otherwise, for chronically ill people in particular, the idea that "my illness is of my own doing on the level of body and soul" becomes almost unbearable.

NH That would be very inadequate. It is basically something tremendously promising when you get the chance to make up for a defect or a debt. The problem is that we usually don't see that with our senses. We must become very cultivated in our attitude so that we do not bring the least speculation about these things to the patient. It seems to me to be essential that we never use the term karma in the missionary sense or project our own ideas into the understanding of life or the self-conception of the other person.

3. Biographical aspects of the nursing profession

When we talk about the role of illness in people's lives, it is logical to wonder about the people who come near to patients during the time of illness—nurses. In contrast to relatives, for example, nurses initially have a relationship to the patient because it's their profession. Nevertheless, nursing work is often experienced as a vocation as well as a profession, as people become increasingly close to those whom they are caring for. If we consider that nursing, when aspiring to be holistic, also engages the wholeness of the nurse—i.e., with all his or her human abilities—this gives new significance to the question of the relationship between the profession and the personal vocation.

3.1 What motivates young people?

NH What is "future-oriented" regarding the question of profession? Is it a gift of grace or atavism when someone still discovers a vocation in their profession today? And what about the many, many people who also work tirelessly day after day and by no means discover a personal vocation and yet still work for the world? It must be borne in mind that the vast majority of humanity is not in a position to feel the meaning of work directly, yet they still do work for others in an incredibly selfless manner, for example at a machine, on an assembly line or in the service industry. A lot is being done for the world without any personal satisfaction for the doer.

RH The word "vocation" means "summons" or "calling." Whether you experience this summons as pleasant or as unpleasant is not decisive at first. Vocation has nothing to do with personal desires. Whether we want it or not today, we are being drawn into isolated, specialized professional activities due to existing social conditions. Even the classical professions of doctor, teacher, or priest are not exempt from this alienation in work life.

This does not mean that this work is pointless in itself if you look at the context in which it takes place. Vocation is experienced when I recognize my isolated position in the overall context as essential and tied to my individual commitment. Strength grows from our awareness of the context in which our personal, perhaps strongly alienating work stands.

Today people are confronted with the task of either pulling themselves inwardly out of work that does not directly give them satisfaction and thus becoming soulless machines themselves, or seeking a conscious connection to their activity.

NH This trend does not stop at the social professions, which at first glance appear to be so close to life. Activity no longer nourishes a person's soul of its own accord. We ourselves must actively seek the inner connection to our profession and establish it anew every day. When this does not happen, we find listlessness, emptiness, the feeling of having to give without getting something in return. Even a so-called ideal profession does not offer any guarantee for a satisfying professional life, because it does not exempt the person from releasing its fruits for themselves and the community.[8]

What motivates young people to enter the nursing profession today?

RH Normally, young people enter the nursing profession around the age of 20. They often do this with the idea that nursing is a non-specialized profession that is close to life. The activities do not appear to be defined to the same extent as in other professions. In nursing you are a bit of a doctor, a bit of a priest, but above all you are human. This idea of the nursing profession deeply meets the need for authentic life experience—experiences of death, birth, pain, illness, love and responsibility for other people. This need burns very strongly at this age. People seek their own experiences and not a second-hand life as it is so dazzlingly presented in the media.

Many young people starting their careers state the desire to help others as a motive for their choice of career. Others are looking for a way to experience themselves in the nursing profession. The encounters with life's borderline situations and one's own abilities and inabilities largely corresponds to this desire.

In this form, however, the motive of self-experience does not go beyond a certain stage of life. Around the age of 28, when the years of travel and apprenticeship are over, so to speak, the desire to shape something concrete in the world comes to the fore. Now the unspecialized character of the nursing profession, apparently limited to just working with people, which made the nursing profession seem so interesting to the young person coming out of school, has become an obstacle. If the person was not able to experience a specific, unmistakable task in nursing during the years of professional activity, rather feeling only that they were providing unspecific assistance, they are now emphatically faced with the question of how to take hold of their own life's task in a more concrete way. Without this concretization, there is the feeling of constantly investing forces in a bottomless pit and not getting through to the personal questions of life.

Many colleagues in this search for their own life's task transfer their attention to professions that they have become acquainted with during their nursing activities. They become therapists, doctors, social workers or specialize as nursing teachers, nursing managers, operating room nurses, or transfer to areas that require qualifications and specialization but where they only apply their nursing skills indirectly.

NH Young people who enter the nursing profession in their fourth seven-year cycle take on a very great responsibility for this time of life. Whether they are actually able to carry this depends to a large extent on their previous path. If what they seek in the helping profession is the satisfaction of their own, often unacknowledged need for help, this would be a very problematic entrance ticket for the nursing profession.[9]

The fourth seven-year cycle is actually still a time of self-discovery. It would be nice if this biographical rule were taken into account by somewhat older members of a nursing team in their cooperation with younger ones. Space for inability should be created so that younger colleagues can test their abilities and assume responsibility in line with their abilities. After all, there is often an immense responsibility weighing on the shoulders of these people. They are confronted with death and birth, with the great threshold experiences of life. Actually, this age is the time in which one wants to experiment with oneself in the world, the time of travel and apprenticeship. If during this time there is the feeling of always having to be there for others without being able to consciously do something for oneself, then this is a very questionable situation. Since many do not see how much they are overexerting themselves, it is the responsibility of older colleagues to make sure that 22-year-olds are not expected to deal with the same load as 40-year-olds.

RH What do you mean by space for inability?

NH Spaces for inability are areas in which a nurse can test himself and gain his own experience without constantly being instructed in a know-it-all manner. Ideals must not be killed by a dismissive know-it-all. It may not be easy for an experienced colleague to see another making mistakes that he himself would avoid. The idealistic young worker has often not yet suffered the discrepancy between what is desirable and what is actually feasible. What he knows and what he wants has not yet been put in relation to what he is really able to achieve.

One can trust, however, that reality itself will separate the legitimate ideals from the illusionary ones. The frail nature of reality presents hurdles that objectify what is feasible. The enthusiasm that an ideal can trigger is tremendously creative. The experienced person could use his knowledge to prepare the ground for the ideal to be realized to the best extent possible.

Another thing is that many, especially young colleagues deal with the big questions of life in a very personal, emotional way. For instance, it cannot be taken for granted that a person of a certain age will maintain an objective distance to the death of a child. This wealth of sensations is a very special treasure, but it can put a considerable strain on the work processes of the nursing team when it is lived to the extreme, for example if the necessary distance to a patient is not maintained. Nevertheless, we must not simply move on to the day's business if a colleague is unable to deal with an upsetting situation. It would be completely wrong to offer comfort in a way that everyone can see that it comes from personal resignation or because your aim is to get the colleague back to work as quickly as possible.

We also create space for inability by making ourselves aware that in certain biographical situations other things than the professional task are also important. Life experience, relationships with the most diverse people in the most diverse areas of life belong absolutely to a rich biography. In the end, they will also flow into professional life as new abilities.

If we respect these spaces of inability, our colleague will not feel: I am only wanted here for my labor. Rather: I am accepted as a whole person with my abilities and needs. Only this feeling of acceptance frees us to develop our own creative powers. At the same time, it provides a model for loving relationships with patients. Ultimately, it also motivates the work on one's own inabilities.

Paying attention to the internal situation of colleagues is just as much a yardstick for the professionalism of nursing as our professional, loving treatment of patients.

In the long term you can only provide nursing care if you have an excess of strength. Up to about the age of 35 you need your soul forces largely for the development of your own personality. A person who has adopted a predominantly giving attitude very early on is always at risk of neglecting her own inner nourishment. The feeling of having missed something, the feeling of being starved and burned out, which often only occurs years later, is an expression of this neglect.

3.3 Work and leisure

RH Many nurses reach the limits of their mental and physical strength in their profession and, despite their great commitment, experience that their profession ultimately does not fulfill them. In their free time, they look for recuperation on the one hand, and compensation for their possibly unsatisfactory professional situation on the other. How can the relationship between work and leisure time be reasonably structured?

NH First of all, it can be said that the time we work in addition to the time in which we pursue our physical needs and our social obligations makes up a large part of our lifetime. We work eight, twelve or sixteen hours a day over a period of about fifty years.

RH According to labor law, a maximum of ten hours is permitted and many people work part-time or do not work at all. A working life of fifty years is probably also a rare exception today. What do you mean by work? What do we do when we're not working?

NH When I feel that what I do in my profession represents a biographical motif that I am expressing in the world, I will always aspire to establish my motif qualitatively, and not only through the time I spend in that function. Then I will spend my free time in such a way that it takes into account what I expect from life. I don't just use my free time to recuperate for my job, that would be too restrictive, I use it to develop in areas that I'm not using in my job, for example artistically. A particularly broad spectrum of experiences must be provided, especially between the ages of 21 and 28 years. When someone seeks a personal life task later, their questions to the world become concrete. What used to be geared to breadth and variety now gets depth and purpose. Experiences become life experience. Then I don't spend my free time in such a way that I ultimately lose more strength than I gain, but I also look for the relationship to my life's motif in my free time. Everyone who is responsible for people will have to find their own style. From this point of view, the separation of work and leisure seems artificial and inconsistent with life. No one will be able to be a different person privately than in their profession, both are shaped in such a way that they have an inner connection.

RH That sounds very tiring! The distinction between work and leisure is clearly artificial. Nevertheless, we need a balance between times when concentration and speed are needed and times when creativity and peace are needed, sometimes even the blessings of deep sleep. It is interesting that burnout does not usually result from overwork, but from a loss of meaning and relationships. Those who find the meaning of life only in a certain task, for example in nursing and devotion to the problems of others, are at risk of neglecting sides to themselves and needs of their own. When you ask people at the end of their lives what they would have spent more time on in life, nobody says—more time on work! But many miss the time of being together with other people or developing their artistic potential.

Finally, let us mention what Rudolf Steiner said about the relationship between selflessness and selfishness, which is much discussed in the helping professions: "I am filled with deep mistrust of people who talk a lot about selflessness, about altruism. It seems to me that it is precisely these people who have no right feeling for the selfish gratification that comes from selfless action. People who claim that one should not stick to the accidental, the insignificant, the temporal side of existence, but strive for the necessary, the essential, the eternal: they do not know that the coincidental and temporal do not really differ from the eternal and necessary. And ingenious behavior is this very thing: to conjure up everywhere the necessary, the significant from the accidental, the insignificant. Truth is where a person's personal interest, subjectivity, selfishness are so ennobled that he does not have an interest in his own person alone, but in the whole world. When someone is so petty that he can only attend to the great undertakings of the world by denying his personal interest, his subjectivity—then he is living in the worst lie of existence [...] Expand your self to the world-self, and then act incessantly selfishly. Be like that hawker woman who sells eggs at the market. Only don't take care of your egg business out of egoism, take care of the business of the world out of egoism! [...] But the truth is that a person's selfishness can become so refined that he gains interest not only in his own affairs but in those of all humanity. Do not preach to men that they should be selfless, rather plant in them the highest interests so that their selfishness, their egotism clings to those higher interests. Then you ennoble a power that really lies within the human being; otherwise you're talking about something that can never exist, but that can make liars out of people."[10]

4. Encounters between patients and nurses

We have talked so far about the situation of destiny into which the patient comes as a result of his illness. This outlined a dimension of disease that is often unconscious in the patient. This dimension seems to us to be indispensable for understanding the course of illness. The powers that enable us to wrestle lovingly with even seemingly "senseless" situations of destiny, such as the fatal illness of a child, arise from the knowledge of meaningfulness. Even if the details of the disease's meaning remain hidden from us, it is precisely this certainty that nourishes our comprehensive commitment to the patient. It does not lead to a fatalistic attitude towards the ill or towards fate. We have already drawn attention to the difficult situation of nurses, who are often faced with great inner hardships in dealing with human suffering. We have seen how conscious handling of one's own abilities or inabilities and understanding support from experienced, expertly working colleagues contribute to the fact that a person reaching his limits does not give in to resignation, dullness or falling ill. When boundaries are experienced as being surmountable or are accepted as spaces of inability for a certain period of time, the nurse experiences himself as being in a process of becoming, as progressing in his own biography. Only from this point of view, it seems to us, can nursing care be taken up as a life task.

In a third step, we want to show how the relationship between patients and nurses can be seen as an intersection of two destinies. It starts with a conversation.

4.1 The nursing conversation

The first question that concerns us is to what extent does a nurse's conversation differ from that of a physician, psychotherapist or pastor?

RH It makes sense to see the differences in the respective profession and the skills developed in them. The physician, psychotherapist and nurse are of course equally called upon to conduct the conversation with a high level of human understanding, i.e., with honesty, warmth and clarity, setting limits if necessary. A division of labor in the sense that the physician is responsible for medical information, the psychotherapist for inner soul suffering and the nurse for translating and mediating between these two and the patient would make a caricature of the human and professional tasks and abilities of everyone involved. We can differentiate between the attitudes and topics by looking at the intentions in the questions of the patient. An outwardly identical question can be based on different intentions, depending on the person to whom it is addressed. The patient's question: "Would you have this operation if you were in my place?" applies to the doctor, the pastor and the nurse in different ways.

Obviously, the patient does not expect a yes/no answer from any of the respondents. He is seeking help in making a decision, the consequences of which he cannot foresee, which he may fear, but which he ultimately has to bear himself. The personal formulation: "Would you, if you were in my place..." indicates that the patient is not only asking for a general statement, but a subjective one, one to which he may even attach particular importance, for his own judgment.

The physician, psychotherapist and nurse are not only being asked for their specialist knowledge in this question, they are called upon to test that knowledge in relation to their own conscience. The answers found by the three people in different professions must therefore be personalized if they are to appear credible to the patient. Their specialist knowledge must be individualized. How could this look for you as a psychotherapist?

NH The patient's question in your example has several aspects. Ultimately, this question is about the need to consider the pros and cons of surgery. The patient wants to become more confident and judicious in his decision. I would try to give him an inner space in which he can express all his fears, misgivings and ambivalent feelings. By speaking of his inner misgivings, he will experience Viktor Frankl's (1905–1997) insight that talking about our suffering with others already diminishes it. The patient's appeal could be formulated as follows: "Give me your time, your interest, so that I can make my decision."
The nurse should also form such a vessel in which the patient's personal decision can mature. In a way it is easier for her than for the psychotherapist or the doctor. The patient may be more impartial towards her. He often behaves towards the psychotherapist as if the latter always wants to decipher a hidden layer behind his statements. That's why he mostly wanted to talk to him: he wants counseling to become aware of his own unconscious will impulses.

RH The patient seeks answers to his questions depending on where he sees the competence of his conversation partner. He expects the physician to initially know the facts of his medical condition. In the wording given in our example, he expects not only factual medical information, but the personal opinion of the physician. The doctor initially looks from the present into the past. He proceeds from the medical history to a diagnosis. He regards the current symptoms as the culmination of the causes of the disease from the past. By resolving this culmination in the healing process, he opens the way for the future. Insofar as the prognosis is based on personal or general experience, i.e., statistics, it ultimately also stems from a look into the past.

If the patient addresses his question to the psychotherapist, he is probably looking for the psychological reasons for his situation ...

NH ... for future aspects. What will happen after the procedure? How will my future social conditions evolve? Questions that go beyond the purely medical. As psychotherapists, art therapists or physiotherapists, we work concretely on the future abilities of the patient, whether they are of a mental or physical nature.

RH As nurses we are completely in the present moment of the patient. We are involved in his suffering and impairments. We stand by him, we accompany him. When talking to us, the patient primarily seeks understanding and support, and of course advice on how to deal with nursing problems. This attitude often gives the conversation something mediating, optimistic, comforting. The nursing conversation usually happens unplanned in everyday situations. Only rarely does the patient explicitly request a consultation with a nurse. There are no fixed times for talk, in contrast to the doctor or the counselor. Conversations occur during washing, eating, going to bed, sleepless nights. Usually it is everyday problems, minor or somewhat more important experiences, memories, wishes, grief, joy, pain, the visit of relatives or simply the need for encounter that give the occasion for a conversation. Only to a lesser extent are problems discussed or deeper life issues addressed. This, too, demonstrates the strong relevance of nursing care to the present moment. The conversation is largely a medium for cultivating human relationships, just like the numerous non-verbal encounters and nursing activities. Whereas therapeutic conversations require effort from the patient, the nursing conversation opens, clarifies and organizes. It is salutary, but not conversation "work" in the therapeutic sense.

NH Many nurses feel the need of more time to talk with patients. One would like to sit beside the bed and listen in peace. It is often overlooked that an immeasurable treasure of non-verbal conversation is hidden in the nursing activities themselves. To exaggerate a little: one nursing attitude consists in working as quickly as possible so that there will be time for a conversation afterwards, the other gives so much attention and warmth to the nursing action itself that an additional conversation is no longer necessary. Of course, this does not have to mean renouncing a conversation if a situation demands it.

RH The verbal and non-verbal conversation should lead to the patient feeling strengthened, encouraged, relieved, confident. It wants to reach the patient in his life forces. The therapeutic conversation, in contrast, must seek discussion, it wants to awaken awareness, stimulate self-knowledge, point out developments. It works with the patient's consciousness. The nursing conversation nourishes, the therapeutic one digests.

4.2 Insurmountable difficulties?

RH I would like to address another important area in encounters with patients. Every nurse has probably experienced that working with certain patients is relatively easy, while almost insurmountable difficulties arise with others. The difficulty can be characteristics that the patient has or certain clinical problems that arouse dislike, fear and disgust. Another phenomenon of this problem is the experience of repeatedly having to face the same or similar situations or being confronted with one's own shortcomings.

NH It is strange that the things that make me furious can be experienced as completely harmless by a colleague, for example. When something bothers me in a human relationship, be it in the relationship with a patient, my spouse or a neighbor, then there is always a deficit also in me.

Everything that is unresolved in our own soul, that we do not want to look at, which is the other side of our white vest, so to speak—we carry all that within us. Carl Gustav Jung (1875–1961) called these unmastered or unredeemed soul aspects the "shadow," anthroposophic spiritual science speaks of the "double."[11]

If we meet a person and have a problematic reaction, then it could be that we have discovered in him exactly the aspect that we have not mastered in ourselves. Instead of fighting it in ourselves, we fight it in others. The "enemy" stays outside. In such a situation it always makes sense to ask: am I seeing an image of myself that is extremely unpleasant for me, mirrored in the patient? Am I fighting something in the other that I have to transform in myself?

RH Perhaps it could be summed up like this: by suffering through encountering the other person, I gain knowledge of what needs to be transformed in myself.

NH Often difficulties between people cannot be clarified in conversation. Too great are the blockages that prevent a free encounter between one 'I' and the other. This is no reason for resignation if we take the following insight seriously: thoughts and feelings are deeds. If a situation cannot be clarified at first, I can direct my thoughts and feelings in a direction in which the situation is at least not exacerbated. Thoughts and feelings transformed in inner struggle become a real source of strength for future action.

> *"When we take people as they are, we make them worse. When we treat them as if they were what they should be, we take them where they should be taken."*
>
> J. W. von Goethe (1749–1832)

4.3 The social impact of an ill person

RH Let us also talk about another experience that represents a star moment in everyday nursing care: a patient with a serious illness meets a nursing team. Her destiny with the illness moves everyone she meets. The people involved are committed to this person in an extraordinary way. Everyone feels close to her in a very personal way. They experience themselves directly as witnesses of a significant, individual destiny.

We often encounter this situation around a person's death. It connects the doctors, therapists, relatives and nurses in a real inner community. The patient seems to have a strong social impact. How can we understand that?

NH Especially the fact that the situation you describe often occurs in encounters with people who are dying indicates that all participants have become aware of their closeness to the spiritual world. When a person is in danger, when he reaches a threshold as it were, we are highly activated. In a sense, we breathe "threshold air". We feel that our conventional knowledge and skills have reached a limit, just as the patient is at a limit. If we do not shy away from this limit with resignation, we immerse ourselves in the atmosphere surrounding the patient's fate. Experiences of existential powerlessness form the inner ground for an encounter with the spiritual world, namely with Christ.[12] Everyone who has the opportunity to experience such a situation feels touched in his innermost being. This touch gives you the strength to go beyond yourself and your limitations.

Everyone's highest abilities are needed now, and this connects the people working together in the therapeutic community. It is as if the spiritual world were calling for a new, future quality of community; a community that works beyond mere functioning together and feeling good together.

RH Actually it should be possible to open our view to the spiritual aspect of a disease even when the patient is not in such a threshold or destiny situation. What is given to us as a gift from the outside in threshold situations must be worked out more and more from the inside, through our real interest in other people. The future task for a therapeutic community lies in uncovering the spiritual aspect of disease.

The relationship between the person nursing and the one being nursed, and also the relationships between the colleagues of all professional groups cooperating together are transformed through their awareness of what is spiritual in the other person.

Category	Example learning objectives	Recommended learning path
Relationships	You conduct nursing conversations with understanding.	B
Your own learning objective		
Knowledge	You are familiar with the concept of karma as it is understood in anthroposophic spiritual science.	C
Your own learning objective		

References

1   Steiner, R. *Theosophy. An introduction to the supersensible knowledge of the world and the destination of man.* Rudolf Steiner Press, London 2005.
2   ibid., p. 74.
3   ibid., p. 79.
4   Treichle,r R. *Die Entwicklung der Seele im Lebenslauf.* Verlag Freies Geistesleben, Stuttgart 2012.
5   Steiner, R. *The spiritual guidance of the individual and humanity. Some results of spiritual-scientific research into human history and development.* SteinerBooks, Great Barrington 1992.
6   Steiner, R. *Occult science: An outline.* Chapter "Sleep and death." Rudolf Steiner Press, London 2013.
7   Steiner, R. Lecture of May 16, 1910. *Manifestations of karma.* 4th revised ed. Rudolf Steiner Press, London 2000.
8   Steiner, R. Lecture of November 12, 1916. *The karma of vocation.* Revised, SteinerBooks, Great Barrington 1984.
9   Schmidtbauer, W. *Die hilflosen Helfer.* Rowohlt Verlag, Reinbek bei Hamburg 1998.
10 Steiner, R. *Methodische Grundlagen der Anthroposophie 1889–1901* (GA 30). Rudolf Steiner Verlag, Dornach 1989.
11 Steiner, R. *Occult science: An outline.* Chap. "Knowledge of higher worlds." Rudolf Steiner Press, London 2013
12 Steiner, R. *Death as metamorphosis of life.* Anthroposophic Press, Great Barrington 2008.

CHAPTER V
Nursing as a Path of Development

ROLF HEINE

Every human being passes through a process of personal development during his or her lifetime. Specific learning tasks also arise for us in professional life. Finally, humanity itself develops gradually over the course of different eras and cultural epochs. As individuals, we stand within this threefold process. This chapter will describe exercises that promote personal and professional development. They will be based on the supplementary exercises that Rudolf Steiner gave for people pursuing a path of esoteric training.

→   Learning objectives, see end of chapter

"O Human Being! Know Yourself!" Ancient mystery wisdom

Our individual life task is the place where we can learn to overcome our inabilities and act in an increasingly realistic manner.

For centuries, characteristics such as devotion and a sense of duty were thought to be more important for practicing the nursing profession than professional knowledge and skill. Adherence to moral standards was authoritatively demanded. Such moral standards were gradually lost with the secularization of nursing care in the 19th and 20th centuries and with the trend towards scientific medicine. Today, nursing performance is rated largely on professional know-how.

Any nursing-care ethics as a basis for the training of inner abilities can therefore no longer rest content with establishing a general, divinely ordained system of values. It must rather take its starting point from nursing care itself. It must be developed out of the profession itself and not imposed from outside. Only then will nurses be able to freely evaluate the training of inner abilities without being patronized.

This chapter will thus begin with a phenomenological treatment of nursing. From this will follow information on the inner and professional prerequisites for working in the nursing profession and freely assuming responsibility for one's personal path of development.

1. Nursing as a cultural task

1.1 Maintaining things

Everyone is a caregiver. There is something needing care in all areas of personal life and culture. Caregiving is an integral part of everyday life. It is rhythmical, ongoing, and inconspicuous.

Care or maintenance is needed for inanimate objects, clothing, household items, machines, buildings, roads, in short, for all objects that the human mind has thought of creating. These things are testimonies to humanity's creative power and cultural expression, which go beyond mere acts of nature. Maintenance and care serve to preserve the *form and function* of objects. Unmaintained machines lose their functionality after a time; their form gradually changes due to wear and tear. In an unmaintained environment, such artfully crafted pieces of work revert to an unfinished state and finally become raw material. Well-groomed objects, on the other hand, retain their shape and function for a much longer period. They are constantly being snatched away from their natural tendency to disintegrate and are returned to their place in the world of people. Through care and maintenance, they remain part of human culture.

Cultivated objects become familiar to us.

The person caring for an object connects himself more and more deeply with it, by immersing himself in its functional attributes. Well-groomed clothes, a well-kept house, become increasingly the person's own, because of his actions upon them which go beyond mere use. As time goes by, they carry ever more clearly the intangible signature of the one caring for them. The well-cared for object thus gains a value that goes beyond mere use. The caregiver can, like an inventor or manufacturer, confront his own creative, maintaining activity in the object. Thus, a well-groomed object, through its well-preserved form and functionality, also appears to outsiders as an expression of diligence, perseverance and inner connection. Perhaps antiques exert an often-irrational attraction in terms of their usefulness because of the care that has been lavished on them, in a time in which care is so lacking.

Care creates a relationship with the object being cared for.

The more frequent, regular and conscious the acts of caring for an object are, the more intense the relationship becomes. Anyone who wants to replace a well-groomed piece of clothing that has been worn and maintained for many years, knows how the relationship quality interferes with utility considerations.

Not all objects invite the user to create such a relationship to the same extent. This includes items made of inferior material—unattractive or impractical objects and disposables (compare veneered chipboard furniture with an oak cabinet, for example). Disposables are said to require no care. In fact, it is difficult, for example, to develop a relationship with a disposable syringe that is any different to the one that arises from simply using the syringe. One encounters this object only once. It is distinguished by the fact that nothing, no thought, no feeling of sympathy or antipathy enters between the object and its function. The object does not demand a relationship, it is discarded after use. On closer inspection, however, we find that disposable articles also require care. This starts with their existence as trash. The need for care only ends when the object, freed of every human impression, has again become a pure natural substance and can be incorporated into the natural environment.

The ecological crisis of our time thus appears as a very great problem in the care sector. Where man-made creations are not cultivated, they fall into the realm of the non-human. This inhumane character of waste can be seen everywhere today. It is the consequence and expression of a careless culture. In its various forms it is a destroyer of all of nature's kingdoms.

Training a basic attitude of caring for things created by human beings, as well as caring for nature, proves to be a contribution towards overcoming the planet's ecological crisis. Care does not make nature more natural, but more human.

The outer prerequisite for the care of man-made objects consists in having the ability to properly use and maintain them. In doing so we must consider the physical properties of their construction and material. The knowledge required for this can be acquired objectively, based on physical and chemical laws. A radio can't take water, glass will shatter when subjected to a sudden change in temperature.

The internal prerequisite in this area is to acquire a responsible relationship to the object or raw material. This is a difficult task in a culture like ours that is so full of material goods. Any individual, concrete object seems to be interchangeable at almost any whim. It takes increased moral strength to value the object as it deserves, despite this. Developing this takes effort and goes against the habitual thinking and behavior of today.

1.2 Tasks in the plant and animal realms

When dealing with man-made objects, nursing staff are tasked with preserving their form and function. Other necessities exist within the plant and animal realms.

Plants receive their form out of their own forces. They grow and transform their form in accordance with the laws of the species. They germinate, grow upwards, form leaves, flowers and new seeds. In addition to these inherited form-giving laws, plants are subject to the conditions in their environment. Specific soil, water, light and temperature conditions are prerequisites for a plant's species-appropriate development. People constantly intervene in the plant's environment, knowingly or unknowingly, thereby modifying the plant's opportunities for growth and reproduction. Breeding and genetic engineering have a direct influence on the inherent laws governing the formation of plants. The selection of soils, irrigation, the combination of species which grow well together are interventions in the environmental conditions of plants.

While breeding basically relies on one-off interventions, maintenance of species-appropriate environments requires ongoing effort.

> The aim of plant care is to preserve vital forms and produce fruit for people.

In this sense, farmers and gardeners are caregivers. They rhythmically and steadily ensure soil, water, air, light and temperature conditions, crop rotation and plant communities. The aim of this work is the fruit that is gained for human beings, i.e., the surplus that is not needed by the plant to preserve its species. In this sense, felled trees are fruit of the forest, for example.

The task of providing care is different again for the animal realm. Animals are partly independent of environmental conditions since they can seek out the environmental conditions appropriate to them. They can do this because of congenital or learned behaviors. These behaviors must be considered when taking care of animals, over and beyond any environmental conditions. Wild animals only need to be cared for by human beings when their habitat has been changed so much that adapting their behavior is not enough to ensure their survival. The decimation of game populations to an ecologically viable level appears to be basically a caregiving task, as is the protection of endangered species.

We'll call the surplus from the animal kingdom gained through the care of human beings *"service."* Animals benefit human beings not only as beasts of labor or nourishment. As components of the ecosystem they play an essential role in preserving the functionality of the environment, which serves to preserve the human habitat. From this point of view, the work of farmers appears to be one of caregiving.

The external prerequisite for the care of plants and animals is to have knowledge of their laws of growth, environmental conditions and species-appropriate behavior patterns.

> The aim of caregiving in the animal realm is to preserve vital, ensouled forms and place them in service to human beings.

The inner prerequisite for the care of plants and animals appears to be the ability to build relationships to plants and animals that go beyond their superficial use value. It is a merit of ecological research, that it has shown the importance of each animal and plant species for the conservation of nature and the human habitat. If such knowledge does not remain abstract, if it awakens a feeling of respect and reverence for each individual being, this can develop into a completely new relationship with the animal and plant realms. The fate of plants and animals then appears to be joined to ours in the most intimate way. So, they are not to be judged based on whether we find them pleasant, useful or likeable, but *independently of sympathy and antipathy,* treated in accordance with their own being and ecological connections.

Human beings need the most comprehensive care of all living beings. In the animal realm the ability to nurture the young, for example, is anchored as an instinct. Such instincts have largely withered away in human beings. There is a great demand for advice on baby care and raising children, which shows that instinctive and traditionally transmitted capacities to care for the young have been lost. The delegation of caregiving activities from the family sphere to separate facilities such as hospitals and nursing homes can also be taken as an indication of this loss. The ability to provide care must therefore be learnt anew, developed further and anchored as a bulwark of culture.

Additional prerequisites are needed in the care of people as compared to the care of the other realms of nature. All biological and psychological characteristics of a human being are shaped by that person's individuality. Our care of a human being must therefore not rest content with merely preserving their ensouled and living form. We must rather enable the person to develop their free individuality. Education in this sense is care of individualities.

> The outer prerequisite for nursing a human being is to understand their bodily, mental, social and spiritual nature. The inner prerequisite results from the person's individuality as their spiritual core.

The spiritual aspect of human nature is not visible, it reveals itself in a person's deeds and biography. Biographies are open-ended towards the future, which means that it is not at first possible to ultimately grasp the person's full individuality. The principle of freely shaping one's own biography, as well as the possibility of entering the biographies of others, implies the unpredictability of human action. Space for the free development of individual impulses must therefore be created in every human relationship. Care of a mortally ill person that is solely concerned with physical decay and psychological destruction falls short of the reality of that person as being capable of development to their last breath. Having a sense for this potential is one of the prerequisites for caring for human beings.

> Caring for a human being is geared to their future. To do this, you must recognize and encourage the seeds for the future that slumber in each person, regardless of their biographical context.

Particular care must also be given to cultivating relationships between people. All social relationships are rooted in this. Connections between people arise instinctively wherever we require the help of others to satisfy our own needs, whether our needs are physical, mental or social in nature. This drive towards human encounter falls away when such mutual needs are not present. However, dependency cannot be the basis for a free human relationship. Free relationships arise only out of brotherly interest in the other person. Contrary to instinctive self-interest, we need to be active in initiating and cultivating our relationships with our fellow human beings. *Directing our unbiased attention towards* the other person is thus the foundation for caring for social relationships. Only then can the other person express himself out of his own being.

Human beings connect with the created world by caring for the three realms of nature below them. By cultivating social relationships, they reach beyond themselves. As spiritual beings, they seek a relationship to the spiritual world. Every spiritual exercise, every ritual gesture lives through rhythmic repetition. It is done voluntarily, contrary to external necessities, and creates a bond between the person and the spiritual world. It is literally religion (to re-unite, lat. religare = tie, fasten).

Realm	Maintains	Prerequisite
Lifeless nature	Form and function	Consideration of physical and chemical laws
Plant realm	Living form and fruits (for human beings)	Care of the environment
Animal realm	Living, ensouled form and service (to human beings)	Care of behavior in relationships
Human being	Living, ensouled, 'I'-endowed form and freedom	Creation of opportunities for development
Social community	Human relationships	Interest from one person to another
Spiritual world	Awareness of the spiritual world	Spiritual practice, ritual

Chart: Human caregiving tasks

1.4   Caregiving tasks and the inner and outer capacities needed to fulfil them

The preceding description showed how care is needed in all realms of nature, to preserve human and natural creations and protect and encourage development. Without care, the objects, plants and animals raised into the human cultural sphere sink back into an uncultured state. Human beings, too, only reach the full height of their humanity through taking care of their development. Even such seemingly natural characteristics as upright walking, speaking and thinking require care, and this is not restricted to the rehabilitation of seriously ill patients.

The unique human capacity to actively relate to all beings of the sense-perceptible and spiritual worlds makes human beings responsible for the created world.

2. Nursing as a relationship

2.1 First exercise: proper thinking—concentration

The relationships that we create with objects and creatures of nature raise them above their mere existence. The impulse for caregiving comes when we have formed such a relationship, over and above mere superficial utilitarian considerations. The deeper this relationship is, the more obvious the essence of the objects and creatures becomes. A table, a rose, a horse and a person now reveal themselves in their own value and in terms of their place in the world. The value of a person only comes to our consciousness when we place ourselves into a living relationship to him and to humanness in general. Everyday superficial encounters do not convey this intrinsic value to us. It is only in getting involved with another person that we begin to sense the source of their specific manner of self-expression.

In everyday life we encounter a multitude of people and objects. We would certainly be overwhelmed if we wanted to enter into an equally conscious relationship with all of them. If we were to renounce every concrete relationship to avoid this overload, our lives would remain entirely superficial. Especially in our daily encounters with people and objects we have an immeasurable opportunity to establish an ever more extensive and deepening network of relationships. A prerequisite for such a relationship is to pay attention to and concentrate on what comes to meet us. This is only possible if we manage to extract ourselves ever anew from the flow of everyday occurrences and encounters, *creating moments of reflection*. This temporary withdrawal from our usual activities must be wrested from everyday life.

Reflection on the people and objects entrusted to our care will only lead to realistic relationships if we succeed in refining our ideas and prejudices through proper thinking. Things must be allowed to "express" themselves, without being deformed by arbitrary notions and opinions. This requires careful monitoring of our own thinking.

Exercise

Rudolf Steiner gave an initially simple exercise to train such thinking as a foundation for spiritual development:

"Whoever overcomes himself to turn his thoughts to an everyday object, such as a pin or a pencil, every day for at least five minutes over the course of months, and during this time avoids all thoughts that are not connected with this object, has done a lot in this direction [...] Anyone who asks himself: what materials is a pencil made of? How are the materials prepared to make the pencil? How are they then joined together? When was the pencil invented? and so on: such a person is adapting his ideas more to reality than someone who thinks about the ancestry of humanity or reflects on what life is. One learns proper thinking through simple mental exercises [...] more than through complicated and learned ideas. Initially it is not the aim to think about this or that, but to think properly, out of your inner strength."[1]

Anyone who undergoes such practice soon notices how much the inwardly strengthened power of thought enables us to grasp real relationships with the people and things around us. The exercise—after a certain period of quiet, persistent practice—can also be used for professional purposes. For example, a patient review can begin with only discussing things which are directly connected to the *physical appearance* of the patient.

- How tall is the patient?
- What color are her hair and eyes?

Then we look at her *psychological expressions*:

- What typical gestures does she have?
- What are her facial expressions?
- What habits does she have when eating and washing?
- How does she walk?
- How does she express pleasure, irritation or sadness?

We consider her *biographical and social relationships* in the same way:

- How did she experience her childhood?
- What important events occurred?

Especially during this last part of the contemplation, we need to ensure that no speculation of any kind flows into our portrayal. Only truly known facts should be mentioned, and these of course only with the permission of the patient. A truly factual portrayal avoids violation of the patient's sphere of privacy. This kind of patient discussion should always be done as if the person were present in the room. It trains our observation of the patient's expressions and generates a deep impression of her unmistakable individuality. It helps those involved to place themselves into a lively relationship with problematic patients.

3. Nursing as a process

3.1 Second exercise: initiative

An activity becomes a nursing activity through being carried out continuously and rhythmically. We cannot speak of "care" when something only happens once. When care is given to an inanimate object, this is to extend its "life" cycle. Language thus assigns a quality to the object that is a biological impossibility. It is an expression of the feeling that objects possess a kind of "life" for as long as they are being used by people. Care and maintenance maintain this life, when regularly given. We wear a pair of shoes for years, from time to time we clean and polish them. Medical instruments are disinfected, cleaned, packed and sterilized. Individual actions require a certain measure of knowledge, concentration and skill. After some practice, though, most of these actions can be carried out completely unspectacularly and uniformly, without paying much attention. The caregiver seems to immerse herself in the life cycle of the object.

Acts of care become habits in everyday life.

This can be seen from the fact that full awareness is not applied. The activity has left the alertness of the head and become "flesh and blood."

Everyday life consists of many such semiconscious routine activities. Everyone takes care of their own body care throughout life—routinely, flowingly. Nothing stands out. Who remembers washing themselves on a morning three days ago, a week ago, or last year?

This changes abruptly when the usual course of action is disturbed. A razor cut, blunt dissecting scissors, a torn-off shoe sole inevitably rouse us from our semiconscious habits. The flow of actions is interrupted, we cannot continue as usual. Now it is not care that is needed, but repairs or therapy.

In the same way, illness interrupts the rhythmic flow of life, awakens us from what we are used to, calls familiar activities into question. The interruption causes suffering and pain, presses us to overcome it, to recover the flow of life, to find healing. The ill person wakes up and consults a specialist. The interruption has stimulated awareness and interest, it creates consciousness.

Nursing care happens in the polarity of uniformly rhythmic everyday life and extraordinary disturbances.

Nurses participate consciously in this polarity in different ways. Consciousness has a dreamier quality when everyday life continues in endless repetition of similar activities. There is little need for a conscious mind when we are immersed in the stream of actions, playfully compensating for fluctuations, and sometimes it can be more of an interference.

When the flow of actions is interrupted, then concentrated waking knowledge replaces the sense of flow. There are different conceivable reactions to this awakening. Displeasure arises for those who are awakened from their habitual sleep at the wrong time, creative self-confirmation for those who can diagnose the disorder and act accordingly. Each attitude belongs to a particular understanding of nursing care.

In the first scenario the nurse experiences himself completely immersed in the flow of actions, dutifully caring, inwardly closely connected to what he is caring for. Reflection on this nursing activity is rare, usually the person acts intuitively out of traditional or self-acquired experience. This attitude can be characterized as pre-professional. Opposite to this is the view that nursing is a process of solving problems. Since the late 1970s there have been models, also in German-speaking regions, that want to lift nursing out of unreflective, one-sided action and make it accessible to alert, knowing consciousness. A control system formulated by Fiechter and Maier describes nursing as: the collection of information, formulation of problems, resources, objectives and measures, planning of nursing care, implementation, evaluation and renewed assessment.[2]

On the one hand, the term "process" refers to the fluid character of nursing care, and on the other hand, elements are introduced that raise awareness through formulating problems and goals, as well as through planning and evaluation. This certainly justified approach one-sidedly prioritizes the knowledge pole of awakening from a "disturbance" over the rhythmical action pole. It ignores the everyday reality of nursing care that takes place below the problem threshold. When nursing care is understood as a problem-solving process, this only describes part of the nursing care process. In fact, many nurses therefore reject the formalized "nursing process" idea.

Example:

A 65-year-old woman with a stable, conservatively treated fracture of her right upper arm receives a thoracic abduction splint. Her disability is obvious. It goes without saying that she requires help with eating, excretions, dressing and undressing, washing and other things, and guidance on regaining independence. Both result directly from the medical findings as well as from the aim of the patient and the nurse for rehabilitation. A listing of the nursing problems, e.g., "the patient cannot dress or undress herself due to the fixed upper right arm," the resources, e.g., "the patient is left-handed," and the aims, e.g., "the patient can wash herself," appear superfluous. A documentation of measures and progress is absolutely sufficient to ensure the continuity of care.

We should only speak of a nursing care problem when the patient and nurse are facing a situation that they truly cannot cope with initially. If no such question comes up it is a pseudo-problem.

The construction of such pseudo-problems is an attempt to bring consciousness into the everyday flow of nursing activities. This basically laudable intention misses the actual nursing activity in its flowing, processual element, if the awareness awakened by the disturbance is seen as the only form of conscious nursing activity.

We have characterized two nursing attitudes: the pre-professional one that loses itself in the flow of activity, and the self-aware one that awakens because of problems. Both attitudes are expressions of the polarity of process and problem. To delve into nursing as a rhythmically flowing process we need to initially strengthen our attention and power of awareness. Our attention must not be restricted to superficial observation of symptoms that have disease value.

Here, it has proven helpful to apply the exercise to develop proper thinking, along with the strengthened ability to concentrate gained by it. This awakens an inner mood for the importance of small everyday matters. When this mood spreads through our everyday work, we repeatedly create moments of waking up out of uniform routine activity.

Any exercise lives from repetition. Especially where it wants to overcome unconscious everyday routines and train better habits, it requires ever-renewed initiative and effort to implement.

Initiative is awakened will—in contrast to routinely sleeping will. Only a conscious, awake deed overcomes the feeling of having to constantly, passively react to external demands. If each of our everyday actions were to be inspired by such an active impulse, there would be no disinclination or boredom. We would find ourselves in every deed. Our own will impulses interrupt the flow of actions that would otherwise passively flow through and past us. We create awareness in the nursing process not just through undergoing disturbances pressing us from outside, but from our own impulses to act from within.

Another exercise given by Rudolf Steiner as a prerequisite for spiritual training has the aim of training initiative power: "One tries to think of any action that one would certainly not have done in the ordinary course of one's life so far. You now make this act your daily duty. It will therefore be good to be able to choose an action that can be performed every day for as long a period as possible. Again, it is better to start with an insignificant act, which one must force oneself to do [...] After some time, a second of the same kind of act should be added to the first, later a third and so on, as much as one can handle while maintaining all one's other duties."[3]

While the first exercise aims to strengthen *thinking*, the second strengthens the *will*. This second exercise can also be practiced in a professional setting after a period of personal practice. The point is to think of actions for which there is no external reason, which come entirely from one's own initiative.

Everyone knows this situation: a patient constantly rings the bell for no apparent reason and then only needs small or minimal assistance, which he could have mentioned during the nurse's previous attendance. Neither a friendly nor an energetic response by the nurse changes this. The patient soon experiences rejection in the impatience or irritation of the nurse and forces renewed attention through even more frequent ringing. If we assign ourselves the task of visiting the patient regularly, at frequent intervals, especially when he does not ring, to ask him if he needs anything, then we break the vicious cycle by our own initiative. Now a relationship of trust can develop, which enables the patient to wait.

It is precisely acting beyond our obvious duties that frees us to shape our own day. This can be practiced in innumerable ways. It succeeds in major things if we develop our capacity to do it in minor things.

Nursing as a process only becomes conscious when we actively shape our everyday work. This provides necessary augmentation to using nursing problems to awaken us to the processes in unconscious everyday activities. Through your own initiative you interrupt the routine of daily duties and complement them with deliberate moments that you have shaped yourself. As a result, everyday nursing appears in a brighter light in some places: we experience ourselves more and more as acting, and less and less as merely reacting.

4. Nursing between closeness and distance

4.1 Third exercise: serenity

Usually we determine closeness to a person by the degree of sympathy that we feel for her. We feel attracted to her, we seek her out and we experience her presence as pleasant.

In antipathy we experience distance. We avoid contact with people we find unsympathetic; we feel repulsed and we rebuff them. Sympathy appears to be an emotional *power of attraction*, and antipathy a *repelling power*. In sympathy the soul goes out of itself and devotes itself to the world, in antipathy it returns to itself and closes itself off.

If we base the relationship between closeness and distance on sympathy and antipathy, our relationship with a person remains marked by desire and reluctance, by the joy and pain that he brings us. Our feelings thus become our measure for evaluating the world. Genuine understanding of the other person cannot grow on this basis because we do not recognize the other person as he truly is, we only see how he affects us. Can closeness to someone be determined by something other than sympathy and antipathy?

Two examples

Let us first look at two people in conflict: a nurse gives a subcutaneous injection. The injection is painful, and the patient accuses the nurse of dilettantism, while the nurse accuses the patient of self-pity. Each feels a high degree of antipathy. From the outside, however, both parties have an extremely close relationship with each other. They lack distance in viewing both the procedure and their relationship with each other. Another example: a nurse gains the trust of a patient with anorexia. The patient's refusal to eat appears all too understandable considering her biographical situation. The nurse believes that he will break this trust if he tells his colleagues of what he knows of the patient's secret misuse of laxatives.

In this case the relationship between the patient and the nurse is marked by forces of sympathy. But they are both dangerously far from truly understanding each other. Sooner or later, the sympathy will turn into antipathy or even hatred when the illusionary character of the relationship becomes apparent.

Closeness occurs when we approach a person, when we begin to understand them. Distance occurs when we believe we have understood someone, that is, when we have finished forming a judgement.

We experience closeness in approaching each other and distance in insisting on our judgement of the other person. Thus, the degree of comprehension determines the actual distance between two people. Real understanding can only be achieved independently of sympathy and antipathy, which ultimately give us more information about our own state than that of others. Sympathy and antipathy cannot be turned off when encountering other people, but they must be controlled.

> "The pupil must develop the ability to behave towards things and people in accord with their unique individuality, to accept each one of them according to their own value and significance. Sympathy and antipathy, inclination and disinclination must receive completely new roles. There can be no question of eradicating them [...] we must take up pleasure and pain with composure, then we stop losing ourselves in them, then we start to understand them [...] Inclination should only be a sign for me that there is a quality in the thing that is suitable for causing inclination. I should learn to recognize this quality [...] This does not make the researcher dull to pleasure and pain; he lifts himself above them, so that they reveal the nature of things to him. The eye can only serve the body by becoming an organ for sense impressions to pass through; inclination and disinclination will develop into organs of the soul when they stop having relevance only for themselves and begin to reveal the other to the soul."[4]

The equanimity exercise should be done at least once a day. There are many opportunities to do this in everyday nursing life. This exercise trains the ability to understand and feel the condition of the patient in a selfless way.

Witnessing and compassion add a further source of perception to cognitive understanding.

It is only out of compassion that we become conscious of the diagnosed findings in their consequences for the patient. "It is only with the heart that one sees rightly," said Antoine de Saint-Exupéry (1900–1944), thereby describing the necessity of training compassion and transforming it into an organ of perception. This lends substantiation to the historical call for *compassion* in nurses.

Example

When we settle a patient, we are initially led by the medical findings. The patient lies motionless and infirm, possibly unconscious, in the bed. He presses heavily against the mattress. We recognize the need for relieving pressure, and we roll him over on his side—taking his condition into account. The necessary gentleness does not come from the medical finding alone, but quite essentially from our feeling for the state that the patient is in.

Stabilizing him in a 30-degree lateral position follows our knowledge of how to provide optimal relief for pressure-endangered parts of his body. Our comfortable adjustment of his body by making fine corrections to the position of his trunk, limbs and head occurs to a large extent out of our empathy with his anatomical condition.

> The result is nursing care that is not only correct in a professional sense, it is also beautiful.

The well-positioned patient is not only relieved of pressure, he also feels comfortable in his situation. His body appears to have been lifted out of heaviness. The findings (pressure), the patient's condition (uncomfortable position) and the overall condition (heavy) have changed in equal measure. Empathy and compassion have become necessary tools for proper nursing, far from any emotional, subjective arbitrariness.

When we observe the nurse in this activity, we find her in constant inner dialogue with the patient. We notice how she experiences the position of the patient in herself and inwardly transforms it into the desired outcome. This comprehension and progression does not happen in her thoughts alone, it affects her body too. For example, when we observe a patient having difficulty swallowing, where a bite of bread lies motionless in their mouth or is pushed from one cheek pocket to the other, we will feel the impulse ourselves—if we are inwardly involved in the laborious swallowing process—to more or less forcefully swallow to simulate the process that is disturbed in the patient. This does not happen in the case of distanced waiting or impatient pleading with the patient. The inwardly involved nurse seems to immerse herself in the life processes of the patient. Her nursing technique can become artistically shaped action.

> The relationship between closeness and distance determines the quality of human relationships.

Just as a dancer feels and picks up the movements of her partner and integrates them into her own movement, the nurse responds to the life expressions of the patient. The relationship between closeness and distance—in body and soul—is a vibrant dance, a rhythmic moving towards each other and apart.

In this sense the nursing process is an artistic process, which establishes a playful balance between the medical findings and the intentions of the nurse [→ Chapter "Rhythm"].

5.   Nursing and hope

5.1   Fourth exercise: positivity

The three forgoing exercises strive for control of our thoughts, will and feelings. Training these abilities enables masterful handling of our soul forces. It is the prerequisite for nurses to be able to bring themselves like a kind of remedy into the nursing process. We have already pointed out how nursing care, through the training of proper thinking, is able to grasp nursing in a realistic way and establish an objective, valid relationship with it. Mastery over our will forces through the practice of free initiative leads to awareness in the nursing process and creative shaping of everyday nursing life that is otherwise determined by external demands. The transformation of sympathy and antipathy into inner perception enables objective compassion with the patient and a feeling for his condition. It is the foundation for shaping nursing as an artistic process.

An exercise given by Rudolf Steiner that links thinking and feeling is "...to acquire the quality that one can call positivity. There is a beautiful legend that tells of Jesus Christ passing a dead dog, while walking with several people. The others turn away from the hideous sight. Christ Jesus speaks admiringly of the animal's beautiful teeth. One can practice maintaining such an attitude of soul as this legend reveals. The erroneous, the bad, the ugly shall not deter the soul from finding the true, the good and the beautiful everywhere where it is present [...] One cannot find the bad good, the wrong true; but one can make it so that the bad does not deter one from seeing what is good, and error does not prevent one from seeing what is true."[5]

We live in a world in which negativity threatens to get the upper hand over what is constructive, future-oriented and hope-giving.

Environmental destruction, war, isolation and loneliness often influence even children's perception of the world today. Daily confrontation with incurable illnesses, pain and suffering can cause even the most dedicated nurse to sometimes doubt the meaning of her modest assistance. Those who can only look at the dwindling life, the hopelessness of a biographical situation, the never-ending pain, are in danger of resigning or becoming deadened in their feelings. Even someone who is convinced of the meaning of this critical situation must ask themselves what the constructive next steps to overcoming the crisis might be. This is often hard to do when faced with the overwhelming problems to be tackled.

The exercise of positivity strengthens our ability to discover seeds for the future dormant in every situation, no matter how hopeless. These are to be encouraged. It is not the illness that must be eliminated, rather we want to stimulate the healing forces already within the organism. Ultimately, our recognition of a patient's resources encourages the quality of positivity. The person then grows into his possibilities. It is only these and not his inabilities that give cause for justified hope. Often a patient's hope appears illusionary: the cancer patient hoping for a "miracle injection" that will save him at the last moment, the dying person wanting to go on one more journey, the lonely person dreaming of salvation through a "fairy tale princess."

How can we be so sure that such hopes are illusionary? The picture that the ill person wraps their hope in may appear unrealistic. Does this give us the right to doubt their future possibilities?

When we succeed in recognizing the positive, future-oriented element in every condition of the ill person, then it becomes possible to transform illusions into justified hope: belief in a "miracle injection," as longed-for help from outside, is transformed into the confidence to be able to courageously survive the course of the disease from one's own inner strength, or a journey desired by a dying person can become an inner affirmation of leaving the body.

Discovering what is good and beautiful beneath the surface of what is negative or ugly gives us a starting point for encouraging and developing future-oriented resources. It supports the self-confidence of the person troubled by illness. It is also a ferment for fruitful cooperation in the therapeutic community. The social climate will be poisoned if we confront our colleagues one-sidedly with their shortcomings. A positive attitude enables us to individually encourage colleagues and assign tasks in a way that suits each person's capabilities.

The practice of positivity "is connected with what is called refraining from criticism [...] There is a point of view that lovingly enters into the foreign or outside being and asks everywhere: how does this other being come to be this way or do these things? Such a point of view strives of its own accord more towards helping what is imperfect, rather than merely admonishing and criticizing."[6]

6. Learning in day-to-day nursing care

6.1 Fifth exercise: impartiality

"Thinking in combination with will undergoes a certain ripening when one tries to never let anything that one experiences or has experienced rob one of unbiased receptivity for new experiences. This thought should lose all meaning for a student of higher knowledge: "I have never heard of that, I don't believe it." For a certain time, he should seek everywhere to allow every thing or being to say something new to him at every opportunity. One can learn from every breath of wind, every tree leaf, every babbling of a baby if one is prepared to apply a point of view that one has not applied before [...] One should judge what one experiences in the present according to one's experiences of the past. These are placed on the scales; on the other side of the scale is placed the spiritual student's readiness to always learn something new and, above all, the belief in the possibility that new experiences can contradict the old."[7]

Learning in day-to-day nursing care does not consist exclusively in the piling up of knowledge.

Rather it requires a questioning, researching basic attitude towards patients, colleagues and all one's own actions, to allow new experiences to find their places next to the old. Each nursing act should therefore be carried out like an (unspoken) question to the patient.

Example

We were told during the handover that a bedridden patient could not get up. That must not hinder us, if there is no contraindication against it, from asking him to sit on the edge of the bed with the inner question, "can you do that?" If the patient is not able to do it, we could reverse this action without endangering him. If the new position is stable, we can try to stand the patient in front of the bed with the same inner question. This is followed by the same check to see whether this effort is reasonable. This step too can easily be reversed. This is followed by turning the patient to the waiting armchair, where he can sit in a stable position.

Each step in mobilization was accompanied by a question. The response of the patient, either verbal or behaviorial, led to the next action.

Expressions of pain are also to be tested without prejudice. Even when an organic cause has been ruled out, the pain remains as a sign of how the patient feels. Unbiased listening, particularly to the communication of confused and psychotic patients, can be valuable. This is not to allow an obviously absurd content to revise our picture of reality, but because a facet of the patient's personality or illness is speaking to us through even the strangest expressions.

> Learning in day-to-day nursing care is a general necessity for maintaining and developing professional competence. The exercise of impartiality creates the inner prerequisite for this.

This path avoids always assigning our impressions of the world to the same categories ("putting them in drawers"). We receive everything new with wonder, without immediately assigning a concept to it. By a conscious effort of will, we inhibit the ordinary connection between perception and concept, which usually happens of its own accord in our thinking. It is as if a pause is inserted between thinking and acting, which holds back the two combined soul forces and strengthens them.

7. Practicing in day-to-day nursing care

7.1 Sixth exercise: inner balance

The objection could be raised against the exercises presented here that it is not necessary for a nurse to train himself in this way, since everyday nursing routine demands and trains the described characteristics anyway. As justifiable as this objection appears, self-reflection shows to what extent we have really mastered our soul forces. Even the most gifted artist practices regularly and systematically, to remain at the height of his art and continue to develop his skills. Artistry in the field of nursing also requires deliberate training of inner capacities, as does the training of manual dexterity. The exercises explained here require a deliberately chosen training plan.

The exercise of *proper thinking* comes first, followed by the exercise of *initiative*, etc. Each exercise should be done for a certain time, such as a month, with special attention. Yet the previous exercises should not be neglected. "Whoever has devoted time to consecutively practicing acquiring these qualities will then need to bring them into a harmonious accord in his soul. He will have to practice them two at a time, then three and one, etc., to achieve harmony."[8]

This inner harmony is necessary to counteract any one-sidedness in the person's development.

Integration of the exercises into the daily work of nursing care should be done circumspectly, as the patient remains the aim of nursing.

Striving for personal development must in no way interfere with the task of nursing. If this were to happen, the training would be harmful as a subtle form of egotism. If the nurse remains lovingly directed towards the patient and at the same time committed to some self-imposed exercises, this can contribute significantly to increased human and professional competence.

8. Outlook on the anthroposophic path of development

8.1 Nursing quality

The reason for describing these exercises is the training of qualities of soul that are needed in nursing. Mastery over one's own soul forces is a prerequisite for securing and enhancing the quality of nursing. In this extended concept of quality, the nurse herself is considered to be a healing factor in the therapeutic process. In this way, the approach offers an alternative to today's widespread tendency towards supposed quality assurance by standardizing a materialistic and scientific understanding of nursing care.

8.2 Path of development

Work on one's inner capacities presupposes a free decision by each person. It cannot be demanded from outside. Usually biographical crises confront people with the necessity of setting out on a conscious, self-chosen path of inner development. Insight into the prerequisites for professional competence can also ripen to a decision to actively begin a path of inner development [→ Chapter "Meditation in Nursing Care"].

8.3 Our view of the human being—thinking as the point of departure

The anthroposophic view of the human being is based on Rudolf Steiner's research findings. It was his contribution to depict knowledge of the foundations of human existence and the cosmos that is not accessible to the senses.[9] Such information appears to be pure speculation to a scientifically oriented view of humanity and the world, because science acknowledges statements about nature and humanity only if they come from methods of knowing that are limited to the sensory world.

Steiner refuted this view many times.[10] He explained how human beings can develop their inner capacities in such a way that they become like sense organs for the non-sensory world.[11] The training of supersensible organs of perception starts with the soul quality in which we are most conscious: thinking. In this, Steiner's approach differs substantially from other consciousness-expanding methods, such as Eastern or mystical ones. Those methods take their starting point from feeling or willing.

If we delve down into the region of our feelings, the brightness of consciousness dims, we find ourselves in a dreamlike world of pictures that is susceptible to suggestion and autosuggestion. When our search for an expanded consciousness takes will as its starting point, this dims consciousness to dreamless sleep. Our will impulses become conscious only in our thinking. It is only there that we become able to judge good and evil, truth and error. Without this thinking and judging of waking consciousness, we act instinctively and are almost defenselessly at the mercy of external influences.

Since the anthroposophic path of development can be thinkingly understood at every point, every kind of suggestive influence is avoided.

8.4 The exercises

Rudolf Steiner gave the exercises described as the fundamental prerequisite for esoteric training, i.e., for gaining knowledge of the supersensible world. This chapter has looked at these exercises in close association with practical nursing. Through the way in which they are portrayed, the aspect of inner hygiene comes to the fore over the esoteric. Their universal value lies in the strengthening of thinking, feeling and willing as soul qualities ruled over by the 'I', even if esoteric development is not the primary goal. If you would like to work your way into a comprehensive understanding of this matter, please refer to Rudolf Steiner's many descriptions of it.[12, 13] Day-to-day nursing care is an inexhaustible field of practice for the main prerequisites of esoteric development. The constant nearness to the threshold to the spiritual world in birth, illness and death is a special opportunity for nurses to encounter the powers and beings of higher worlds.

8.5 Where are human beings headed? —Nursing as a cultural task

Our starting point was a description of the cultural task of caregiving. Caregiving proved to be a first-rate factor in cultivating and maintaining culture. However, this alone does not say much about the groundbreaking goal of this task. We already indicated that human beings raise up and "humanize" nature in caring for it. But where are human beings headed—can they themselves become more human?

According to a Christian understanding, human beings only achieve a higher stage of existence when they connect themselves with the *Christ Being*. This does not require professions of faith; it asks us to be aware of and act from the power of love that came into the world with Christ. In this sense the anthroposophic path of development is a Christian path of initiation. It is not a path to self-redemption, as is often assumed, but a preparation for an ever deeper grasping of Christ's healing work. The six exercises described, given by Rudolf Steiner as preparation for esoteric development (called supplementary exercises in *How to Know Higher Worlds*) are part of a Christian path of development. They serve the purification and strengthening of human soul forces, so that the soul can stand firm when encountering beings of higher worlds.

Everyone active in nursing care, privately or professionally, maintains the world and its people in a state capable of development and transformation, wresting them from their tendency to sink down into mere natural and inhuman levels. It is as if the nurse offers what has been entrusted to his care to the spiritual world for transformation. His care creates a way for the transformative, spiritualizing, healing element to fall on fruitful ground. Lovingly cared for objects are ready to become carriers of immaterial values. A lovingly cared for invalid will experience the effect of treatment more sustainably than would be possible in cool, distant surroundings.

Nursing care understood as a cultural task paves the way for the influence of the spiritual world in the earthly course of development. Without this care and preparation, the sense world is in danger of losing its living connection to the spirit. Work on our soul forces strives for the same thing on our individual path of development that a nurturing culture will mean for the development of humanity as a whole.

Category	Example learning objectives	Recommended learning path
Skill	You are practicing the exercise to control your thoughts.	A
Your own learning objective		
Relationships	You are intensifying your relationships to patients using the exercises described.	B
Your own learning objective		
Knowledge	You see nursing as a cultural task and path of development.	C
Your own learning objective		

References

13   Steiner, R. *Occult science: An outline.* Rudolf Steiner Press, London 2013.

14   Fiechter, V.; Maier, M. *Pflegeplanung. Eine Anleitung für die Praxis.* Recom Verlag, Basel 1985, p. 27 ff.

15   Steiner, R. *Guidance in esoteric training. From the esoteric school.* 3rd ed. Rudolf Steiner Press, London 1998.

16   Steiner, R. *Theosophy. An introduction to the supersensible knowledge of the world and the destination of man.* Rudolf Steiner Press, London 2005.

17   Steiner, R. *Occult science. An outline.* Rudolf Steiner Press, London 2013.

18   Steiner, R. *Guidance in esoteric training. From the esoteric school.* 3rd ed. Rudolf Steiner Press, London 1998.

19   ibid.

20   Steiner ,R. *Occult science. An outline.* Rudolf Steiner Press, London 2013.

21   ibid.

22   ibid.

23   Steiner, R. *Riddles of the Soul.* Mercury Press, Spring Valley 1996.

24   Steiner, R. *How to know higher worlds—a modern path of initiation.* Anthroposophic Press, Great Barrington 2002.

25   Steiner, R. *Occult science. An outline.* Rudolf Steiner Press, London 2013.

CHAPTER VI
Meditation in Nursing

ROLF HEINE

All spiritual and religious movements and schools that focus on achieving personal spiritual experience are likely to describe meditation in one form or another. To meditate is initially a method and meditation itself is a stage on a spiritual path. Thus, "right concentration" is the eighth stage of the Buddha's eightfold path, and is prepared by "right effort" and "right mindfulness." Meditation on the "most beautiful names of God" in Islam is embedded into the everyday lives of active people, just as immersion in the words of the Lord's Prayer or the Beatitudes of Jesus Christ can be at the center of an active spiritual life.

1.   Aims of meditating

The different needs, goals, and motives to begin a spiritual path are summarized in the chart on the following page. These good and justified aims stand opposite darker, less noble motives, and even genuine distortions of spiritual development. The darker motives make it clear that these necessary steps in human development can be misguided when they act as unconscious drives. For instance, the necessary impulse to acquire self-control can be projected into the lust for power and the desire to control others. Or it may happen that a desired side effect of inner work becomes its main purpose, namely personal health. Likewise, vanity can be fostered when the conscious impulse to "make oneself a better person" is distorted into an addictive need to win affirmation and admiration from others.

Initially, the subject chosen for meditation will be the sublime, wise words of the sacred writings of humanity. But pictures, signs, and symbols can also be used to direct the human mind toward a sphere which is inaccessible to the physical senses. The significance of mantric words goes far beyond their conceptual content. They are like archipelagos of spirit, places of refuge and transformation in the sea of the trivial. The world of sounds and tones, rhythms and harmonies, even without conceptual content, also has the power to lead the meditator from the sensory world into the adjacent etheric world. Ultimately, any phenomenon of nature—a plant, light, or any phenomenon of social life such as love or freedom—can become the subject of meditation when a person's consciousness rests on it. Meditation in this sense is a way to expand our consciousness beyond the life of soul that is bound to the sensory world.

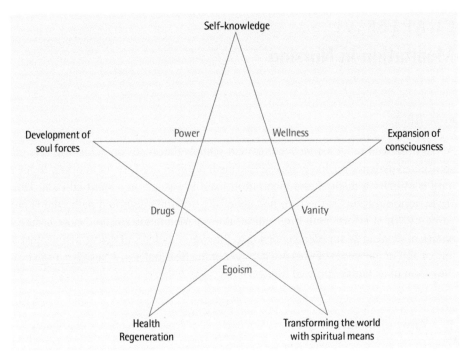

Fig. 1: Needs, goals, and motives on the spiritual path

1.1 Expansion of consciousness

There are numerous occasions to seek such transformation of consciousness in the nursing profession and to push toward that unadulterated reality which stands behind the suffering, behind the illness, behind the confused and tragic fates of our patients and our involvement with it all as nurses. However, these occasions alone are not enough to find a way to expand our awareness in the nursing profession. Rather, we must apply what Rudolf Steiner said about the "seeker after human wisdom": "only they can be anthroposophists who feel certain questions on the nature of humanity and the universe as an elemental need of life, just as one feels hunger and thirst."[1]

For nurses, it is not only the mysteries of illness, destiny, and death that motivate us to take up such a search. It is often the everyday life of nursing work which, like hardly anything else, repeatedly threatens to freeze into routine and to become exhausted in seemingly irrelevant auxiliary activities, precisely because repetition, rhythmic recurrence, helping, and serving belong to the essence and the task of nursing care. Time and again, in everyday life, it is necessary to revivify that which tends to freeze up and become sluggishly exhaustive. The following meditation recommended by Rudolf Steiner in a course for young people effectively supports this transformation of everyday, routine activity:

Feel in fever's measure
Saturn's gift of spirit
Feel in the pulse's count
The sun's soul strength
Feel in the weight of matter
The forming power of the moon:
Then you will see in your will to heal
Also the need to be healed of the earthly human being[2]

This meditation calls on the middle quality of feeling in three everyday activities of nursing care: measuring fever, counting a pulse, weighing a patient. Our alienation from sensory experiences of the qualities of fever, pulse, and weight that results from the measuring instruments that we use today (ear thermometers, pulse oximeters, electronic scales, etc.) stands opposite the feelings needed in meditation. Meditating on this verse therefore definitely requires sensory preparation. It is important to become aware of the sensation that occurs when you touch a feverish body. You experience, for example, a glowing forehead, the fleeting, thin warmth of the hands and the cool lifelessness of the feet up to the calves. We can acquire a sense for differentiations in the patient's warmth organism in the following way, for example: we observe warmth that accumulates in the head and has withdrawn from the limbs. Later on, the fever shows a different picture. The whole body is hot. The warmth is pushing outwards. Beads of sweat appear on the forehead and trunk. The temperature drops. Soon the patient will be shivering in his wet nightshirt. The warmth now appears in its temporal form. Fever is warmth differentiation in space and warmth fluctuation in time. Warmth appears as an organism, as an entity. In this entity we measure what is "too warm" or "too cold," the centralized or peripheralized existence of warmth. Fever becomes a phenomenon in which warmth can be imagined as an independent organism. In the verse, the imagination of fever, pulse, and weight sounds together with an inner view of the planets Saturn, Sun, and Moon. The planets call into the consciousness of the meditator the harmony of the spheres sounding in the rhythmic course of time and the planetary stages of the development of the Earth. They allow our imaginative image of the warmth organism to be attuned to inspired knowledge of world development. Imagination and Inspiration prepare the ground for the intuitive act of healing, in which the task of the healer is one with the need and question of the person in need of help. The path of transformation of everyday consciousness through Imagination, Inspiration, and Intuition is a longing and incentive for many people in this age of the consciousness soul.

1.2   Health—Regeneration

Every meditation begins with directing one's attention to the object of one's meditation. This focusing of attention is also a turning away from the soul mood of everyday life, which tends to be determined more by external impressions.

"Create moments of inner peace for yourself, and in these moments learn to distinguish the essential from the non-essential."[3] In this attention turned towards one's inner soul, towards a spiritual saying, a prayer, a sound, or a movement, the meditator gradually creates an inner space that can expand into a source of concentration, strength, and joy. Meditation is initially the creation of a "pause," a damming up of the flowing stream of consciousness. In contrast to mere "unwinding" or "resting," the meditator remains in calm alertness. The meditator actively shapes a bright space of consciousness, which she enters with her own soul mood:

> *Find yourself in Light*
> *With your own soul's tone*
> *And tone disperses*
> *Becomes color-form*
> *   In the Light*
> *Light-Divine-Being.*
>
> *Tone disappeared*
> *Restored again within him*
> *   Speaking through him:*
>
> *   You are*
>
> *Your own tone*
> *In the light of the World*
> *   Sound illuminating*
> *   Illuminate sounding.*

This verse,[4] given by Rudolf Steiner to his physician collaborator Ita Wegman (1876–1943), which she then spoke with nurses at the Clinical Therapeutic Institute in Arlesheim over many years, describes in a moving and enigmatic way how people can enter a space of attention in which they may come to themselves. The empty silence that is experienced in the middle of that space is the turning point from which our attention is transmitted to the world again, shining and sounding. The "pause" in light and sound has a refreshing, invigorating, and healing effect.

1.3   Transforming the world with spiritual means

Despite all the rational interpretations provided by scientific models, the healing of a human being remains a mystery. In particular, we are amazed by healings that go beyond the effects that substances are known to have on body and soul. We call them miracles—and the scientific side excludes their existence. In miracles, the physical-sensory world is changed by spiritual means. Numerous phenomena that were once regarded as "spiritual and supersensible," such as the occurrence of epidemics and natural disasters, have been clearly explained through the disenchantment of the world since the Age of Enlightenment. They have been attributed to predictable cause-effect mechanisms. Nevertheless, our amazement at the healing power of a mild gaze, a good word, a warm hand, a prayer or a medication whose material substance has been potentized out of it, brings back to our soul—unimpressed by rationalizing explanations—the miracle, the "magical influence" of spirit upon matter.

Prayer and intercession are well-known ways that spirit influences matter. Decades before the establishment of scientific psychoimmunology, Rudolf Steiner explained in his "Samaritan course" the effect of consciousness on the immune reaction in the process of wound healing, as an example of the "magical effect" of consciousness on matter: "Today we say: the good spirits send us these healing forces," (such as the migration of leukocytes into the area of a wound) "and today a person must be injured if they are to appear and be effective. What will be normal in the future must today be evoked through such a wounding. When, however, we really take up into ourselves the power of the Spirit, then we shall be able to evoke these forces ourselves."[5] To support this process of strengthening the power of consciousness, Rudolf Steiner gave the following mantram:[6]

Well up, O blood
And in the welling work!
Quickening muscles
Quicken the seeds!
May loving care
Of a warming heart
Be healing breath!

Obviously, this verse—like the others mentioned above—is difficult to grasp by pure intellect. Regular repeated meditation on these words and thoughts, cultivated over a longer period of time, reveals ever new layers of meaning. Ultimately, it is not just the conceptually comprehensible word contents, it is also their phonetic and rhythmic, figuratively interwoven surfaces of meaning which gradually reveal themselves. In this process, we transform the intellectually interpreted verse into a space of meditation that we imbue with feeling. This space condenses into a spiritual point—it becomes a mantram.

1.4 Developing our soul forces

The aim of meditation can also be to develop individual human abilities. Our willingness to put ourselves in our patient's shoes, to perceive the need for care and to help lovingly and effectively is an everyday challenge for every nurse. The meditation called the "meditation for nurses," which is described in detail later in this chapter, develops the area of the heart as a place of light and warmth. Starting from there, we combine the power of the individual with the power of the community of colleagues, because nursing care is always a shared task.

All motifs ultimately lead to the question of self-knowledge. "O Human Being! Know Yourself!" stands as a challenge and a promise before the soul of every seeking individual. Self-knowledge is neither an act of initiation nor one of enlightenment. It happens neither at a certain time nor in a certain place, neither while awake nor asleep, not even during meditation. Partial insights into our soul's depths, into biographical threads, constellations of fate or karmic necessities can be luminous landmarks, encouraging, and sometimes shattering; they are not yet complete self-knowledge. Self-knowledge is the ever more conscious, continuous process of change that accompanies people through life and death and through incarnations.

Meditation promotes this process of transformation. It is a cultural treasure to be integrated into everyday duties and pleasures such as eating and drinking, work and rest, waking, sleeping and dreaming, art, and habits. Like those life processes, meditation has effects on the whole person. It can become a source of conscious transformation of one's life. The mood of meditation, the inner posture during meditation, and what is discovered in meditation affect the outer layers of our being (soul body, etheric body, physical body) and the core of our being. This work is entirely voluntary. In contrast, it is the task of every nurse, doctor, and therapist to work on the outer constitutional layers. What happens to the patient through our respective professional techniques needs an inner balance in the nurse, doctor, or therapist. The medications prepared and used for the patient lose their effectiveness if the therapist uses them for him- or herself.[7] In this sense, it is unselfish self-care to meditate on the remedies and the powers of the soul and mind used for healing. It makes the therapist authentic because in meditation one has spiritually experienced what the patient suffers physically and mentally. Meditative practice, in this sense, is a necessary condition for Christian healing care.

2. Practical meditation for nurses

The need for places of rest, silence, regeneration, and inner development arises from the manifold occupational stress and borderline situations of nurses. As a rule, these places of rest are not to be found in the physical world. And even when the sun is shining warmly on our backs and contemplation of the clouds fills our minds, or the laughter of a child or a conversation makes us happy, these "gifts of the moment" are worth nothing if we do not consciously involve ourselves with them, if we are not "present" in the moment. It is also important to let them go again, so that looking back on them longingly does not bind the power gained. Where are these places of rest and regeneration? How can the three steps of opening oneself, lingering, and freeing oneself succeed? The practice of an inner path often begins with these questions. "Create moments of inner peace for yourself, and in these moments learn to distinguish the essential from the non-essential."[8] Some people master this ability on their own. They can quiet themselves down and come to themselves through contemplating nature or a work of art or in prayer—in an activity that fills them and in which they are completely present. Others, when they visit a quiet room, first become aware of how much their inner restlessness, chatter, fears, omissions, and compelling will impulses disturb their peace of mind. Quite often silence can be experienced as oppressive, as a threat. The person leaves it hastily and is glad to dive back into places of diversion again.

Whoever withdraws for a certain time—initially five minutes—from external sensory impressions and tries to bring to rest memories, thoughts, and feelings related to the events of the day, can find support in a word meditation. Words and sentences from the wise teachings of humankind are suitable, such as the Bible, the Bhagavad Gita, the aphorisms of Novalis (1772–1801), and prayers and poems. It is particularly helpful to choose a word or phrase yourself. During the meditation your attention rests as well as possible on this sentence and its words. With a phrase like "Wisdom lives in the light"[9] it is not (only) important to think about the content, we need to dwell with our consciousness on or in the sentence. When thoughts, memories, and ideas appear that do not belong to the meditation, one returns to the task one has set oneself without annoyance, but determinedly again. Over time, it becomes increasingly easier not to lose the object of one's meditation from one's awareness. Then it begins to become brighter, more differentiated, warmer, more colorful. Inner movements emerge. In this phrase "Wisdom lives in the light," for example, the small word "in" can lead into a sense of the inner space of meditation.

As with all exercises, after an initial period in which the object of our meditation reveals certain new sides that had been inaccessible to mere imagination and reflection, it will then lose this initial attraction too. What can be experienced in the meditation will then appear familiar, almost self-evident; it will lose its liveliness. Faithfulness and constant, relaxed perseverance, even playful earnestness, can revive the meditation. A very simple object of meditation can still help, even after years and decades, to make someone aware of something new and important for the here and now.

This immersion in a meditation creates a space of consciousness into which one enters again and again, with some practice. It has become a place of retreat, relaxation, and refreshment. This space is created by the inner activity of the meditator. The content of the meditation accommodates this activity and forms *its own* peculiar shape in the consciousness of the meditator. In this way, insights into the world beyond the senses mature, like pearls.

Like every place, the space of consciousness created by meditation needs to be cared for. This space is maintained by good habits, such as rhythm, earnestness, wonder and reverence. Habits integrate things into life, into our daily routine. The activity becomes self-evident, familiar, and relieving. We "live" in it. If the "dwelling" becomes too small or too big, we move, we look for a home that better suits us in this moment. Habits arise when you repeat something rhythmically over a certain period of time. But what is it that is to be repeated? Where should one meditate? When should one meditate? How should one meditate? These practical questions often arise at the beginning of consciously starting meditative training.

Where: The outer place is not essential for meditation. It can be done anywhere—even in the most turbulent bustle of everyday life for experienced meditators. However, a quiet place that is free of distractions supports concentration. A quiet room, which we visit regularly, facilitates our inner self-collection. Meditation in nature requires more concentration than meditation in a closed space. An upright sitting position and relaxed posture allows the consciousness to rest on the object of meditation better than a horizontal position in which it seems to be harder to resist falling asleep. (One can experience, though, while meditating lying down, what a good sedative a thought-supported meditation can be. This has helped some patients with sleep disorders.)

When: The time of day for meditation depends on the requirements and duties of everyday life. Those who are well awake early in the morning and can arrange to meditate in peace will have a good start to their day. Those who are not too tired in the evening can practice distancing themselves from the impressions of the day and directing their gaze to something essential as they meditate. Meditations that refer to the seasonal festivals and the course of the year (such as Rudolf Steiner's Soul Calendar[10] or the monthly virtues[11]) bring one's inner experience into harmony with the rhythms of nature and the cosmos. Some meditations are given especially for a certain time of the day, because they take into account the respective mood of consciousness of that time of day (e.g., the point-circle meditation).[12] The duration should not bring the meditator into conflict with his or her tasks and daily duties. Many practice for a total of between 5 and 30 minutes a day. A daily rhythm strengthens the effect of meditation. It is also helpful to take a few minutes between waking up and falling asleep, for example in the middle of the day, and briefly reflect on what is essential for you in life.

Alone or together: "Those who walk to the truth, walk alone, no one can be brother to another."[13] This is how Christian Morgenstern (1871–1914) characterized the spiritual search. During meditation the physical presence of other people is neither needed nor sought. It is like the physical place of meditation—without meaning. When people meditate together in a room, however, a very intense atmosphere can develop which increases concentration. Since such an intense atmosphere is not the goal of meditation, but at best a strengthening consequence of meditating together, joint meditation has no special value in itself, unless you deliberately agree with a group of people to meet for a particular spiritual task.

How: Like every processual event, meditation has a preliminary part, a main part, and a conclusion. External preparation creates the conditions for undisturbed meditation. Inner preparation opens the consciousness for that which will show itself in the space of meditative awareness. Finally, though, we need to consciously end the meditation.

Preparation: Outwardly we isolate ourselves from outer disturbances and turn our attention completely to the inside. This opening of our soul is related to the mood of amazement—with the difference that amazement is usually directed outwards to the sensory world. In this mood you are completely devoted to what you are experiencing. Usually people are amazed by impressive natural phenomena or artistic skills. In amazement[14] their consciousness is attracted by what they behold in the sensory world. To evoke such a mood in oneself, without there being any reason to be amazed, one needs an active inner strength, which can be generated solely from one's own activity. All one's senses open up without anything concrete being perceived.

We set a limit to our devotion in amazement: to inwardly withdraw again in loving contact with what amazes us is nothing other than *reverence*.[15]

As with the deliberate awakening of amazement, the easiest way to evoke reverence is to first *remember* a situation in which one felt reverence, for example, before meeting a person whom one has great respect for. The exercise will have the strongest effect if it succeeds in creating "reverence" even when there is nothing "awe-inspiring" present. Steiner describes the activation of a mood of devotion—awe, reverence, humility—as a prerequisite for any healthy spiritual training. It opens one's inner sense for the significance of the true and the sublime.[16]

After creating a receptive, devotional inner movement in "amazement" and invoking a humble, inner gesture of "looking up and bowing down" in "reverence," we proceed to the main part of the meditation.

Main part: Rudolf Steiner characterized the state of meditation in his introduction to the "rose cross" meditation:[17] *"By calling to mind the concept of memory, we can begin to grasp what it means to immerse ourselves in a visualized image. For example, if we look at a tree and then turn away from it so that we can no longer see it, we can reawaken the mental image of the tree out of our memory. The mental image we have of a tree when it is not actually present before our eyes is the memory of the tree. Now let's imagine that we retain this memory in our soul; we allow the soul to rest on this memory image and attempt to exclude all other images. Then the soul is immersed in the memory image of the tree. But although the soul is immersed in a mental image, this image is a copy of something perceived by our senses. However, if we attempt the same thing with an image that we insert into our consciousness through an act of free will, we will gradually be able to achieve the necessary effect."* As already in the preparatory steps of generating *amazement* and *reverence*, the meditator actively builds up an inner image out of his or her own free will. This demands concentration and strength.

Conclusion: The main part of the meditation can end, for example, with adopting two more inner postures in the soul. Looking back at the space of meditation and looking forward to everyday life, we call up the mood of "feeling in harmony with the phenomena of the world."[18] This is necessary in order to bring together the extraordinary disparity of the sensory and everyday world compared to the inner soul-spiritual world of meditation, to find oneself and act in a coherent reality of physical world, soul, and spirit. This mood is created by an inner movement that is horizontal, expansive, and affirmatively balancing.

Meditation can also end in a different mood, namely in "devotion."[19] We consciously place ourselves into a framework that encompasses both ourselves *and* the world. This transforms all urgent aspiration and wanting to press ahead, instead creating an open, patient, affirmative mood. Steiner did not tire of emphasizing the importance of patient waiting as an essential prerequisite for the anthroposophic path of development. The mood of devotion consciously puts one's own will, one's own searching and pressing forward, into a larger context.

3. The central meditation for nurses: transforming the verse into a mantram

We shall now explain the most important meditation that Rudolf Steiner gave for nurses.

It stands next to many other exercises and mantras which people work with in anthroposophic nursing care.[20] It occupies a central position, since it is Rudolf Steiner's only specific instruction for professional nurses.

> *Within the heart there lives*
> *In shining light*
> *The human sense of helping.*
> *Within the heart there works*
> *In warming might*
> *The human strength of love.*
> *So let us bear*
> *The soul's whole will*
> *In heart-warmth*
> *And heart-light*
> *Then we work to heal*
> *Those in need of healing*
> *Out of God's sense of grace.*

Ita Wegman received the verse for nurses from Rudolf Steiner on December 2, 1923, with the condition that it should only be passed on to the nurses at the Clinical Therapeutic Institute in Arlesheim, near Basel, Switzerland, when there was good cooperation and a genuine feeling of community among them. Steiner had promised to hold a course for nurses in 1925. This was no longer possible due to his death in March 1925. The course was finally given in May 1925 under the direction of Ita Wegman. On that occasion, she handed over the verse to seven selected nurses who were also members of the First Class of the School for Spiritual Science founded by Rudolf Steiner. At the same time, this group was admitted as a "subdivision" of the Medical Section, one of the eleven departments of the School for Spiritual Science. Until its publication in the 1990s, the verse for nurses was only passed on to members of the First Class of the School for Spiritual Science. In this context it was meditated on in order to train the heart forces in the professional community and in nursing practice. After the verse was published, those who work with this meditation agreed to meditate on it every Sunday in the first half of the day. They wanted to create a worldwide spiritual bond between the nurses. The deceased who had lived and worked in the spirit of this meditation can also be included in the meditation.[21] This strengthening of their inner work thus made the meditation publicly known and accessible.

3.1 Working with the verse for nurses

The following describes a personal work cycle with the verse for nurses in seven steps. Each step is divided—as described above—into a twofold preparation, the main part, and a twofold concluding mood. The first five steps describe a path to Imagination. Steps six and seven point the way to Inspiration and Intuition, based on Rudolf Steiner's descriptions.[22]

Preparation	Main part	Conclusion
Amazement	Building up a picture	Feeling in harmony with the laws of the world
Reverence	Resting in the picture	Devotion

Chart: The course of a meditation

First step:
After you have prepared and induced the moods of "amazement" and "reverence," read the verse slowly out loud. Before listening to it a second time, let it reverberate in you, in the way that you would reflect on an experience that has just ended.

When reading it out loud for the second time, it is helpful to pause after each line and visualize the meaning of what it says. Anything incomprehensible or contradictory is to be noticed as such without dwelling on it. After this second reading, let the verse reverberate again in silence. In a third reading you follow the rhythm of the verse's language and at the end you linger again in the echo of what you heard. The meditation ends with you engendering the two closing moods of "feeling in harmony with the laws of the world" and "devotion."

Second step:
After the preparation you speak the verse out loud. On the second reading you build it up line by line, together with inner pictures of the respective motifs. These images in your imagination, for example the "heart" or the "shining light," should appear lively and colorful. Some try to create a vivid image of the flow of blood in circulation, of the rhythmically beating heart, or of the feeling heart. It is not a matter of working with other people's images, but of creating an image from one's own perception or

conceptualization. Then you rest your attention again for a while on each picture before moving on to the next. When reading the whole verse for the third time, you recall the images thus formed as you (slowly) speak. Let the rhythm and images resonate before concluding the meditation with the two final moods.

Third step:
Amazement and reverence initiate the meditation. The experiences of the first two steps resonate as you speak the verse. The mood of amazement maintains your openness to progress in practice, without dwelling too long on the past and without the pictures losing their intensity. When speaking the verse a second time, you look more closely at words or contexts whose meanings remain mysterious and which therefore do not evoke inner images. The words "the human will to help" and "sense of grace" could, for example, raise puzzling questions.

Meditation is not about explaining or judging the content in its meaning. It is important to perceive one's own opinion and differing ideas or experiences without continuously resorting to them. Rather, one can investigate *in which sense* the verse's statements are true. It has the greatest value when such questions remain without a quick answer. Living with the question creates a mood of closeness to the spiritual world. In your third speaking of the verse, you try to hear it as if it were a possible answer to your unanswered questions. The third step concludes with the final moods "feeling in harmony with the laws of the world" and "devotion."

Fourth step:
Special attention should be paid to the creation of the preparatory moods. When speaking the verse for the first time you try to place the whole verse before your soul with all the intimacy, vividness, and mysteriousness gained so far.

When speaking the verse for the second time, you give special attention to the words "within," "in," "the," "so," which you perhaps heeded less up until now. It is hardly possible to develop images in your mind from these words. "In" and "within" hardly differ in their meaning, but they do in their logical context. They can be experienced as inner movements. A different kind of inwardly experienced picture can be generated by noting the rhythm of brighter and darker vowels or the mirroring of similar words, such as "sense of helping" and "sense of grace" (in the German original: "*Helfersinn*" and "*Gnadensinn*"), as well as "heart-warmth" and "heart-light." In the second step it was still possible to easily imagine the pictures. The aim was to create new inner pictures of one's own, in contrast to the old existing ones of others. The task now is to transform abstract, logical connections into living constellations and movements.

When speaking the verse for the third time, it is important that you have the entire verse in front of your mind's eye right from the start. Beginning, middle, conclusion and intensification sound together. The final moods emerge automatically from this contemplation.

Fifth step:

The fifth step results from your efforts so far: you have created a picture of the heart. Blood from the veins of the metabolic organs, limbs, and sensory organs flows into the right atrium of the organ of the body's middle. The left atrium simultaneously receives the oxygen-enriched blood from the pulmonary circulation. In the relaxation phase, diastole, the blood flows into the heart chambers. From there it flows in systole (the tension phase), into pulmonary circulation and body circulation. The polarities of diastole and systole, of lung and body circulation, of right and left heart, of atria and ventricles, shape the anatomical and functional events of the heartbeat. Between heart and lung, as well as between pulse and breath, there is a rhythmic ratio of 4:1.

The verse for nurses consists of thirteen lines, which can be divided into four stanzas of three lines each. The seventh, middle line of the thirteen ("So let us bear") differs linguistically from the rest both by its culmination of dark vowels (German: "*So lasset uns tragen*") and by its invocative, refreshing character. It also divides the entire verse into an inward first part and an outward second part, oriented towards a community:

1: *Within the heart there lives*
    In shining light
    The human sense of helping.

2: *Within the heart there works*
    In warming might
    The human strength of love.

    So let us bear

3: *The soul's whole will*
    In heart-warmth
    And heart-light

4: *Then we work to heal*
    Those in need of healing
    Out of God's sense of grace.

	So let us bear	
1	*Within the heart there lives* *In shining light* *The human sense of helping.*	*The soul's whole will* 3 *In heart-warmth* *And heart-light*
2	*Within the heart there works* *In warming might* *The human strength of love.*	*Then we work to heal* 4 *Those in need of healing* *Out of God's sense of grace.*

Fig. 2: Surprising perspectives through giving a new configuration to the verse for nurses

In Figure 2, the four stanzas appear as that which fills the right and left half of the heart (stanzas 1 and 2 or 3 and 4). Stanzas 1 and 3 form the level of the atria, stanzas 2 and 4 the level of the chambers. Functionally, after filling the atria, the flow of blood stands still for a moment. All heart valves are closed in this moment. Now the heart becomes an organ of perception. It awakens in luminous brightness the human will to help (right auricle) and the soul is filled with warmth and light (left auricle) after being refreshed by a breath ("So let us bear"). The contracting chambers in their effective force are polar to the atria, whose main functional work is the will that rests in perception. In the right chamber "The human strength of love" works outward in the direction of soul breathing. In the left chamber, the soul connected to the outside world places itself into the active, healing working ("Then we work to heal") of the entire human organization. The quiet, resting character of the first and third stanzas (the two atriums) with the soulful "lives" and the lush "whole" contrasts with the stanzas two and four (the two chambers) with their mobile, active "works" and "work." The third stanza without a verb not only summarizes the stanzas one and two, it increases the polarity of calm and power. It is as if it has placed the verb, the action word, outside of itself in the line "So let us bear," so that it is filled with full, yet resting will.

Another relationship becomes visible when we compare the first stanza with the fourth (right atrium and left chamber). It is not only the link between the meaning of the "human sense of helping" and "God's sense of grace," it is also the formative use of the consonants "H" and "L" in the middle lines ("*In leuchtender Helle*"; "*Das Heil den Heilbedürft'gen*"), as well as the identical rhythm and number of syllables of the first lines ("*Im Herzen wohnt*"; "*So wirken wir*"), which refers to an almost musical reference between beginning and end. The beginning of the first line ("Within") and the beginning of the last line of the mantram ("Out of") express the pulsation of internalization and externalization, of receiving and giving in the simplest way.

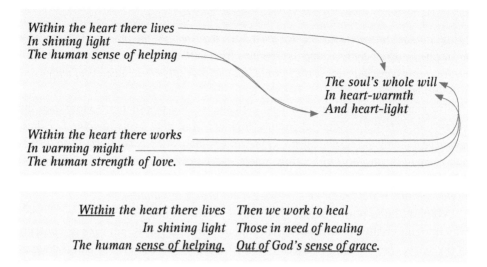

Within the heart there lives   *Then we work to heal*
In shining light   *Those in need of healing*
The human sense of helping.   *Out of God's sense of grace.*

Fig. 3: Interrelated references of meaning within the first three stanzas* of the verse for nurses

The meditator is now delving into a self-created image. Individual concepts such as "warmth," "light," "the will to help," and "sense of grace" are given a new depth when seen together with the functional reality of the heart. The meditation has now also arrived at the physiological reality of the heart. The rhythm of individual perception of a person's need for help (will to help) and of a "work-oriented love" (force of love), which a collegial, sisterly-fraternal community seeks and needs, and which experiences confirmation through being looked at from the spiritual world (God's sense of grace), appears real right into one's own physicality. This meditation thus reveals the heart character of the verse for nurses. Here, form and content form poles in an organism. They intertwine in the outer peace of meditation and the inner activity of image-creating reflection.

The final moods of "feeling in harmony with the laws of the world" and "devotion" are of particular importance for this fifth step, both to sober up any premature, not yet sufficiently tested images, and to connect the feeling of happiness and freedom created in meditation to a sincere attitude of seeking the good.

Sixth step:

After the preparation you meditate on the verse. You are now familiar with it. Now you try as hard as possible to extinguish the resulting pictures. The goal is to establish empty consciousness. Rudolf Steiner described this as follows: *"when a person's sense-impressions have been gradually shut off; when all is dark around him and he can see nothing; when all noise is shut out so that he hears nothing and even the day's impressions are suppressed, he falls asleep. This empty consciousness, that comes to anyone on the verge of sleep, now has to be brought about at will. But while all conscious impressions, even those self-induced, have to be blotted out, it is most important*

---

*   Stanzas 1 and 2 are summed up in stanza 3. Linguistically, "lives" from the first line corresponds to "whole" in the first line of the third stanza. "Works" from the first line of stanza 2 corresponds linguistically to "will" in stanza 3. "Light" and "will to help" from stanza 1 appear in stanza 3 as "heart-light"; while "power" and "force of love" from stanza 2 appear as "heart-warmth" in stanza 3.

for the student to remain awake. He must have the strength, the inner activity, to keep awake while no longer receiving impressions from without, or any experiences whatever. An empty consciousness is thus produced, but an empty consciousness of which one is fully aware."[23]

The empty consciousness fills itself with silence. But this silence is more than the absence of external or internal sounds. Steiner: *"And now let us imagine [...] there would be not only the absolute peace of the zero-point of silence, but it would go further and come to the negative of hearing, quieter than quiet, more silent than silence. [...] When, however, we arrive at this inner negative of audibility, [...] we are then so deeply in the spiritual world that we not only see it but hear it resounding."*[24]

Warmth, light, power, sense, grace, love, salvation and other things work their way into this empty consciousness. They do not work as words, not even as contents of the verse. They resound as effective force fields. They are at the same time sources of inspiration and interpreters of the verse, which only now is acquiring its meaning through them. In the concluding mood you experience "devotion" and "thankfulness" especially intensively.

Seventh step:

In the preceding steps, we developed the verse for nurses into a meditation for nurses as a pictorial description of nursing ideals. Images, rhythms and sounds gained importance and strength in the meditation. The meditator discovers a mantram in the verse. The mantram unfolds its effectiveness in life. This is the seventh step.

The meditative preparation, the main part, and the conclusion of the mantram now form a unity which in turn represents the preparation for the seventh step. Meditation has brought the mantram to life. It unfolds pictures, sounds and meaning. The soul finds itself in a world full of light and silence, full of warmth and power. It is important to carry this mood out into the world, upright and awake. To recognize earthly needs, to feel compassion for the suffering of others, to understand every sensory impression, every encounter as the revelation of a self-expressing being, trains our ability to act with presence of mind. For Rudolf Steiner it is the "ability to love" that enables human beings to act intuitively fully consciously—that is, with presence of mind.[25] The seventh step concludes with a review of the day.[26]

3.2   Other practical aspects

"One should not have any "mystical" ideas in connection with meditation, nor indeed imagine that it is an easy thing. Meditation must be something completely clear, in the modern sense. Patience and inner energy of soul are necessary for it, and, above all, it is connected with an act that no man can do for another, namely, to make an inner resolve and then hold to it. When he begins to meditate, man is performing the only completely free act there is in human life." Rudolf Steiner said.[27]

This principle stands before every meditative exercise. It also applies to the steps proposed here for working with the verse for nurses. Each step must be repeated for as long as it is experienced as being fruitful. If stagnation occurs, this should spur you on to increase your effort to do the exercise and overcome the dry spell on the one hand, and on the other hand, such an obstacle can be a justifiable reason to move on to the next step.

One's systematic reflection on the verse and its coming to life in meditation sets inner development in motion. Sense and meaning in the meditation go beyond the pure message of the mind. Even if one intuitively grasped the full meaning of a verse, it would not have the effect achieved by persistent practice. Only through practice do sustainable skills develop. An exercise carried out over a longer period of time creates a personal familiarity in which the essence of the verse can appear. The verse has been raised to a mantram.

3.3   The mantram for nurses and the activation of heart thinking

The seven-step structure of the above meditation gives an idea of the complexity of a path of development. It seems to oppose the need for simplicity, relief and tranquility that often establishes the need to meditate. Let us therefore try a new, more leisurely look at the verse for nurses:

Within the heart there lives
In shining light
The human sense of helping.
Within the heart there works
In warming might
The human strength of love.
So let us bear
The soul's whole will
In heart-warmth
And heart-light
Then we work to heal
Those in need of healing
Out of God's sense of grace.

The heart appears and resounds as the organ of compassion and active love when we read and hear the verse in a reflective manner. Here we recognize the bond with a community of nurses as a source of healing, blessed work. The verse expresses an old nursing ideal and encourages us to carry out our daily work in this mood. If it were not for the unusual words "sense of helping" (*Helfersinn*) and "sense of grace" (*Gnadensinn*), one might tend to regard these beautiful words simply as confirmation, refuge, comfort, and goal. This is also necessary, because constructive, encouraging words are a true elixir of life in an everyday working environment in which we can often no longer recognize the meaning in providing nursing care. On the flipside, a person could develop antipathy and resistance to a view of nursing care that puts ethical ideals in the foreground instead of professional competence and professionalism. Those who think so will rebel against an image of nursing care that no longer seems to fit in with our times.

These two attitudes of soul can also be the starting point for working with the verse for nurses. It can be in the form of an (inner) dialogue, which is perhaps oriented towards the following questions:
- Why is the heart an organ that reveals a person's need for help?
- Is there really a sense organ for a person's need for help?
- Why is the heart called the organ of love?
- How can something healing for the patient arise from something that happens in the soul of the nurse—a uniting of light and warmth in the will of the nurse?
- Is healing due to grace or to a complex biological-medical event?
- What is the relationship between working with a verse like this and the necessary professional competences needed for assessment ("sense of helping"), implementation in a team ("strength of love"), and evaluation (effect on the person who has "need of healing")?

At a certain point of such questioning and reflection, the impulse to act arises, for many things cannot be answered in thought alone. It will be noticed that in practice one's powers are not sufficient to act only from one's existing will to help and one's available forces of love. It is precisely the lack of these forces or the exhaustion of them that is the starting point for an inner search. How can the will to help, the force of love and the sense of community be strengthened in such a way that they are strong enough to cope with everyday life and actually heal those "in need of healing"?

You can find a way of doing this in the "six supplementary exercises"[28] [→ Chapter "Nursing as a Path of Development"]. Rudolf Steiner described them as a way to expand and strengthen one's ability to perceive with the heart and to act with the forces of the heart. We open the "heart chakra"[29] by doing such exercises. The supplementary exercises strengthen thinking, willing and feeling and bring these soul forces into harmonious relationships with one another. These are exercises for:
- Control of thought (thinking exercise)
- Initiative training (will exercise)
- Equanimity training (feeling exercise)
- Positivity (connecting feeling and thinking)
- Open-mindedness (connecting thinking and willing)
- Equilibrium of thinking, feeling and willing.

Here they shall only be explained in their connection to the verse for nurses. Obviously, the will to help, with its quality of light, develops from an intensification of thinking. In the exercise to gain control of one's thoughts one learns to focus on essentials.

The force of love comes from the sphere of the will. It combines with the warmth pervading everything. Our will, which usually works deep in the unconscious, becomes concentrated in the initiative exercise and aligns itself with a self-imposed goal.

In the exercise of equanimity, we subordinate our unconscious will impulses—which reflexively determine our feelings—as well as any paralyzing, slowing thought impulses to the judgement of our 'I'. It is precisely community life and the sense of community that thrive when initiative and structural forces work in a balanced relationship.

The forces of hope cultivated in the positivity exercise can alleviate any situation, no matter how hopeless it may be. This is how healing arises, even if healing in the physical sense is not always achieved.

The miracle of healing springs from the divine grace that meets the human struggle for healing. The verse for nurses concludes with an open-mindedly practiced ability to consider the miracle of healing.

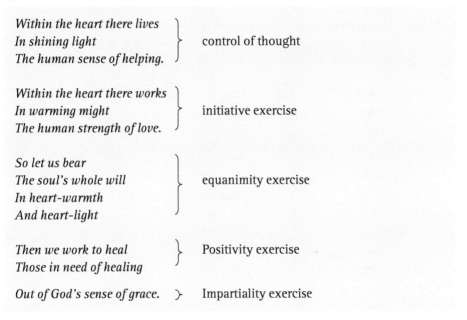

Within the heart there lives
In shining light   control of thought
The human sense of helping.

Within the heart there works
In warming might   initiative exercise
The human strength of love.

So let us bear
The soul's whole will   equanimity exercise
In heart-warmth
And heart-light

Then we work to heal   Positivity exercise
Those in need of healing

Out of God's sense of grace.   Impartiality exercise

Fig. 4: Assignment of supplementary exercises to the verse for nurses

The sixth exercise summarizes the qualities already practiced. It finds a symbol in the twelvefold structure of the mantram. It passes through the zodiac from Aries to Pisces, with the last, thirteenth line representing the circumference from whose source all creation originates. The following figure illustrates this connection.

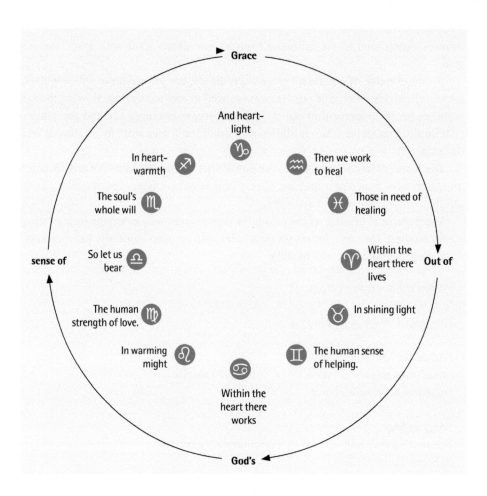

Grace

And heart-
light ♑

In heart-
warmth ♐

The soul's ♏
whole will

So let us ♎
bear

The human ♍
strength of love.

In warming ♌
might

Within the
heart there
works ♋

Then we work ♒
to heal

Those in need of ♓
healing

Within the ♈
heart there
lives

In shining light ♉

The human sense ♊
of helping.

sense of

Out of

God's

References

1   Steiner, R. *Anthroposophical leading thoughts. Anthroposophy as a path of knowledge. The Michael Mystery.* Rudolf Steiner Press, London 2007.

2   Steiner, R. *Meditative Betrachtungen und Anleitungen zur Vertiefung der Heilkunst* (GA 316). Rudolf Steiner Verlag, Dornach 2008. p. 202. Translated by Christian von Arnim, in: *Leadership questions and forms of working in the anthroposophic medical movement.* Verlag am Goetheanum, Dornach 2016, p. 114.

3   Steiner, R. *How to know higher worlds—a modern path of initiation.* Anthroposophic Press, Great Barrington 2002, p. 25.

4   Steiner, R. *Mantrische Sprüche. Seelenübungen II* (GA 268). Rudolf Steiner Verlag, Dornach 1999, p. 115. Translated by Astrid Schmitt-Stegmann, in: Glöckler M., Heine R. (eds.). *The anthroposophic medical movement. Responsibility structures and modes of work.* Verlag am Goetheanum, Dornach 2010, p. 90 f.

5   Steiner, R. *The Samaritan course.* Lectures given in Dornach, August 13–16, 1914. *Thoughts for the times on the destinies of individuals and nations,* Berlin, September 1, 1914. Mercury Press, Chestnut Ridge 2014, p. 17.

6   ibid, p. 10. Translated by Anna Meuss, in: Glöckler M, Heine R (eds.). *The anthroposophic medical movement. Responsibility structures and modes of work.* Verlag am Goetheanum, Dornach 2010, p. 91.

7   Steiner, R. *Understanding Healing. Meditative reflections on deepening medicine through spiritual science.* Rudolf Steiner Press, Forest Row 2013.

8   Steiner, R. *How to know higher worlds—a modern path of initiation.* Anthroposophic Press, Great Barrington 2002, p. 25.

9   Steiner, R. *Die Sendung des Geistes* (GA 214). Lecture of August 20, 1922. Rudolf Steiner Verlag, Dornach 1970, p. 127.

10 Steiner, R. *The Calendar of the Soul.* SteinerBooks, Great Barrington 1988.

11 Steiner, R. *Soul exercises. Word and symbol meditations.* SteinerBooks, Great Barrington 2014.

12 Steiner, R. *Education for special needs. The curative education course.* Rudolf Steiner Press, London 2015.

13 Morgenstern, C. *Wir fanden einen Pfad.* Zbinden Verlag, Basel 2004.

14 Steiner, R. *The world of the senses and the world of the spirit.* Rudolf Steiner Press, London 2014.

15 ibid.

16 Steiner, R. *How to know higher worlds—a modern path of initiation.* Anthroposophic Press, Great Barrington 2002.

17 Steiner, R. *Occult science. An outline.* Rudolf Steiner Press, London 2013, p. 291.

18 Steiner, R. *The world of the senses and the world of the spirit.* Rudolf Steiner Press, London 2014.

19 ibid.

20 Heine, R. Anthroposophische Pflege. In: Glöckler R, Heine R (eds.). *Führungsfragen und Arbeitsformen in der anthroposophisch-medizinischen Bewegung.* Verlag am Goetheanum, Dornach 2015. Translated by Christian von Arnim, in: Glöckler M, Heine R (eds.). *Leadership questions and forms of working in the anthroposophic medical movement.* Verlag am Goetheanum, Dornach 2016, p. 124. The original German verse in its entirety:

> *Im Herzen wohnt*
> *In leuchtender Helle*
> *Des Menschen Helfersinn*
> *Im Herzen wirket*
> *In wärmender Macht*
> *Des Menschen Liebekraft*
> *So lasset uns tragen*
>
> *Der Seele vollen Willen*
> *In Herzens-Wärme*
> *Und Herzens-Licht,*
> *So wirken wir das Heil*
> *Den Heilbedürft'gen*
> *Aus Gottes Gnadensinn.*

21 Tittmann, C. Erste Anfänge der Anthroposophisch orientierten Pflegebewegung. In: de la Houssaye, E.; Heine, R. (ed.). *Beiträge zur Entwicklung der Anthroposophischen Pflege 1921–2003*. Medizinische Sektion am Goetheanum, Dornach 2005.

22 Steiner, R. *Occult science*. Anthroposophic Press, Great Barrington 2009.

23 Steiner, R. *The evolution of consciousness as revealed through initiation knowledge*. Rudolf Steiner Press, London 2006, lecture of August 19, 1923

24 ibid., lecture of August 20, 1923, p. 51 ff.

25 ibid., p. 59 ff.

26 ibid., p. 60 ff.

27 Steiner, R. *The spiritual ground of education*. SteinerBooks, Great Barrington 2004, lecture of August 20, 1922.

28 Steiner, R. *Aus den Inhalten der Esoterischen Stunden 1903–1909* (GA 266a). Rudolf Steiner Verlag, Dornach 1995, p. 201 ff.

29 Steiner, R. *How to know higher worlds—a modern path of initiation*. Anthroposophic Press, Great Barrington 2002.

CHAPTER VII

The Concept of Nursing Gestures as a Model for Nursing Care

ROLF HEINE

The concept of nursing gestures describes the importance and effect of a nurse's inner attitude. This subjective or personal side to nursing care greatly influences the condition of the person being cared for. The twelve gestures developed here form the basis of all nursing care procedures, irrespective of the nursing specialty.

→   Learning objectives, see end of chapter

1.   What are nursing gestures?

Like any human activity, nursing care includes an external aspect, such as washing, mobilizing, or conducting conversations. In addition, nurses carry mental and spiritual motives within themselves, and moods such as respect, sincerity, patience, and cheerfulness. These moods have a more or less clear effect on their nursing activities. They make a mobilization gentle or rough, a washing respectful or mechanical. The nursing action shows the nurse's mindset, in which their inner attitude appears as a gesture. Action and attitude, deed and expression merge in the gesture. Every nursing activity needs its gesture of expression, every inner attitude requires an action to appear in the outer world. We call gestures that arise from empathic perception of the patient "nursing gestures." They are archetypes of nursing care.

Example

A frequent, basic nursing activity is to provide food. It is supported by the intention that the patient should ingest, digest, and make the food his own. This intention is accompanied by an attitude of benevolence and caring. The activity, intention, and attitude combine in a gesture of *nourishing*. This gesture can be found wherever substances are prepared in such a way that they can be absorbed, digested, and transformed into the body's own substance. If we trace back the flow of nourishment to its origins, we find sunlight, air, and water at the beginning of substance formation. They form the plant substance that undergoes a process of social and cultural transformation, beginning with harvesting. Plants and animals are brought to the human metabolism via commercial trade in food, preparation during cooking, and, finally, the presentation of the food. The simple activity of providing food reveals a process of light and social life. It is actually only our daily routine that separates us from this magnificent process. When we become aware of this, we find that serving a small spoonful of vegetable soup becomes an action with a sublime background. Contemplation of such processes can be a remedy for the loss of meaning that lurks in daily routines [→ Chapter "Nursing as a Path of Development: First exercise"].

We can distinguish between twelve basic nursing gestures. How do these gestures work? How were they found? What is their significance in the daily practice of nursing? This chapter will examine these and other questions.

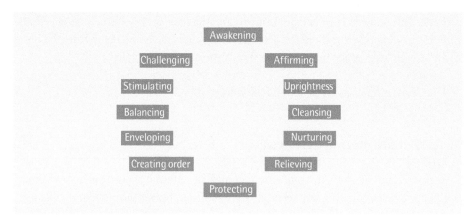

Fig. 1: The twelve nursing gestures

1.1   Nursing activities and inner attitude

Nursing care is concrete. It comprises a wide range of tasks that depend on the context [→ Chapter "Nursing as a Path of Development"]. While activities such as dressing, washing, skin care, feeding and diaper changing meet the primary requirements of healthy infants, a ventilated patient in intensive care may require medically induced actions such as monitoring their circulation and respiration, monitoring infusion times, changing bandages, and tube care, which can take up more attention than body care. In psychosomatic care, the focus shifts to conversing and organizing the day. If we compare activities such as conducting conversations and changing bandages, it is apparent that the concept "bandage change" already covers the purpose and content of the procedure pretty well. The word "conversation," at best, tells us something about the form of communication, but nothing about its content or purpose. This requires a more precise definition, such as "informative conversation" or "valuing conversation." "Informative" and "valuing" are essentially inner attitudes. These inner attitudes shape the quality of the conversation. They often have a stronger effect than the words spoken. A patient only experiences themselves as being valued if the nurse really means it. Inner attitudes are also the basis for all seemingly unambiguously defined nursing-care actions. An infusion can be changed correctly and hygienically. The nurse's inner attitude while changing the infusion is characterized by confidence and clarity. The aim is to avert danger from the patient. Inner attitudes are not just a reality within the person's own soul. Rather, they can be experienced directly by those who are receiving care, as well as by third parties observing the interaction. An inner attitude that has become visible is a nursing gesture. The inner attitude of the nurse *appears* within it. There is an intention behind every nursing activity and its inner attitude can be discerned in the way that it is carried out. In this sense the gesture stands between the nurse's inner attitude and the nursing activity.

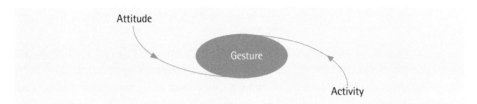

Fig. 2: Gestures are found between attitude and action

An inexhaustible abundance of gestures appears in nursing care. Each nursing activity is individualized by them. No subcutaneous injection, no change of dressing, no washing, no help with food is the same, no matter how standardized the procedure. Indeed, it is precisely the attempt to eradicate the individual signature from an activity, so that only the thing itself, only the standard is applied, that spreads a cold, unapproachable atmosphere.

The concept of nursing gestures serves on the one hand to describe qualities in the intentions behind nursing care. On the other hand, these gestures can become a path of training and development for nurses when they practice and reflect on the inner activity involved.

2.   How did the concept of nursing gestures arise?

The concept of nursing gestures was first presented to the public during an international nursing conference at the Goetheanum in Dornach in 1998. It owes its development to nursing case studies, self-observation and external observations of nurses in everyday working life, as well as philosophical and phenomenological considerations about the nature of nursing care. It combines these findings with the results of anthroposophic spiritual science.

The concept evolved from the observation of patient discussion meetings among nursing staff and in therapeutic teams. A colleague would present a patient at a meeting, while questions and observations from colleagues complemented the presentation. A picture of the patient's problems and resources was created. Solutions to problems often arose spontaneously from the professional knowledge and experience of the nursing staff. For example, incontinence was met by a series of measures ranging from toilet training and protective pants to skin care.

However, before clear nursing care measures, therapies or medicinal products could be identified in these discussions, people used more descriptive terms and judgements, such as, "This patient has to learn to distinguish himself more from his environment" or "His metabolism has to be stimulated." These statements proved to be extremely fruitful because they described the therapeutic intention in a multidisciplinary manner and at the same time allowed each individual discipline to concretize its specific contribution. For example, "stimulation of the metabolism" meant for the doctor a prescription of a bittering agent, for the eurythmy therapist it meant work with the sound "R," and for the nurse it meant the application of yarrow liver compresses.

If we look at a larger problematic context, such as can be found with bedridden somnolent patients, we can see that their skin is endangered by pressure, their lungs by infection and their joints by stiffening. Instead of assigning an action to each problem immediately, we try to find an overarching term for the direction of the pending nursing care measures. In our example, we might consider *averting* hazards in the respective area or *stimulating* skin circulation, lung ventilation or limb mobility. Such terms denote intentions, which still have to find their concretization in an action. They are pre-stages of the therapeutic measure. We can also say that they reveal the immanent goals of an action.

We found about fifty commonly occurring and sometimes similar terms in nursing care:

> Enveloping, averting, providing, helping, supporting, accompanying, mediating, cleansing, awakening, protecting, defending, nourishing, feeding, entertaining, distracting, setting limits, encouraging, tidying up, creating order, balancing, comforting, hoping, confirming, relieving, making demands, uprightness, showing respect, mobilizing, being of service, organizing, stimulating, prompting, renewing, dressing, awareness-raising, sympathizing, harmonizing, warming, creating space, leading, taking an interest, mirroring, practicing, training, promoting independence, etc.

Some of these terms primarily characterize the mental attitude, personal moods and values of the nurse. They do not directly relate to the patient's actual need. In the above list such terms are: being of service (mirroring for the patient)—mediating—sympathizing—taking an interest—leading—organizing—accompanying. In contrast to nursing gestures, these attitudes are referred to as "basic nursing moods."

Nursing gestures do not form a self-contained system. Rather, a wide variety of metamorphoses, overlaps and interpenetrations are possible.

If we consolidate terms from the list (see box) that have similar intentions, such as *averting, protecting, defending,* the number is further reduced.

This reduction results in the following groups:

1. Enveloping, setting boundaries, dressing, warming
2. Averting, protecting, defending
3. Providing, nourishing, feeding
4. Helping, supporting, relieving
5. Cleansing, renewing
6. Awakening, making conscious, asking questions
7. Entertaining, stimulating, enticing, prompting, distracting
8. Tidying up, creating order, creating space
9. Compensating, harmonizing
10. Comforting, hoping, confirming, encouraging, showing respect
11. Making demands, mobilizing, practicing, training
12. Uprightness, promoting independence

Of course, there can also be other terms describing nursing intentions. However, they can usually be assigned to one of these twelve groups. It is not a question of assigning definitional classifications, but of finding indications of internal movements that express the intentions of nurses engaged in providing nursing care.

3.   How do we find a gesture?

In the abundance of inner attitudes two types can be distinguished. The first originates from the personal moods and values of the nurse. Mindfulness or inattentiveness, respect or disrespect, joy or grief determine the quality of our work. These attitudes are connected with the nurse's spiritual and ethical attitude. The second type of attitude arises directly from empathic perception of the patient and his needs. These attitudes developed in interaction with patients are called nursing gestures. They can be found by the nurse experiencing the distress of the person in need of care and first of all activating a compensating gesture in herself. Two examples may explain this: when we hear someone speaking with a husky, hoarse voice, we usually feel an involuntary need to clear our throat. Or we give someone a spoonful of porridge to eat and notice how we swallow too, as if we could assist the patient by doing so. A neuroscientific explanation of such phenomena involving imitation can be found in Giacomo Rizzolatti's discovery of mirror neurons. However, in our examples the nurse not only imitates the behavior of the patient (hoarse voice or aimlessly moving food in their mouth) but develops a semiconscious, physical reaction (clearing of throat, swallowing) to eliminate the problem. Many gestures arise spontaneously from our empathic perception of inner movement. They must be raised to consciousness and translated into professional action.[1]

Example

After chemotherapy, a patient develops a pronounced inflammation of the oral mucosa. She is hungry, but every meal and every mouth movement causes her pain. The need to abstain from eating food in order to avoid pain conflicts almost insolubly with the need for food and drink. The nurse who empathetically enters into this situation intends to both protect the patient (the oral mucous membrane) and find suitable nourishment to satisfy the patient's hunger and promote physical recuperation. This is to both *protect* and *nourish*—gestures active in all nursing measures. Caring for the oral mucous membrane with marshmallow tea mouthwash is an expression of the protective gesture. Marshmallow tea contains a neutral-tasting mucilage that lines the mouth mucosa and buffers acids. Procurring tasty, liquid food and administrating it in small portions with a rounded teaspoon are expressions of the nourishing gesture.

These examples illustrate the process of finding nursing gestures: empathic perception stimulates an inner movement in the nurse. He forms an often unconscious counter-movement that balances the one-sidedness of the one perceived. We may assume that during the course of a working day we continuously carry out such internal balancing movements, not only to restore our own homeostasis, but to synchronize physiological processes in other people. The inner balancing movement is itself a gesture—the gesture of *compensating, harmonizing, synchronizing.* It is this gesture that helps us find all the other nursing gestures. We use an enveloping gesture towards a chilled, anxiously shy person, we use an erecting gesture towards a depressed, discouraged person, we use a protecting gesture towards an unconscious person or one receiving artificial respiration, and so on.

Further assistance in finding nursing gestures arises from knowledge of the basic tendencies of human illness—hardening and dissolution—whereby the gestures can create a harmonious equilibrium [→ Chapter "The Anthropological Foundations of Nursing Extended by Anthroposophy: Functional threefolding in health and illness"].

3.1   Hardening and dissolution as human disease tendencies

The above-mentioned patient is suffering from the loss of her bodily boundaries. Her oral mucous membrane is dissolving, she is losing weight and is acutely susceptible to infection, due to leukopenia as a side effect of chemotherapy. The gesture of *defending/averting* results in a counterbalancing movement against the tendency to dissolve.

In the following example, mental and physical hardening are the main focus. After three strokes, a 68-year-old man suffered from hemiplegia on the right side and vascular dementia. His muscle tone was hard, his paralysis was spastic. He appeared withdrawn in himself and usually rejected any attempt to address him. He rarely accepted care of his body and defended himself with blows against such attempts. Rigidity and hardening characterized the situation. We counteracted the solidification with warm hand baths and later foot baths. These "sounding baths" [→ Chapter "Variations in Whole-Body Washing"] led to a significant softening of body tension, reduction of spasticity, and above all, his mental resistance decreased within his sphere of trust. So it was the gesture of *enveloping* that brought about a decisive change in the situation of excessive hardening.

Every nursing gesture can be indicated for both sclerosis and dissolving tendencies. It can balance the extremes. The following questionnaire compares typical polar opposite hardening and dissolving conditions. The respective nursing gesture is to be used if the hardening or dissolving tendency has been evaluated with three points on the scale. This is usually the case with two to three nursing gestures. These gestures are helpful in real situations. If none of the gestures reaches three points, the highest scores are used. A person who is in equilibrium between hardening and dissolution has no need for care.

The Twelve Nursing Gestures						
Dissolving						**Hardening**
unprotected			Enveloping			armored
3	2	1	0	1	2	3
downcast, hunched, aimless			Upright-ness			stiff, supported from outside, fixated
3	2	1	0	1	2	3
weak			Relieving			strong
3	2	1	0	1	2	3
exuberant, overdoes it			Challeng-ing			anxious, demands too little of themselves
3	2	1	0	1	2	3
chaotic			Creating order			overly formed
3	2	1	0	1	2	3
vain			Afffirming			self-doubting
3	2	1	0	1	2	3
sensitive, irritable			Stimulating			dull, heavy, motionless
3	2	1	0	1	2	3
undernourished, underfed			Nurturing			overly nourished, overly fed
3	2	1	0	1	2	3
dark, muffled, hidden			Cleansing			sterile
3	2	1	0	1	2	3

strong one-sidedness			Balancing			mediocre
3	2	1	0	1	2	3
putting oneself in danger			Protecting			unnecessary defense
3	2	1	0	1	2	3
sleeping			Awakening			too wide-awake
3	2	1	0	1	2	3

Required gestures	Practical measures	
1.	a	b
2.	a	b
3.	a	b

Chart: Questionnaire to determine the required nursing gestures

4. Nursing archetypes

Motherliness and fatherliness, brotherliness and sisterliness appear as the human archetypes of nursing care. Family blood relationships and self-chosen communities are sources of personal and social caregiving.

If we immerse ourselves further into the archetypes of nursing care, we find the paradisiacal state of being completely cared for by our surroundings during embryonic development. This is the starting point for a phenomenology of nursing care and nursing gestures.

After the fusion of egg and sperm cells, the embryo develops, embedded in its embryonic envelope in the uterus. It is connected to the maternal organism via the umbilical cord and placenta. There, the unborn child lives in a unique world. Weightless in the amniotic fluid, surrounded by the warmth and sounds of its mother, it develops without the conscious participation of the mother or the outside world. The child develops according to its abilities in the protective space and strength of the maternal body. It leaves this space at birth. Now nothing is what it was. Bright light is everywhere, noises, sounds and words reach its ear unmuted. It is cold. Its small body has become heavy. Rhythmic lung breathing replaces the regular supply of oxygenated blood from the umbilical cord. The flow of nutrients must now build up the child's organism from the outside via the mouth, esophagus, stomach and intestines. All this is no longer happening by itself. The baby's mother, together with the human community into which the child was born, helps him, warms and feeds him, creates a space for him and cleanses him from his excretions. Care of him begins with his first breath. Human culture now complements what used to happen in the uterus solely because of the forces of growth and differentiation, because of nature alone. In contrast to animals, which instinctively care for their broods as a continuation of a natural process, human beings arrange the care of their children according to cultural traditions and personal feelings, concepts and goals.

The care of a newborn infant goes in two directions. On the one hand, we regulate the environmental conditions of the respective habitat—warmth and air, food and excretions, sensory impressions—in accordance with human requirements. Without this adjustment, the newborn infant would not be viable. On the other hand, the child needs a connection to an attachment figure, he needs active love and attention to survive. Only in encountering others does he learn to walk, speak and think. He is not born with these specifically human abilities. He develops them by imitating his caregivers. Only in an intimate relationship with other people does he learn to be human [→ Chapter "Nursing as a Path of Development"].

To find an imaginative picture to express these two basic principles of caregiving, we might describe the shaping and regulation of environmental conditions as a protective mantel, a nest, a cocoon or a two-dimensional circle. Helping people to become self-reliant, to acquire speaking and thinking, requires that they leave the nest, experience a separation and acquire a self-aware upright stature. The archetype for this is the free, upright confrontation between two individuals.

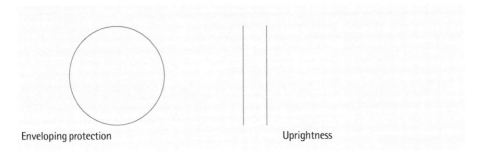

Enveloping protection   Uprightness

Fig. 3: Gestures of enveloping and uprightness

4.1   Substituting and activating gestures

Gestures such as *protecting* and *nurturing* belong to the family of enveloping gestures, which we characterized with the symbol of the circle. *Cleansing*, whose gestural power consists in making the essence of a thing appear, is also an enveloping gesture, as is *relieving* as an expression of assistance. The seventh nursing gesture that the nurse makes for the patient and within which the patient is cared for is *organizing* or *creat-*

ing space. Enveloping gestures replace a power that is not currently available to the patient.

In addition to substituting gestures derived from the enveloping gestures, patients also need assistance with regaining independence and uprightness. *Raising upright* is the archetypal activating gesture in nursing care. A characteristic feature of this category of nursing gesture is that it only has a limited external effect. The actual activity comes from the patient himself. Independence cannot be done for the other person. For example, stimulation (of the circulation) with cool water can only be successful if the organism has sufficient powers of its own to respond to the stimulus with an increase in blood circulation. *Stimulating* gestures must therefore always wait for the patient's ability to react. Other gestures with this peculiarity are *challenging* and *awakening. Affirming* also belongs to this group of gestures, because only the patient is able to generate the sense of self-worth or self-esteem associated with an affirmation.

We therefore have seven substituting or enveloping gestures and five activating or uplifting gestures:

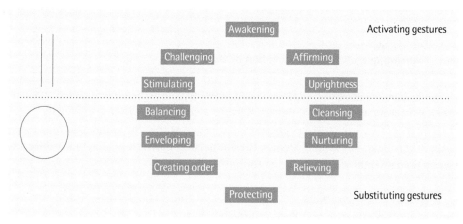

Fig. 4: Substituting and activating gestures

4.2   Gestures as inner movements

Substituting and activating gestures are by no means a closed system. Rather, a wide variety of metamorphoses, overlaps and interpenetrations are possible. For example, the gesture of *protecting* has a slightly different character than shielding or repelling. Nevertheless, the basic internal movement remains intact: when *defending* and *protecting,* our attention is focused entirely on the threatening object. The object to be protected is almost forgotten. It is located "behind" the defender. Seen externally, the gesture of enveloping could also be understood as a protective gesture, because enveloping forms a layer of protection. However, the difference between enveloping and repelling becomes immediately clear when we consider how the nurse surrounds what is to be enveloped and forms a unity with it. Nursing gestures arise from this inner movement, which follows the flow of consciousness.

In the gesture of *creating order,* for example, our attention is not fixed statically on the chaotic objects to be brought into order, but oscillates back and forth between perception and movement. The objects are placed into relationships with each other. In this rhythm, order is created as a kind of force field. The amount of energy required to bring order into even simple matters (for example, when tidying up a desk) shows that the actual challenge is not the activity itself, but the calling up of one's inner ordering power.

5.   Gestures in typical areas of nursing

The concept of nursing gestures will now be presented in relation to four typical nursing areas—the nursing and upbringing of children, the nursing of elderly and demented people, the nursing of the dying, and the nursing of cancer patients. The concept proves fruitful for all areas of nursing.

5.1   Nursing gestures in the education of the child[2]

Nursing gestures permeate all interactions between children and their caregivers, parents, educators and pediatric nurses. Raising a child is caregiving, especially in the first years of life. The creative processes that began within the womb continue in the care of the child. For Rudolf Steiner, the connection between healing and education was a fundamental idea of Anthroposophic Medicine.

> *It was in ancient times,*
> *That there lived in the souls of initiates*
> *Powerfully the thought that*
> *By nature every human being is sick.*
> *And education was seen*
> *As a healing process*
> *Which, as they matured,*
> *Gave children the health*
> *To be complete human beings in life.*[3]

Both anthroposophic education and anthroposophic medicine see themselves as supporting development [→ Chapter "Illness and Destiny"]. Nursing care enables development. It lends duration to therapy. It creates space, so that the child has time to develop and the sick person has the environment to be able to live through and heal his illness. This enabling becomes visible in the nursing gestures, especially in the care of the child.

Cleansing	
Newborns	When a child is born, we remove amniotic fluid and mucus from the respiratory tract, wipe off secretions, and remove meconium, urine, umbilical cord remains and gneiss.
Babies and toddlers	We remove stools, urine, sweat, food residues, dirt, etc. The child is washed, bathed, his nails are cut and his teeth are brushed.
Kindergarten children	Kindergarten children increasingly perform body care independently. However, some aspects, such as dental care, should continue to be supervised by adults. Children develop dexterity when they are supported in their independence, that is, they mainly need time to carry out the individual steps involved in washing. Kindergarten children are happy to try cleaning each other or dolls in play. In this way, they also mimic caregiving as a social activity.
What is important when cleansing?	Cleansing is done in a well-prepared changing area. The ergonomic height of the changing table protects the caregiver's back and facilitates communication with the baby. A border provides protection and prevents the baby from rolling off the changing table. The mother, father or nurse announces every single step of the washing process with calm words. Their gestures say the same thing as their spoken words. The baby is turned over only from his side and not pulled upwards by his legs. Turning over from the side corresponds to his natural development of movement and prepares his active participation; he will be able to turn himself over onto his side in about half a year.
What does the child "learn" when being cleansed?	The naming of activities, the concordance of word and deed promote language acquisition. The gestures and facial expressions of the child and caregivers mirror each other. The experience of what is pleasant and unpleasant can be noticed immediately. Movement development is promoted by allowing babies to experience the dimensions of space in relation to their own bodies, and by not anticipating developmental steps (no passively sitting the baby up before she has done so on her own; no placing the baby on her feet before she can stand up on her own, etc.). Cleansing as care for the body is to be practiced as social interaction, as a model of self-care and help for others.

Nurturing	
Newborns	Breastfeeding is the appropriate form of nourishment for newborn babies. In breastfeeding it is not just the nutrients (the mother's milk, with its optimal composition for the child at every stage of development) that are important, it is also the time devoted to the child, the rest, physical closeness and attention. This is all mixed in with the breast milk. Mental, emotional, spiritual and physical nutrition still form an inseparable whole in breastfeeding. Breastfeeding is one of the most important factors in mother-child bonding.
Babies and toddlers	Nutrition with other dietary substances gradually replaces breastfeeding after four to six months. While breastfeeding was largely limited to the mother-child relationship, eating together at the family table is an important social event. The nourishment is shared. Patience and mutual consideration must be balanced with the driving forces of hunger and thirst. The taste of the different foods arouses sympathy and antipathy.
Kindergarten children	The kindergarten child eats largely independently. He needs help with the selection, quantity and composition of food. The social rhythm of meals and snacks replaces the endogenous rhythm of breastfeeding. The mother's preparation for breastfeeding is transferred to the preparation of the food (possibly together with the child) and the preparation of the dining table. The intimacy of the relationship with the breastfeeding mother is replaced by rituals (cooking, setting the table, washing hands, grace). Physical nutrition separates from mental-spiritual nutrition. Here too, helping or cooking for dolls, sharing and giving away are essential steps in the training of social competence.
What is important when nurturing?	Impatience and despair must be avoided if food is refused in the form offered, that is, cannot be ingested. It is also harmful to overfeed in order to enjoy the feeling of doing something "good" for the child. Mental-spiritual needs (nearness, affection, relaxation) should not be compensated by food and addictive substances (sweets). High-quality foodstuffs (e.g., biodynamic foods) offer numerous taste differentiations without using additives.

What does the child "learn" when being nurtured?	In the rhythm of hunger and satiation, the child experiences the basic model of interlocking physical and social rhythms. She learns that the world means well. She experiences satisfaction in satiation and gratitude for the "gift" of food. Eating together develops the ability to share, to assert oneself, to balance one's own needs and the needs of others. Table manners should therefore be imparted through the good example of the parents and not through disciplinary measures when eating. Only in this way does gratitude and a basic mood for the religious life arise from the ritual of eating (together).

Carrying, relieving, helping	
Newborns	A newborn baby cannot survive without the help of an adult. The adult takes care of the baby's needs. With this help, the infant develops physically, mentally and emotionally. The baby's dependency is particularly visible when the location is changed. In the womb, the infant was always with the mother. After birth, there are naturally more or less long separations. The newborn baby must be lifted and carried by an adult. This overcomes gravity and spatial separation.
Babies and toddlers	The infant's movement development has advanced. He crawls, sits, stands, walks. On the one hand, independence of movement reduces dependence on the adult and on the other hand, the child's radius of movement must be limited to a safe area. The (movement) intentions of the child contrast more often with the intentions of the adult. It is now necessary to allow the impulses of the child and his intentions to explore the world and discover his own physical, mental and social abilities. The gesture of *helping–carrying–relieving* retreats compared to the gesture of averting danger. Consideration must be given to the child's area for play and movement.
Kindergarten children	The kindergarten child increasingly acquires the competence to carry out simple everyday activities (washing, dressing, walking, carrying...) in a purposeful manner in pursuit of objectives. But everything she does is play. Achieving a goal can and should be promoted by the adult without frustrating the child's own effort. This could be the case if the child is corrected, criticized, interrupted or overtaxed, or if the adult thinks that the child is not capable of doing anything.

What is important when carrying or relieving?	One danger is to paralyze the independence of the child through excessive care and thus keep her dependent. It is easy to overlook impulses for independence.
What does the child "learn" when being helped?	In being carried (as with any kind of support and assistance) the child learns that her own impulse can be furthered and brought to the goal by others. She learns to ask for help, to accept help, to cooperate. In her dependence on help, however, the child also encounters the topic of "power." This touches on central themes of social coexistence: we depend on the support of other people throughout our lives. I have to coordinate my own intentions with the intentions of others. I learn to cooperate, to dominate or to submit.

Protecting	
Newborns	The newborn infant loses the protection of the womb. He is exposed to a wealth of new, rapidly changing sensations and cannot escape them. They have a profound effect on his corporeality. In addition to protecting against the major threats posed by the environment (cooling, overheating, suffocation, infections...), an important task of educators is the protection against excessive sensory impressions (noise, careless contact, harsh light, changing caregivers, hecticness...).
Babies and toddlers	When the child expands his range of movement, sources of danger must be secured in the environment (outlets, unstable furniture, easily swallowed objects, electrical appliances...). The basic rule is to set up the environment in such a way that you don't have to prohibit the child from doing anything.
Kindergarten children	The kindergarten child will gradually be able to recognize and avoid sources of danger. As the radius of action increases, the adult's foresight is needed to remove "protective barriers" and create space for the child's urge to explore.
What is important when protecting?	Preventing all contact with anything "harmful" and thereby isolating the child should be avoided. The danger here, too, is that of paralyzing the independence of the child through excessive care and thus keeping him dependent. It is easy to overlook impulses for independence.
What does the child "learn" when being protected?	The child feels safe and secure in a sheltering space. This certainty gives him the leisure and confidence to follow his urge to explore and overcome limitations.

Creating space, tidying up	
Newborns	Pregnancy is already a place of preparation and space creation. The mother "creates space" in her own body. An outer environment is prepared for the child. With the birth of the baby, the temporal structure of the day must also be adapted to the infant's needs and brought into line with the rest of the social life around her. Rhythm is order in time. The healthy newborn baby strives for a rhythm of breastfeeding, sleep and wakefulness, solitude and being with her mother. Adults must get involved in this rhythm and bring it into harmony with the surrounding conditions.
Babies and toddlers	A certain temporal and spatial structure has been established in the infant. The child demands temporal rhythms, but tends to bring chaos to spatial conditions. As with the infant, the adult must arrange for the rhythmic order of the day, and also for order in the play area.
Kindergarten children	The kindergarten child is increasingly adapting to the rhythms given by the outside world. Shared meals, bedtimes, play and rest periods are possible. The child now also shows the need for clear order in space. He knows the places where items are stored. It is fun to organize things in a playful way and to dissolve order again. However, he is not in a position to plan the use of space and time on his own. Creating space and bringing things into order initially remain the task of the adult. The child likes to participate in a playful way, especially if he experiences that adults are happy to tidy things up.
What is important when tidying up?	Order does not come about on its own. It requires considerable creative power. Pedantic order, inflexible planning and rigid ideas are to be avoided.
What does the child "learn" when living in an orderly environment?	The result for the child is familiarity, security and clarity. Habits are encouraged. She finds her place, feels welcomed and wanted. Lively rhythm and order are a source of well-being. Initially provided from the outside, order awakens the child's sense of beauty, proportion and measure. The adult's living arrangement of spatial and temporal order is a preschool for the child's musical and mathematical abilities.

Enveloping	
Newborns	The unborn child grows in a perfect enclosure. He owes his entire development to this covering (embryonic membrane, uterus, mother). Shortly after birth he is wrapped in cloths. His close physical contact with his mother forms a new protective covering. Cloths and clothes cover the newborn baby just as caregiving and body care should.
Babies and toddlers	With each step in development, the child sheds a layer. At first it was the womb from which the child separated. Gradually he leaves the small enclosure of the cradle. With walking, speaking and thinking he emancipates himself from his social "nest." Until he has stripped away his physical and social protective layers, he needs warmth, attention and clothing as a space for physical and mental development and growth.
Kindergarten children	The kindergarten child leaves the shelter of her primary caregiver and forms new social bonds. The more securely she was connected to her first reference person, the easier it will be for her to enter into new relationships with confidence. In the course of the first few years of life, the child increasingly acquires "self-care competence." She begins to take care of her own outer layers of protection, to wash herself, dress herself and withdraw. In play she cares for, washes, combs, dresses dolls, in role play she covers herself and others with cloths and clothing.
What is important when enveloping?	Enveloping things creates a warm and structured interior. This should not become too cramped. Since the gesture of enveloping usually happens with great sympathy, there is a danger of suffocating the child in the enclosure, crushing him, getting into symbiosis with him or even enjoying the dependency of the child. Clarity and matter-of-factness protect against emotional overload from the protective mantle.
What does the child "learn" when being enveloped?	The child matures in his physical and social environment. He experiences a safe, "benevolent" habitat through warmth, air, food and boundaries. The relationship mantel with his mother or another primary caregiver allows him to widen the radius of the mantel and establish his own relationships. Only a person who has been enveloped (loved) can envelop (love) others.

Balancing	
Newborns	Immediately after birth, the newborn infant must adapt to completely new environmental conditions. She is neither able to regulate her body temperature completely independently, nor to move about or regulate her excretions. For this adaptation the infant needs caregiving. The parents caring for her compensate when there is too little or too much of something (satiating, warming, moving, cleansing).
Babies and toddlers	The toddler shows his needs more clearly than the newborn, but as a rule he is not yet able to compensate for them. Here it is important to pay attention to the child's expressions and intentions and to lend a hand as the adult.
Kindergarten children	Even in kindergarten children, not all self-regulation skills have been mastered. They do nevertheless increasingly take an active part in balancing activities. Games that develop balance (climbing, balancing...) are very popular.
What is important when balancing?	Balancing creates relief from stress. Needs and tensions must, can and should sometimes be endured. If adults cannot tolerate extremes (e.g., fever), they are more likely to regulate their own needs than those of the child. Static, preconceived average values, or a "falling from one extreme to another" should be avoided.
What does the child "learn" when experiencing balance?	When parents and educators are even-tempered, the child experiences what it means to be able to swing around one's own center with alert flexibility. She builds up the confidence that no extreme, no suffering and no joy last forever.

Stimulating	
Newborns	Breathing, circulation, warmth, food intake, and even the excretions of the newborn baby are stimulated by direct physical contact with the mother (nursing, bonding). This direct body contact is gradually replaced by contact during body care, dressing, playing, stroking or Rhythmical Einreibung.
Babies and toddlers	In toddlers, physical and mental stimulation is added to their experience of nature. Walks in the woods, in meadows and fields make it possible to encounter wind and weather, sun, light and shade. In particular, encounters with other children are physically and mentally stimulating.

Kindergarten children	Discovering plants, animals and soil stimulates development of the child's imagination, movement, speech and thinking. The child's interest and curiosity require wide, safe fields of activity. Fairy tales connect the experience of nature and the social environment with the inner space of the child's soul.
What is important when stimulating?	Stimulation can easily lead to overstimulation, especially if parents or educators are impatient. The effect of a gesture always depends on the dose. *"Life thrives on stimulation. The stimulus itself is something very vulnerable—i.e., it must not be too strong or too weak. Weak stimuli lead to the development of organs, medium stimuli strengthen them; strong stimuli inhibit, and excessively strong stimuli destroy."* Hugo Kükelhaus (1900–1984)
What does the child "learn" through stimulation?	A child who receives deliberate encouragement and stimulation understands the world as a field of learning and experience, ultimately even as a remedy. He learns a kind of "therapeutic attitude" which is expressed in every human action, and in every profession.

Challenging	
Newborns	The newborn infant is confronted with existential challenges as she becomes accustomed to her new environment. To master these, she receives support from her parents (relieving gesture). Nevertheless, it is not possible to relieve the child of all strains or save her from every confrontation with her environment. It is important to observe where the child herself takes the initiative to solve a problem or overcome resistance. Searching and sucking movements, which are early breastfeeding signs indicating that the child wants to drink, indicate an activity that the mother should accommodate.
Babies and toddlers	Seen from the adult's perspective, toddlers have ongoing frustrations. Their ability to get around and their fine motor skills are often not sufficient to accomplish the goal that they have set their sight on. At the same time, we observe the willpower with which they overcome "failures" again and again, until they gradually attain skill and certainty in moving, walking and speaking. Here it is important not to undermine the eager (sometimes impatient) efforts of the child by offering overly hasty "help."

Kindergarten children	The older the child gets, the higher the adult expectations of certain abilities and achievements becomes. Parents compare their children's "abilities" with those of others and they worry if their own child does not walk, is not yet toilet trained, does not speak in whole sentences, does not yet dress himself independently or does not yet sleep through the night. Legitimate concern for the child's health is often overwhelmed by the projection of adult-world performance thinking into the nursery. "Give me time" is therefore the most important maxim of early childhood education. Overwhelming the child with inappropriate performance requirements and simultaneously expecting too little of him, which happens when people limit their child's activities, because he is still too "clumsy" and "takes too long," as well as unjustified rules of obedience and behavior (e.g., making him hold your hand in places that are not dangerous) often characterize the daily life of the kindergarten child.
What is important when challenging?	Planned exercise, training and practice programs are unnecessary if there is no need to compensate therapeutically for congenital or acquired one-sidedness. Healthy children are generally confronted with strengthening challenges in the course of their socialization process. From this point of view, health can be defined as the ability to train the forces to overcome stress and resistance through dealing with stress and resistance.
What does the child "learn" through being challenged?	The child strengthens his will through meeting demands which enable him to develop his forces. Continued disappointments and frustrations due to excessive demands weaken self-confidence. Having too little demanded of him and having obstacles that he can overcome cleared away paralyzes his will.

Awakening	
Newborns	Newborn infants sleep for more than two thirds of the day. They absorb innumerable sensory impressions while awake, but they are unable to either process them consciously (understand) or react directly to them. Thus, sensory impressions have a very strong effect on their bodies. It is important to make sure that the newborn baby can stay as close as possible to her mother (her first reference person), that sensory impressions reach her eyes and ears in a moderate fashion, and that everything hectic, garish, loud and violent is avoided. According to Rudolf Steiner, "mother's milk arouses the sleeping spirit in the human being."

Babies and toddlers	Toddlers increasingly learn to seek out sensory impressions, explore their sources and also distance themselves from them. Everyday objects and toys that are simple, transparent and stimulating for a wide range of sensory experiences awaken initial recognition and understanding. Technical and electronic toys are therefore unsuitable.
Kindergarten children	With the first beginnings of I-consciousness, discernment awakens in the child for relationships with mother and father, brothers and sisters, relatives, and people in the neighborhood. The child begins to awaken to the social space around him. Role-playing and trying out clothing broadens the spectrum of play.
What is important when awakening?	It is important to feel intensely into the child's state of consciousness. We gently and patiently introduce the child to the world of the senses. This is a wellspring of joy in each lighting up of consciousness, e.g., in smiles, eyes, first sounds and words. Avoid overstimulation and early awakening of the intellect. Pictorial descriptions and lingering in colors and forms promotes an awakening to the world.
What does the child "learn" through being awakened?	The child learns to discover, the joy of recognizing things, she experiences inner light, the discovery of her own self.

Affirming	
Newborns	The more attentive, devoted and loving the infant's daily care is, the more accepted, valued and loved he feels. This attitude, which affirms the child's essence, permeates all gestures and facial expressions, the sound of language, every physical touch. This may seem self-evident, but it is difficult to maintain when feeling impatience or aggression against a screaming, "headstrong" baby, or when the desired mindful, comforting and hopeful basic mood is lost in everyday routines.
Babies and toddlers	Experiences of success and failure characterize the everyday life of a toddler. His will and curiosity help to transform failure into new effort. Here the child needs confirmation and sometimes comfort. Adults are particularly effective at providing comfort and affirmation when they themselves have no doubt that the child has the ability to overcome obstacles.

Kindergarten children	The child becomes increasingly receptive to praise and criticism. Since he fully identifies with his actions, any praise or criticism of the "matter at hand" also has a strong effect on self-perception. The child has the right to experience esteem even if he has done something "wrong" or "evil" in the eyes of the educator. A reprimand can be given without hurting the child's self-esteem.
What is important when affirming?	Inflationary praise is to be avoided, as is perfectionism or criticalness. Praise as a reward for the adult's fulfilled expectations is less affirmative than when the adult expresses joy in something beautiful or unexpected, when discovering one of his child's traits.
What does the child "learn" through affirmation?	Affirmation and recognition strengthen the child's I-forces.

Uprightness	
Newborns	The movement development of infants is already based on the upright gait. However, it takes twelve to eighteen months for the child to take her first steps. For this development to happen, the child needs the example of upstanding caregivers. From the supine position she turns over onto her side, then onto her stomach.
Babies and toddlers	The toddler belly crawls, sits up and "bear crawls" before he pulls himself up on objects, takes his first steps while holding on, and then walks free. This work to become upright is an expression of autonomy achieved through the child's own initiative.
Kindergarten children	Upright walking is the physiological precondition for the child's head to gain an overview of his surroundings and his hands to be free. Deliberate, intentional action is now possible. The child acquires manual skills.

What is import-ant when model-ling uprightness?	The gesture helps with becoming upright. Physical uprightness is out of place for newborns. The gesture remains predominant-ly in the caregiver. He or she is the source of uplifting forces. The child seeks orientation and finds it in the uprightness (sincerity) of his caregivers. Human beings stand between heaven and earth. They are rooted in the spiritual and connect themselves with the earth. In their uprightness, they are free, and thereby responsible. Just as uprightness is anatomically based on the feet, the human hand is an expression of free creative power.
What does the child "learn" through experi-encing uprightness?	Uprightness conveys an awareness of human dignity. The child experiences his transcendence and uniqueness. The newborn and toddler experience their own striving for humanness even in their very first steps in developing movement, in the obsta-cles and joyful successes associated with this. Uprightness is the basis for feelings of freedom and responsibility.

5.2 Nursing gestures in the care of the elderly

Nursing care of elderly people and dementia sufferers is polar opposite to the care of children. It is precisely this polarity that demonstrates the general validity of the concept.

5.2.1 Cleansing

Elderly people in need of care often find it difficult to have their bodies washed by strangers or relatives. Feelings of shame in cases of incontinence, for example, or traumatic memories of assault (abuse, rape) are common causes for defensive behav-ior, as are lifelong cleansing rituals or the fear of opening the cover of one's own clothing, body odor and body heat. The nursing gesture of cleansing takes this de-fense into account. The caregiver's gaze is directed at the "pureness" that lies under-neath what has become old or foreign, and not at impurities such as sweat or urine. The body is only unclothed as far as absolutely necessary, any nakedness is always immediately covered with a towel. The wash water has a pleasant temperature, the nurse's touches are respectful and gentle. Every action is announced verbally or by an initial touch.

For dementia sufferers who fight verbally or physically against washing we can build a bridge to more extensive cleansing by means of a "sounding bath." We wash only the face at first, with gentle touches, followed by a hand bath of the right and then the left hand, then a foot bath of the right and then the left foot [→ Chapter "Variations in Whole-Body Washing"]. This treatment refreshes without tearing open any protective coverings. It creates trust and enables access to more intimate areas.

5.2.2 Nurturing

Elderly patients often suffer from malnutrition and the associated impairment of energy balance, muscle maintenance, wound healing and defense against infections. The main causes are protein, vitamin and trace element deficiencies due to a one-sided diet (porridge), poor tooth status, loss of appetite, difficulty swallowing, constipation or social factors such as not getting enough help with food preparation and eating. The latter is an urgent problem in homes for the elderly and hospitals. Medical interventions such as parenteral or enteral (tube) nutrition often fail because of the patient's rejection, or they do not achieve the desired effect if the given food substrates are not sufficiently metabolized. Side effects of dietary therapy—such as diarrhea, water retention and sugar metabolism disorders—can be treated, but sometimes affect the quality of life to an extent that is not tolerated by the patient. From this point of view, nutritionally balanced food and liquid quantities rarely correspond to the person's actual possibility to take in food and digest it. The composition and quantity of the food should in any case reflect a realistic relationship between what is medically desirable and the person's actual metabolic situation. The relationship to food changes in elderly people. The following simple grace aptly expresses this in words:

> *Bread does not nourish you;*
> *What nourishes you in the bread*
> *Is God's eternal Word,*
> *Is Love and Spirit.*
> Angelus Silesius (1624–1677)

It is important for nurses to eliminate external causes of a qualitatively and quantitatively inadequate diet and arrange for an atmosphere in which patience and empathy create the possibility for the absorption and digestion of food. This attitude is reflected in the gesture of nurturing. Just as a breastfeeding mother connects with her baby physically and mentally, so is it important to build up a "nurturing" attitude towards elderly people, one that has metamorphosed into an attitude of soul and spirit. The most important key points for this are:

- Preparation of customary food (have it brought from home)
- Presentation of meals in small, aesthetically appealing portions (e.g., finger food)
- Ergonomic cutlery, plates and cups
- Three main meals, three snacks, frequent offers of tasty drinks
- Fresh, soft, and balanced food

- A pleasant atmosphere when eating, preferably together with others
- Appreciation of food

5.2.3 Relieving—Challenging

The increasingly unwieldy weight of the physical body requires a counterforce. If stimulating the person's life forces and encouraging their will do not suffice, then comprehensive help from the nurse will be required. Relief from the weight of the body through positioning and movement, relief from pain through appropriate pain therapy, or relief from worries through the regulation of the person's social conditions. Every assistance of this kind is supported by a gesture of relieving. The aim is to liberate the person from any heaviness so that there is room for inner and outer activity. The person's inner gaze can now be filled with other content, their remaining power can flow into artistic activity or encounters with important people. When a person requires nursing, it means that they are dependent on the help of others in carrying out daily life activities. This assistance should never be an end in itself. Assuming responsibility for washing, feeding, help with walking or communicating with relatives always requires a concrete goal. What forces should be released in a person in need of care when I relieve him? What am I relieving him for? Pressure relief for bedsore prophylaxis, which a paralyzed person cannot provide for himself, does not only protect him from bedsores. It also enables him to release his consciousness from his body, to pursue thoughts and feelings without the constant fixation on painful or endangered body surfaces.

On the other hand, mere provision of relief prevents necessary perception of the body. The relief therefore needs a counterweight, it needs a burden, a challenge, a demand.

Making demands is the nursing gesture that underlies every mobilization and every exercise. The art of nursing care for the elderly is to combine every provision of relief with stimulation or exercise. For example, a person who is brought to a certain place in a wheelchair can be stimulated by a conversation. Even the care of a somnolent, dying patient can be seen as relieving the body, so that the soul can collect itself within itself, untethered by pain and illness.

5.2.4 Protecting—Enveloping—Creating order

Increasing fragility of the body, along with diminishing sensory perception, coordination of movement, heat sensation and memory, detract from a person's safe and adequate orientation in space and time. A number of protective measures are therefore necessary to compensate for impaired sensory function. The biggest resource is a familiar environment. Any disability-friendly reorganization of an apartment should always ensure that the usual paths and objects are preserved. Nursing homes for the elderly are strongly advised to allow people to bring some of their own furniture.

ANTHROPOSOPHY AND NURSING

From this point of view, hospitals are the most unsuitable places for elderly people who are confused and in need of care. Unknown people, rooms, furniture and daily routines unsettle even patients who are largely independent in their usual surroundings. Few hospitals have introduced structured protection and guidance measures for this growing group of patients. A few hospitals in Germany have created special care services and facilities for dementia patients. From the point of view of health policy, the principle of "outpatient before inpatient treatment" has hardly been implemented as poorly in any other patient group. There is a lack of medical and nursing capacity to adequately carry out diagnosis and therapy at home or in nursing homes.

The gesture of protecting is directed outwards. The gesture of enveloping creates a physically, mentally and socially warming space which is crucially important for an elderly person in need of care. People who have cold extremities or who are physically and mentally "thin skinned" require warm, enveloping clothing (e.g., made of virgin wool, mohair, angora or wool-silk blends), usually room temperatures above 22°C (71.6°F), warming foods (carbohydrates, fat, boiled fruit, warm drinks), as well as enveloping touching via Rhythmical Einreibung with oil blends such as *Solum oil* (WALA) or *mallow oil* (WALA). Sources of warmth in the social sphere are integration into social contexts, visits and joint celebrations of festivals. Very old people in need of care, who close themselves off within their own inner soul space, often have little inclination to seek social interaction. Nevertheless, even "just being present" also creates a social mantle of warmth. Rituals, prayers and worship create a warm environment. In this warm space the soul prepares itself to leave earthly life.

The "disorder" that can be found in the homes of many elderly people is often an expression of their "need of protection," similar to their neglect of personal hygiene. In this case, tidying up and organizing is only possible after protection, warmth and trust have been established. Trust is created through reliability, regularity, and good habits—which are signs of order in time.

5.2.5 Confirming—Awakening—Uprightness

Decreasing physical mobility in old age is often accompanied by a hardening of the person's conceptual life. Typical dangers of aging are fixed habits, loss of orientation in unusual situations, stereotypical ways of speaking, unchangeable opinions and even the proverbial stubbornness of old age. Corrections and criticism do not lead to greater inner flexibility or to changing fixed opinions in either dementia sufferers or well-oriented patients. Gestures of affirmation do not mean that you are sugarcoating untruth, ugliness or evil. Rather, they have to do with discovering and appreciating the intentions and hopes that are behind an opinion. Other possible behaviors in old age are refusing to believe in upcoming changes, such as an inevitable move to a home, and suppression of evidence of the nearness of death. Interested, serious questions can lead the person's consciousness into these fearful, tabooed areas of the soul. "What if your daughter-in-law falls ill and can't take care of you?" The gesture of awakening leads the person from the night of unconsciousness into the light. In this sense, awakening is also the most important gesture in accompanying dying people.

Awakening and affirming find bodily expression in the gesture of uprightness. It is important to help the elderly person in need of care to overcome physical and psychological gravity again and again. Any straightening of the upper body, even lifting the head or a hand, is an expression of self-assertion against the processes of deterioration of old age. Regular straightening upright supports the 'I' force in the body and thus acts as a prophylaxis of bedsores, pneumonia and thrombosis.

5.2.6 Balancing—Stimulating

How much activation does an elderly person need? Relatives and nurses ask themselves this question in the face of the lethargy and desolation that often characterize the mood in institutions of inpatient care for the elderly. Limited human resources deepen the discrepancy between the ideal of activating care and the reality of "fed and washed" care. On the one hand, we know that physical exercise and mental challenges, such as memory and concentration exercises, as well as the cultivation of rituals, are decisive factors for maintaining physical and mental health. On the other hand, we observe the need of elderly people for peace and quiet and reflection. Deliberately shaped rhythms bring the two poles into balance and are the key to well-being: daily rhythms, with body care, meals, encounters, movement, reflection or contemplation, weekly rhythms, with cultural events and visits, yearly rhythms with encounters with nature, festivities, commemoration days. A spiritual, religiously oriented lifestyle has a strong effect on physical and mental balance: times of prayer and meditation, participation in religious worship and preparation for death through reflecting on what is essential, eternal and meaningful.

As a rule, stimulation for a spiritual way of life can only succeed if the person can connect with religious, spiritual experiences and encounters such as those experienced particularly intensively in childhood. Alternatively, we can evoke an intimation of a world beyond the person's everyday experiences with familiar warm pictures that hold memories of stirring moods and human closeness. People who do not have access to such experiences can nevertheless encounter something authentically "true and good" in the people around them (nurses, relatives, neighbors), even if they reject all religious and spiritual intentions.

In this sense, it is important to stimulate processes of warmth, breathing and nourishment on the physical level, to support the capacity for perception, memory and concentration on the mental level (the gesture of challenging) and to ask the question of the value and meaning of life on the spiritual level (gesture of awakening).

5.3   Nursing gestures in the accompaniment of people who are dying

[→ Chapter "The Accompaniment and Care of the Dying and the Deceased"]

People who are approaching death pass through different phases. They are surrounded by a special atmosphere that is characterized by physical, mental and spiritual questions. A nursing gesture is assigned to each of these phases.

5.3.1 Creating space—Creating order

Anyone who encounters a dying person enters a special space. You can hardly escape the moving atmosphere. The entire drama of being human appears condensed in an individual destiny. We want to enter the room with reverence, unfamiliarity and awe, it is a place where external circumstances often contrast strangely with the inner reality of the dying person.

THE OUTER SPACE: Perhaps a room at home, perhaps in a hospital, a home or a hospice, perhaps a room in the house of relatives or friends, each with its own peculiarities, dependent on its time, culture, architecture and furnishings—with useful objects and decorations, luxuriant or sparse, pictures.

THE INNER SPACE: Perhaps not yet wishing to accept death or protesting angrily against the inevitable, perhaps arguing and negotiating with God and fate, perhaps frozen in depression, perhaps having found peace, filled with clarity and hope for what will come, with peace behind every expression of soul, questioning or affirming.

Whoever cares for the dying stands in the midst of these changing outer and inner spaces and yet remains outside, if he or she is not allowed in by the dying person and is not prepared to change along with them.

Creating space—this gesture refers to the establishment of a physical, social and spiritual place where the "birth" into the spiritual world can take place. Just as pregnancy is marked by a mother's creation of space in her body, her life of soul and by preparing the physical place of birth and the child's first habitat, so the dying person arranges his possessions, clarifies relations with the people connected to him and seeks to summarize his understanding of the events and stations of his life. Initially, caregivers regard this ordering process from a wait-and-see distance. No pressure, no premature mediation (no matter how confused the circumstances may at first seem) can or may force the dying person to accelerate this often quietly maturing process of creating order and resolution. Patiently describing the situation and clearly identifying what still needs to be taken care of creates the necessary clarity and openness in which inconsistencies, contradictions, hopes and fears can be expressed and questions of fate can mature.

Where the ordering forces of the 'I' fail, it may be justified for nurses or companions to directly mediate, to sort out external circumstances in the service of the dying person. In the case of an exhausted or unconscious person, essential nursing tasks based on the gesture of creating space include setting up a suitable room for the ill person, keeping order in this room, acting as a mediator for encounters, and providing spatial and temporal orientation through word and deed.

5.3.2 Affirming—Comforting—Hope

This gesture is part of every nursing action. Any activity would be pointless without the hope that accompaniment and care will lead to good results. Actions and words affected by this gesture radiate confidence, no matter how severe the pain and suffering of the dying person may be. It is the gesture of affirmation of destiny. The dying man's hope that perhaps destiny will still turn and allow him to heal, that the pain will be relieved, that death will come quickly and as a liberation, his struggling and wrestling and even his wanting to remain true to himself—unreconciled and proud—all this can be understood and affirmed by the gesture of affirmation. Affirmation of fate, affirmation of hope does not mean that you comply with what is seemingly inevitable, does not mean speaking of illusionary ideas, does not mean empty, unfeeling consolation, it means recognition of the difficult path that the dying person will take between lust for life and longing for death.

Nothing justifies the nurse in disillusioning someone, in taking away the person's hope for a miracle, their hope for a further period of life. On the one hand, experienced companions have seen many "miracles," have witnessed how deathly ill people have regained their health, or have received another span of life that is decisive for them. On the other hand, the desires and hopes of the dying often conceal insights into body-free, spiritual existence. Healing does not always mean physical recovery, it may often be the longing for purity, freedom and wholeness. The conviction of a debilitated patient, tormented by pain, that their next holiday in the warm south will bring back the vital forces so urgently needed for recovery, can also be a symbolic code for the redemptive lightness of the body-free state or a deep premonition of the forces that will flow to the person after death.

In the gesture of *creating space*, the nurse works from her spirit self and has an ordering effect on the 'I' of the dying person; in the gesture of *affirming—comforting—hoping*, she works from her 'I' and has an effect on the suffering and longing of the soul that is preparing to let go.

5.3.3 Stimulating

The life forces retreat in a dying person. This can be seen in the loss of respiration, warmth, nutrition, excretion, maintenance, growth and reproduction. These processes require appropriate stimulation by the nurse to counteract the agonizing heaviness of the physical body. Faltering, irregular breathing, cold extremities, loss of appetite, the drying up of secretions with dry mouth, constipation and water retention, tormenting weakness, inner retreat and the loss of creative powers require support.

Life process	Symptoms of weakening
Breathing	irregular breathing, breathing pauses, shortness of breath
Warming	cold or marbled extremities, chills, hot flashes
Nourishment	loss of appetite, food is not ingested, vomiting, diarrhea
Secretion	dry mouth, water retention, diarrhea, constipation
Maintenance	weakness, powerlessness, no regeneration through sleep
Growth	retreat, involution
Reproduction	the dwindling of creative powers

Chart: Weakened life processes in those who are dying

The use of water as the epitome of life is a gesture in itself. Moisturizing the lips, gently wiping out the mouth, washing the face and body, giving a hand or foot bath have a releasing and invigorating effect at the same time. It is not the physical purification that is indicated here, but the lightness and warmth or cooling power of the water. The water itself becomes the archetype of the nursing gesture. Anyone who nurses from out of this gesture makes themselves into a mobile, clear, light, well-tempered instrument of life forces.

On a psychological-spiritual level, the dying person needs stimulation through simple, light-filled pictures that liberate their life of emotions and thoughts (which may be laden with worries, perhaps broodingly bound to the physical) and lift their inner life into the light. The symbol of the caterpillar withdrawing into its cocoon, with its subsequent unfolding and resurrection as a butterfly, may be one such valid, liberating and uplifting image.

5.3.4 Nurturing

"To nurse" means to care for, to feed, and to nurture. To nurture means to weave earthly materiality into the organism that absorbs this substance. The dying person's need for food is generally low. Old people—or those approaching death—make less and less effort to feed themselves. Thirst and hunger are hardly present among their needs anymore. Their life organization is no longer able to integrate the physical substance into their organism. Diarrhea and edema are expressions of this. Sudden cravings for familiar or exotic food and drinks, just as women know from pregnancy, occur more rarely. The delight of relatives and nurses when they perceive this need, which is so much aimed at earthly life, is usually clouded by the minimal amount of food that is actually eaten. Often it is enough to look at the food just longed for a moment ago, to take away the dying man's courage and strength to eat it.

Nevertheless, the lovingly prepared and patiently administered food will act as a gesture of union between soul and body, in which an earthly quality appears once again in smell and taste—or perhaps only in the memory of it.

All food that the living organism no longer digests and assimilates becomes a plague. If it can be assimilated, though, then tube feeding or infusion therapy seems to be appropriate. In this case it does not disturb the dying process. The art of nursing care can be shown precisely in the fact that it is possible to administer drip feeding out of full respect for its upbuilding forces, and in amazement at the will of the organs to connect with the physical world—using a nurturing gesture.

As the need for physical nourishment usually decreases in the dying person, so too does the need for mental and spiritual stimulation. The habits of everyday life stabilizing the soul, regularly cultivated interests, prayer and meditation sometimes lose their former meaning for the dying person. Not only has he lost the strength to practice these things—they are becoming foreign to his life of habits, like physical food. Often, small reminiscences of a familiar daily routine, such as a certain sequence of body care or the first words of a prayer, the soft reminder of a joyful life event, are enough to satisfy the need for inner nourishment. Here too, in the gesture of nurturing, we find the weaving of the forces through which the soul finds its place in the body and in life.

5.3.5 Challenging—Encouraging

To accompany a dying person is to accompany life until the last breath. Life includes the confrontation with death as well as caring for the body and shaping the world. To those who are approaching death it may seem like an anachronism to be creative, yet we can only realize our humanness by engaging in external or internal actions. In this, the dying person needs encouragement and support. To make demands means to expect and believe in that which is still within the dying person's power. The dying man doesn't have to spare himself. He is allowed to consume his strength and himself, even if it is only to get up out of bed, maybe even just to open his eyes. In every slightest self-willed and self-aware effort, he overcomes the negating, Ahrimanic power* that continually wants to prove to us the powerlessness and futility of human will. The least effort of will is a victory of the spirit over death. In this gesture, motivation as an inner movement and mobilization as an outer movement seem to be almost imperative. It goes without saying that a mechanical training concept would not be appropriate, and there must be proper space given to the opposite gesture, that of providing relief.

---

* Anthroposophic spiritual science distinguishes between three spiritual adversaries (Lucifer, the Asuras, and Ahriman). Ahriman is the force that seduces human beings into mechanical solidification, into devotion to practical constraints and prevailing circumstances. He is called "Mephistopheles" in Goethe's *Faust*.

5.3.6 Relieving

The increasingly unwieldy weight of the physical body requires a counterforce. If stimulating the person's life forces and encouraging their will do not suffice, then comprehensive help from the nurse will be required. Relief from the weight of the body through positioning and movement, from pain through appropriate pain therapy, or relief from worries through the regulation of the person's social conditions. Every assistance of this kind is supported by a gesture of relieving. The aim is to liberate the person from the burden of the body and everyday life, so that there is room for inner and outer activity. Her inner gaze can now be filled with other content, her remaining power can flow into artistic activity or into encounters with important people (see challenging).

5.3.7 Uprightness

The interaction between making demands on oneself and getting relief is realized in the upright form of the human being. Starting from a will impulse, human beings need about two years to learn to walk upright. This frees their arms for creative activity, it releases their arms from the supporting and carrying function that these limbs have in animals. The head rests at the uppermost point of the vertical form—in a free, surveying view of the world—and achieves self-awareness in thinking. Assistance with uprightness is another nursing gesture.

The child attains uprightness by imitating upright people. The upright gait and the self-awareness associated with it cannot be trained from outside. To educate is to "help someone up" in the best sense of the word.

In a dying person, the 'I' has left an almost complete impression on the body. The body has become an expression of the deeds of the self. This can be seen in a special way in the sublime uprightness that often runs through a corpse, and it becomes clear that uprightness is not found solely in the dimension of physical verticalness. It also appears psychologically and spiritually. In the upright sincerity of nurses and companions it can be a point of reference for the dying person, who may be losing courage and self-confidence.

Sincerity is called for, for example, when a dying person asks how long he has left to live, or whether he will suffer pain or suffocate. It is distressing for the questioner when he feels that the answer is evasive or heartless. To tell the truth with love means to describe the dying process objectively and, if you have a certain spectrum of personal experience, to give examples. Your description should relate as concretely as possible to the situation of the dying person and should not contain any generalizations.

Returning the question, asking " ...and what do you think—do you feel close to death...?" makes it clear that the dying person is always ahead of us in his knowledge of dying, despite all the experience we may have, through his individual situation.

Returning the question can at least open up the emotional and experiential layer that may have resonated in the depths of the question.

The dying person's companion may also express her own hopes and uncertainties. She should not, however, flood the dying person with her own emotions. A will-oriented response is also justified. "If you are in pain, I will stand by you..." or "If you die, be it in a short time or much, much later, there will always be someone with you, if you wish it..." The one who is dying can find orientation in the inner uprightness of the nurse, who is poised between what is spiritual and what is earthly, between what is light and what is heavy. Even the straightening up of the body from the sickbed, lifting the person's head, treating his back with simple swabs, gently rubbing his feet, awakens uplifting forces. A clear, uplifting thought supports the uprightness from the spiritual side. To tell the truth with love creates sincere, uplifting encounters between free people.

5.3.8 Enveloping

A germinating physical human embryo develops in its mother's womb. It creates its own embryonic membrane that surrounds it—nourishing it and forming its organs until birth. This protective membrane is abandoned at birth, and outer nature—with warmth, light, air, water, and earth—takes over this function, mediated by the social protection of the infant's parents. In caring for and educating the child, the parents continue the formative work of the creative forces.

Providing enveloping protection through nursing care is another gesture that is used in the most varied ways—wrapping, dressing, embracing, and therapeutic applications.

In a dying person, the physical body requires enhanced enveloping as the 'I', soul body, and etheric body detach. We already discussed warm clothing and rhythmical oil applications in connection with the gesture of stimulation. However, it is not uncommon for dying people to have the need to undress themselves, push a blanket to the side or ask for something cold (a cold room, cold drinks). This often happens together with restlessness and an urge to move. This is an expression of the longing to free oneself from the body. It is precisely in this situation that the provision of enveloping protection is important. Applying lavender oil to the feet (*lavender 10% oil* (Weleda), *Moor lavender oil* (Dr. Hauschka)), hanging a canopy over the bed, a light blanket, perhaps just a sheet, creates a protective layer without imposing too much on the patient.

A quiet holding of the patient's hand is an enveloping gesture, or a comforting and affirming gesture, depending on the nuance that the nurse gives to it. In the social sphere, the presence of friends or relatives can form a protective sphere in which the dying person feels well safeguarded. If, as is often the case, he seeks his time of death when he is alone, this can be understood as a necessary departure from his social sphere.

Prayer to the angel of the dying person, or to Christ, or thoughts that seek the core individuality of the dying person, form a protective sphere for the 'I' and give it strength, both for its release from the physical body and for its entry into the spiritual world.

5.3.9 Helping the essence to appear—Cleansing

The word "decay" ("*verwesen*") has a strange double meaning in the German language. On the one hand it means the decay of organic matter, on the other hand it means a return to being, "becoming being." "Earth to earth, dust to dust"—this traditional funeral formula states the sober truth about the mineral essence of the physical body. The only imperishable part of the human being is the 'I', precisely because it constitutes the actual essence.

The gesture of "helping the essence of something to appear" is also the gesture of cleansing. In physical and symbolic-cultic purification, we separate the insignificant from the essential. A layer is discarded, the new can appear. To accompany a dying person is to assist with a birth into the spiritual world. Reverence for the bodily home from which the spirit is born is just as important as patiently expecting the moment of birth in which the 'I' will liberate itself. Our cleansing and washing of a dying person and also of a corpse have a gestural character in this sense when we appreciate the essence of the bodily home and the birth of the spirit in equal measure.

5.3.10 Balancing

We have repeatedly made references to incarnation and excarnation as the basic forces in the relationship between body and spirit. Every day a rhythmic alternation between incarnation and excarnation takes place in waking and sleeping. Incarnating forces predominate in childhood and adolescence, excarnating forces predominate from the middle of life onwards. On a soul level, they appear in the polarity of awakening and fatigue, as *joie de vivre* and world-weariness. The 'I' swings between these two poles. This oscillation between connecting and releasing is often disturbed in the dying process. Fears or organic causes can prevent someone from letting go, exhaustion and fears make it difficult to connect. Nurses and companions often conclude that the dying person cannot let go. Sometimes even a slight reproach or impatience accompanies this statement. What should the dying man let go of, and why? Isn't there probably a good reason for him being held there or holding onto something? Experienced companions of the dying know that it is often precisely people who feel completely ready to die, who even long for death, who have to stay in their bodies for a long time still. On the other hand, we can observe again and again that dying people may suddenly seem to feel better, they make every effort to get up again, to receive or visit friends, and then they die after just a few hours or days. Just as sleep can only come after fulfilled activity, so also death only after the 'I' and soul body once again dive deeply into the physical body and then take the etheric body with them into the spiritual world.

Balancing as a nursing gesture in this sense means paying attention to the rhythmic swinging of connecting and releasing occurring in sleep and wakefulness.

In physical care, this succeeds particularly by means of a rhythmic daily routine or through rhythmic rubbing of oil into the arms and legs, or through a whole-body treatment with Rhythmical Einreibung, for example with *Solum Oil* (WALA) or *lavender 10% oil (Weleda) or Lavandula, Oleum aethereum 10%* (WALA). Rhythmical Einreibung with gold ointment (*Aurum/Lavandula comp. cream* (Weleda)) in a five-pointed star, as an archetype for the human form and the main etheric currents* has proven its worth in the work with dying people.

On the level of soul and spirit, it can have a balancing and harmonizing effect to behold the beauty and uniqueness of the sensory world, and to be reminded of the constant presence of the spiritual world.

5.3.11 Averting—Protecting

Every threshold crossing is dangerous. In the past, to die fully conscious was thought to be ideal. Unprepared death was feared, because the dying person was in danger of having to enter the spiritual world without spiritual support or the forgiveness of sins. Preparation for death was therefore an important part of life. Today, most people wish for a sudden, rapid death, if possible in their sleep. This attitude corresponds to our culture's repression of death and its mania for youthfulness. The long decline and the need for long-term care experienced by many elderly people today arouse anxiety in those for whom independence and youthfulness are the determining ideals of their lives. The impending loss of autonomy is then considered to be the biggest problem of dying. The call for self-determined dying and the discussion about death-on-demand have their origins in this. The loss of memory, of the ability to think, of consciousness, joie de vivre, the courage to live, mobility and continence cannot be equated with the loss of human dignity. Nurses and companions of the dying experience the lovable, autonomous essence of suffering and dying people as a luminous center that motivates their work, giving them strength and meaning. If this view is lost, doubts arise concerning the meaning of life and of nursing care. Only then will shameful, insulting and painful situations arise for the dying person, ultimately resulting from the overstrain of the nurses or therapists involved. Now the patient in need of care needs protection—protection from overstrain of relatives and nurses. It is not the autonomy or dignity of the dying person that must be protected, which are actually inviolable, but those around the dying person whose pain, fear or hard-heartedness obscures their view of the light-filled essence of the person.

---

*   According to Rudolf Steiner, there are five main ether currents in the human etheric body, which flow from the head to the right leg, to the left arm, to the right arm, to the left leg and back to the head. He also described the pentagram as the "skeleton of the etheric body."

ANTHROPOSOPHY AND NURSING

Advance personal healthcare directives are intended to protect dying people from degrading treatment. However, these must be drafted with care and preferably with medical advice. Otherwise, the patient is at risk of being left untreated or unattended to, even though treatment could be the most urgent concern in an acute situation.

The gesture of protecting and defending is completely directed towards the periphery. On the physical level, it keeps pressure or skin irritation away through softness and repositioning. It averts stress caused by sensory impressions and regulates the visits of friends and relatives. On the soul level it rejects envy, resentment, jealousy, greed and falsehood, regardless of whether they emanate from the dying person or from his environment. In the spiritual-social sphere, conversations between nurses and relatives, understanding listening, mutual clearing of blame, and seeking for an understanding of the individuality of the dying person form a protective wall against inhuman attacks.

In this sense, the inability of an unconscious person to articulate his own will does not require abstract protection of his presumed will, but rather an increased sensitivity for the expressions of the essence of the deeply unconscious person. We are often perplexed by a question that concerns, for example, the further treatment of an unconscious person. The person accompanying him can live with this question and address it to the dying person calmly and openly. Again and again, we find that suddenly a self-evident point of view can emerge from our own life of thought, or we hear it expressed by a colleague or relative, or the dying person himself gives a clear sign. This method proves to be particularly effective when we consider the question calmly and vividly before falling asleep at night, and then the next morning are attentive to receiving an answer. Certainty in the answer and protection against hasty judgments can be found through talking with the people around the dying person.

5.3.12 Awakening

The origin of the gesture of awakening is found when a sleeping person enters waking consciousness. Every morning we wake up for the world of the senses. In the case of people who are dying, we can speak of an awakening for and into the spiritual world, because death is ultimately a maximal increase in consciousness that penetrates beyond the sensory world. Accompanying a dying person is an awakening for the spiritual world in this sense. Like the waking of a sleeper in the morning, it is best done by gently using the person's name, gently touching them and looking forward to what the day will bring. In the gesture of awakening, the nurse's accompaniment connects with what would be the work of a priest. Just as a priest prepares the way to the spiritual world through the sacraments, so the nurse by shaping everyday life. All nursing care gestures for dying people eventually lead to the gesture of awakening. Death is the great awakening.

[→ Chapter "Anthroposophic Nursing Care in Oncology"]

As nurses, we do not treat illnesses, we treat people who are in certain circumstances. Every life situation has its own specific need for care and requires nursing gestures attuned to it. Even if our trained nursing eye looks for and promotes health in people, we encounter illness as a force that marks the people affected by it. A diabetic person appears very different from someone who has rheumatism, a stroke patient is different from one who is suffering from multiple sclerosis. Diseases, especially life-threatening diseases, affect people physically, mentally and spiritually, depending on their type. Just as an exhausted person needs enveloping, protecting and relieving gestures, so too can we look for gestures typical of a person suffering from cancer. Even if the life situation of each cancer patient naturally requires specific care and appropriate gestures, a typical nursing gesture can still be found as a guiding principle.

Despite the successes of modern oncology, it is still shocking to receive a diagnosis of cancer. It is not only the uncertain prospect of recovery that seems to be the reason for this shock in individual cases, or the probable life expectancy and restrictions on the quality of life under the recommended therapy, or the progress of the disease. Rather, it is the feeling of powerlessness towards the cancer, shaped by the imagination of the malignant process developing in your own body, which occupies your body, consumes it and tortures it with pain. Unlike bodily injury or illness, cancer appears to be accompanied by an existential insecurity in your own readiness for life and health. Life itself has caused the disease. Life no longer serves the self, but has become a threat, an enemy. Life is called into question, not only by a bad prognosis, but by life itself.

The spectrum of the first psychological reactions to a diagnosis of cancer ranges from unconscious inner numbness, to not wanting it to be true, to agitation and panic.* There may also be the feeling of having experienced a truth that was already suspected in the depths of one's soul, a sense of gaining insight into the illness, and affirmation of fate, or trusting hope in the help that will come.

Inner numbness characterizes the pole of exaggerated holding fast mentally, while panic is an expression of exaggerated mental agitation. In between we have all the individual nuances of mental processing, with affirmative, hope-borne insight into illness as a dynamic inner center. Some patients also experience the state of being "at one with oneself" immediately after the diagnosis. However, this is seldom maintained and usually quickly gives way to a desperate alternating rollercoaster of numbness and panic. During the course of the disease or the healing process, the cancer patient passes repeatedly through the entire range of these attitudes of mind, as well as experiencing the phases of death described by Elisabeth Kübler Ross. Ultimately, all mental processes push for inner balance, for peace with oneself and the

---

*   Elisabeth Kübler Ross distinguishes between five phases in people who live in the expectation of death: not wanting it to be true, negotiating, anger, depression, hope.

world. However, the way there is often painful and marked by internal and external crises, conflicts and struggles.

As modern research into the origins of health or salutogenesis has shown, a health-promoting factor is to have an active inner attitude that successfully processes the illness. It is a force to inhibit the progression of the disease, if not even to cure it. Aaron Antonovsky (1923–1994) described this health-promoting inner attitude as a "sense of coherence." According to Antonovsky, a perception of an inner coherence with one's own destiny is characterized by having an understanding of the situation (comprehensibility), experiencing its meaning (meaningfulness) and being aware of effective possibilities for action (manageability). Conceptual comprehension, a sense of meaning and purposeful action create strength in the life of soul that is also healthy for the body. Arousing this power is the essential prerequisite for the cure of cancer. Patients who do not gain a deeper understanding of the disease process within them, who do not find a sense of perspective or who fall into lethargy without their own impulses for action, slip down into indifference, despair and powerlessness. This soul mood also wears down and weakens the body's health. This is in no way intended to propagate uncritical, calculated, optimistic "positive thinking." Rather, it refers to an often slow, discontinuous process of awakening to the whole context of one's individual fate.

The motif of "awakening" also has a further meaning, which is immediately understandable from the tumor process. If we look at tumors as a dominance of the substance-upbuilding processes that normally prevail in sleep, which the conscious formative powers of the day are not strong enough to counter, then "awakening" also becomes a leading therapeutic thought on a biological level. [→ Chapter "From the Question of the Meaning in Cancer to the Care of the Senses"].

Accompanying an individual's awakening in the physical, mental and spiritual sense is thus a paramount nursing task. It becomes effective as the nursing gesture of awakening in various measures. To explain its quality, we shall consider the archetypal process of waking up from sleep.

5.4.1 How do people wake up?

A variety of sensory impressions approach the sleeping person as if from far away. Usually sounds are the first to become conscious, initially as pure, nameless perceptions. Only with further awakening do we assign a concept to them. Smells and sensations of touch also approach us in this way. We wake up in a special way when this is caused by a voice speaking our name softly. We open our eyes and now find orientation in space, mostly through our sense of sight, and orientation in time, through perceiving daylight. Memory sets in. We feel ourselves, come to ourselves. Pleasure and disinclination, joy and anxiety gradually fill the soul. The pulse accelerates, the blood pressure rises. We move our limbs, stretch, touch ourselves. Awakening spreads from the senses concentrated in the head, to the rhythmic system and the limbs. The awakening is complete only when these three areas are harmoniously permeated.

We are only really awakened, even for a fact of life, when it can be adequately perceived, thought through, felt and lived. There seems to be no limit to the depth and brightness of awakening. Rather, it progresses from stage to stage. The highest form of awakening is self-knowledge, which is inseparably linked with gaining conscious knowledge of the world.

5.4.2 What do cancer patients awaken to?

The diagnosis of cancer is itself a rude, drastic moment of awakening. The tumor, which has long since formed in the subconsciousness of the body, enters consciousness. Questions arise. How could this happen? Why didn't I notice anything? Am I going to die soon? What treatments am I going to have to deal with? How will my relatives, friends, colleagues and neighbors react to this? Will I suffer? Why has this disease come to me, of all people, even though I have never been seriously ill and have always lived in a healthy way? These and similar questions surface. They are based on deeper questions, and there will follow experiences that raise new questions. Ultimately, it is the four topics presented in the chart below that characterize the questions of cancer patients. They often have an external cause, but at their core they are endogenous, and they affect everyone.

Life topic	External cause	Internal disease context
The question of death	Prognosis of the life-threatening disease.	Parasitic life (of the tumor) kills integrating life (of the organism).
The question of pain	Reports of other cancer patients.	Displacing or infiltrating tumor growth.
The question of the meaning of life	Necessary lifestyle changes due to therapy and disease progression.	The randomness of tumor growth overgrows the purposeful development of the organism.
The question of the 'I'	Isolation through the withdrawal of relatives, neighbors, etc.	The body becomes idiosyncratic. It is no longer suited to the 'I' as an instrument. Through its identification with the body, the 'I' is also threatened with death.

Chart: Life topics of cancer patients

5.4.3 How can external and internal processes of awakening be accompanied by nursing care?

If you want to waken someone, you must put yourself in their current state of consciousness. This cannot be achieved without personal experience. Everyone should be familiar with the experience of waking up from sleep. However, only those who know many nuances and ways of awakening become "wake-up artists." The life questions of a cancer patient, as general human questions of existence, require individual valid answers. Just as one cannot wake up from sleep on behalf of another, one cannot answer the life questions of another from outside. The questioner can only find the answers himself. The nurse supports him in this by asking questions herself. Only people who have questions can ask them. Those who do not wrestle with the above-mentioned life questions will therefore not be able to help the patient. They fall short of the other person's misery and power of transformation. This is perhaps the greatest isolation of the cancer patient if he does not find someone who shares his questions, who understands him, that is, who is ready to awaken to a new state of consciousness.

As with bodily sleep, spiritual awakening begins in the periphery. It begins with quiet sounds, rarely with loud confrontational ones. We ask questions from different perspectives and consider them on the level of thoughts, emotions and will. The right time and context of the questions is crucial. It is our interest in the other person, apart from all curiosity, that paves the way for awakening.

Thought sphere	What does the disease mean to you? What do spiritual things mean to you? What do you think about death?
Emotional sphere	Are you afraid of ...? Do you remember a happy experience from your childhood? What do you want most?
Will sphere	Which big or small tasks do you see for yourself? What would it mean for you if the disease took a different course than you had hoped for?

Chart: Sample questions to awaken

Awakening has two opposite directions. Usually we associate the term with an incarnating process, a taking hold of the body by the soul and spirit, with a simultaneous increase in the brightness of consciousness. This process can be accompanied by deliberately touching the patient's body by administering a Rhythmical Einreibung treatment. Thereby, something can be released in the treated organ or organ system, which leads to relaxation on the bodily level and an opening up on the emotional level. Often emotional content buried in the body is released by Rhythmical Einreibung and now appears free of the body as pain, fear, longing, warmth, courage. In particular, rhythmical oil applications to the back, legs and feet have a deep incarnating effect. Letting go of the body, excarnating as an awakening for something spiritual, also results in a maximum increase in the brightness of consciousness. In nursing this is prepared by means of compassionate questions, gentle searching and references to the reality of the spiritual world that leave the person free. Ultimately, accompanying a dying person is permeated by this nursing gesture of awakening.

Application	Attitude of the nurse	Indication
Rhythmical Einreibung of the feet, with strong sole strokes	Firmness, uprightness, concentration, carefulness	Strengthening perception of the body and will, relief for the head
Rhythmical Einreibung of the legs, with special emphasis on joints	Powerful, controlled mobility	Strengthening perception of will forces, stimulation of blood circulation and excretion metabolism
Rhythmical Einreibung of the back	Rhythmic, harmonious, quasi musical swinging, empathetic attention	Stimulation of respiration and circulation, release of tension in the shoulder/neck area, mediation of thought and will activity, strengthening the center.
Application	Attitude of the nurse	Indication
Rhythmical Einreibung of the arms	Careful lightness	Promoting upbuilding metabolism, e.g., in cases of cachexia, relieving breathing
Rhythmical Einreibung of the abdomen	Release in the area of the solar plexus, consolidation in the left lower abdomen	Promoting intestinal activity, relaxation in cases of agitation and pain

Chart: Examples of external applications that awaken

6. Nursing gestures in typical activities

All nursing activities can be carried out in the various gestures. This gives them an individual form. Every nursing activity has a certain closeness and relationship to typical nursing gestures, which we referred to as their overall character. The more consciously we live with these gestures, the more differentiated and effective our nursing care becomes. The following examples should explain this.

Gesture	Rhythmical Einreibung: whole body	Wash: whole body	Mobilization	Compress
Cleansing	In cases of severe sweating, incontinence, or after chemotherapy, cleaning (showering) the patient's body prior to treatment is recommended.	Removal of impurities, skin remnants, sweat, loosening with water, fresh clothes, fresh bed linen.	Possibly a change of protective pants for incontinent patients.	In case of heavy perspiration after an application or fever, rinse off, especially in the skin folds, if necessary remove substance residues from the skin (e.g., after a farmer's cheese compress).
Nurturing	Use of skin-care substances that give the patient a feeling of well-being.	Use of skin-care substances as bath additives or with Rhythmical Einreibung.	"Reward" after mobilization.	If necessary, use of skin-care substances after an application to promote well-being.
Relieving	Back support, knee roll to relieve the abdominal wall, guided support of the limbs, avoid active movements of the patient, relaxed silence during treatment.	Comfortable and expedient positioning, helping the patient according to the person's strength and orientation.	If necessary, administer painkillers before moving, use supports, mobilization or walking aids if necessary.	Back support, knee roll to relieve the abdominal wall, guided support of the limbs, compress removal.
Gesture	Rhythmical Einreibung: whole body	Wash: whole body	Mobilization	Compress
Protecting	Close the door, close the window, if necessary screen from view, possibly switch off the telephone.	Close the door, close the window, if necessary screen from view, possibly switch off the telephone.	Eliminate sources of danger on the way, check the function of the aids, possibly use fall protectors.	Close the door, close the window, if necessary screen from view, possibly switch off the telephone.
Creating space— Creating order	Inform patients, prepare room, ventilate, take the time you need, clarify the time frame with the patient, prepare oil and cloths.	Inform patients, prepare room or a bath, ventilate, take the time you need, clarify the time frame with the patient, have washing utensils ready.	Inform patients, take the time you need, clarify the time frame with the patient, dress them appropriately, possibly comb their hair	Inform patients, prepare room, ventilate, take the time you need, clarify the time frame with the patient, prepare oil and cloths, prepare the compress.

Enveloping	Cover with warm cloths, cover treated areas of the body well again, gentle, enveloping touch, use of a warming oil.	Remove bed cover and clothing only at the areas to be treated; dry, dress and cover any treated, moist areas of the body.	After mobilization, create a relaxed environment, possibly cover the patient carefully.	Enveloping application of the compress, after applying it and after the patient's rest, tuck the patient in, if necessary use skin-care oil after the treatment.
Balancing	Rhythmic binding and releasing of the hands, proximity and distance, uncovering, covering, dynamics of movement.	Movement control as with Rhythmical Einreibung, proximity and distance, uncovering, covering, dynamics of movement.	Find the middle between making demands and relieving. Transfer the patient's position safely step-by-step to the next one, include rest breaks along the way, allow rest afterwards.	Two-phase application rhythm: sensory stimulation then relaxation during post-treatment rest, waking and sleeping.
Stimulating	Use of essential oils, impulsive quality of touch, post-treatment rest.	Use of water, choice of water temperature, use of a bath additive, rubbing with a washing glove or towel.	Possible washing of the face, a foot rub before mobilization, or medications to support circulation.	Effect of the substance and medium.
Gesture	**Rhythmical Einreibung: whole body**	**Wash: whole body**	**Mobilization**	**Compress**
Challenging	The patient must accept relaxation and emerging feelings, tolerate touch and movement for the duration of the treatment.	Asking for the patient's own activity according to their potential strength and orientation, independence training.	Asking for the patient's own activity according to their potential strength and orientation, discussing the training workload, formulating exercises.	Patient must allow the application.
Awakening	Evaluation of the treatment with the patient, questions about health and experiences, awakening awareness for warmth and the body's boundaries.	Evaluation of the treatment with the patient, questions about health and experiences, awakening awareness for warmth and the body's boundaries.	Awakening awareness for the sequence of movements, for the possibilities and limits of the demands that can be made, evaluating the treatment with the patient, questions about health and experiences.	Evaluating the treatment with the patient, questions about health and experiences.

Affirming	Gentle, respectful, attentive touch, careful approach and release of the hands. The hands say, "You're good!"	Gentle, respectful, attentive touch, benevolent commentary on achievements of independence training.	Benevolent commentary on the achievements.	Confirmation of the effect; motivation to tolerate unpleasant side effects (e.g., burning sensation during mustard compress).
Uprightness	Paravertebral strokes, sole strokes.	As upright as possible (sitting), paravertebral strokes during washing.	Make eye contact, paravertebral strokes, support of the back, possibly guidance with the hand on the patient's sacrum, guidance from in front (holding both forearms).	Help with sitting up, putting on and removing the compress.
Overall character of the treatment	Enveloping, compensating, affirming	Cleansing, stimulating, relieving—challenging	Challenging, uprightness, affirming	Stimulating, enveloping

Chart: Nursing gestures in typical nursing activities

7. Nursing gestures and external applications

The nursing gestures listed below describe the nursing process from the assumption of nursing responsibilities through to supporting the patient in regaining independence. This is reflected in external applications. The gestures trace the mode of action of external applications in a very concrete way.

Gesture	Application	Experience / Reaction of the patient
Relieving	Do everything possible to ensure that the patient can be fully involved in the application: position the patient comfortably, have them empty their bladder before treatment, the patient may relinquish control of what is happening.	Regression; from the upright to the horizontal; 'I'-forces are freed from the encounter with the outside world and immerse themselves in metabolic processes.
Protecting	Protect the space and time from interference (switch off the telephone, put a sign on the door, screen if necessary, etc.).	Surrender of control and outward orientation by the patient presupposes the assumption of these functions by the nurse.
Creating order	Preparing the materials, scheduling the application into the daily routine, informing patients about the application.	The order that occurs later inside is initially established outside—in space and time.

Enveloping	Laying and wrapping of compress cloths, applying the hot-water bottle, enveloping gestures during Rhythmical Einreibung, wrapping the patient after a bath, covering, tucking in the bedclothes	Peripheral forces at work in the elemental world are introduced to the body in the gesture, substance, material and medium of the application.
Balancing	Adapting the application to the patient in terms of duration, dosage, temperature; if necessary, varying the application during a series of treatments.	Proximity and density of the envelopment must be adapted to the situation and constitution of the patient.
Stimulating	Selecting the substance, medium and type of application with regard to the patient's ability to react; ensuring post-treatment rest.	The patient responds with all members of his fourfold nature to being introduced to the elemental substance—especially in the post-treatment rest, the "night side" of the application.
Challenging	Transferring responsibility back to the patient: self-care, lifestyle changes, continuation of treatment with external applications at home.	The patient experiences and asserts himself in this response, in the creation of "a life of his own" as opposed to the given environment. This is the starting point for consciously taking hold of his own body.
The circle of gestures now runs in the opposite direction, from providing relief towards making demands.		
Nurturing	Allow the patient to take part in as many steps of the application as possible (preparing tea, taking out tea herbs, filling the hot water bottle, preparing the compress, preparing the room, etc.); "celebrating" the application.	Understanding the concentrated, lovingly done procedures prepares a feeling of respect and reverence. This is part of the treatment and creates a feeling of acceptance.
Cleansing	Take care of excretions after the treatment (sweat, urine, stool, tears) and if necessary remove them together with the remnants of the compress. Take note of what the patient wants to "get rid of."	The application creates a feeling of renewal, freshness and new beginning.
Uprightness	Always also see the healthy "whole" person in the patient. Meet him sincerely and truthfully.	In true therapeutic encounters, the patient experiences himself as a partner. This is a prerequisite for self-awareness and self-responsibility.
Affirming	Undivided attention to the patient before, during and after treatment.	In undivided attention the patient feels perceived and taken seriously. He experiences himself lifted beyond himself.
Awakening	Awakening awareness for the patient's own body by asking questions about warmth, lightness, heaviness, light, mood, etc., within the framework of the evaluation of the application.	Perception of one's own bodily state and the experience of giving it language are prerequisites for self-regulation. Attracting consciousness to "underexposed" areas of the body increases vitality (warmth, light) and completes the circle of the challenging gestures.

Chart: Nursing gestures in external applications

8. Nursing gestures and the zodiac

We have looked at nursing care as a kind of mediation between the human being and the natural and social world that surrounds him. The human being stands at the center of a stream of forces acting on him through nature and culture. Enveloping, substituting gestures aim to integrate, while uplifting, activating gestures aim to ensure autonomy and freedom. There is an anthropological explanation for the enveloping gesture: when a human being physically originates from the fusion of oocyte and spermatozoa, a spherical cell cluster forms during the first few days, in which an initially single-celled layer develops that divides the sphere into two halves. The surrounding cell envelope is called a trophoblast, the middle cell layer is the embryonic disc or embryoblast. The child born after nine months develops from the embryoblast, while the trophoblast is the nutrient-providing perimeter of the embryo. The embryo appears as the nucleus and its embryonic envelope develops from the same cell material, genetically identical to the child. In this phase it is still identical to the human being growing there.

It is not just the embryo that is surrounded by its embryonic envelope; the trophoblast is also enclosed in the uterine mucosa. It is completely embedded in the uterus, which in turn is embedded in the mother's abdominal cavity. The mother forms the protective organism for the child. But even the mother is not an autonomous being. Like all human beings, she remains dependent on an even larger protective organism; she depends on light, air, warmth, water and soil—we are essentially surrounded by the "great Mother Earth," as ancient peoples called it. And Earth itself is inserted into an even larger cosmic context. Earth's ability to provide all the conditions for human life is due to the sun, the moon and the other planets. But the solar system itself is also embedded in the even larger organism we call the Milky Way, or—as seen from Earth— the fixed stars, the horizon of the zodiac. Even astrophysicists today speak in categories outside of space and time when they think about what is beyond the perceptible and measurable universe. They encounter a background that can only be grasped mentally and spiritually. In the context of Christianity, this background is called the first beginning, the Logos.

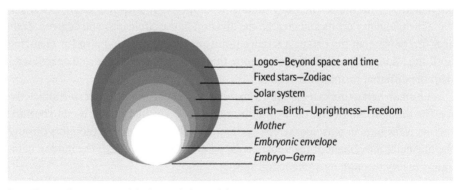

Fig. 5: The enveloping layers of the human being and the cosmos

Let us once again consider the embryo as the center of these enveloping layers. Something dramatic happens at birth. The embryo gives up this position at the center of the world. The enveloping layers die, he leaves his mother and steps onto the earth. In this way, the born human being has a completely different relationship to his environment. He is no longer the center of a world that surrounds him. He is excreted from the mother who surrounded him. He looks into her eyes. The layers of protection become a person opposite! This juxtaposition increasingly develops into independence. The enveloping organism abandoned at birth must now be replaced by a new one, a new life-giving environment. It is caregiving that brings the child into a relationship with the warmth, air, liquids and gravity of Earth. Caregiving conveys the four elements to the child and thereby creates a new enveloping context [→ Section "Substituting and activating gestures"]. But neither through these forces of nature nor by inheritance do human beings gain their specific abilities (their upright gait, speech and their ability to think)—only human beings can support the development of someone into a human being [→ Section "Substituting and activating gestures"].

A THINKING EXERCISE: Imagine a nurse taking care of a bedridden patient for several hours. The patient's bed is in the middle of the room. There is an invisible thread on the wrists of the caregiver. At certain times the nurse enters the room and takes care of her patient. At the end of the day the invisible thread is made visible. We see an exact image of the nurse's movements. It expresses the actions and character of the nurse. The visualized movements form a cocoon that surrounds the patient and makes his recovery possible.

Rudolf Steiner described the forces that act from the enveloping organism of Earth and the cosmos as peripheral or formative forces. Their archetype has been the zodiac since ancient Babylonian times (about 6000–4000 BC). Human beings of that time lived in a kind of mystical consciousness, experienced themselves as being looked at by the gods out in the universe. They felt that forces from the cosmos radiated onto the earth, shaping the bodies of human beings and their destinies. Babylonian culture combined this mystical-clairvoyant view of these forces with a close study of the movements of the stars. The Babylonians developed mathematical models to determine the planetary orbits and created the division of the circle into 360 degrees. Zodiacal forces were an important reference point for astronomy, and also for medicine, until the Middle Ages. Rudolf Steiner took this picture of the zodiac and correlated it with the different formative forces.

A human being thinks a thought. The thought comes from an inner spiritual activity. The thought comes into the world through *a deed*. The instrument used to perform this act is the human musculoskeletal system. Speech also expresses thoughts through the muscular movement of the vocal cords, palate, tongue and lips. The human being enters reality through movement and speech.

The speaking person's thought thus finds its corporeity. It incarnates itself into the word. Based on this principle, Steiner developed eurythmy as an art of movement which makes speech visible. He divided the consonants into twelve groups, which he assigned to the zodiac. He discovered the vowels, as carriers of soul expression, in the rhythmically moving, harmonious world of the planets.

We encounter the principle of twelvefoldness in different contexts. In everyday experience, we encounter it by dividing time into the twelve hours of the day and the twelve months of the year. In Christian tradition we speak of the twelve apostles, while anthroposophic spiritual science differentiates between twelve senses [→ Chapter "From the Question of Meaning in Cancer to the Care of the Senses"] and Rudolf Steiner described twelve world views.[4]

Twelvefoldness expresses a wholeness whose parts each represent an aspect of the whole. Thus, the world of appearances can be grasped with every sense organ, but the respective sense conveys only the qualities that are accessible to it. The world appears to the eye as light and color, to the ear as sound. Each worldview interprets the world but focuses only on a certain meaning or thought form. The zodiac is the sum of the cosmic forces that shape the human being and human destiny. The twelve apostles represent the typical characteristics and social tasks found in a human community.

Twelvefoldness is not an empirically counted quantity. The number of Christ's disciples was significantly higher than the twelve designated apostles, the number of cosmic formative powers is by no means limited to twelve, not even the number of possible worldviews is limited to twelve, and even current physiology of the senses now counts more than twelve of them. The number twelve represents a certain quality which is expressed in mathematical peculiarities. Twelve is divisible by the numbers 1–2–3–4–6–12. As a result, on a circular surface that is divided into twelve parts, there are again clear whole-number units: the day (12 hours), the morning and afternoon (2 x 6 hours), the quarter day (4 x 3 hours). By multiplying twelve by five, the only number which twelve cannot be divided by, we obtain the familiar unit of the hour, with its 12 x 5 = 60 minutes. Sixty can now also be divided by 5–10–15–20–30, with all the advantages of the clarity that we value so much on a clock face. 12 x 30 days results in a year with 360 days, which corresponds to the division of the circle into 360 degrees. 360 can be divided 24 times into whole numbers.

In the twelve nursing gestures, the wholeness of nursing appears in twelve inner movements. From these movements, all further nursing gestures can be derived as transitional or hybrid forms, or can be expressed in one of the seven basic nursing moods. This results in several gestures in practice. The nurse's personality shapes each gesture. His personality ultimately shapes his relationship with the patient. The archetypes from which this individual relationship is derived can be found in the gestures of nursing care. Rudolf Steiner once described worldviews as thoughts that high angelic beings think. People think in thoughts—these high angelic beings think in worldviews.[5]

When people act as nurses, they use cosmic creative powers. These are described in the twelve nursing gestures.

A relationship between the gestures of nursing care and the zodiac results from the zodiac's archetypal images. The zodiac offers pictorial expressions of forces that can be found in nature, in the inner space of the soul and in the formation of the human form. This is the indirect correlation that is meant when gestures are assigned to zodiacal forces. There is no deterministic cause-effect principle, as simple astrology postulates, at all. The concrete assignment of nursing care gestures to individual zodiac images is illustrated by the relationship between the gestures of sounds and the forces of the zodiac discovered by Rudolf Steiner. The gestures used in eurythmy show a surprising relationship to the inner movements expressed in the nursing gestures. Since gestures are the language of the hands and the body, resorting to eurythmy as "visible speech" seems to make quite obvious sense.

9.   The basic nursing moods and the planets

Just as the planets move within the horizon of the zodiac, so does the inner mood of the nurse modify the nursing gestures. These basic inner moods are described below.

In the language of eurythmy, the soul moods correspond to vowels and vowel combinations A (pronounced "ah," Venus—sympathizing); E ("ey," Mars—guiding); I ("ee," Mercury—mediating); O ("oh," Jupiter—organizing); U ("oo," Saturn—accompanying); AU ("aw," Sun—being interested); EI ("ahy," Moon—serving).

9.1   ⊙ Sun quality—Being interested—Vowel AU

If we look at the circle of nursing gestures, we find that terms such as love, compassion and companionship are missing. You can't find them, because love is not a gesture. There is a quality of love when you are really interested in a person. Light and warmth are woven into your interest. In this sense, interest—not curiosity!—is a metamorphosis of love. It forms the basis for all gestures as a spiritual force. Love and interest permeate the whole zodiac like the sun.

9.2   ♂ Mars quality—Leading, Guiding—Vowel E

Mars works in courage, strength and will. It represents the quality of doing something purposefully up to the end, e.g., when we show a patient a way forward during a crisis. Mars knows the way. Leading is the Mars quality in nursing care. When you apply a mustard compress, you need to know exactly what will happen. If the patient thinks it is burning him in the first two minutes, we need to know: no, there won't be any burns. And we need to know when to terminate the treatment.

9.3 Venus quality—Sympathy, Empathy—Vowel A

Venus is the opposite of the Mars quality. Venus wants to be open, to listen and to understand what is going on in the patient. It wants to pay full attention to his condition. Empathy is a Venus quality. It connects with the patient more strongly than the power of interest. It doesn't go ahead, it waits.

9.4 Jupiter quality—Organizing—Vowel O

Zeus-Jupiter is the father of the gods, enthroned on Mount Olympus. He represents the quality of having an overview, combined with creative power. In nursing care, this is the quality of organizing: we shape events from an overview, planning nursing care, coordinating staff, perceiving what the individual needs, always keeping an eye on the whole.

9.5 Mercury quality—Mediating—Vowel I

Mercury is the god of doctors, thieves and merchants. It stands for flexibility and mobility. Mercury is the messenger of the gods, who puts people in relation to each other and mediates between the heavenly and the earthly world. Wherever mediation occurs, this element is at work. This mood is particularly pronounced among young staff members. Example: a patient rings the bell. The nurse comes to the patient's room. A thermos jug is on the table, the patient wants fresh tea. The nurse takes the thermos flask; the neighboring patient waves and needs the bedpan. The nurse puts the thermos jug back down, picks up the bedpan, pushes it under, wipes it off, takes the bedpan in one hand and the thermos jug in the other, opens the door with his elbow, puts down the thermos jug, places the bedpan in the sink, heats the water for the tea, and answers the bell in room seven. He then takes the bedpan out of the sink, puts tea bags in the teapot, etc.

9.6 Saturn quality—Accompanying—Vowel U

Saturn, the outermost planet of our solar system visible to the naked eye, takes 28 years to go once around the sun. In Roman mythology, he is portrayed as the Janus-faced god, with one face that looks towards the past and one that looks towards the future. In the Saturn mood, we trust in development because we know about the forces that work in our patients, in illness and in destiny. From this certainty we gain the ability to accompany our patients. This accompanying is more than just taking someone to the toilet. Respect, attention and consideration are the most important qualities of Saturn. In the Saturn mood, the will to heal is characterized by perseverance and seriousness. Knowledge of the various routes is the basic prerequisite for being able to accompany someone. Accompaniment has a different temporal dimension than the Mars quality of leadership. When leading, the nurse is very active. In the Saturn mood, there is already confidence that doors will open.

9.7 Moon quality—Mirroring, Serving—Vowel EI

The moon reflects sunlight. In nursing care there are two forms of mirroring—sympathetic and antipathic mirroring. In sympathetic mirroring, you don't notice that you're mirroring the patient. This is the case, for example, when you suddenly fall into using the patient's dialect or when you believe that you recognize symptoms of illness in yourself which you have discovered in the patient. It is a very important ability to be able to participate in the life forces and emotional state of the other person, but when it happens unconsciously it can lead to a source of illness in the helping professions due to the lack of boundaries.

We know antipathic mirroring as a method of conducting conversations. We reflect the patient's point of view or tell him how he has affected the environment. This mirroring is antipathetic because it does not adopt the intention of the other person. It throws the other person back on themselves.

Antipathetic and sympathetic forms of mirroring can be transformed. Then the mirroring turns into service. We contribute it as a tool for the person. We lend him a hand, our ear, we listen to his intentions. We do whatever he needs. The transformation from mirroring to serving happens through a conscious decision.

For many nurses, these seven basic moods of nursing care sound more familiar than the terms we used to describe the gestures. They are closer to us because we experience our inner moods more intensely and consciously than the formative powers of the zodiac.

The basic nursing moods complete the cosmic image of nursing care. The sun's quality permeates the entire zodiac. Only interest, only love makes all nursing gestures visible. Love conveys and strengthens the power of each gesture.

There are gestures that harmonize particularly well with certain basic moods of nursing care. For example, the Mars force supports stimulation. Awakening and affirming can be carried out in the Saturn mood. Schematically, the assignment of the planetary forces to the zodiacal gestures can be illustrated as follows:

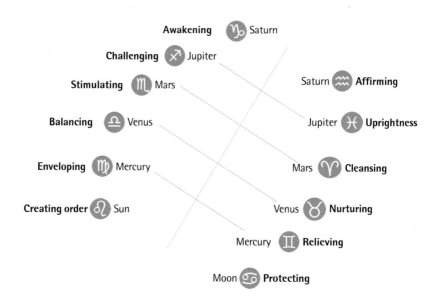

Fig. 6: The planetary forces and their correlation with the zodiac

10. Overview of nursing gestures

Aries ♈ W	Cleansing
Other terms	Removing impurities (feces, sweat, urine), wound cleansing, clarifying conversation
Examples for cancer patients	*Body* • Physical cleansing, oral hygiene, intimate hygiene • Wound cleansing, e.g., for ulcerating wounds • Cleansing after heavy sweating, chemotherapy, etc.	*Soul and spirit* • Letting the patient express themselves • Allowing tears • Consciously leaving the old behind, letting go • Reviewing the day's essentials • Previewing the day after waking up • Morning toilet as a ritual to prepare for the day

Activities relative to the human fourfold nature	*Physical*: removing impurities. *Etheric*: recognizing the pure, the new, the shapeable. *Soul*: catharsis (allowing crying). *'I'*: "confessing," forgiving.
Character of the gesture	Attention is paid to the cleanliness that lies below any contamination. Residues that conceal what is essential are carefully removed. The cleansed area now appears in its own light. It emerges from concealment.
The gesture as a force field	When an item has been washed properly, it is clean again and can be reused. Washing as part of body care protects against skin infections (gesture of *protecting*), stimulates the circulation (gesture of *stimulating*) and ideally restores the self-image of the washed person (gesture of *affirming*). In the gesture of cleansing, the purified area is freed from everything that does not belong to its true nature. In this way, its possibilities reappear.
Mood	Joyful expectation of what is appearing. Sober distance or objective interest in what is to be removed. Controlled, careful, guided and precise action.

Zodiac mood	In spring buds break open and new life appears. The snow thaws and nature blossoms again. It is the time of the equinox, the time when the new appears. From this mood we look at cleansing. Washing not only aims to remove dirt, it also intends to bring out the underlying new. The symbol for Aries can be interpreted in two ways. On the one hand, we recognize the horns of the ram, the power, the pushing, the breaking out, and on the other hand, we can see it as two opening cotyledons from which the new appears. The caring hand removes the old to help the new appear.
What is to be avoided?	Superficial "wiping around," "whitewashing" of impurities, ruthless scrubbing.
Self-care	To be able to deal with a situation in a new and unbiased way, I must leave the old behind. My attention is then only focused on the new. A good way to get rid of the old is to wash one's hands or take a shower or bath after work. Any conversation that I conduct in such a way that I am allowed to express the past, a matter that is troubling me, without holding on to it, also clears my eye for what is to come. If disgust overcomes me in the cleansing process, it helps to keep the filth or pollution factually distant, while looking with pleasure at the underlying purity that wants to appear.
Meditation	*"Now imagine the green sap flowing through the plant as an expression of the chaste forces of growth which lack any passion. And then imagine how the red blood flows through the human being's veins as an expression of the urges, desires and passions. All this is conjured up before the soul as a vivid thought. Then imagine further how the human being is capable of development in that he can purify and cleanse his urges and passions by working with the higher capacities of his soul. Imagine how what is inferior in these urges and passions is destroyed and then brought to birth again at a higher level. In this case the blood can be imagined as an expression of the cleansed and purified urges and passions. Look at the rose and say to yourself: 'In the red sap of the rose I see the color of the green sap transformed into the red; and the red rose, like the green leaf, follows the laws of growth which lack any passion. So may the red of the rose become a symbol for me of the blood in the human being which is now an expression of the urges and passions that have been purified, that have laid aside their lower qualities and in their chasteness now resemble the forces which are at work in the red rose.'"[6]*

Taurus ♉ R	Nurturing
Other terms	To nurse = to feed an infant—nurturing, encouraging, helping, nourishing
Examples	Preparing food, serving food, doing something (materially) good for someone. Reading fairy tales or poems as "soul food"; prayer or meditation as "spiritual nourishment."

Examples for cancer patients	*Body*	*Soul and spirit*
	• Suitable selection and preparation of food for cancer cachexia or opiate nausea • Considering preferences • Administering small portions in an appealing way • Administering digestive medication (e.g., *Amara drops* (Weleda) or *Gentiana comp. pillules* (WALA))	• Dignified administration of food, including tube feeding or parenteral nutrition • "Soul food," e.g., via conversation, reading (fairy tales!), literature recommendations • "Spiritual" nourishment, e.g., communion • Grace

Activities relative to the human fourfold nature	*Physical*: serving food, feeding. *Etheric*: ensuring the quality of the food, providing it at rhythmic intervals, shaping the surroundings and ensuring tranquility; sensory impressions (smell, taste), images. *Soul*: considering the person's expectations. *'I'*: sharing, community, communion.
Character of the gesture	Everything that establishes mankind's material connection with the earth belongs to this gesture. We take into account not only the nutrients, but in particular the type of preparation and administration as well as the conditions under which optimal digestion and incorporation into the body can be achieved. Time, warmth, silence, calmness and attention are as if woven into the nourishing substances.
The gesture as a force field	The administration of food ensures the building up of and preservation of the body. The gesture of nurturing establishes a relationship between the substances—as they are formed in the plant kingdom from light, water and carbon dioxide—and the social process of sharing.

Mood	Giving pleasure. Respect for the food. A feeling for the foreignness of food and for the difficulty of the (unhealthy) person to accept it and make it his own. Patience with the patient's digestive processes. "Love goes through the stomach." "Human beings do not live on bread alone."
Zodiac mood	Cattle, as archetypal metabolic animals, transform plant matter into milk (cow) and muscle meat (bull), which they give to human beings in abundance for nutrition. Oxen carry loads, plow the soil and multiply human power. Plants receive light from the cosmos... The light is condensed in animals which absorb plant matter. With their body formation, animals make this cosmic power of light more similar to human beings. With their physical strength, they help mankind to cultivate the earth. The eurythmy gesture for Taurus is 'R'. Eurythmy therapy uses this sound to treat many metabolic diseases.
What is to be avoided?	Impatience, despair, if food is refused in the form offered, that is, cannot be ingested. Overfeeding, in order to enjoy the feeling of doing something "good" for someone.
Self–care	When I realize that nutrition gives me strength for the preservation of my body, I don't eat just for the pleasure of satisfying a need, but I learn to feel gratitude and responsibility for the quality of food. This is expressed in most mealtime prayers. This attitude avoids unrhythmic, habitual eating, as well as eating out of boredom or frustration. I look for non-material nourishment when I become aware of something lacking in my soul. Alternating between lack and abundance of food teaches me to share.
Meditation	*The sun gives* *The plants light,* *Because the sun* *Loves the plants.* *So does a human being* *Give soul light* *To others,* *When he loves them.*[7]

Gemini ♊ H	Relieving
Other terms	Relieving somebody of something, substituting, doing what the other cannot do, helping
Examples	Exploring the person's needs. Doing anything for patients that relieves them. Bed rest. Warming up, giving food, cleansing, dressing, establishing relationships, etc.

Examples for cancer patients	*Body*	*Soul and spirit*
	• Relief from physical exertion or if there are limitations due to metasta-sis, pain • Relief after surgery • Relief during and after chemotherapy or radiation therapy • Pain therapy	• Releasing from convention • Assuming obligations • Reminding the person of appointments • Decreasing or redefining responsibility • Reallocating tasks • Forgiving

Activities relative to the human fourfold nature	*Physical*: relieving someone of a physical burden. *Etheric*: lifting something into lightness, clearing something up, lightening a load. *Soul*: relieving someone of a worry, dealing with something for someone. *'I'*: representing someone, taking responsibility.
Character of the gesture	The all-round neediness of a sick, injured or handicapped person calls forth the gesture of wanting to help from great depth. First, we need to recognize the areas where help is necessary. They are found in physical, mental/emotional and spiritual realms. The nurse's inclination to help comes into play. The gesture pervades all care activities. Similar to the gesture of nurturing, it conveys to the person in need of help that he is being cared for and that he can use his power for healing and regeneration or for reflection and cognitive activities.
The gesture as a force field	When you relieve someone of a burden or help them, you reduce the effort that they have to put in. As a gesture, relieving is a social bond that allows the recipient of the help to use previously bound forces for something else. This gesture forms the basis for a society based on division of labor.

Mood	A cordial and joyful willingness to act for the needy, taking all the person's needs seriously. Selflessness, matter-of-fact actions, working love. Bearing warmth and light in your heart and bringing to the needy what they need.
Zodiac mood	A warm, cheerful spring atmosphere. Nature is mild, kind to human beings. Ease. Everything grows, blossoms, seems to want to go beyond itself. Nature produces excess forces. It makes people inclined to look beyond themselves. Hearts open. When you try to make a relieving gesture, you will in some way move your arms and hands away from you, maybe throw them into the air. This is the eurythmic gesture for the sound 'H'. You need strength yourself to relieve someone. You need firm ground to stand on to make a radiating gesture or make things lighter. The figure of the twins impressively shows how one supports the other and both pursue a common goal. This mood is created when you offer natural, joyful help to someone.
What is to be avoided?	Paralyzing the patient's independence through excessive care and thus keeping them dependent. Helper syndrome. Overlooking impulses for independence. Ignoring real needs and achieving "peace" via distractions or substitute satisfaction.
Self-care	The danger of the gesture lies in overestimating one's own strength. Only if I am mindful of my physical, mental and spiritual condition can I help without becoming a burden or danger to myself and others. Only when I am firmly rooted in my own body, soul and spirit do I find the strength to turn away from myself and be selflessly there for others. Only if I know my strengths and weaknesses can I relieve others. Being fixated on one's own powers is more of a hindrance. It usually leads to overestimation or underestimation. By recognizing and showing my own need for help, I become a social person. When I realize what I owe to others, a sense for the neediness in others awakens in me.

Meditation	*Within the heart there lives* *In radiant light* *The human will to help.* *Within the heart there works* *In warmth-giving power* *The human force of love.* *Then let us bear* *The soul's whole will* *In heart-warmth* *And heart-light* *Then we work to heal* *Those in need of healing* *Through God's sense of grace.*[8]

Cancer ♋ F	Protecting	
Other terms	Defending, shielding, averting, keeping outside	
Examples	Keeping stress, disturbances and irritations away from the patient. Disinfection, wearing a mouthguard, pressure relief for bedsore prophylaxis. Screening, closing doors, cancelling appointments, switching off the telephone, maintaining visiting hours.	
Examples for cancer patients	*Body* • Hygiene, wound disinfection • Isolation for patients with weakened immune systems (e.g., after cytostasis, radiation therapy) • Pressure relief for bedsore prophylaxis • Acid buffer for ulcer prophylaxis	*Soul and spirit* • Allowing visits only in agreement with the patient • Representing the interests of the patient to others • Maintaining data protection, confidentiality • Enabling privacy
Activities relative to the human fourfold nature	*Physical*: avoiding hazards (prophylaxis), keeping something at a distance. *Etheric*: informing the patient and radiating confidence. *Soul*: thinking ahead. *'I'*: being a guard.	

Character of the gesture	Our attention is directed outwards. The thing to be protected moves almost entirely out of our consciousness. We work exclusively on the environment. The thing to be protected is at the center, the nurse turns her back towards it and creates a boundary. She represents the interests of the patient externally. The patient should not have to apply his strength to isolating himself.
The gesture as a force field	Protection preserves limits. Defense against dangers ensures existence. Warding off as a gesture creates a field of undivided attention towards the surroundings. It forms the guardian's field of action, where security and peace are possible.
Mood	The nurse does not have a direct relationship with the patient. The work of "defense" absorbs him. He lives in danger of forgetting his inner relationship with the patient and dealing only with external matters. There is the problem of forgetting and endangering what is to be protected in the zeal of providing defense. Level-headedness is required in this zeal.
Zodiac mood	The summer solstice. The air shimmers in the sun's heat. The heat makes you dazed. You travel far away, make new acquaintances, open yourself up to the new. You exhale yourself, you're outside and not much within yourself. Your attention is completely devoted to the periphery. The crab is an impressive symbol of fending off, with its armor plating and simultaneous hypersensitivity to vibrations and shadows. We find this mood in our foresighted recognition of what might endanger the patient.
What is to be avoided?	Fear of disturbances or danger. Restricting care to only this gesture of protecting, out of fear of all kinds. Attempting to prevent any contact with what is "harmful" and thus isolating the patient.
Self-care	Anything weak and undeveloped needs protection. I put it at risk in the heat of the moment. When I put armor around it, it is in danger of suffocating. Most of all, fear ruins my defenses. If I want to protect or defend something, I must always be aware of the appropriateness of the means. Often, I harm myself or the one I want to protect when I blindly destroy my opponent or a disturbance. The best way to protect myself is to go my way calmly, compassionately and decisively. It is not by fearfully trying to assert myself that I protect myself, but by relying on the forces of renewal that form a firm but dynamic boundary from within.

Meditation	*(Thinking of my left foot)* *My I carries me* *(Thinking of my right foot)* *My I holds me* *(Thinking of my left hand)* *My I protects itself* *(Thinking of my right hand)* *My I defends itself* *Carrying power* *Holding power* *Protection and defense* *I make these four* *Into one* *In my heart.*[9]

Leo ♌ T D	Creating order	
Other terms	Creating space	
Examples	Preparing the patient's room, the nursing facilities, tidying up, sorting. Dealing internally with upcoming changes. Making plans.	
Examples for cancer patients	*Body* • Patient-friendly furnishing of the hospital or other room • Timing of the daily routine, taking into account therapies, social contacts and solitude • Maintenance of all sensory areas through the shaping of the premises	*Soul and spirit* • Imagining physical and mental-spiritual wholeness and integrity in relation to the "space requirement" of the tumor, being fragmented by metastases, being mutilated by organ amputation or being "poisoned" (chemotherapy, radiation therapy) • Finding your own middle ground between setting limits and devotion
Activities relative to the human fourfold nature	*Physical*: tidying up, arranging, creating space. *Etheric*: shaping, beauty, aesthetics, rhythm. *Soul*: systematizing, formulating rules, setting priorities. *'I'*: ruling without force.	

Character of the gesture	Our attention wanders from the details to our surroundings and back again. Space is created between the center and the surrounding area. Things have their place or will be put in their place. Order is the harmonious relationship between the parts and the whole. Rhythm creates order in time. The result for the patient is familiarity, security and clarity. Habits are encouraged. The person finds their place, feels welcomed and wanted.
The gesture as a force field	Tidying up and making plans are tasks of organizing. They provide clarity and reliability. When order or space is created, a force field arises as a gesture which shapes a place in such a way that people involuntarily let themselves be guided by this order in their actions. In contrast, a disorderly environment makes things chaotic.
Mood	"Blazing enthusiasm." The lion who rules his territory with strength and power. Rule as the ability to connect the whole with the individual.
Zodiac mood	In the gesture of creating space and order, we are alternately in the periphery with our consciousness and then again at the point where we stand. We encounter this mood when we shape things from an overview and with creative joy. Contemplation and action are in a harmonious relationship. We act artistically, aesthetically and creatively. We create an active and appropriate order in this way.
What is to be avoided?	Pedantic order, inflexible planning and rigid ideas.
Self-care	When I don't see any room for shaping things myself, I feel unfree. My actions are then determined by the outside world. When I only live in the future or in my ideals, I cannot shape the present. My circumstances get into disorder. I can strengthen myself when I fill myself with an ideal and take the first step immediately. Looking back on the day, I realize what I have created and what has remained in disorder. I widen my gaze and start every day anew with small and definite steps. When I find order in myself, I create space for new things.

Meditation	*Point and circle*
	 In the evening
	      In me is God
	 In the morning
	      I am in God[10]

Virgo ♍ D	Enveloping
Other terms	Protecting, enfolding, warming, building a nest, incubating
Examples	At birth, the child leaves the protective mantel of the uterus. She comes into the care of her parents. She is picked up in their hands, wrapped in cloths, taken into their arms, dressed. Cover the patient, treat him with Rhythmical Einreibung, hold him. Create an envelope of warmth.
Examples for cancer patients	*Body* • Full-body Rhythmical Einreibung for the patient to have an intensified experience of his own body boundaries and physical wholeness. • Providing an enclosure of warmth via external applications and clothing for constitutionally weak or rigid warmth organisms • "Reading" the patient's needs "in their eyes."	*Soul and spirit* • Security through friendly, warm and interested attention • Carrying the patient in your mind
Activities relative to the human fourfold nature	*Physical*: enveloping, clothing, embracing, wrapping. *Etheric*: loving, patient, tolerating, allowing to thrive, getting used to, warming up. *Soul*: making an interior, taking something inside. *'I'*: faithfulness, responsibility.
Character of the gesture	In the gesture of "creating space," the patient receives a place where he can be and develop. The gesture creates space for development. In the virgin's mantle are the forces for growth and development. This is a prerequisite for organ maturation, regeneration and growth.
The gesture as a force field	Enfolding, embracing, building a nest are activities that provide for warmth and protection, and they prepare space for development. The gesture of enveloping does not have a mental effect, but rather creates forms and shapes. It is a kind of "creation," similar to when we scoop water from a spring with our hands, thereby creating something separate from the general flow of water.

Mood	The gesture comes from the middle. It is usually carried out with great sympathy. Rudolf Steiner called it "sensible disillusionment" to characterize the gesture in eurythmy. This matter-of-factness protects against too great a mental overload of the protective mantel. The nurse perceives her own boundary and includes the patient. The power for this comes from her own relationship with her surroundings. Zodiac mood
Zodiac Mood	The virgin bears the fruits of the earth in her arms. She receives what has come to earth from the cosmos. Her abdominal cavity is a protective enclosure in which the child, having come from the spirit realm, can thrive and mature.
What is to be avoided?	"Smothering" the patient with enveloping protection. Getting into symbiosis with him. Enjoying the dependence of the patient. Seeing him as property.
Self-care	I can only give someone enveloping protection when I feel surrounded by beings and forces that sustain and strengthen me. The care of my own mantle of protection is therefore a prerequisite for giving others warmth and security. My protection is cultivated by being attentive to my health, to purity in my soul and by cultivating a living relationship with the spiritual powers to whom I owe my existence.
Meditation	*May my love be the sheaths* *That now surround you—* *Cooling your heat,* *Warming your cold—* *Sacrificially woven in!* *Live borne by love,* *Light-gifted, upwards![11]*

Libra ♎ c	Balancing
Other terms	Harmonizing, making rhythmical, regulating
Examples	Adapting clothing to body heat, compensating for lack of fluid, keeping waking and resting phases in balance. Draining congestion. Creating a primal image of "living equilibrium" by means of Rhythmical Einreibung.

Examples for cancer patients	Body	Soul and spirit
	• Rhythmical daily routine • Balancing out physical overreactions (sweating, chills, permanent fatigue, insomnia, loss of appetite, cravings, etc.)	• Finding a rhythm between being alone and being with others • Rhythm between concentration and relaxation • Rhythm between thinking and acting
Activities relative to the human fourfold nature	*Physical*: weighing, measuring, replacing. *Etheric*: finding the right (human) measure, complementing. *Soul*: justice, finding a just balance, mediating. 'I': finding your individual center; knowing when to act and when not to act.	
Character of the gesture	Removing something where there is too much—adding something where there is too little. Any one-sidedness is inwardly imitated and increased until awareness of a countermovement arises. The path of perception is empathy, the gesture appears as an inner "complementary afterimage."	
The gesture as a force field	Balancing activities create balance. The result is temporary rest and satisfaction. As a gesture, maintaining uprightness keeps the nurse in a state of constant attention and movement. Just as standing upright is a continuous, semi-conscious balancing activity of the muscular system, this gesture creates a kind of dance field in which one's own point of view, actions and rest are continuously renewed in relation to the other dancers (the therapeutic team and the patients).	
Mood	Compassion, balancing out one-sidedness and creating a dynamic center.	
Zodiac mood	The autumn equinox. Libra aims to compensate for any polarities. Scales do not produce the center itself, but rather display it. Harmonies, well-proportioned conditions, peace and justice emerge from this mood.	
What is to be avoided?	Not being able to endure extremes (e.g., fever). Aiming for static, predefined averages. Sudden emotional roller coasters. Falling from one extreme to another.	

Self-care	Only when I find my way back again and again to my own center can I lovingly recognize one-sidedness in others and create a balance. When I lack my center, then I tend to project my own ideas and needs onto others. How do I find my center? I find it by becoming acquainted with extremes and experiencing that I can assert my essence in the oscillation between devotion and egoism. I nurture my center in mindfulness of the rhythms of my body, soul and spirit.
Meditation	*If you want to know yourself,* *Look into the world in all directions.* *If you want to know the world,* *Look into all your own depths.*[12]

Scorpio ♏ S SH	Stimulating	
Other terms	Irritating, suggesting, provoking	
Examples	Washing the face, hands, feet or the whole body should be stimulating. The gentle sensation of touch, the water, the temperature, the rhythm of movement, the smell of a bath additive stimulate the circulation and warming of the skin. External applications stimulate life processes. Consciously managed conflicts can stir up mental processes.	
Examples for cancer patients	*Body* • Stimulating the body functions with washing, baths, compresses, Rhythmical Einreibung according to need (acute or constitutional), e.g., in the area of respiration • Body warmth • Nourishment, digestion • Excretions • Wound healing	*Soul and spirit* • Asking personal questions • Confrontation, reflection of problematic behavior and ways of thinking • Suggestions for stimulating literature (e.g., biographies or fairy tales)
Activities relative to the human fourfold nature	*Physical*: setting external stimuli. *Etheric*: giving impulses through thinking. *Soul*: stimulating through feeling. *'I'*: using the transformative power of an event.	

Character of the gesture	Using targeted, intentional, often selective gestures (movements, touch) to evoke a certain reaction. Our consciousness is directed outwards. The gesture comes from the outside and provokes a reaction from within. "Friction generates heat."
The gesture as a force field	Irritations and stimuli trigger reactions. The more targeted the intervention, the more predictable the result. Stimulating as a gesture generates attention and sets into motion what was at rest. It bears the signature of the soul, which provokes rhythmic movement in the etheric like the wind stirring up waves.
Mood	Alert, precise observation and targeted, measured action. Attentive, patient waiting for a reaction.
Zodiac mood	When you apply a mustard compress, administer an injection or say something ironic, such "stimulation, irritation, provocation" is initially based on a slightly antipathic tendency, even if you mean well. There is always a mild poisoning in such a gesture of stimulation, which is justified only because we are aiming at the patient's metabolic response. The stimulus is followed by a reaction, the provocation by a change in behavior. This is aptly portrayed in the image of the scorpion as a creature armed with a venomous stinger. In ancient times this zodiac sign was called the eagle. The eagle embodies all-embracing, "heavenly" intelligence. Falling to the earth, it transforms itself into the poisonous power of the scorpion, the image of the materialistic intelligence of our age bound to the earth. The scorpion and the eagle are both creatures of the senses. They sharply sense any sensory stimuli, and when a stimulus threshold is exceeded, they respond with a targeted, reflex-like reaction. The scorpion stabs, the eagle falls on its prey. There is no emotional weighing. Their attention to the targeted object seems perfect. The accuracy of their reaction is precisely calculated and measured out. Eventful, rhythmic life seems to be pushed out of this process. It appears cool, mechanical, dead. The zodiac sign appears as a dragon on the north portal of Chartres Cathedral, and in the Judeo-Christian tradition it symbolizes a fallen angel. In nature, life dies in late autumn. The landscape and nature appear in cool colors. Light and warmth are created in the human soul.
What is to be avoided?	Acting out of emotion. Pleasure in the effect and the prompt reaction. Too frequent use of the gesture.

Self-care	An inner motive has the most stimulating effect. Movement arises from it. Since I form the motive myself, the activity is all mine (gesture of awakening). When I look for external stimulation, e.g., cool water, hot coffee, an inspiring book, I nurture myself.
Meditation	*Victorious spirit* *Flame through the faintness* *Of hesitant souls.* *Burn up ego's self-craving,* *Ignite compassion,* *So that selflessness,* *The life-stream of mankind* *Will surge as the source* *Of spirit's rebirth.*[13]

Sagittarius ↗ G K	Challenging
Other terms	Expecting something, encouraging
Examples	Activating care, mobilization, training, exercises, overcoming resistance and obstacles. Gaining strength through overcoming.
Examples for cancer patients	*Body* • Expecting physical activity (offering relief in the acute phase! In the convalescence phase, balance between challenging and relieving. In the rehabilitation phase making demands within the patient's limits.) • Sports • Demanding independence • Training	*Soul and spirit* • Expecting someone to deal with tabooed topics • Expecting socially adequate behavior • Expecting an independent search for self-help groups, personal perspectives, etc. • Expecting someone to fulfill their commitments • Practicing
Activities relative to the human fourfold nature	*Physical*: demanding physical exertion from someone, expecting something of them. *Etheric*: trying something unfamiliar, changing habits. *Soul*: going to the limits, accepting and withstanding conflicts. *'I'*: taking on tasks, setting one's own limits.

Character of the gesture	The patient is believed to be capable of something. We expect him to do what he can do on his own. For this purpose, it is necessary to know the limits and resources of the patient.
The gesture as a force field	Mobilization, exercises and training maintain, promote and strengthen existing resources. As a gesture, making demands acts as an expectation and preparatory force. There is a mood of new beginnings.
Mood	Confidence in the patient's abilities—courage, patience.
Zodiac mood	To challenge a patient, we must know how much strength is available to him and what the purpose of making the demand is. The relationship between strength and target is very well expressed in the zodiac image of the archer. Greek and Persian mythology depicts these two aspects in the image of a centaur: a human being who uses his mind and aligns his arrow with the goal, and a horse's body which symbolizes will and power. This mood can be encountered in the feeling of playfully using energy, in the act of practicing and gaining competence.
What is to be avoided?	Mobilization without a motive. Training without a goal. Overstrain caused by toughening. Unreflected transferring of performance standards to the patient. Creating time grids. Demands and expectations of the patient. Convenience ("He can do that himself!").
Self-care	Every day I experience myself limited in my abilities and powers. If I acknowledge these limits as unalterable, I am in danger of stagnating. If I run blindly against these boundaries, I'll use myself up. Patience, level-headedness, cheerfulness and trust in the goal enable me to train all the skills and powers that I really need. If not today, then tomorrow.

Meditation	*The wishes of the soul are springing,* *The deeds of the will are thriving,* *The fruits of life are maturing.* *I feel my destiny,* *My destiny finds me.* *I feel my star,* *My star finds me.* *I feel my goals in life,* *My goals in life are finding me.* *My soul and the great world are one.* *Life grows more radiant about me,* *Life grows more arduous for me,* *Life grows more abundant within me.* *Strive for peace,* *Live in peace,* *Love the peace.*[14]

Capricorn ♑ L	Awakening	
Other terms	Preparing transitions	
Examples	Awakening in the morning. Helping the patient understand his disease. Bringing new possibilities of experience to him through sense impressions, pictures or thoughts. Asking questions. Accompaniment through various biographical phases and dying. Giving the patient time to wake up.	
Examples for cancer patients	*Body* • Making the patient aware of their body (false and favoring postures) • Interpreting body signals	*Soul and spirit* • Awareness of body, soul and spirit • Asking questions • Discovering what is hidden • Promoting understanding of the disease • If necessary, addressing painful and distressing issues

Activities relative to the human fourfold nature	*Physical*: waking the person up from sleep, helping him fall asleep. *Etheric*: awakening thinking. *Soul*: awakening feeling. *'I'*: awakening willing.
Character of the gesture	It is about accompanying and conveying the way out of the unconsciousness of sleep into an awake consciousness of the world and oneself. Sense impressions slowly approach the awakening person from the periphery. It is the way out of the darkness of unconsciousness into the light of the world of the senses and the world of thoughts. It is important for the person waking up to come step by step to himself and not only partially, like a morning grouch.
The gesture as a force field	The activity of awakening generates consciousness. It creates a field of attention for different degrees and levels of consciousness. It is like a quiet question: "What inner place are you in?"
Mood	Strongly feeling the patient's state of consciousness. Joy in the lighting up of consciousness. Patience. Equilibrium of thinking, feeling and willing. Self-knowledge.
Zodiac mood	In the language of the zodiac, the image for the process of awakening is the ibex. It is an animal that climbs from the depths of the lush, green valleys up to the bright mountain regions. The theme is: from darkness to light. This zodiac sign represents the winter solstice. The outer light disappears and inner light rises up. In old paintings the ibex is sometimes depicted as a hermaphrodite or with a reptilian tail. This symbolizes the change from an unconscious earthbound state to the bright consciousness of awakening.
What is to be avoided?	Impatience, causing irritation. One-sided intellectual demands.
Self-care	Being interested in the world, in other people, in the big context and in the small things of everyday life is the mood in which I find myself. When I wake up for the world, I come to myself. Knowledge of the world becomes self-knowledge. Looking back at the past, I wake up for the forces that have shaped me. When I look to the future, I see the possibilities that the world holds.

Meditation	*In pure beams of light*
	Gleams the Godhood of the world
	In pure love for all beings
	Shines the godliness of my soul
	I rest in the Godhood of the world
	I will find myself
	In the Godhood of the world.[15]

Aquarius ♒ M	Affirming	
Other terms	Comforting, hoping, blessing, taking along the other person from wherever he stands.	
Examples	Accepting the patient as he is. Focusing on his questions and needs and responding in a friendly manner. Fostering courage, consolation. Being consistent.	
Examples for cancer patients	*Body* • Body contact (greeting, holding hands, hugging)	*Soul and spirit* • Consciously perceiving the patient, taking an interest in him • Reaffirming hopes. • Comforting
Activities relative to the human fourfold nature	*Physical*: judging positively, affirming. *Etheric*: seeing opportunities for development *Soul*: formulating criticism constructively and positively. *'I'*: addressing the 'I'.	
Character of the gesture	It is a trinity. Comforting refers to the past aspect, hoping relates to the future and affirming addresses the present. Every action should be based on the conviction that it makes sense. No condition remains the same for all time. The present is the starting point for development. The gesture gives actions optimism and openness to the future. The past is affirmed and viewed from the perspective of change.	
The gesture as a force field	Affirmation, consolation and hope as mental activities are empty of content, for there is nothing said about what is affirmed or what one should hope for. As a gesture, *affirming–comforting–hoping* work precisely because the content is left open. It is not the content, not praise for a particular merit, nor the hope of a probable or probably not occurring outcome that works in the gesture, but a force integrating the past (comfort), present (affirmation) and future (hopefulness), which touches the spiritual origin of the human being.	

Mood	You experience yourself in balance. Faithfulness, empathy. An optimistic mood towards life and destiny.
Zodiac mood	When you affirm or confirm something, you say "hmm." So, benevolence and confirmation can be heard in the sound 'M'. Affirming, hoping and comforting are the tasks of a being that is often portrayed in the zodiac as an angel: the Water Bearer. Cosmic light pouring down on the earth. The angel affirms the human being's free and self-responsible deed.
What is to be avoided?	Inflationary praise. Unfeeling, superficial comfort. Lip service. Sugarcoating. Criticalness.
Self-care	Hope is trust in the future. *"Hope is not the same as optimism. It is not the conviction that something will go well, but rather the certainty that something makes sense, no matter how it ends up."* Václav Havel (1936–2011) I cannot affirm myself, but I can be mindful of what I owe to others. In thankfulness I am aware of the benevolence and confirmation that has been given to me.
Meditation	*The Lord is my shepherd; I shall not want.* *He maketh me to lie down in green pastures:* *he leadeth me beside the still waters.* *He restoreth my soul:* *he leadeth me in the paths of righteousness* *for his name's sake.* *Yea, though I walk through the valley of the shadow of death,* *I will fear no evil: for thou art with me;* *thy rod and thy staff they comfort me.* *Thou preparest a table before me in the presence of mine enemies:* *thou anointest my head with oil; my cup runneth over.* *Surely goodness and mercy shall follow me all the days of my life:* *and I will dwell in the house of the Lord for ever.*[16]

Pisces ♓ N	Uprightness
Other Terms	Raising upright, lifting up
Examples	Lifting up when mobilizing. Back position. Rhythmical Einreibung of the back, with an emphasis on vertebral strokes. Seeking your counterpart. Eye contact. Consciously addressing the person, using their name.
Examples for cancer patients	*Body* • Upright posture in conversation • Going to eye level • Positioning that leaves the view unobstructed • Regular straightening up of a weakened patient *Soul and spirit* • Looking for the free inner core of the person • Being sincere, lovingly telling the truth • Biography work (being interested in the person's intentions, life goals) • Aiming for higher goals
Activities relative to the human fourfold nature	*Physical*: raising the body upright. *Etheric*: pointing towards lightness, striving towards the light. *Soul*: orienting yourself towards ideals. 'I': being sincere, trusting in the victory of truth and goodness.
Character of the gesture	The gesture helps with becoming upright. Like all five of the "activating gestures," raising upright requires activity by the patient. The patient can only erect himself.
The gesture as a force field	In raising themselves up, human beings lift themselves off the ground. Their heads rest paramount on their shoulders, gaining an overview. Their arms and hands are released from the supporting function that these limbs have in four-legged creatures, and are free for gripping, carrying, working. In uprightness human beings experience their 'I'. To be "upright" is "to stand by the truth."
Mood	Awareness of human dignity. Deeply moved by the transcendence and uniqueness of each person and their goals in life. Awareness of a spiritual world. One's own quest for humanity. A feeling of freedom and responsibility.
Zodiac mood	Human beings stand between heaven and earth. They are rooted in the spiritual and connect themselves with the earth. In their uprightness, they are free and thereby responsible. Just as uprightness is anatomically based on the feet, the human hand is an expression of free creative power. The feet and hands are associated with the zodiac sign of Pisces.

What is to be avoided?	Overstrain due to physical raising up of weakened patients. Talking about the patient instead of with him.
Self-care	With every turning to the patient, with every enveloping gesture I move out of my center and my own uprightness. If I do not keep returning to this center, I will lose my own point of view. I can't be a free counterpart to anyone anymore. My muscles become tense if I don't find my uprightness from within. I break when I'm simultaneously driven in two different directions. By being truthful and sincere, I find my direction between necessities and ideals.
Meditation	*From my head to my feet* *I am the image of God,* *From my heart into my hands* *I feel the breath of God.* *When I speak with my mouth* *I follow the will of God.* *When I behold God* *Everywhere, in mother, in father,* *In all dear people,* *In animal and flower,* *In tree and stone,* *Nothing can fill me with fear,* *But only with love for all* *That is around me.*[17]

11. Nursing gestures in practice

The daily routine of nursing is interwoven with gestures. They are always happening. Just as one cannot "not communicate," it is impossible to act without these gestures. They form the focus of nursing care. Each patient needs different gestures. The constant confrontation with new situations, the building up of a force field of order, security and rhythm all demand the nurse's strength. The concept of nursing gestures makes these forces conscious and creates an instrument of professional communication about topics that are otherwise barely discussed. Up to now, the nuances of nursing attitudes have rarely been discussed in teams. They are considered to be "private," and to depend on personal moods and talents. Conflicts arise again and again when one colleague administers a wash more from the gesture of cleansing, another from the gesture of stimulating, a third from the gesture of averting danger, a fourth one without conscious inner orientation, simply as a routine task. Nursing gestures are therefore an important means of vocalizing and agreeing on such matters. This can be done during handovers, patient discussions, ward rounds and in documentation once the concept has been introduced in a team.

To introduce the subject, each month can be given a gesture as a motto. For example, if the gesture of creating order is the "*gesture of the month*" the team can look at order, overviews and conflicts about different views on order. The month can be used to implement reorganizations in learning curve management, logistics or the daily structure. We can congratulate each other on successful order and on newly created space for shaping things.

A broader goal would be to introduce the concept within the framework of nursing planning. The gestures to be applied to the patients can be determined using the questionnaire presented at the beginning of this chapter. Responsibility for defining gestures and the type of documentation should be determined in advance.

But an application of gestures is possible even without conceptual introduction in the team, e.g., by focusing on your inner attitude during a handover. "When caring for this patient, I attach particular importance to making him feel enveloped and protected." Such a statement is usually understandable even for colleagues who do not yet have a conceptual understanding of gestures. Speaking like this will improve the quality of care in the team, because it raises awareness for a hidden level of action.

Another possible application of the gesture concept is to deepen nursing quality and effectiveness individually. "How can I increase my powers of enveloping, uprightness, organizing and giving rhythm to my daily work?" is the question to use in working with nursing care gestures. This path begins with becoming aware of the gestures in our daily work. Only when I discover which gestures I am currently working with can I consciously develop them further (see learning path B). The second step is to choose a gesture and practice it by characterizing an activity, such as washing, Rhythmical Einreibung or giving food. A third step can be meditation on the gesture. This sustainably strengthens the power of the gesture.

The discovery of the qualities described in the gestures is also a useful tool for nurse training. Here, too, there is no need for a formal introduction to the concept. Rather, it can suffice to draw the attention of nursing staff in training to the protective, challenging, awakening or stimulating quality of a particular nursing measure and to name and practice it in concrete terms.

Last but not least, the nursing gestures are a source of strength for nurses themselves. Responsible handling of one's own body, soul and spirit not only sets an example for patients and colleagues. It strengthens physical and mental health. We should not treat ourselves any worse than our patients or the people we look after. (Also not better!) A nurse can have no enveloping effect if he himself is living without a mantle of protection. A chaotic person will hardly have an ordering effect on their environment. In a state of lassitude, you can't be stimulating. A sleeping person does not awaken anyone.

Each simple activity for the patient, be it brushing teeth, tying shoes, each everyday encounter can be lifted into the big context of the zodiac. The more consciously we do everyday things for the patient, the more effective these formative forces become. Creation has not ended; it arises every day anew. We work with these forces of creation in nursing care.

We have looked at two basic nursing gestures: the circle and its counterpart (uprightness). We know the circle (enveloping protection) as the archetype of the human being in the womb. We have seen how a new principle is added after birth: the principle of the person opposite, which leads to the new human being not remaining woven into the context of nature, but leaving it, confronting the world, thinking about it, making it his own and shaping it. This is the decisive difference between human beings and animals. When an animal is born, it does not confront the world, it remains integrated in the whole of nature. The forces of creation continuously shape the animal until it is fully grown.

Human beings develop differently. With them, the creative forces retreat at birth. They leave people free. A human being learns to walk, speak and think not from nature, not from angels, but only from other people. As parents or nurses, after a child is born, we take over part of the work that nature does for animals. When we use these shaping forces consciously, we learn from the cosmos. In this sense, to provide nursing care is to preserve and complete creation. When people don't cultivate the land, when they don't cultivate it continually, when the objects around us are not cared for, then they return to their natural state.

Thus, caregiving has a huge task for the development of the earth, for individual people and for our social community. The significance of nursing care is often misunderstood because it seems to be commonplace and ordinary. We only recognize it when it is lacking—or when we encounter someone who loves nursing.

Category	Example learning objectives	Recommended learning path
Skill	You can identify nursing gestures using the "Twelve Nursing Gestures" questionnaire.	A
Your own learning objective		
Relationships	You can practice one or two gestures in your own daily nursing practice.	B
Your own learning objective		
Knowledge	You know how the nursing gestures are assigned to the zodiac.	C
Your own learning objective		

References

1   Compare Heine, R. Die Klingende Waschung–Das dialogische Prinzip ihrer Wirkungen. In: Bertram M. (ed.). *Entwurf eines ökologischen Modells therapeutischer Prozesse.* Springer Verlag, Berlin 2016.

2   Compare Heine R. Heine I. Pflegen ist Erziehen–Erziehen ist Pflegen. In: Glöckler M, Grah-Wittich C (ed.). *Die Würde des kleinen Kindes. Vereinigung der Waldorfkindergärten in Deutschland,* Neustadt a. d. Weinstraße 2010. p. 112–126.

3   Steiner, R. *Mantrische Sprüche. Seelenübungen II.* Rudolf Steiner Verlag Dornach 1999 (GA 268). English translation: Steiner R, in: Glöckler M. Heine R. (eds.). *Leadership questions and forms of working in the anthroposophic medical movement.* Translated by Christian von Arnim. Verlag am Goetheanum, Dornach 2016, p. 114.

4   Steiner, R. *Human and cosmic thought.* 3rd facsimile ed. Rudolf Steiner Press, London 2015.

5   ibid.

6   Steiner, R. *On meditation. Spiritual perspectives.* Translated by J. Collis. Rudolf Steiner Press, London 2011, p. 39.

7   Translated from: Steiner, R. *Wahrspruchworte* (GA 40). Rudolf Steiner Verlag, Dornach 2005, p. 334.

8   Steiner, R., in: Glöckler M.; Heine, R. *Leadership questions and forms of working in the anthroposophic medical movement.* Verlag am Goetheanum, Dornach 2016, p. 124. Translated by Christian von Arnim.

9   Translated from: Steiner, R. *Mantrische Sprüche. Seelenübungen II* (GA 268). Rudolf Steiner Verlag, Dornach 1999, p. 183.

10 Steiner, R. *Education for special needs. The curative education course.* Rudolf Steiner Press, London 2015.

11 Translated from: Steiner, R. *Mantrische Sprüche. Seelenübungen II* (GA 268). Rudolf Steiner Verlag, Dornach 1999, p. 205.

12 Translated from: Steiner, R. *Wahrspruchworte* (GA 40). Rudolf Steiner Verlag, Dornach 2005, p. 159.

13 Translated from: Steiner, R. *Mantrische Sprüche. Seelenübungen II* (GA 268). Rudolf Steiner Verlag, Dornach 1999, p. 73.

14 Translated from: Steiner, R. *Wahrspruchworte* (GA 40). Rudolf Steiner Verlag, Dornach 2005, p. 174.

15 Translated from: Steiner, R. *Seelenübungen I* (GA 267). Rudolf Steiner Verlag, Dornach 1997, p. 188.

16 Psalm 23.

17 Translated from: Steiner, R. *Wahrspruchworte* (GA 40). Rudolf Steiner Verlag, Dornach 2005, p. 319.

Elements of Nursing Practice

CHAPTER VIII
Rhythm

ANNEGRET CAMPS

Rhythm is a fundamental element in nursing care. The human rhythmic system mediates between hardening and dissolving tendencies in the human being. This chapter will point out the importance of rhythm for all life and all healing processes, as well as give practical suggestions for using rhythm in nursing care.

→   Learning objectives, see end of chapter

1.   The phenomenon of rhythm

When Rudolf Steiner was once asked, "What is life?" he answered: "Study rhythm! Rhythm carries life."

Where there is life, development does not happen as if pressed out of a tube, it happens in rhythms: permeated through and through by movement, rising and falling, decelerating and accelerating, etc. The word "rhythm" (from the Greek) means symmetry. The symmetry in rhythm has to do with the fact that rhythm is organized, i.e. it is based on a beat which represents the principle of order for the respective segment. The beat sets milestones in always identical repetition, it sets the timescale. Rhythm moves between these "time posts" and unfolds its activity in lively variations.

Wilhelm Hoerner (1913–2013), who gave a wealth of suggestions on this topic in his book on time and rhythm (*Zeit und Rhythmus*), designated inhalation and exhalation as a primal rhythm and clearly explained the difference between rhythm and beat:

> *"Compared with processes in the field of mechanics and machines, one must be more careful and thus more objective when using words than is generally the case. If one calls subsequent, exactly identical revolutions of a machine wheel repetitions of the first revolution, then this same word should not be used in the area of the living. It should be replaced by a more accurate term. One could then describe an inhaled breath of air as a living resurrection of the preceding one—or better yet, as a renewal. Nevertheless, the thing being renewed is not exactly the same as the one before, it is only very similar. In life, no leaf of a tree is exactly the same as another, they are just similar. Only in manufacturing do we demand complete uniformity of the products. A machine must produce an exact repetition of the same thing in all its parts. Every engine must run to the designated beat. This is not so in the realm of life."* [1]

A rhythm that loses its connection with the beat turns into disorderly, rather random movement. A beat that is not taken up by rhythm remains monotonous, boring, dead.

The concept of renewal is the key to understanding the invigorating revival that a healthy rhythm makes possible.

The fact that each repetition is accompanied by a small change is what makes development possible, it gives refreshment and variety through the appeal of the new. It also gives us the opportunity to build on what we know, because each change picks up on what came before. This allows us to experience rhythm as a force that gives us support:

> Rhythm carries us by means of what remains the same within it, rhythm refreshes us by means of variations of the same.

When I have found my way into a rhythm (gotten the feel of it) it can carry me along; when I do not fully enter into it, I come to a standstill and cannot resonate with it in my experience. In music we experience the following: the more similar the recurring rhythmic elements are to one another and the more often they are repeated, the more irrelevant the piece can be, as we know from trivial popular music. The rhythm there is very strongly bound to the beat. The music can be easily recorded and sung along with, but also quickly loses its charm. That is why pop song producers must ensure a constant supply of these short-lived products.

Military music is similar in nature. Military music reinforces the beat so emphatically with drums and timpani that one can no longer even speak of entering into it, one seems almost forced to subordinate oneself to it with every step. How difficult it can be to walk out of sync when listening to marching music!

More sophisticated music is characterized by the fact that it plays around the beat much more yet does not ignore it. Delays, accelerations, stretches, syncopations, changes of time and variations are elements that enrich a piece of music and bring in something new (refreshment). In contrast, repetitions, ongoing or recurring rhythms give security and let both—the listener and the musician—resonate in the rhythm once recognized (recovery). We find unrhythmic music immediately disturbing, even if it is a piece that we have never heard before.

The beneficial effect of music does not come only from melody and harmony, it has to do with the way in which both appear in a living rhythm, one that neither disintegrates into all too liberal arbitrariness through inserting too many—albeit clever—changes, nor bores us to death with the mundane uniformity of a constant beat.

2. Rhythm in the human being

All natural processes happen periodically in rhythms that are embedded in the great cosmic rhythms of the stars (the sun above all), which determine life on earth in the course of the day and year. Countless different rhythms work together, side by side and superimposed on each other, to form—as long as we do not disturb them—a harmonious whole: the tides of the oceans, the growth phases of plants, the life cycles and behavior cycles of animals.

We humans, too, are embedded in these rhythms, but we emancipate ourselves somewhat from them by arbitrarily creating our own individual laws of time. Lamps, indoor heating and clocks make us independent of daylight, climate and the course of the stars. The achievements of civilization allow us to live according to our personal needs and tastes, regardless of where we live or the time of year.

These interventions in the rhythms of nature are the result of human conscious-ness. On the one hand, they are a prerequisite for civilization, on the other hand they also promote pathogenic, destructive tendencies. Many organic rhythms, such as heartbeat, respiration or sleep, can temporarily compensate for disturbed rhythms. However, in the long run they cannot escape the effects of an unrhythmic lifestyle. Many diseases of civilization, such as cardiovascular disease, diabetes mellitus and sleep disorders, are direct or indirect consequences of an unrhythmic lifestyle. Yet our relationship to rhythm need not be restricted to problematic interventions. We can also make conscious use of natural rhythms by aligning our lives a little bit with them and thus letting their supporting and invigorating power take effect.

Research has shown that certain exercises that strengthen and deepen breathing, for example, can promote heart rate variability: a healthy heart increases its frequen-cy during tension and strain and slows it down during relaxation and recovery. The heart can deal flexibly with the changing demands of life when people maintain a healthy balance of challenging and relieving it. Heart rate variability is high. But when people subject their heart to chronic overload or inactivity, the heart rate may "freeze" in constant monotony. Heart rate variability is then low. Chronic overload (too much stress, too little sleep, irregular meals, etc.) can be life-threatening. But even constant inactivity is an unhealthy condition. Heart rate variability is also re-ferred to as a biomarker for "willpower reserve." Rhythm promotes willpower and helps us to stand healthily in life.

In looking at the functional threefolding of the human organism Rudolf Steiner developed the term "rhythmic system" for the middle of the human being, represented by the chest area above all, with the heart and lungs.[3] *The rhythmic system* stands as a balancing element between the polarities of the neurosensory and motor-metabolic systems. Functional threefolding is not to be understood as a threefold division, but as an expression of various functional effects that interlock in such a way that they cannot be separated from each other, yet nevertheless find their respective focus in three different organ systems.

The neurosensory system has its center in the head and is connected to the rest of the organism via the spinal cord and the cranial nerves. The motor-metabolic system is found mainly in the organs below the diaphragm and in the limbs, but it is also ef-fective throughout the body.

Nerve tissue is very differentiated and well-formed, it has little vitality, is highly sen-sitive and seems with its low capacity for regeneration to be just short of dying. Ru-dolf Steiner referred to the neurosensory system also as the "form pole". This part of the organism, when confronting the outside world, rejects material substance and takes in "form."[4] We use it to perceive and understand information, i.e., things that are non-material. Nerve activity serves as a basis for consciousness, whereby structuring and degenerating forces are in the foreground. It is different in the motor-metabolic system, which absorbs substance and destroys form.[5] These are processes that occur largely unconsciously in healthy people. The digestion of substances once absorbed consists of the organism making the substances its own by gradually dissolving their external and internal structures. Substances that do not completely lose their form are not absorbed and have a disturbing effect on the organism, which may resist with vomiting, for example.

The organs of the metabolic system have a strong vitality and regenerative power in comparison to the neurosensory system. The metabolic organs are considered belonging to the substance pole, which ultimately serves upbuilding processes in the human being. They are constantly moving, surging up and subsiding. Standstill in the metabolism would be as harmful as turbulence and swelling in the nervous system [→ Chapter "The Anthropological Foundations of Nursing Extended by Anthroposophy"].

2.1 The rhythmic system

In the activity of the rhythmic system we find the balance between the described polarities, which would collide harmfully without a mediating bridging quality.

If one places a stethoscope on the three body cavities skull, thoracic cavity and abdominal cavity (this is unusual on the skull, because one knows that there is nothing to hear there, even during intensive brain activity), then one can observe how the middle organs alternate rhythmically between complete rest and constant movement, at a ratio of 1:4 (inhalation and exhalation; systole and diastole). This area absorbs neither non-material nor coarse material from the outside world, only finer substances. Its processes of upbuilding and degeneration are reflected in arterial and venous blood or in carbon dioxide and oxygen in the air that we breathe. Tension and release are in constant change, in a living balance. Thus, we recognize this middle of the human being as the area from which harmonization and health emanate. Already Paracelsus (1493–1541) called the heart the "doctor in the human being." It is the place where extremes can be compensated for. Apart from congenital heart defects, the heart rarely gets sick on its own, it happens mostly because of irregularities in the rest of the organism. The heart is also the organ which, as a rule, is the only one that remains free of cancerous growths and allergies.[6]

Strengthening the middle is always conducive to recovery. Before diseases become diseases, they are first physiological abilities. Amplifications or exaggerations of the two polarities appear as "hardening" or "degeneration" and "dissolution" or "inflammation." Physiologically, these processes tend to be found in the neurosensory and metabolic systems. The human being is healthy when both functional focal points find their right equilibrium, which happens again and again anew due to the working of the rhythmic system.

The three organ systems described provide the basis for both physical functioning and mental and spiritual activity. Thus, we find in the neurosensory system the instrument for our awareness and thinking, in the motor-metabolic system the prerequisite for action and in the rhythmic system the basis for our feelings swinging back and forth between antipathy and sympathy, which accompany our thinking and actions.

Of course, rhythmic processes are not only to be found in the middle organs of the human being. Today, medicine and human biology have developed differentiated views on the specific rhythms of each organ and have observed that these have effects on human performance. This has led to the widely used term "biorhythms." The rhythmic system is emphasized because the activity of circulation and respiration is the basic rhythm underlying all other processes.

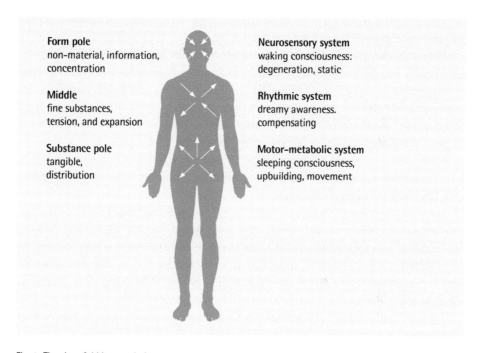

Fig. 1: The threefold human being

3. Leeway as an opportunity for freedom

"The human being plays only where he is a human being in the full sense of the word and is fully human only where he plays.

Friedrich Schiller (1759–1805)

Summing up we can say that life always happens in rhythms. A living rhythm is neither rigid nor chaotic, it adheres to the measure of the beat and plays around it in ever new variations.

Although this is certainly also fundamental for other artists too, it is especially true for musicians–they play! They play a piece of music; they play it on their instrument. And it is musicians who deal with rhythm in a special way.

What do we generally mean by 'play'? Play is not an expression of absolute arbitrariness. Every game has its rules, and only the mastery of the rules makes free play possible. Even small children, when they play with each other, make rules without adults having to advise them, often without the adults even noticing. The playing child is the epitome of the developing human being, the epitome of new possibilities.

"If you do not become as children..."

Gospel of Luke 18.3

We learn the most when we're at the age in which we play. Even with animals you can see this–as long as they can play, they can learn.

Play is the possibility of free development within the limits respected by the players. We also use the term "leeway" to refer to freedom granted to us by other people, by circumstances or by our schedule. We even use "play" as a technical term applying to steering wheels, meaning the same thing: freedom of movement between fixed points. A reference to freedom can even be found in the fact that there are "dangerous games," "forbidden games," and games that "end badly."

Having leeway in rhythm refers to the phase in which something new is at work, it is the moment between two beats that can bring a turn. Play is the way that we deal with laws without overturning them.

Is nursing perhaps nothing other than "play" in this sense? After all, there is an etymological connection between the English word "play" and *Pflege* (the German word for "nursing" or "caregiving"). Think of the many different ways in which one and the same action can be performed, or of the rules for treating certain diseases which we apply to each patient in a different way. Just think of the "eternal monotony" in nursing care, which can undergo renewal every day and needs to!

Playing is something very human. Nursing has a very playful aspect. "Caregiving is like dancing in the sun."[8] To care for something means to accompany a process beneficially.

When we succeed in leaving leeway for free development, then the words "Medicus curat, Deus sanat" can become a reality. Freely translated, it means: the person working therapeutically does not heal–he or she creates the conditions so that God can heal.

Caring for something generally also means doing something over and over again. The words "I've been in the habit of" mean: "I usually do" this or that. This indicates another nuance of nursing activity:

In addition to the free element of playing, there is also a need for the caregiver to be committed to a willingness to do something again and again. That is the point in doing it. You can't wash or feed someone just once, you can't dress a wound just once or administer a single external application. Nursing care lives from repetition. In other words, we must also associate nursing with terms that seem old-fashioned to our

ELEMENTS OF PRACTICAL NURSING

emancipated, politically sensitive ears: faithfulness and duty. "Duty" here is understood as a task, whose fulfillment one cannot (or does not want to!) escape, because it results from a genuine necessity. This does not have to mean self-sacrifice to the point of self-abandonment. It can be understood as a sober affirmation of what is necessary.

Nurses can ensure that this awareness of their inner commitment does not become a "bitter" or "begrudging" duty by not losing sight of the playful side of their activity, in line with the well-known fact that "service by the book" sooner or later becomes "deadly" for one's work. Nursing care lies between duty and play: this, in turn, shows the general humanity of our profession and touches on the existential question of the relationship between necessity and freedom that has occupied philosophers. This means that what has been said here applies not only to nursing care, it concerns human action in general. The nursing profession makes us particularly attentive to it: that people are cared for is a necessity; *how* they are cared for—this is an expression of free creative ability.

4. Rhythm in nursing

4.1 Basic patterns in nursing care

We often encounter great wisdom in simple circumstances, and many an insight goes unnoticed because it appears in the garment of a "truism."

A basic pattern of nursing care, which we already learned at the beginning of our training and which has not left us since then, is the sequence of preparation, implementation and follow-up. Whatever model of nursing care we have in mind, whatever idea of humanity guides us, whatever field of specialization we turn our attention to: we always come back to those three steps.

The work of a nursing team consists of a continuous chain of repetitive actions, where each one following depends on the one before. This is a rhythmic element, and if caring for something is "like dancing in the sun," then it is a dance in three-quarter time.

With every *preparation* we build on the past. We select what we need from the available material. The knowledge we have acquired in the past gives us an idea of what material we are using and how to best organize our work. Our knowledge about the patient and his illness is also a prerequisite for carrying out our nursing action. In the *implementation* phase we are entirely in the present. Prepared from the past, in the moment of action we must do exactly the right thing, be completely alert, possibly deviate from what we had planned, because the current situation demands this, and at the same time already be aware of the future and what our action should lead to. So, while our knowledge was very important during preparation, it is our ability that is required during implementation. This phase can be mastered with skill, presence of mind and a sure hand.

The *follow-up* is oriented towards the future: Yes, the materials should be properly put away, so that the next person can continue working, but we especially want to ensure that the patient can experience the healing effect of our treatment during his or her post-treatment rest.

This last segment of nursing action is often in danger of not receiving enough attention, due to how busy we are. Yet it gives us the basis to learn from our work by becoming aware of the consequences of our treatment and it enables us to think ahead to future activities based on this experience.

These three phases of work structure our time, giving our action a beginning and an end, with the end forming the prerequisite for the next beginning. This can be found in big things as well as small, and we can even read it from every movement in the rhythmic oil applications of Rhythmical Einreibung, a central activity of anthroposophically oriented nursing care [→ Chapter "Rhythmical Einreibung According to Wegman/Hauschka"]. Rhythmical Einreibung incorporates a three-step process.

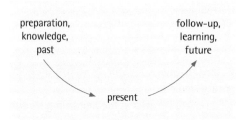

Fig. 2: Basic patterns in nursing care

1. Initiating contact: The first touch does not happen too softly or too violently, whereby the hand becomes the organ of perception for what presents itself to it as form, texture, temperature etc., receptive to what has become what it is from the past until today.

2. Accentuation: Taking into account what we perceived, we intensify the contact, so that touching intensifies into accentuation.

3. Letting go: The hand lets go by loosening the contact without letting go completely, and without giving up the chosen direction ("letting go without leaving").

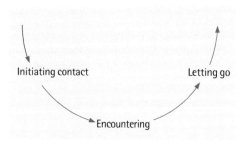

Fig. 3: A basic gesture in nursing

A slight swinging out in the pause leads us back to a beginning and enables us to delve in again. The three steps are repeated as described. What happens during Rhythmical Einreibung can thus become a picture for the basic gesture of nursing care in general.

ELEMENTS OF PRACTICAL NURSING

We find rhythm in the process: as we rhythmically work, we take up the familiar, which we trustingly engage with, and at the same time we anticipate what is to come in joyful readiness.

4.2   The importance of time frames

The knowledge of these three steps alone, however, does not constitute rhythmic working. This can only be achieved if recurring activities are repeated in the same way and at the same time. Whether it is an external application at a certain hour or ordering materials on a fixed weekday: everything that is done out of habit happens a bit "by itself" and thus saves a lot of additional energy, because rhythm replaces strength. Room care, group work and primary nursing are forms of work which favor the creation and maintenance of rhythms in a special way, because any changes to the primary nurse should be kept to a minimum. Nurses and patients "tune in" to each other. Ideally, patients and nurses will feel trust and security when both feel carried by a common rhythm. Rhythm in nursing care is not only beneficial for patients, it is also something that supports the nurses.

Let us briefly refer here to an aspect of anthroposophic anthropology which can give us ideas for a new division of labor. The elaboration of this approach to nursing should be seen as a task for the future.

Rudolf Steiner distinguished between four rhythms in his discussion of the four-fold human being: the year, the month, the week and the day. The annual rhythm inscribes itself into the physical body, where we set an accent by celebrating birthdays. Life processes are embedded in the rhythms of the moon, i.e., in the course of about four weeks. The strongly changing colorful life of soul is influenced by the rhythm of the week, with its seven days that have different qualities. In the shortest rhythm, finally, the alternation between day and night, the human 'I' finds expression: brightness of consciousness is wrested from sleep every morning and subordinates itself to it again at night, when the wakeful work of day has caused fatigue.

There are also numerous other rhythms for human beings. These are embedded in the four main rhythms that underly our calendar year, which survives all reforms.

What conclusions can be drawn from this?

The *rhythm of the year* can give us reason to look at what has become. Like sometimes on the occasion of a birthday or New Year's Eve, we can look back on what we have achieved so far, on what we have been able to physically manifest. We make New Year's resolutions to correct mistakes, maintain our successes and try something new. We can set ourselves a period of about *four weeks* or a multiple of that to develop a new habit, train new members of staff or become familiar with new types of treatment. This is often difficult to achieve in hospitals, as the shortened length of stay of the patients has led to increasingly short-winded nursing care. This makes it all the more important to focus on processes that are independent of the time that the patient spends there. When habits carry us along in our everyday working life, which have become stable because they have been allowed to develop over a reasonable period of time, then a peace can enter the work that also affects patients who spend only a few days in the hospital. All too often, however, the effort to introduce a particular style of care or even to tackle a single activity in a new way is discarded before it has been given time to develop properly. "Let's try this for four weeks and then see" is wise advice that we can give each other in this regard. Also, the time for a restful annual vacation should not fall below four weeks. Everyone knows that everything takes time: letting go of the daily work, arriving at the holiday resort, settling in, discovering the new, and finally the anticipation that marks the beginning of the work to be resumed.

Weekly rhythms give us a basic framework for planning the staff roster. This is a difficult undertaking, as long as shift work is our pacemaker! This type of service (as "practical" as it may seem) has a destructive effect on everything rhythmic and is to be regarded as questionable, especially when it comes to rotating shifts. In some places, there is at least an attempt to make early and late shifting more continuous by keeping staffing levels constant, although it is always difficult to find people who are willing to work in the afternoons all the time. Where this has been achieved, there are reports of greater job satisfaction, fewer sick days and lower fluctuation. The staff develop a stable rhythm of life in the broadest sense. Regularity in waking and sleeping, mealtimes and maintaining social contacts, family time, leisure time and learning has a healthy effect on people.

Adventurousness, creativity and perseverance will certainly take us even further along the path of planning a new staff roster, for example in the direction of considering a real seven-day week: we can give the different days points of emphasis or coloring corresponding to their respective quality, into which we can integrate the regular periods of service of the nurses. For example, individual staff members may be entitled to five different days of work, as well as one for rest and one for celebration. It is in the nature of things that this will not be Saturday and Sunday for everyone at the same time, but it can be assumed that with otherwise stable working hours, changes to free weekends planned well in advance do not have to disrupt the planning. The courage to take risks and to try things imaginatively can certainly lead us to completely different ways of doing things, the correctness of which will have to prove itself in life.

The weekly rhythm also sets accents in therapy. In Anthroposophic Medicine, for example, this can be found in the term "therapeutic pause." A treatment that is interrupted regularly once a week has been given a temporal structure. After the day of rest, it resumes with a new impulse. Something that applies to habits in general comes into play here. To deliberately omit something once, not out of forgetfulness or lack of time, invigorates a habitual act and enhances its value. This brings us closer to the significance of the individual *day*, whose current schedule is shaped by the 'I'. I must decide what I will do today, regardless of all the obvious routines, which, if they are not personally taken hold of, have a soporific effect. ("We have always done it like this.") Our shaping of the day, its beginning, its middle and its end, comes from the alert consciousness that should rule all our actions. So that we do not lose ourselves dreamily in unimportant things, or let ourselves be hectically driven to disordered doing for the sake of doing, we ourselves are the instance that lets us pause from time to time to gain a clear overview. Even "not being able to start" and "finding no end to the work" can be overcome by the 'I'. Finally, we should mention the importance of pauses. *Pauses* in our work, with the possibility of receiving new impulses, act as resting points, similar to pauses in therapy for patients.

We often consider pauses to be short interruptions, in which we are still hanging on to what we have done just before and at the same time are thinking about continuing the work after. Perhaps we may use them to quickly do something else in between. Looking at its meaning from the Greek, we find that "pause" equals "stop." Whether it is short or long, it is important that for a moment it gives freedom from what has happened before and what will come after, without pulling us completely out of the context of our activity. A pause is already given with the hand washing that we do so often, which is thereby lifted above the mere cleansing function into a moment in which we wash away with the "dirt" also everything which still clings to us from work just done. We wash our hands to complete an action and free them, so that they can take hold of something new. For some, the cigarette break may also fulfill such a function, although it is important to make sure that nothing of the haze of this break still clings to us during our next nursing action.

A breakfast break in which we do not talk about work all the time allows us to let go and become free for what we will do afterwards. This does not exclude the possibility that a short meeting may take place at the end of this break, but then the break is over.

The break is very important, especially when there is a lot to do. Pausing between two activities saves us from infectious hecticness. How often does it happen that we start many actions at the same time and do not properly finish any of them, resulting in a concert of dissatisfied patients ringing their bells!

Nursing care, like all action, consists in doing and in not doing. Usually only doing is recognized as a real achievement, just as in the heart only contraction is described as a working phase. But just as the heart can only do this work when diastole has preceded it with a very short standstill, so the more rhythmic and accentuated our actions are, the better and more persistently we will work. Signs of burnout should cause us to ask: "How is our work rhythm? How about our habits and breaks? Can changing our habits help us to become more serene?" However, this requires patience, which can be rather far from us in times of stress. Four weeks as a measure for practicing new habits may seem too long to us, when the need seems so great right now. But this too is like with living organisms: development needs time and rhythm. We require special perseverance and care, especially when our rhythm gets off track.

In the recognition of letting go lies a possibility to become attentive to the reaction after our action, to learn from our completed action. The job title "lady in waiting" (German "*Wärterin*") comes from the "dark ages" of nursing care and has a negative connotation for our current understanding. Liberated from its historical context, though, it is basically a beautiful word that points to the ability to wait. Acting and then consciously letting go can give lively rhythm to our work every day anew.

Category	Example learning objectives	Recommended learning path
Skill	You consider aspects of rhythm when organizing work processes.	A
Your own learning objective		
Relationships	You relieve your forces and the forces of your colleagues by ensuring meaningful breaks.	B
Your own learning objective		
Knowledge	You understand the importance of rhythm for all life processes.	C
Your own learning objective		

References

1   Hoerner, W. *Zeit und Rhythmus.* Verlag Urachhaus, Stuttgart 2006.

2   Leonhard, K. *Biologische Psychologie.* Hirzel Verlag, Stuttgart 1993.

3   Steiner, R. *Riddles of the soul.* Spring Valley: Mercury Press, 1996. Chap. Physical and spiritual dependencies in the human being.

4   Dumke, K. Biologische Individualität—Aspekte zur menschlichen Dreigliederung und das Immunsystem. *Die Drei* 1987; 57 (5).

5   ibid.

6   Fintelmann, V. *Intuitive medizin.* Hippokrates Verlag, Stuttgart 2007.

7   ibid.

8   van der Star, A. *Über die Pflege der Sinne. Vortrag bei der Pflegetagung des Verbands anthroposophisch orientierter Pflegeberufe.* Velbert 1992.

CHAPTER IX

The Human Warmth Organism and Its Care

ADA VAN DER STAR

Warmth provides the physical basis for the human 'I'. This chapter will describe phenomena of warmth in nature and the human organism, as well as present therapeutic warmth applications. The main emphasis will be on influencing warmth via clothing, nutrition, and the environment.

→   Learning objectives, see end of chapter

Warmth is more than a physical phenomenon. Its psychological aspect is evident when we think of terms such as "warm welcome" or "warm hospitality." But warmth also has a spiritual dimension, and only all three aspects together form a complete picture—at least when considering warmth in the human being.

The typically human aspect of spiritual warmth becomes clear to us when we consider the special position of human beings compared to the other living beings on our planet.

1.   Earth's climate and living things

Not every living thing has its own constant body temperature. In principle, plants produce hardly any heat of their own. They depend on the temperature surrounding them. In spring, however, we can observe how the very first delicate plants melt their way up through the snow. The strongest heating up happens inside germinating seeds and in flowers.[1]

External temperatures are an important factor for the functioning of life processes in *plants*. Many plants die when the temperature drops below 0°C (32°F), some require the presence of cold for their seeds to germinate, and in winter they must even "freeze through" properly to develop the following year. Other plants only thrive in high temperatures. For this reason, some species can only be found in certain climatic zones. In general, however, it can be said that plants need a temperature of at least four degrees Celsius for the fertilization process to take place. There is hardly any vegetation in areas of the earth where this temperature is not reached.

Animals create their own specific heat during metabolism. They also have various mechanisms for dealing with temperature. Some animals are completely at its mercy, e.g., cold-blooded animals, whose body temperature is only slightly higher than that

216

of their environment. A snake that gets too cold stiffens completely. The snake has no fur to retain body heat like the more advanced mammals. Mammals also have other ways of surviving periods of cold, such as hibernation. During this time, all bodily functions are reduced to a minimum and stored fat is sufficient to supply energy for the most necessary life processes.

Bird migration is another way to survive. The birds which escape winter show us this particularly clearly. In autumn, when the migrating flocks of geese from cold regions fly past us overhead, we know that the cold periods of winter are imminent. It is all the more hopeful when the same birds return in early spring, because then the end of the cold season is in sight.

Birds do not choose their travel times voluntarily or use conscious measurements. Their whole organism reacts to the position of the sun, the rise or fall in temperature. The animal must migrate, whether it likes to or not. Birds that are too weak or sick stay behind and certainly don't survive. The whole organization of the animal is aimed at securing its vital functions. For example, no goose will make a "detour" during the migration to explore new areas! Animals have fixed life patterns that can only develop in certain climatic zones. Animals are fully integrated into these geographical and climatic contexts.[2]

1.1   The human warmth organism

With human beings we can observe other conditions, people live almost everywhere on the planet. Nevertheless, it is true that the regions where survival is very difficult are much less populated than those where the climate is more favorable. In the cold of the polar regions, it is still necessary to have a sophisticated survival system, taking special care with food and clothing, despite many easing resources that were mostly developed by people in the temperate zones.

In extreme cold, people need almost all their energy to keep their life processes going. The inhabitants of the polar regions live in small groups. Social life is shaped by the circumstances of life. Art unfolds on a small scale, their thinking results from living with nature. The experience of these people is directed strongly inwards.

In tropical regions, where people still live directly in nature, life is characterized by other dependencies. Unlike in the polar regions, they are not packed in a good layer of insulation. They remain almost entirely naked. In their fight for survival they must protect themselves from predators, poisonous animals and infectious diseases and push back the variegated vegetation to the benefit of their own habitat. Social life is diverse, happening in large communities. Impressive works of art are also created, which depict the supernatural aspects experienced in nature as a source of life-giving power. People give themselves completely to nature.

In temperate zones we experience these two polarities in attenuated form throughout the year, according to the position of the sun and the corresponding temperatures: in summer we are more outward oriented in casual social life, e.g., in street cafés. In winter we are turned inward and retreat to closed, mostly heated rooms. Spring and autumn provide transitions between the two extremes of summer and winter. However, they do not take place in flowing uniformity. Rather the fire of summer is extinguished, and a time of turning inward is necessary. This was formerly celebrated in the St. John's festival at the summer solstice. The other turning point is still celebrated today at Christmas time.

Many people in the industrialized countries of the temperate climate zones have no connection to these turning points, they are hardly affected by them. If it is hot in summer, for example, air conditioning brings relief. In winter we turn on the lights and we may take a trip to warmer countries to forget the gloom of the darkest season. Civilization has emancipated itself from nature through technology.

This independence means that human beings must no longer spend all their energy just ensuring the continuation of their life processes. Enough surplus forces remain for inner maturation of their personalities, for individuality, and for development of social, economic and spiritual life in society. The result of this independence is culture.

It is important to create the right "climate" in oneself: to live and work as an alert, conscious person in harmony with spiritual laws, to shape one's own life and thus a piece of the world.

The human being is the only living being who can create this "climate" himself, to emancipate himself from external thermal conditions. He can create the physical, mental and spiritual warmth conditions that he needs to exist as an organism, independently of nature.

Greek mythology depicts this phenomenon in the story of Prometheus, who creates the human being and teaches him everything: Prometheus brings to mankind fire that he has stolen from the gods. But the moment that mankind becomes acquainted with fire, Zeus sends Pandora with the horn of plenty. It is a jar containing all evil and suffering. Pandora opens the jar and releases the possibility to err. Only hope remains in the jar—a pictorial representation of the exclusively human ability to control one's warmth forces or to internalize the divine spirit and to deal with it on one's own responsibility.

Nancy Roper (1918–2004) designated body temperature regulation as one of the twelve "life activities" and described the complicated physiological processes necessary to constantly measure, increase or decrease body temperature. She also explained which physical measures are to be applied in nursing care to compensate for temperatures that are too high or too low.

The right body temperature is not only physiologically important, it is also necessary for mental and spiritual presence.

This aspect must be borne in mind if we are to provide holistic nursing care. We are referring to the life activity of "keeping warm" in a broader sense, in that we are not only referring to body temperature but are understanding human warmth as a warmth organism.

With the term "warmth organism" we mean more than temperature regulation. It is the force with which the warmth is kept at a constant level despite fluctuating outside temperatures, which can vary between plus and minus 60°C (140°F) in extreme cases. The warmth organism is a differentiated structure (think of the different organ temperatures and warmth zones) and can maintain its independence from the outside world:

> *"He carries this uniform warmth area through the changing environment and only then becomes a world of his own, a microcosm. Of course, he is in constant connection with the surrounding space because he constantly gives off warmth to it. The boundaries of the warming organism are therefore not as sharp as those of the physical body, but still there is a rather sharp drop in body temperature against the environment [...] Here the warmth organism continuously dissolves into the environment. Necessarily, it must be formed anew continually from within. This 'exchange of heat' is just as characteristic for it as 'metabolism' is for the solid organism."*[3]

Body heat serves to enable biochemical processes to take place in the body. At the same time, these processes generate heat ("combustion") in the human body. One requires the other. The question arises as to whether the processes themselves are the ultimate goal or whether an ordered, well-regulated warmth organism is in fact the overall carrier of a higher function.

At the beginning of this chapter it was shown how human beings pursue their goals in balanced warmth, independent of nature, and use the energies thus released for inner and outer development:

> *"The connection of 'I' and will lives in the element of warmth. There is physical warmth that accompanies all physical activities, but there is also an original, spiritual warmth that develops when the 'I' develops enthusiasm for something beautiful, valuable, true, good, etc. The 'I' lives in warmth. It is a youthful warmth that is created by 'I' activity, a product of enthusiasm. 'I' and will come together when this enthusiasm leads to action."*[4]

An individuality requires warmth that fluctuates within a certain temperature range. The human 'I' needs the warmth organism with a certain body temperature to grasp the body and express itself in it, to develop. Spiritual warmth can be ignited in connection with human ideals and goals, an area that is often weakened, especially in the sick, and is closely related to their ability to recover. The use of language shows many examples of degrees of commitment, from "cool disinterest" to "flaming enthusiasm." The word "interest" comes from the Latin "inter-esse," in English: to be between. If someone is too cool, his 'I' cannot be comfortably in his body, it cannot incarnate well, i.e., "be in the flesh." Human encounters, where the participants may not immediately reveal their individualities, first require a mutual "warming up" so that the people "thaw." When they really "warm up" to each other, enthusiasm often arises: they discover the other person as a being of soul and spirit behind the façade of external physicality. However, the warmth can also become too intense, which can be observed, for example, when children play together with great enthusiasm at a birthday party: soon they get red faces, start sweating, and the experienced mother or teacher knows that now a small accident can easily happen due to the overshooting of the childlike, untrained forces. If the child's body temperature were to be measured on this occasion, it would be above the upper normal value of 37.5°C (99.5°F).

Over the course of a person's life, temperature fluctuations decrease as they learn to take control of themselves. Gradually, an equilibrium of 36 to 37.5°C (96.8 to 99.5°F) is reached, although this can vary individually by a few tenths of a degree. Thus, we also find various "mental climates" ranging from distant cool cynicism to overflowing "warmth of heart." In medicine, these two tendencies are reflected in the "cold" and "warm" diseases [→ see Chapter "The Anthropological Foundations"].

2. Perceiving warmth

Over the centuries, various physical methods were developed to determine heat in measurable units. Finally, the definition according to Celsius (C) became accepted, in which boiling water is defined as 100°C (212°F) and freezing water as 0°C (32°F). But when we dip our hands into water, for example, we do not perceive the temperature in degrees, but only in relation to our own body temperature. Thus, we feel a moderately heated apartment to be warm when we enter it frozen from a long walk in icy cold. After a while, though, when we have warmed up a little, we experience the same room temperature as being too cold to sit still in. If we then have a sumptuous meal, we would like it to be cooler. It may be that we find bath water on our hands quite pleasant, but if we step into the tub with our feet, the water is much too hot for us. Our sensation of heat is therefore not an exact temperature measurement. Regarding our sense of movement, we agree on the terms "downwards" and "upwards." This is different for our sense of warmth: what is already cool for some is still warm for others.

When cold penetrates a person, he contracts both externally and internally. His soul is compressed. At first this causes a clear alertness, but in the long run numbness sets in and consciousness disappears. Thus, cold can be used as an anesthetic. However, people can also dispel a feeling of cold if they are enthusiastic about their thoughts. In literature there are numerous examples of people escaping death from freezing because they tried to think inspiring thoughts, that is, to bring spiritual warmth to meet the external cold. The English polar explorer Robert F. Scott (1868–1912) and his companions defied all deprivation and cold as long as they were motivated by the thought of being the first people on earth to reach the South Pole. When they were not the first to reach that much desired place (a Norwegian expedition had arrived a month earlier), they were so disappointed that they went to sleep exhausted and died of cold.

Warmth is felt in the soul in such a way that one has the feeling of being able to flow outwards. The soul expands and connects with the warm environment. It becomes more flexible. Only when equal warmth prevails inside and outside is there no difference to be felt. Temperature can therefore be felt especially in the transition when something flows from the inside to the outside or vice versa. The corresponding sensation is a mental quality, not the measurement of a certain numerical value.

To perceive the world around you, with whatever sense, you must be ready: you must open yourself, and something must move between you and the outside world. The basis for this is warmth. Every sensory perception first needs warmth, human warmth, human interest. The 'I' flows in the warmth to the outside world, whether it is a mountain range shimmering on the horizon, the sounds of a violin reaching our ear, or the person opposite who is talking about something.

The right warmth must flow in an encounter between two people if it is to become a meeting from 'I' to 'I'. In nursing care, warmth is a wide field, in which there is still a lot to discover.

3. Warmth in nursing

According to Rudolf Steiner, human beings originated from and were created by the highest hierarchies (angelic beings) who sacrificed their substance in the form of warmth to form a basis for the human 'I'.[5] This warmth, the human warmth organism today, still provides the basis for individuality. From this point of view, there is an important task for any kind of nursing care, be it for children, the sick or the elderly, and for the care of one's own body: ever new provision of balanced warmth, so that the person being cared for may live in their body in a way fit for a human being, as present as possible. One method to prevent this is to inhibit warmth, for example as a punishment or—even more extreme—as torture. A beginning has already been made if you make a child stand outside in the cold hallway as punishment.

A newborn baby does not yet have a mature warmth organism and must therefore be protected from heat loss. Sensitive areas such as the head must be covered, at least as long as the fontanels are open and the head is not yet protected by a thick layer of hair. A child must always feel nice and warm on their whole body, even their hands. Their whole body is then grasped and individually shaped by their 'I'. Febrile teething troubles help to individually remodel the body inherited from the infant's parents. A child who is allowed to have a childhood illness with a corresponding fever usually grows quite a bit after this illness. Not only outwardly, but also inwardly the child seems to become more "himself." Of course, such a childhood illness must be accompanied, and the temperature must be regulated in such a way that no damage is caused by overheating.

In adulthood, people who suffered childhood illnesses generally show greater assertiveness against disease-causing factors. During childhood and adolescence, the warmth organism becomes more stable and differentiated. Certain parts of the body, such as the armpits and groin, develop sweat glands to release heat, others require special protection against heat loss. Fat covers organs such as kidneys and digestive organs in a gender-specific manner, so that in adulthood the shape of men and women differs considerably. It is interesting to note that the organs whose products are intended to serve another organism selflessly during reproduction, i.e., the mammary and semen glands, are located outside the trunk and thus in cooler areas.

Regions that are particularly sensitive to heat and where warmth applications can be applied well are the throat, neck, upper abdomen and kidneys. The muscle areas of the calves as well as the wrists are well suited to cool applications to extract heat. Cold areas, such as cold feet, a cold kidney region, a cold neck or too cold a head, often result in illness: if the warmth organism does not completely penetrate the physical body, the body functions get confused. A cold can be the result. In this sense, cooling calf compresses should not be used to reduce fever when the feet are cold: the cool compress would increase the tendency of the warmth organism to accumulate in the head area. The well-intentioned compress would then have the opposite of its intended effect.

3.1 Temperature extremes and illness

Today we are seeing an increase in "cold" diseases, especially in industrialized countries. "Cold" diseases arise when the formative forces flowing from the neurosensory system begin to control the organism excessively. These patients tend more to coolness, objectivity, and to suppression of their personality. They try to control themselves, to adapt to the norm, and are often proud of not having had feverish childhood diseases in their youth. They prefer order and objective thinking, which is oriented as much as possible towards things that are externally visible[6] and they suffer from arteriosclerosis, cancer or multiple sclerosis, for example. Their disease is based on the fact that the body becomes "too hard" at one place or another and thus impermeable to life processes. Knots, hardening, deposits, etc., occur with all their consequences. Any fever that may occur in these cases must be seen as an attempt to overcome the cold processes. Therapeutic nursing care consists in stimulating and supporting the warmth organism in its efforts to dissolve the hardenings. Oil is used as a heat-carrying medium in external applications (baths, compresses, Rhythmical Einreibung), as described in more detail in the chapter "Compresses." However, the nurse can do even more and encourage the patient to understand his individuality by asking about his biography and working with him on it.

Febrile infectious diseases are generally regarded as "warm" diseases. They used to be more common. "Warm" diseases present the following picture: patients are often very flexible and restless both internally and externally. Their movements appear not well guided, also their thoughts are often characterized by a rich imagination, which can increase to fever fantasies when their body temperature is very high. Their body is very warm and rather moist, as if the whole person is dissolving. Their life forces swell uninhibitedly in their metabolic system. Therapeutic nursing care strives to not let the temperature overshoot, to create order, to give shape and to convey a sense for the surrounding reality when the person's fantasies get out of hand. Here too, external applications can provide targeted support and help with structuring, for example, by using cooling preparations. Instead of oil, we use fat-free preparations such as gels and essential oils.

The standing human being is comparable to a column of heat. Most of the heat is generated by the metabolic system, which reaches the outermost tips of the feet via the bloodstream. In the same way, the heat flows upwards, although it radiates away from the chest and head. The head should always be slightly cooler than the torso; in summer it helps to wear an airy hat. While the clothing on the neck and upper front thorax is often opened to release heat, the neck is particularly sensitive to cooling, even if this is not immediately noticed. Neck tension with headaches is often the result. The thorax must also be protected from cold.

Another area at risk of cold is the kidney area and, especially in women, the area above the iliac crest. These cold zones are in constant danger of being undersupplied with warmth due to ready-made clothing and underwear fashion. Nature tries to protect these areas by thickening the layer of fat.

From below, the cold creeps upwards from the soles of the feet, especially when the feet are not moving or when there is no friction in the callus areas, e.g., when very fine stockings are worn in smooth-lined shoes or the soles of the feet have been excessively covered with greasy substances. The large muscle areas of the calves give off a lot of warmth. In cool weather, knee socks already ensure that the warming organism is less overtaxed.

If the body is adequately protected in all places—in winter by a shirt with a neckline and long underwear or tights and warm shoes—the outerwear can be adapted to the prevailing circumstances. Whether to wear a cotton tunic, sweater, blouse or vest, for example, must be decided according to need, taste and fashion.

Since nurses are doing physical work, they find a room temperature above 20 to 22°C (68 to 71.6°F) very warm, despite their light working clothes. From their point of view, therefore, it makes sense to open windows and turn down the heating. Here, caution is always required so that elderly and sick people are not thoughtlessly exposed to room temperatures that are too cool for them. This also applies to centrally regulated heating when it switches from nocturnal back to daytime heating. It should be done early enough so that the rooms are already warm before people get up and attend to their personal hygiene.

Sometimes, for reasons of practicality, patients or the elderly are only lightly covered with a blanket of synthetic fibers and dressed in a rough hospital gown. This lack of attention to the warmth organism takes a lot of strength away from the patient. The aim is to dress these people with an undershirt and bed jacket, to cover their genital area with a towel if underpants or diapers are not suitable, and to provide them with wool socks. Especially in nursing homes you can experience how a tense and apathetic elderly person will suddenly respond to his environment in a friendly way, regain his appetite and thirst, and his stiffness will dissolve into movement.

Particularly in old age, people gradually lose their ability to generate sufficient warmth; they need additional protection especially in parts of their bodies that are susceptible to cold. It is also important to ensure that the materials from which their clothing is made are suitable for the climate and the season.

Despite the excellent properties of many modern textile fibers, especially in terms of durability, crease resistance and washability, *wool* remains the unsurpassed material for the cold season. It retains body heat but is breathable, so that the person doesn't sweat. The better the quality of the wool, the less care it requires.

Cotton is very washable and absorbent, but does not retain air or liquid, so it has no warming properties. On the contrary, when someone sweats, cotton releases moisture so quickly that it has a cooling effect.

Silk, an animal protein product like wool, stands between wool and cotton. Especially rough-structured bourette silk is a good warmth balancer in summer as well as in winter. Densely woven silk leaves little air on the skin and offers protection from the wind. Knitted silk lingerie balances the body's temperature regulation the best.[7]

When wearing underwear made of high-quality materials, everyone can observe that this creates a feeling of emotional well-being. Since many people have never heard of this topic, it is the task of the nurse to enlighten them.

If we want to establish the above-mentioned well-being as support for healing processes, we must pay particular attention to the bed climate of our patients. While hundreds of thousands are spent on expensive medical equipment and drugs, the beds are often sparsely equipped. Only a sheet separates the patient from the thin cotton or synthetic mattress protector that covers a sweat-impermeable foam mattress. The covers are made of synthetic material. Freezing patients do not find warming protection in this climate; feverish patients experience a pressing accumulation of heat. Wool bedding and duvets create the right balance of warmth. Unfortunately, hygiene regulations hardly allow the use of natural products in hospital beds. Nevertheless, many a patient would be much helped if they could bring their own things from home.

It is important that the transition to warm clothing be *gradual*. Otherwise the attempt could fail because the suddenly warmed person cannot cope with the physical and mental changes, becomes anxious and rejects the whole thing, citing their unwillingness to suffocate in such unbearable warmth.

3.3 Further aids to stimulate and regulate the warmth organism

A suitable bed climate and appropriate clothing should be a matter of course for everyone. This could be counted among the "human rights." In addition, further aids are available to nursing staff: the simplest is the hot-water bottle, which serves as a local heat source. However, hot water bottles must not be used on body parts with sensory disturbances, as the heat on the skin is then not perceived, the hyperemia required for convection is not activated and dangerous blisters may develop. This also applies to paralyzed or anesthetized body parts. Unfortunately, hot-water bottles are rarely found in modern medical and nursing facilities.

Another possibility is to rub the skin with oils that provide special warmth. Oil usually only forms in plants after the plant has flowed into the cosmos in its flowering process. The oil forms as a "response from the cosmos" and then collects mainly in the maturing seed.

Other plants send their oil deep into the root area or into the fruit. These peculiarities give the oils their healing powers. Most edible oils are obtained from seeds.[8]

Depending on the plant's signature, the oil may be more or less suitable for the care of the skin and the warmth organism. Essential oils may possibly be added, and they give a special quality.[9] Oil, carefully applied to the skin, forms a thermal envelope around the body. However, it must not stand on the skin, as it then has an excessively closing effect.

Essential oils are quickly absorbed into the blood capillaries and transported further by them.[10] This is how external warmth transforms into internal warmth. If one also considers that it is precisely blood that is the organ that carries the 'I,'[11] it makes sense that Rhythmical Einreibung treatment with vegetable oil can be an immediate aid to incarnation. Our knowledge of this fact and our respect for the individuality of the patient—apart from experienced and warm hands—are indispensable prerequisites for giving such treatment.

Care products based on crude oil are unsuitable. Unlike vegetable oils, which originate from living organisms, mineral oils are produced by decomposition processes and are preserved underground for millions of years.[12] Although they give the skin a beautiful, shimmering sheen, they are not absorbed by the skin and reduce its breathability and metabolism, which leads to dry and itchy skin.

3.4   Nutrition and warmth

Another way of directly stimulating the warmth organism is nutrition. Seasoning food with plants from the Lamiaceateae family, e.g., rosemary, thyme, marjoram, melissa and savory, helps because of the special warmth quality of these herbs[13, 14] [→ Chapter "Preventing Bed Sores, Pneumonia and Thrombosis in Severely Ill Patients"]. They should be available in every ward kitchen. Fats and oils have a special relationship to heat, as already mentioned. With the current fears about slimness and cholesterol levels in the blood, care must be taken to ensure that fat intake from food is not neglected. Of course, fried foods do not replace good quality, unsaturated edible oils (safflower, sunflower or olive oil). Another suitable fat, moderately consumed, is cream, which can be added to chopped fruit or compote, for example. This makes it easier to absorb fat-soluble vitamins.

Ripe fruit also stimulates the warmth organism.[15] Fruit is well suited as a snack or as a refreshment for people suffering from fever. Visitors who want to do something good for sick or elderly people can be encouraged to bring fruit. However, it should be ripe, otherwise it consumes too much heat when being digested.

For healthy people, raw food and bulb vegetables pose a challenge to the warmth organism. Weakened people, however, no longer have the required energy, which manifests in flatulence and diarrhea.

Instead of cold mineral water, we can offer warming herbal teas (e.g., caraway, fennel, thyme, peppermint, basil and lavender). It is important that they be prepared correctly and served fresh. Too strong tea, and tea left standing for too long have no effect and are often rejected. Generally speaking, herbal teas should be thin, transparent and fragrant.

3.5   Shaping the environment

A remarkable factor in the care of children, the sick, the elderly or other people in need of help is the color of their surroundings. If possible, it would make sense to use colors that form a protective covering, e.g., pink or a light orange, for people in need of warmth. Cooler colors, such as light blue, are more suitable for fiery people. Although the walls of the room cannot be repainted for every patient, it does not make sense to keep them white or toxic grey, or grey yellow-green. When applied moderately, a color will contribute more to well-being than a soulless white. Glossy, smooth surfaces intensify the impression of cold.

Bed linen in different colors is relatively easy to obtain. It is up to the nurse to report appropriate needs to the person responsible for purchasing. In the nursing profession in particular, people are often still far too uncritical of the patient's external circumstances, which are usually designed by (albeit well-meaning) people who are not nurses. Rudolf Steiner apparently once said that the patient should feel better even just by seeing the nurse. The color of the nurse's clothing can also contribute to this effect. As already described, a color conveys warmth or cold. This can inspire us to think about alternatives to the neutral white of our work clothing.

As described, no complex measures are necessary to support the warmth organism, but a keen awareness of the conditions under which warmth unfolds. The external circumstances that we create in nursing care form the basis for how the human 'I' can become involved in the body. Our care of the warmth organism as a support for the individuality helps the patient to find the way to recovery.

Despite all the practical suggestions for supporting warmth, highest priority must be given to human warmth. Politeness, friendliness and a warm interest in the other person are qualities that everyone can develop. In human relationships, it is precisely these qualities that make patients feel relaxed, comfortable, accepted and secure; a prerequisite for healing processes that start from within.

Category	Example learning objectives	Recommended learning path
Skill	You practice methods that care for the human warmth organism.	A
Your own learning objective		
Relationships	You recognize warmth phenomena in encounters between people.	B
Your own learning objective		
Knowledge	You know the importance of warmth for healing processes.	C
Your own learning objective		

References

1   Linder, H. *Biologie—Lehrbuch für die Oberstufe.* J. B. Metzler und Poeschel Verlagsbuchhandlung, Stuttgart 1989.

2   Kipp, F.A. Über den Vogelzug. In: Schad, W. (ed.). *Goetheanistische Naturwissenschaft. vol. 3—Zoologie.* Verlag Freies Geistesleben, Stuttgart 1983.

3   Schwab, G. *Sagen des klassischen Altertums.* Anaconda Verlag, Cologne 2014.

4   Roper, N. *Die Elemente der Krankenpflege.* Recom, Basel 1987, p. 389.

5   Steiner, R. *An Outline of esoteric science.* Anthroposophic Press, Great Barrington 2009.

6   Fintelmann, V. *Altersprechstunde.* Verlag Urachhaus, Stuttgart 2005.

7   Simonis, W.C. *Wolle und Seide.* Verlag Freies Geistesleben, Stuttgart 1995.

8   Hauschka, R. *Substanzlehre.* Verlag Vittorio Klostermann, Frankfurt 2007.

9   ibid.

10   ibid.

11   van Houten, C. *Awakening the will. Principles and processes in adult learning.* 2nd ed. Temple Lodge, Forest Row 2000.

12   Hauschka, R. *Substanzlehre.* Verlag Vittorio Klostermann, Frankfurt 2007.

13   Geuter, M. *Kräuter in der Ernährung.* Novalis Verlag, Steinbergkirche 1976.

14   Simonis, W.C. *Die Ernährung des Menschen.* Verlag Freies Geistesleben, Stuttgart 1971.

15   ibid.

CHAPTER X
Variations in Whole-Body Washing

ROLF HEINE

A whole-body wash aims to do more than just clean the body. It also addresses the patient's vital forces. The atmosphere and the nurse's inner attitude determine the quality of the wash. Standardized or routine washing is not an expression of professional nursing care, rather: patient-appropriate, creative variation of whole-body washing.

→   Learning objectives, see end of chapter

1.   General aspects

Washing is a process that touches body, soul, and spirit equally. Let us look first at the various aspects that can be considered when washing.

When a wash involves the removal of impurities such as sweat, feces and urine, we are primarily considering the *physical body*. The purpose of cleansing is to protect the skin from infection and maceration. In addition, a wash can enliven, refresh, relax, enable the patient to feel their body's boundaries, stimulate sensory activity. This kind of wash addresses the patient's *life forces* and achieves effects that go beyond the physical body.

Washing and nursing care also contribute to a patient's well-being by enabling her to present herself to the people around her in an aesthetically pleasing state. Through the attention bestowed during the washing and the improved appearance of her body there is an effect on her *soul* as well as on her physical body and life forces.

When special emphasis is placed on the patient's own contribution during a wash, this supports willpower, concentration and dexterity. Washing now serves above all to maintain or regain everyday and self-care competence. The wash addresses the 'I'.

For the seriously ill or dying person, washing gains an even deeper quality. In an unsentimental way it becomes an expression of human support, a pure gesture of service. The physical and psychological aspects of washing become less important; the washing seeks the human being as such. This can intensify into purification in the sense of a ritual.

Since washing always affects the whole human being, these aspects cannot be considered in isolation from one another. Nevertheless, knowing what quality we wish to address via the washing can enable us to set priorities in the way we do it. Thus, we do not primarily wash a bedridden, continent patient (such as after a heart attack) in order to remove soiling, but to accommodate his personal habits and his need to feel well groomed. Washing can also aim to relieve cramps and provide a feeling of security.

In an unconscious person, aesthetic aspects take a back seat during washing but do not have to be neglected. Here, it is the stimulation and support of the life forces that gains essential importance.

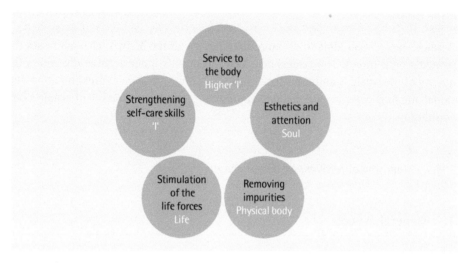

Fig. 1: Qualities in washing

Independence training is usually important when washing a patient with hemiplegia. This seems to be the ultimate way for an awake, practicing person to progress.

For a dying person, apart from relief and refreshment, service to the physical body as the "temple of the spirit" comes to the fore. The nurse remains inwardly oriented towards the person's soul, which is gradually detaching itself from the body. The individual nursing activities appear in a new light in view of the approaching death.

Knowledge of the levels of being that can be reached in washing makes it possible to treat people in need of care in a differentiated way. It extends the merely schematic approach, in which all patients are treated according to a fixed hygienic standard and simultaneously denied exclusive orientation to their wishes. In the following, five qualities are applied to various care situations by way of example. No schematic instructions for washing follow from this. The practical procedure in each individual case must relate to the specific situation of the patient. The basic forms of washing only unfold their effect when they have been individualized by the nurse and are put into practice on the patient.

ELEMENTS OF PRACTICAL NURSING

2. Basic types of washing

2.1 Washing as service to the body

The washing of a person in need of assistance is often regarded as a nursing service. Such an attitude is inclined to adapt the wash to the wishes of the patient. But what if the sick person does not express a need for this, or is indifferent or annoyed by being washed? Do we then follow our own ideas as to whether and how they should receive body care?

When we regard the physical body as an image of the being of soul and spirit, we see it as the result of the individuality working within it. The body-forming activity of the soul and spirit only cease when the body has become a corpse. The body has then reached its final form. The care of the physical body, if we understand its image character, can be carried by our respect for the being of soul and spirit expressed in this body. Respect and devotion allow us to enter into the service of the physical body. We use the elements of washing, i.e., water, temperature, touch, and rhythm, in such a way that they appear as gestures of service given in awareness of the mystery of the physical body. Water becomes the symbol of life. It frees the body from what is foreign and dead. Warmth and touch can be experienced as gestures of encounter between the nurse and the patient, the rhythm of the movements appears as a symbol of the connection and detachment between soul and body.

2.2 Strengthening self-care skills

Care of one's own body is an expression of human independence and autonomy. For many people the idea of being dependent on the care of others is therefore unbearable, especially concerning body care and excretions. The idea of being subject to existential, degrading dependence (on machines and people!) is—besides the loss of consciousness in dementia—a main reason for the death wish behind living wills and suicides.

Fortunately, in the vast majority of cases, when dependence on care occurs, we experience that it is not the feeling of loss of dignity that is in the foreground, but the feeling of relief and liberation from a painful situation. As a nurse, you are dependent on the trust of the person in need of care. This trust can be perceived as a gift, especially if you are aware of the shame and powerlessness of the person in need of care. Being allowed to help and receiving help then creates a super-personal quality of dignity and humanity. It is focusing on this healthy aspect, on what is intact and human, that makes body care one of the special moments of nursing care, despite all the unpleasant smells, the shame and sometimes resistance.

In order not to force people in need of care into the role of dependents and beneficiaries, every effort should be made to support their own activity. Independence is often not promoted consistently and purposefully, especially in inpatient care, because, at first glance, rehabilitative care takes longer than passive care. However, when the patient can move his hands and arms, sit up in bed or stand in front of the sink, this mobilization, this handling of the washcloth, towel, toothbrush and comb activate his life-long habits and life forces. His soul dips into the body in movement and rest, in muscle contraction and relaxation. The 'I' realizes itself in the physical body through this orderly, purposeful washing of oneself, raising oneself upright and facing oneself in the mirror.

2.3   Esthetics and attention as elements of washing

A well-groomed body becomes an expression of the attention paid to it. Neglect is the corresponding counter-image in which indifference towards the body appears. This does not necessarily have to correspond to a general feeling of the patient, it can occur temporarily in states of exhaustion. The need to appear well-groomed then takes a back seat to the struggle for homeostasis (balanced life processes).

In this case the care of the patient's external appearance becomes the task of the nurse. It enables the patient to face the people around him without shame, i.e., in accordance with his self-image; it becomes a visible expression of comprehensive care. In this sense, hair care, shaving if necessary, nail and skin care are not just cosmetic problems. Rather, such care gives an impulse for order and form that contributes significantly to the well-being of the soul in its home, the body.

Example

A young patient wanted to go to the hairdresser one day before her death, which she had been expecting for quite some time. When she came back radiantly with freshly washed and cut hair, we greeted her with admiration and wonder and she responded, smiling: "So that the angels have something nice to look at!"

From the point of view of esthetics, washing and nursing care try to maintain order as appropriate to the patient. They thus take care of something on behalf of the ill person who cannot establish this order herself. It is precisely in paying attention to these "external" things that the patient intensively experiences the nurse's personal attention.

Physical touch and closeness require and create trust [→ Chapter "Rhythmical Einreibung"]. Especially the washing of the sex organs is often a litmus test for the empathy of the nurse. It is important to perceive the shame of the patient as well as one's own feelings of not being at ease. Covering the intimate area with a towel whenever the nurse is not directly involved, even if only to rinse out the washing mitt, is an exemplary gesture of attention and respect. This makes a significant contribution to the patient being able to tolerate the washing, especially when it must be carried out particularly thoroughly from a hygienic point of view. Such a gesture makes it clear that you want to meet the hygienic requirements and protect the patient's private sphere in equal measure.

2.4   Washing to stimulate the life forces

A wash can enliven, refresh and awaken—or relax, harmonize and lead to sleep. It stimulates sensory and metabolic activity or supports the rhythmic balance between them. The appropriate washing technique must be chosen to achieve specific effects.

The following section presents three different types of wash.

2.4.1 Invigorating wash

An invigorating wash is indicated for:

- people who have a hard time waking up in the morning
- those sufferering from heart failure (beware of pulmonary congestion or pulmonary edema!)
- somnolent or unconscious patients
- depressed patients

In a stimulating, invigorating wash, the temperature of the washing water is selected to be at or slightly below body temperature. As the water cools down in the bowl and on the skin, the wash has a cooling effect without the patient beginning to freeze. The addition of rosemary or citrus bath milk enhances the refreshing effect (e.g., *Rosemary Invigorating Bath Milk* (Weleda) or *Lemon Lemongrass Vitalising Bath Essence* (Dr. Hauschka)).

The wash begins on the face, as the body region where we are most conscious. When we wake up in the morning, we first experience our facial area before we perceive and activate our limbs. The wash thus follows the process of awakening from the head region down to the limbs [see Fig. 2].

When washing the face, the washing mitt is thoroughly wrung out, so that no water flows out or is pressed out uncontrollably. The pressure applied to the different regions of the face should allow the patient to experience the boundaries of his body without feeling oppressed.

After the face you wash the right arm. Thus, the wash starts on the "strong", more conscious side. The treatment begins on the forearm in circular movements towards the shoulder, following the movement of blood to the heart. We apply criteria analogous to Rhythmical Einreibung [→ Chapter "Rhythmical Einreibung"].

Then wash the right hand with a little more pressure. The patient often responds to this touch with slight counterpressure or finger movements. We treat the left arm in the same way.

The front upper body is washed in circular movements from the shoulder via the sternum along the rib arches, first on the right, then on the left. The abdomen is treated in a clockwise spiral running towards the umbilical region. The movement thus follows the direction of peristalsis. The patient's sides are stroked down from the lowest rib arch to the hip.

Then the patient is brought upright to wash her back, or she lies on her side. The wash begins—analogous to a back treatment with Rhythmical Einreibung—on the shoulders with circular movements from paravertebral to lateral, first right, then left. The drying of the back accentuates uprightness by moving the towel with light pressure along the paravertebral muscles from top to bottom.

The washing of the legs is done in the same way as the washing of the arms from the ankles to the hips, i.e., towards the heart. The inner thighs are omitted as they are included during intimate care. The washing of the feet is the concluding act in each case.

The pressure exerted by the washing mitt or towel should not cause any tissue to be pushed forward (as with Rhythmical Einreibung): the stimulating effect does not result from firm grips, but from rhythmic movement impulses.

An activating wash should convey as many sensory impressions as possible. The strength of the sensory stimulus is less important than the *targeted stimulation* of the sensory zones.

This can be done by:

- the perception of the body's boundary through touch
- the perception of the effect (stimulation, relaxation, etc.) on the body
- the experience of active and passive movements
- the experience of equilibrium during positioning
- the smell of the bath additive
- the taste experience in oral hygiene
- the optical perception of the washing
- the warmth or coolness of the water
- the sounds caused by the water
- the speaking of the nurse
- the perception of the deliberate order in the series of actions
- the perception of the nurse's personality

In order not to overwhelm the patient with an abundance of sensory impressions and to make orientation easier for him, it is important to announce each step of the wash. Awareness should not be created by stress, which occurs when the patient is unable to anticipate what is going to happen on his body and resists it.

2.4.2 Soothing wash

A soothing wash is indicated for:

- emotionally or physically tense, cramped patients
- excited or anxious people
- patients with, e.g., hyperthyroidism, hypertension or after a heart attack
- pain sufferers

Lavender or spruce needle bath milk is recommended as an additive to the wash water.

■ *Moor Lavender Calming Bath Essence* (Dr. Hauschka)

■ *Lavender Relaxing Bath Milk* (Weleda)

■ *Spruce Needle Bath Oil (Wind und Wetter Bad)* (Dr. Hauschka)

■ *Pine Reviving Bath Milk (Edeltannen Erholungsbad)* (Weleda)

The temperature of the water is about 40°C (104°F), so that the patient feels pleasant warmth, despite the cooling of the water during the process and the cooling by evaporation. The washing mitt is wrung out well so that no water drips off.

The soothing wash begins with treatment of the patient's face. You kind of sculpt the contours of their face with calm movements. The patient often experiences this gentle cleaning as very gentle attention. You do not only feel the surface of their face, it is like a wide landscape through which your hand moves empathetically.

You continue the soothing washing on the right shoulder. From there you move down to the hand, following the muscles of the arm. Without pressure, you wipe the arm down to the fingertips. The washing of the left arm is done in the same way.

You wash the chest area, starting at the shoulders, along the rib arches in calm strokes, then, after the patient has been turned to the side, along their back, right and left along their spine. You stroke the legs in the same way as the arms from the hip to the feet without pressure.

The direction of movement during a soothing wash thus goes from the center to the periphery, from the trunk of the body to the limbs [see Fig. 3]. This releases tense and cramped limbs, which tend to bend closely towards the trunk, and orients them in the direction of expansion and relaxation.

The movement corresponds to the path of the soul as it detaches from the body in sleep, in contrast to the soul's approach to the body when waking up, as described in the stimulating wash, which leads from the periphery to the center.

2.4.3 "Sounding bath"

This wash takes the patient's state of strength into account in a special way. A "sounding bath" is indicated for:

- patients whose general condition is reduced
- patients after major surgery
- polytraumatized patients
- dying people

The weakness of the patient demands a particularly careful handling of active and passive movements that would overstrain him but would be unavoidable during a normal wash. To give these patients freshness, stimulation and relaxation, we reduce the wash to the treatment of the face, plus a hand and/or foot bath.

We begin with the cleansing of the face in the sense of a soothing wash and continue with a bath of the right hand. For this purpose, a wash bowl with a low rim is filled with water at a temperature of approx. 40°C (104°F) and placed on the right side of the patient. The patient's upper body is slightly elevated, so that the person's fingers are comfortably immersed in the water. The nurse now scoops water from the wash bowl with his hollow hand and pours it over the patient's hand, which is half resting in the water. (Do not squeeze out the washing mitt over the hand instead of scooping water!) The resulting slight current and the sound of the softly splashing water (hence the name "sounding bath") have a calming and stimulating effect at the same time. Mostly the patient likes to move her hand and reaches for the washing mitt or the hand of the nurse. The nurse can now easily press the crumpled washing mitt into the patient's palm and gently close her fingers into a fist which involuntarily grips the bundle.

After about one to two minutes, lift her hand out of the water and place it on a prepared towel, cover and dry it with light pressure. Then place the wash bowl on the other side and treat the left hand in the same way.

For the washing of the feet the water should still be about 38°C (100.4°F) warm. Again, we start with the right foot. The lower leg is pulled up to a 90-degree angle and the foot is placed in the water. In most cases, the leg must be supported by the hand of the nurse or suitable positioning aids. As with the hand bath, we pour water several times from our hollow hand over the foot. We dry the foot again after about one to two minutes. We then treat the left foot in the same way.

Hand and foot baths, as well as face washing, whether administered together or separately, give an exhausted patient the feeling of being treated as a whole person. The washing of a small area of the body thus becomes the starting point for mild but comprehensive invigoration.

To avoid the danger of misunderstanding the basic forms of washing as a fixed system, here are some examples which describe modified procedures.

Example 1

One patient suffered from pain all night long and therefore slept only a few hours. In the morning he felt tired and shattered. As several examinations were scheduled on this day, the results of which the patient eagerly awaited, it was not possible to catch up on the missed night's sleep in the morning. He was given a calming wash with lavender bath milk (e.g., with *Moor Lavender Calming Bath Essence* (Dr. Hauschka) or *Lavender Relaxing Bath Milk* (Weleda)), appropriate to his tense overall situation, as well as a foot bath, which provided mild stimulation and enlivening. The patient relaxed visibly during the treatment, slept for about half an hour and woke up strengthened and optimistic.

Example 2

An elderly hemiplegic patient in a depressed mood was sleepy all day long. The morning stimulating wash with rosemary bath milk (e.g., *Rosemary Invigorating Bath Milk* (Weleda)) helped him to greater alertness for only about one hour, then the usual sleepiness returned. The night watch reported that the patient was very active at night and slept little. We countered this reversal of the waking-sleeping rhythm with an activating wash in the evening. Together with a cup of coffee, it led to a brief, bright alertness, as in the morning. After about one hour the patient slept deeply and firmly until about two o'clock.

Example 3

We treated a patient with heart failure with citrus bath milk (e.g., *Citrus Refreshing Bath Milk* (Weleda) or *Lemon Lemongrass Vitalising Bath Essence* (Dr. Hauschka)) in the mornings as part of a complete wash, and in the evenings with citrus arm baths* to support the rhythm between stimulation and letting go during the day. The treatment was later intensified by administering corresponding Rhythmical Einreibung treatments of the legs and arms.

---

*   The patient sits at the sink. Fill the sink half-full with body-warm water and add Citrus Refreshing Bath (Weleda) or Lemon Lemongrass Bath (Dr. Hauschka). Dip both forearms in the water. Application time approximately five minutes, rest for at least ten minutes. This relieves the patient's respiration. A feeling of lightness ensues.

2.6 Cleansing impurities and the procedure for whole-body washing

So far washing has been presented without consideration of physical cleansing. However, this aspect must not be neglected in nursing practice. Given the widespread overemphasis on this aspect, I do not wish to go into it further here. Instead, it must be shown how physical cleansing fits into the process of a stimulating whole-body wash. There are two different forms:

- The washing of a patient who is actively involved.
- The washing of a completely dependent patient.

In both cases the wash must be prepared. After informing the patient (even an unconscious one!), we close the windows and, if necessary, set up a screen to create an undisturbed, protected atmosphere. The room should be warm.

We prepare the equipment required for washing and remove superfluous supports from the bed. We position the patient on her back with a slightly elevated upper body. She remains covered in any case, so that she does not get cold and feels protected and wrapped under the blanket. During the wash, only the areas to be treated are uncovered. Patients who are partly actively involved in the washing process are asked about which areas they require assistance with. Since this is often not verbalized by the patient herself, especially in the area of intimate care, we must form our own opinion about the need for help and suggest appropriate assistance to the patient. The aspects described at the beginning are decisive for making this judgment. Training independence is not always a priority.

For example, the patient's washing habits can be adjusted to the aspect of enlivening, if we gain her consent.

In most cases, partially independent patients are responsible for washing their own face and upper body. They may need help in coordinating a meaningful process in this area also. By washing their back, genital area, and legs, we clean those parts of the body that are difficult to access.

Mouth, nail and hair care, which are the most visible for the person's outer appearance, complete the washing process.

We finish the treatment possibly by changing the bed linen, smoothing the sheets, shaking the pillows and duvet, repositioning the patient and tidying up the washing materials and the hospital room. The outer environment thus also appears well ordered. For patients who are completely in need of assistance, the nurse largely determines the criteria under which washing will be performed. Here it is particularly important to announce each step of the wash. Unconscious patients and patients suffering from disorientation tend to experience activities on their body as a threat if we do not perform our actions calmly and in a coordinated manner. It often makes sense to divide the washing into two or three segments in order not to overburden the patient.

Depending on the urgency, we start with oral or intimate care. In these areas, physical cleansing is usually in the foreground. It often makes sense to use disposable washing gloves for this. The patient is cleaned of impurities, the bed linen is renewed, the sheets are smoothed, the pillows shaken. After a break, we wash with a view to stimulating the vital forces. After another break, during which we tidy up the room, we now attend to the patient's hair, nails and, if necessary, a shave.

This structuring of the wash also makes it easier for the nurse to adjust inwardly to the characteristics of the individual segments. The removal of impurities takes place at an objective distance. Compassion for the weakness, tiredness or tension of the patient and one's impulse to alleviate his discomfort contribute to the stimulation of life forces. Our care for the person's external appearance is based on their search for their self-image and on the effort to make their body appear as an expression of being human. Washing thus serves the whole person in a completely unsentimental way.

Category	Example learning objectives	Recommended learning path
Skill	You confidently practice the three basic forms of therapeutic washing.	A
Your own learning objective		
Relationships	You treat washing as a dialogue between the patient and the nurse.	B
Your own learning objective		
Knowledge	You know the indications for the basic forms of washing.	C
Your own learning objective		

CHAPTER XI

Preventing Bedsores, Pneumonia, and Thrombosis in Seriously Ill Patients

ROLF HEINE

Bedsores, pneumonia, and thrombosis, when they occur secondarily in the hospital, are considered to be nursing errors that can endanger a patient's life. This chapter will show how prophylaxis as a holistic treatment can do far more than just protect patients from secondary complications. The key lies in recognizing the constitutional condition of seriously ill patients. This will expand and relativize the usual pattern of risk factors.

The following assumes a *sound basic knowledge* of *risks* and *prophylactic measures* and does not replace it. Instead of providing a sequence of risk factors and alternative methods for prophylaxis, we shall develop an overarching point of view. This will give the reader the opportunity to critically examine and expand his or her own nursing practice.

→ Learning objectives, see end of chapter

1. Understanding the causes of bedsores, pneumonia, and thrombosis

Bedsores, pneumonia, and thrombosis manifest themselves in three different organ systems: the skin, the lungs, and the blood. Despite the different noxious agents involved, severely ill patients in particular often tend to succumb to all three of these diseases simultaneously. Prophylactic measures must be taken in all three areas. Risk factors may be immobility, old age, clouding of consciousness, and nutritional disorders.

To get a closer look at the common causes of bedsores, pneumonia, and thrombosis, we shall first consider a patient who is obviously at risk in all three areas. We shall begin by only presenting phenomena that are accessible to external observation and we shall disregard data that are not immediately perceptible.

Example

An approximately 50-year-old woman lies in bed with her upper body slightly elevated. The white duvet covers her body up to her chest. The contours of her body are barely visible under the covering. Her cheekbones and lower jaw bones emerge sharply from her pale face. Her eyes are closed except for a small gap in which the white of the sclera appears. Barely audible breath flows through her pale red, slightly opened lips. Her head, with its flattened, brown-gray hair, has sunk weakly to her shoulder. Her upper body is supported by a pillow. Her right hand lies motionless on her breast, which barely rises and falls, but threatens to slide down at any moment, following gravity. Her left arm rests next to her body as if laid aside. Her hands and feet are cool. The patient only notices that someone is with her when she is spoken to. She opens her eyes but does not seek eye contact with the person. Her gaze remains veiled, as if directed into emptiness. Her head rests motionless on the pillows. She tries to moisten her dry lips with her tongue, which is also dry, and ends this futile effort with a faint sigh. After a few minutes she tries to detach first her upper body and then her pelvis from the support, but immediately sinks back to her original position. The sight of this arouses our compassion and an impulse to alleviate her condition.

The patient's consciousness is dulled. She cannot freely focus her attention on the world around her or deliberately turn away from it. In contrast to a healthy sleeper, who awakens to the bright light of consciousness, the seriously ill person in our example remains in a kind of mist of consciousness.

Her movements are powerless, without tension, her limbs are sagging or stiff. She has lost the ability of healthy people to move powerfully and purposefully or stand up. The ease with which even the unconscious movements of a healthy sleeper happen has given way to heaviness. The whole person seems heavy. She can no longer overcome gravity and is at its mercy, without any means to counteract it.

1.1   The importance of the 'I'-organization

Unconsciousness, flaccidity, numbness, and *heaviness* characterize the picture described above. Healthy people, in contrast, have an awake consciousness, mobility and lightness, thanks to their life forces.

The patient cannot overcome gravity with her own power to raise herself upright, cannot overcome inanimate rigidity with flowing, guided movement, cannot replace her dimmed consciousness with inner light. The laws operating in inanimate, inorganic nature begin to dominate the forces of conscious human life. Gravity pulls the body towards the earth without resistance. Where the body rests, anything beneath it pushes itself piece by piece into and beyond the body's boundaries. Consciousness and life have moved a little out of the body. The foreign, outside world has taken their place. Body tissue has died, in necrosis the person seems to partially become part of the outside world.

We recognize the cause for the outside world being able to assert itself within the boundaries of the body—it is the retreat of the forces that maintain bodily integrity. The power that creates and maintains bodily integrity is what we call the 'I'-organization. This penetrates and individualizes the human soul and etheric body and shapes the physical body's upbuilding and regenerating metabolic processes. In the neurosensory system it enables thinking consciousness, while having a degenerating effect [→ Chapter "The Anthropological Foundations"]. The 'I'-organization enables the human 'I' to express itself in corporeality.

All internal risk factors that are important for the development of bedsores are based on a weakening of the upbuilding power of the 'I'-organization in the metabolic system. This is ultimately the reason why the outside world can spread within the boundaries of the person's body.

The torpidity of movement and the slackness of the muscles in somnolent or paralyzed patients are expressions of the weakening or retreat of the soul organization (soul body). Lifelessness of the skin, malnutrition and circulatory disorders show an impairment of the fluid and flowing vital-force organization (etheric body). The 'I'-organization integrates the soul and etheric bodies. Prophylaxis must therefore start with it.

Pneumonia is another disease that can develop when the outside world spreads within the boundaries of the human body. Foreign life penetrates the human organism in cases of viral or bacterial colonization of the lungs. However, this foreign life can only assert itself if the person's own life has receded somewhat from an organ. The inflammatory reaction in the lungs is often an attempt to fight foreign life and restore bodily integrity. Just as the foreign substance of food is overcome and transformed into the body's own substance in the digestive process, so does a parenteral digestive process take place in inflammation.

Thrombosis, too, is to be understood from the point of view of the outside world spreading its influence within the limits of the body. Normally we experience a coagulation process when, after an injury, the blood that has escaped thickens and hardens on the surface of the body, contributing to the closure of the wound. Here, too, the coagulation process happens in the tissue debris and air of the outside world (!) The causes of thrombosis characterized in the Virchow triad can also be understood from this point of view.

Vascular wall damage, if caused by injury, is an external world influence that extends into corporeality. Changes and deposits on the vascular wall are also processes and substances that have fallen out of the blood and thus become foreign to the organism. They act within the blood vessels like a disturbing foreign process or body through which the coagulating activity is activated.

If there are changes in flow behavior, for example due to varicose veins, blood flow comes to a standstill. Congestion and vortexes occur. The blood performs a movement that is actually foreign to it, and the coagulation process begins. The balance between dissolution (e.g., in fibrinolysis) and hardening or blood coagulation inherent in the blood is one-sidedly disturbed in favor of the hardening tendency.

1.2   Excarnation and incarnation

Anthroposophic anthropology describes the withdrawal of the 'I' from upbuilding metabolic processes in the body (the basis for the development of bedsores, pneumonia and thrombosis) as "excarnation," in contrast to "incarnation," which is the connecting of the 'I' with its corporeality. We find incarnation processes when, after conception, the spiritual core of the human being enters into the embryo prepared by the parents and connects itself ever more deeply with it. Such incarnation processes predominate in the first half of life. They cause the body to develop into its own unmistakable, individual shape. Through them the body becomes an instrument of the spiritual being of the person.[1]

In the second half of life, processes of excarnation begin to predominate. The spiritual being, the human 'I' gradually frees itself from its close union with the body and becomes more and more independent of it. The upbuilding life forces are transformed into forces of consciousness [→ Chapter "Illness and Destiny"]. Thus, in the second half of life, it is obvious that degeneration processes predominate over upbuilding ones, causing people to age. Finally, in death, the 'I' and with it the other members constituting the human being detach themselves completely from the physical body and delve into a bodiless existence.

This makes it clear why elderly people, in whom the processes of excarnation naturally predominate, are particularly susceptible to developing bedsores, pneumonia and thrombosis. Very rarely, however, are these diseases found in the incarnating phase of life, in children or adolescents. Only in life-threatening conditions is there a danger of it happening in this phase of life.

The polarity of processes of excarnation and incarnation is also found in the rhythm of sleeping and waking. In the waking state we experience ourselves as being connected with our body. Through our sense organs we perceive the world and our body, show feelings and can act. In sleep, on the other hand, we have no consciousness. If consciousness enters while we sleep, we are already beginning to wake up.

The 'I' and the soul body separate in sleep from the etheric and physical bodies. When the soul body approaches the physical body again during sleep, without being completely connected to it, we experience dreams, a state of consciousness which is subdued compared to waking consciousness. In dreams, body-bound and body-free consciousness mix and cause the chaotic dream images that are not subject to the laws of the sensory world.[2]

In contrast to healthy people, the body of someone who is seriously ill does not regenerate sufficiently during sleep. Degenerating external world influences are no longer completely balanced out, they push into the body without resistance. A disposition to develop secondary problems develops.

2.   General prophylaxis

We have identified the common cause of bedsores, pneumonia and thrombosis as the withdrawal of the upbuilding aspect of the 'I'-organization. This withdrawal allows external influences to start having an effect within the boundaries of the body. As prophylactic measures, we can consider, on the one hand, everything that protects the organism from external influences. On the other hand, we can strengthen the 'I'-organization to prevent the occurrence of secondary damage.

As shown in the chapter *"Warmth,"* the 'I' works in warmth within the human body. Blood distributes the warmth throughout the organism. Fluctuations in the balance of warmth are an expression of the depth with which the 'I'-organization intervenes in its physical corporeality. *Stimulation of the warmth organism* is thus the key to counteracting the tendency of severely ill people to excarnate and the key to supporting the connection of the 'I' with its corporeality.

We need to take into consideration the stimulation of warmth in body, soul and spirit. While warmth in the body expresses itself in measurable body temperature, it appears in the soul and spirit as a non-sense-perceptible quality.

2.1 Warmth in the spiritual aspect

We find the warming element in spirit wherever something grips us so strongly that we become enthusiastic about it. When we connect to something inwardly, we say: "We've warmed to the idea" or "we're fired with enthusiasm." Wherever we must overcome resistance, there is friction and friction generates heat. We have "heated" arguments—or something "leaves us cold" when we do not want to relate to it. Wherever we actively associate ourselves with an idea, a thing or a person, we have a specific, experience of warmth in soul and spirit. This can have a physical effect. People who are enthusiastic about something feel warmth right down into their limbs. Warmth and fire manifest in their whole being.

In ailing people, we often find that this inner fire is lacking. They are apathetic, without a goal, without motivation. When we succeed in leading a patient out of apathy to an occupation with goals and interests, we have stimulated a spiritual warmth quality in him. A patient who develops an interest in his environment, who sets himself tasks and goals, is not only cooperative regarding therapeutic and nursing measures, he also creates in himself a basis for his 'I' to be present in his body. Motivation therefore comes before mobilization. Motivation and willingness to cooperate are essential resources in bedsore prophylaxis and, when they are lacking, also represent factors in determining the risk of bedsores on the extended Norton scale.[3] This also applies to the prophylaxis of pneumonia and thrombosis. It is not enough to inform the patient about the need for prophylactic measures or to make her aware of the consequences of neglecting them. Her intellectual capacity might not be up to that. Rather, the aim is to promote and care for even the smallest interests of the patient. Here we find a starting point for strengthening her willpower and initiative. When this happens, the patient warms up to things in the sense described above.

2.2 Warmth in the soul

Everyday language often relates soul warmth to the heart. In this center of our life of soul we experience the quality of warmth directly. A warm-hearted person is thought to have empathy, richness of feeling, trustworthiness, leniency, the ability to forgive—in short, predominantly sympathetic qualities. We experience a cold-hearted person as being hard, rejecting, unfeeling, selfish, occupied with himself. Antipathetic traits predominate. Whoever experiences a person as being warm-hearted is inclined to confide in him—rather than in a cold-hearted or hard-hearted person. In an emotionally warm environment, we feel comfortable and accepted. When someone gives us a "cold shoulder," we experience rejection. When we encounter soul warmth, we expand; when we encounter mental coldness, we withdraw.

This withdrawal from the environment must be counteracted, especially in the case of the seriously ill. Unfortunately, the hospital atmosphere is not always such that patients feel warmly welcomed and accepted. Functional hospital rooms, which hardly allow for use that suits the patient, uniform daily routines, which take little consideration of the life rhythms of the patient, and nurses and physicians who do not let feelings of inner sympathy develop in themselves, push patients into mental isolation.

Especially patients who are in danger of contracting pneumonia need an atmosphere in which they can open themselves to the environment. People are in constant physical and psychological connection with their surroundings through their breathing. Their respiration participates in emotions as if seismographically. In shock the breath falters; we breathe a sigh of relief when we are delivered from a stressful situation; we breathe in and out calmly, fluently and pleasurably when we feel comfortable. When we feel unwell, our breathing is restrained and halting. In the mentally withdrawn states of depressed, apathetic or somnolent patients we notice an inability to participate in the environment, as well as flat, monotonous breathing that is insensitive to external impressions.

Many common methods of pneumonia prophylaxis do not consider the connection between breathing activity and the person's mood. Even today, slapping the back with a cold, wet solution is still an often-used method of pneumonia prophylaxis. Although it achieves a short-term shock effect due to the sudden cooling and the quick blows to the back, it probably only achieves deep breathing once. Together with the resulting coughing stimulus, this measure is extremely unpleasant for patients, especially if they are in a weakened state. The possible relief or the prophylactic effect that the patient experiences because of this treatment is usually out of proportion to the strain endured. Such a measure certainly does not encourage joyful sympathy for the environment, it rather reinforces the impression of being subjected to a hostile, perhaps even violent human environment.

If you treat the patient's back and chest with Rhythmical Einreibung instead of this, she will feel personally perceived and tended to. The nurse's touching hand reacts sensitively to every movement of her thorax. In addition to the physical warmth that develops, the treatment conveys a feeling of human closeness, inner attention and caring. The patient's breathing deepens during this rhythmical treatment, she is not overwhelmed by an experience of shock, but is lured by the rhythmically moving touch from "being closed in herself" into alertness and participation in her environment. Rhythmical Einreibung of her sides opens her breathing space into the abdomen. Paravertebral strokes create awareness of her upright form [→ Chapter "Rhythmical Einreibung"].

- *Lavandula, Oleum aethereum 10%* (WALA)

- *Lavender 10% oil* (Weleda)

- *Plantago Bronchialbalsam (*WALA)

The use of lavender 10% oil eases and relaxes and is therefore indicated for anxiety, thoracic pain and irritability. Plantago Bronchialbalsam supports the loosening of secretions with sun dew, thyme and narrowleaf plantain, and its beeswax content forms a particularly warming sense of protectedness.

Dead space enlargers such as tubes or other respiratory training devices, which are designed to encourage the patient to build up pressure or suction in the thorax, are as off-putting as back slapping. They usually overtax the ability of a patient who is actually at risk of pneumonia to cooperate. Such measures have their justification for the pre- and post-operative training of vital capacity in conscious patients. However, a mentally withdrawn, weakened or dimly conscious patient remains uninvolved in such proceedings. They do not reach him in his inner mood. What weakened patient can tolerate having their nose closed with a clamp? The breathing difficulty forced by the increase in dead space arouses anxiety and is usually undermined by "forbidden," "normal" breaths. No measure that has only the filling of the lung with air as its goal will reach the patient in his soul.

If, on the other hand, it is possible to make the patient laugh or perhaps just smile, he is able to immerse himself in a warm soul atmosphere, and the deepening of inhalation happens with his inner participation. Even the singing of simple songs with or for the patient primarily seeks inner participation and reaches a deepening of breathing secondarily, but all the more sustainably.

Both Rhythmical Einreibung and singing are effective in the prophylaxis of thrombosis and bedsores, since the patient's soul is stimulated and "warmed through." The ill person begins to feel at home in her body again. She becomes more alert, her mobility increases, her blood circulation revives.

2.3   Warmth in the body

Warmth phenomena in the body play an important role when determining the risk of bedsores, pneumonia and thrombosis.

- Lack of blood circulation in the skin manifests in cold zones perceptible to touch.
- High-risk patients cool down quickly and sustainably when they are not protected by clothing or blankets.
- Fever becomes a risk when it consumes the patient's energy.

- When first-degree bedsores, thrombosis or pneumonia are already present, the organism responds with an inflammatory reaction. In this case we find local overheating besides the other classical signs of inflammation.
- Especially in pneumonia, fever is added to the local heat reaction.

Local overheating and fever are expressions of an attempt at healing. This is a further indication of the prophylactic effect of stimulating and strengthening the patient's warmth organism.

Neander and Birkenfeld showed that passive heat treatment, e.g., via cooling and blow-drying, does not improve circulation in the skin, but worsens it. It is therefore unsuitable for bedsore prophylaxis.[4] Laser Doppler Flowmetry and thermography confirm the observation that heat and cold stimuli applied to the organism from the outside do not automatically lead to an internal heat reaction.[5] Whether a heat stimulus coming from outside is taken up by an internal warmth response depends ultimately on the extent to which the organism is able to rhythmically balance the polarity of heat concentration inside the body and heat expansion into the body's periphery. If it is not possible to attract the heat from inside the body to the periphery, the body surface remains cold.

It has been observed that cold hands or feet of exhausted patients or patients suffering from circulatory disorders, in whom a hot-water bottle did not lead to warming, can still experience a sustained warming of their extremities and/or abdomen by means of Rhythmical Einreibung treatment of their extremities and/or abdomen. Rhythmical Einreibung can therefore be regarded as a suitable means of stimulating warming and blood circulation. An expertly performed Rhythmical Einreibung of the legs warms and enlivens both the lower extremities and the person as a whole [→ Chapter "Rhythmical Einreibung"]. The person's breathing deepens, he becomes tired in a pleasant way, perhaps he falls asleep and wakes up strengthened.

The resulting stimulation of the patient's legs also encourages movement, so that a holistic basis is created for thrombosis prophylaxis as well as for bedsore and pneumonia prevention.

3.   Special aspects

3.1   Bedsore prophylaxis

In bedsores, the skin is the damaged organ. Skin is the most extensive sensory organ on the body's surface, part of the neurosensory system, and provides an entry for the impressions approaching from outside. When this sensory function is lost through local or central disturbances of consciousness, then adequate reaction to a sensory stimulus is no longer possible. The stimulus then does not lead to a conscious impression, but only has a physical effect on the body's outer boundary.

Prophylactically helpful are therefore not only those measures which keep the stimulus away from the body or limit its duration, such as freeing or repositioning, but also all those which promote sensory perception. Washing, Rhythmical Einreibung, conscious touch and guided movements stimulate sensory activity and support the presence of the 'I' in the body.

Regular two-hourly inspection of a pressure-endangered part of the body has more than diagnostic value. On the one hand, it replaces the patient's impaired ability to perceive, on the other it directs the patient's consciousness into those areas that elude his perception. Constant reference to body regions that the patient cannot perceive as belonging to himself has a high prophylactic value in this sense and is a first approach to restoring healthy body awareness. Immobility is the greatest risk factor in the development of pressure sores. However, weakness, loss of consciousness and paralysis not only restrict the patient's mobility, they also force her from an upright posture into a horizontal one. Uprightness is a specific quality for which only the human movement organism is equipped. A child learns to walk upright around the first year of life, before learning to speak and to think. Only in sleep, when the 'I' detaches itself from the body, do we lose uprightness, as well as speaking and thinking, and sink into horizontalness. In uprightness the 'I' reveals itself in its physical form. The horizontal posture prescribed by a doctor or nurse, or forced by illness, relieves the patient of the effort of being upright. Since the immobile bedridden patient is not able to rise from the horizontal without help, she lacks an essential incentive to take hold of her form as an 'I'. Regular setting upright and positioning of immobile bedridden patients, even unconscious patients in bed or on the edge of the bed is therefore an important measure to stimulate the incarnation process, unless there are contraindications. Rhythmical Einreibung of the back and paravertebral strokes emphasize the spine in its upright position and thus additionally support this process.

The repositioning of an immobile patient to relieve pressure should therefore be supplemented at least three times a day with uprightness lasting at least a few minutes [→ Chapter "Geriatric Care as Care for Human Beings"].

This measure, too, helps prevent pneumonia and thrombosis by stimulating respiration and blood circulation. In addition to the regular repositioning of the patient who is at risk of bedsores, essential elements of prophylaxis are hollow positioning and super-soft positioning. As a rule, these measures are only carried out with pressure relief in mind. The nurse's attention remains focused on the outside damaging influence. If, on the other hand, we consider not only the external noxious agent but also the perspective of the patient weighing heavily on the mattress, we discover other perspectives for positioning. The aim is then to move the patient from heaviness to lightness.

In fact, a patient who is well supported, e.g., in a 30-degree position on her side, not only appears to be relieved of pressure, she also seems relaxed, light, as if bedded "on clouds." In this case, the term "light" refers to both the physical facts of "pressure relief" and the condition of the patient. When the caregiver acts with a view to the aspect of "lightness," he will feel inspired to artfully harmonize the physical goal of "pressure relief" with the well-being of the patient as he creates a new situation for her.

The lung, as the organ primarily damaged in pneumonia, is part of the rhythmic system. Just as the neurosensory system forms the bodily basis for conscious perception and conceptualization, so the rhythmic system forms the basis for feeling [→ Chapter "The Anthropological Foundations"]. Pneumonia prophylaxis should take this into account.

It has already been pointed out that all respiratory support measures must involve patients inwardly. Breathing exercises that are merely mechanically done lead neither to the desired ventilation of the lungs nor to the loosening of secretions, nor do they achieve the swinging of the soul that exhales out into the world and then inhales and returns to itself, which is necessary for prophylaxis. Speech and singing as expressions of the soul live in the respiratory stream and are therefore very suitable for deepening and encouraging the rhythm of breathing. They create the connection to the physical respiratory process. This point of view must be considered in all actions directed at the physical body. Thus, the mere prompting to "take a deep breath" seldom leads to a good result. Deep breathing must be learned. Those who are (still) able to do it are generally not at risk of pneumonia.

Intonating a vowel, or later the entire "a–e–i–o–u" vowel series, on a note that is appropriate for the patient, is an exercise that enables him to directly perceive the strength and depth of his airflow. The inhibition threshold for this exercise is relatively low. The situation is different with singing, where often considerable barriers must be overcome by both the patient and the nurse. The vowel exercise is a first step in this direction. If it is possible to sing a small song with the patient, we have obtained a suitable means for efficient pneumonia prophylaxis.

The measures described require a certain willingness to cooperate on the part of the patient. But how do you proceed to deepen the respiration of a *somnolent* or *unconscious* patient? In this case, the following procedure is recommended:

The patient is first placed on his back with his upper body slightly elevated, possibly in a slight stretch. The nurse places her warm hand on the patient's umbilical region. She lifts her hand as the patient inhales, without loosening it completely from the abdominal wall. In the exhalation phase she lowers her hand again. The raising and lowering of the hand takes place in the rhythm given by the patient, with the lowering hand exerting a slight increasing pressure on the abdomen. Usually abdominal breathing (with lifting and lowering of the abdominal wall) occurs after a few breaths. The flow of breath calms down and deepens. Now the nurse reduces the gentle pressure exerted during exhalation until her hand passively follows the lifting and lowering of the abdominal wall.

The treatment lasts until the patient can continue the stimulated breathing rhythm without the support of the nurse's hand. If it is not possible to deepen the patient's breathing in this way, or if the patient retains his thoracic breathing, the exercise can be performed in the same way by applying light pressure to the patient's sides. As a swing is pushed at the reversal point, the caregiver swings into the patient's breathing rhythm and strengthens it.

In addition to inadequate ventilation, another risk of pneumonia is poorly soluble secretions or difficulties in coughing up. Room humidification, inhalations and the practice of an efficient technique of coughing up are the most common nursing pro- phylactics, medically supported by mucolytics and pain therapy if necessary. These measures are complemented by external applications and Rhythmical Einreibung.

The beneficial effect of Rhythmical Einreibung on breathing depth and loosening secretions has already been demonstrated. If you want to increase the warming and loosening effect of the oil used in Rhythmical Einreibung, it is advisable to administer an *oil chest compress.* You heat a cotton cloth dabbed with (thyme) oil between two hot-water bottles and place it on the patient's back and/or chest. You place a slightly larger, previously made and likewise heated cotton pad on top of it and secure the pack around the chest (not too tightly!) with a woolen cloth.

■ *Thymus, Oleum aethereum 5%* (WALA)

The compress should be applied for several hours, but at least 30 minutes.[6] The long-lasting, mild warmth and the pleasant smell of the essential oil have a relaxing, antispasmodic, expectorant effect and alleviate unproductive irritable coughing. If bronchitis is already present, mustard or ginger thorax compresses are useful for deepening respiration and dissolving secretions in cooperative patients who have a stable circulation.[7, 8]

Warm farmer's cheese chest compresses bring relief[9] to patients with malignant pleural effusions. For patients with lungs previously damaged by emphysema, treat their back with Rhythmical Einreibung, using crystalline table salt mixed with a few drops of rosemary 10% oil (*Rosmarinus, Oleum aethereum 10%* (WALA)) in the palm of your hand to form a mush. The latter examples give an idea of how patients with pre-damaged lungs can be treated with external applications in cooperation with a physician.

MUSTARD THORAX COMPRESS: For the mustard thorax compress, sprinkle ground black mustard (1–2mm, available in pharmacies) onto a gauze compress cloth lined with tissue or a dish towel and fold it into a pack. Soak the pack in 40°C (104°F) warm water and wring it out carefully. Apply the compress to the patient's back and leave on for 5 to 7 minutes under the constant supervision of the caregiver. The post-treatment rest period is at least 30 minutes. The pack produces a strong burning sensation and pronounced reddening of the skin. It warms through and has an expectorant and antispasmodic effect. The mustard application may only be carried out by experienced nurses and by relatives after thorough instruction, as burns may occur if used incorrectly [→ Chapter "Compresses" and "Active Principles in External Applications"].

GINGER THORAX COMPRESS: Soak 1 tablespoon of dried, ground ginger root (available in pharmacies) in 300ml of hot water. Soak a triple folded gauze compress cloth in this brew and wring it out as firmly as possible. Apply the compress to the lower part of the dorsal thorax and leave it there for 20 to 30 minutes. The result is a pleasant warmth that penetrates into the depths, often accompanied by moving inner images. About 10 minutes of post-treatment rest.

FARMER'S CHEESE CHEST COMPRESS: Spread about 500g of low-fat farmer's cheese on a single-layer gauze compress. Heat the pack to about 38°C (100.4°F) with hot water bottles or a heat lamp and place it on the thorax. Leave the compress on for about 30 to 40 minutes, as long as it is pleasant. The post-treatment rest period is 30 minutes. The compress has an expectorant and relaxing effect. It is preferable to mustard or ginger applications for pleural effusions and other fluid blockages. Since farmer's cheese releases whey and easily smears, it is necessary to administer it carefully and use bed protection.[10]

3.3 Thrombosis prophylaxis

The risk of thrombosis seems to be the most difficult to assess of the three potential risks discussed here. We detect changes to the skin, as an organ that is completely exposed to the outside world, comparatively early and without great diagnostic effort. Changes in respiration can also usually be detected quickly on close observation. In contrast, processes in the blood and in the vascular system remain hidden from direct perception. This corresponds to the lack of perception that we have for our metabolic processes in general: only when disturbances in the form of pain or functional restrictions have manifested themselves do we become aware of our metabolic processes.

This means that for the indication of thrombosis prophylaxis we cannot fall back on direct observations but are to a large extent dependent on statistically assessing risk according to risk groups. This often results in prophylactic measures (e.g., heparinization, antithrombosis stockings) being applied schematically to people belonging to a risk group. Such an approach should not be criticized, considering the lack of a reliable alternative. However, holistic care should not relate the prophylactic measures solely to risk groups but should see them in the context of the specific overall situation of the patient.

The essential thrombosis prophylaxis measure performed independently by nursing staff is mobilization, including active and passive movement exercises, elevation of the extremities at risk, usually the legs, and compression by means of elastic stockings or wrapping. These measures aim to improve venous return flow by activating the "muscle pump," relieving the venous valves and reducing the lumen of the leg veins. This prophylaxis is therefore essentially justified by mechanical aspects.

If we take a closer look at the patient at risk of thrombosis, we often find that his limbs seem not to belong entirely to him. They appear either rigid and hard (e.g., in diabetes, contractures and spastic paralysis) or unformed, swollen, without tonus (e.g., in varicose veins, heart insufficiency and flaccid paralysis). The limbs are mostly cool, the movements without flowing dynamics.

For prophylaxis, all treatments that lead to invigoration, better "animation" of the limbs are therefore useful. This is particularly the case with mobilization. By actively using his arms and legs, the patient takes hold of what no longer fully belongs to him and makes it his own again. The more actively, i.e., the more inwardly he is involved, the more he penetrates his body. In this sense, mechanically completed exercises are less effective than conscious, guided movements. Rhythmical Einreibung counteracts the tendency towards excessive forming and rigidity, as well as the tendency towards slackening and loss of muscle tone. Rhythmical Einreibung does not, as one might think, "push" the blood towards the heart, but rather balances one-sidedness in muscle tone and stimulates the rhythmic flow of the blood. Rhythmical Einreibung thus leads to an animation (ensoulment) of the limbs and the entire organism.

4. Nursing care substances

The following section introduces some nursing care substances that are used prophylactically, e.g., in Rhythmical Einreibung treatments. Nursing care substances that have a particularly stimulating effect on warmth can be found among *fats* and *essential oils*.[11] Fats and essential oils are not chemically related. What both have in common, however, is that they are the most energy-rich substances that plants form. Fatty oils are found primarily in seeds, i.e., in an organ that is at the very end of a plant's growth process. Plants absorb light and warmth from the cosmos during growth and condense these qualities in their reproductive organs for the next generation. In a germinating seed, light and warmth are seemingly metamorphosed and released again into the newly sprouting plant. Fatty oils used as nursing substances also have this warming and enveloping property.

Essential oils are usually found in the flowers and leaves of plants. They give a plant its characteristic scent. In contrast to fats, essential oils are very volatile and highly flammable. They serve the plant, among other things, as an attractant for the insects which pollinate it. In fragrance and color, plants relate to the animal kingdom. Plants need fatty oils for their own existence, and they excrete essential oils. The following table summarizes the difference between fatty and essential oils. The comparison shows the following aspect for the prophylactic use of the two substance groups:

Essential oils actively stimulate warmth processes. Fatty oils protect and preserve the existing mantle of warmth. The combination of fatty and essential oils as in:

- *Oleum aethereum Lavandulae 10% oil* (Weleda)

- *Lavandula, Oleum aethereum 10%* (WALA)

- *Oleum aethereum Melissae indicum 10%* (Weleda)

is therefore suitable for stimulating and maintaining the warmth organism. Essential oils are also available as components of bath additives, such as:

- *Moor Lavender Calming Bath Essence* (Dr. Hauschka)

- *Lavender Relaxing Bath Milk* (Weleda)

- *Rosemary Invigorating Bath Milk* (Weleda)

- *Pine Reviving Bath Milk* (Weleda)

- *Spruce Needle Bath Oil* (Dr. Hauschka)

- *Citrus Refreshing Bath Milk* (Weleda)

- *Lemon Lemongrass Vitalising Bath Essence* (Dr. Hauschka)

Here it is the activating effect that dominates in combination with the invigorating element of water.

	Fatty oils	Essential oils
Primary localization in the plant	seeds	flower, leaf
Function	reproduction	aroma
Gesture	compacting, preserving, centripetal	dissolving, dispersing centrifugal
Therapeutic effect	enveloping, passively warming, protecting	opening outwards, actively warming, stimulating

Chart: Fats and essential oils

We got to know essential oils as warmth-stimulating substances. Rosemary is particularly suitable for bedsore prophylaxis. Applied externally, it has a stimulating and refreshing effect on the metabolism. As a bath additive

- *Rosemary Invigorating Bath Milk* (Weleda)

it is excellently suited for morning washing. Also, because of its warming and invigorating function,

- *Rosemarinus 10% ointment* (Weleda)

- *Revitalising Leg & Arm Tonic* (Dr. Hauschka)

are suitable for Rhythmical Einreibung of the legs.

In the local treatment of pressure-endangered areas, we must also consider skin care and protective substances in addition to stimulating the warmth organization. This includes the ointment bases or hydrocolloid dressings used. If the skin is dry, use an ointment base that absorbs well and contains oil and water. A protective ointment base with lanolin and zinc is recommended for skin endangered by wetness.

Extracts from Calendula officinalis (marigold), Matricaria chamomilla (chamomile) and/or Echinacea angustifolia (coneflower) have proven effective for prophylaxis and damaged skin. They contain essential oils and several substances that strengthen the skin's resistance. Due to their anti-inflammatory effects, they can also be used for first-degree decubitus ulcers.

As a rule, these creams are rubbed in three times a day or before and after each repositioning.

Skin condition	Ointment base	Suggested preparations
dry, scaly	sesame oil, almond oil, water	*Comforting Body Lotion* (Weleda)
normal	e.g., beeswax corn oil	*Calcea wound cream* (WALA)
danger of wetness	e.g., beeswax, zinc oxide	*Calendula Baby Cream* (Weleda)
strong danger of wetness	–	hydrocolloid dressing
first degree pressure sores	e.g., beeswax, corn oil	*Calcea wound creme* (WALA)

Chart: Calendula applications according to skin condition

Essential oils have an intense, characteristic scent. They stimulate breathing and circulation and dissolve secretions. This makes them particularly suitable for pneumonia prophylaxis. As the scent of essential oils is occasionally perceived to be a nuisance and they irritate the skin when applied in a concentrated form, essential oils should always be used sparingly and mixed with olive or peanut oil.

For pneumonia prophylaxis, we mainly consider plants which concentrate the essential oil in the leaf area, because this area corresponds to the rhythmic system in human beings [→ Chapter "Compresses"]. This is particularly the case with the Lamiaceae. The strict rhythmic structure of their bilaterally united leaves emphasizes the dominance of these organs over the roots and flowers in the plant's appearance. Lavender, peppermint, sage and thyme belong to this plant family and are proven agents for warming through and dissolving secretions.[12] In concentrations of 5% to 10%, these oils are suitable for both Rhythmical Einreibung and packs.

■ *Oleum aethereum Lavandulae 10% oil (*Weleda*), Lavandula, Oleum aethereum 10%* (WALA)	easing, relaxing in patients with anxiety, inner tension, excessive irritation
■ *Oleum Menthae piperitae 10%* (extemporaneous pharmacy preparation)	has a pronounced cooling effect, dissipates heat to the outside, refreshes patients with high fever (do not use when the fever is rising, only use locally, e.g., on the back or chest, never on the whole body).
■ *Oleum aethereum Salviae 10 %* (pharmacy formula)	invigorating, refreshing, especially suitable for heavily sweating patients
■ *Thymus, Oleum aethereum 5%* (WALA)	highly secretion-dissolving

4.3   Thrombosis

The family of Mediterranean Lamiaceae is characterized by its special relationship to the element of warmth.[13] However, its individual representatives show quite varied therapeutic effects. Lavender has a calming effect, sage and thyme dissolve secretions. Rosemary has particularly stimulating, invigorating effects on the metabolism. It is therefore preferred for the treatment of hardening conditions. Since thrombosis is always a risk when the formative forces streaming in through the neurosensory system are not sufficiently counteracted by upbuilding metabolic processes, rosemary is a suitable means of supporting the metabolic side.

When there is a risk of thrombosis due to varicose veins, it is advisable to treat the legs with Rhythmical Einreibung, using

- *Venadoron (Skin Tone Lotion)* (Weleda)[14]

The substances used (e.g., hamamelis) strengthen connective tissue and have also proven their worth as a care product during pregnancy.

Category	Example learning objectives	Recommended learning path
Relationships	You use complementary prophylactic methods creatively, adapting them to the patient.	A
Your own learning objective		
Relationships	You use the patient's resources for prophylaxis.	B
Your own learning objective		
Knowledge	You understand the mentioned secondary diseases as processes of excarnation.	C
Your own learning objective		

References

1   Bühler, W. *Der Leib als Instrument der Seele.* Verlag Freies Geistesleben, Stuttgart 1993.

2   Steiner, R. *An Outline of esoteric science.* Anthroposophic Press, Great Barrington 2009. Chapter "Sleep and Death."

3   Bienstein, C. et al. *Dekubitus, Prophylaxe, Therapie.* Deutscher Berufsverband für Krankenpflege Frankfurt am Main 1990, p. 233.

4   Neander, K-D; Birkenfeld, R. Welchen Effekt hat "Eisen und Fönen" zur Dekubitusprophylaxe? In: *Bienstein C et al. Dekubitus, Prophylaxe, Therapie.* Deutscher Berufsverband für Krankenpflege Frankfurt am Main 1990, p. 148 ff.

5   Risse, L. Institutionelle Bedingungen bestimmen die Form der Prophylaxe – Thermographie kontrolliert den Effekt. In: *Bienstein C et al. Dekubitus, Prophylaxe, Therapie.* Deutscher Berufsverband für Krankenpflege, Frankfurt am Main 1990, p. 108.

6   Eichler, E. *Wickel und Auflagen.* Gesundheit Aktiv – Anthroposophische Heilkunst, Bad Liebenzell 1991, p. 15.

7   Heine, R. et al. *Praxisintegrierte Studie zur Darstellung der Frühwirkungen von Ingwer (Zingiberis officinalis) als äußere Anwendung.* Selbstverlag Filderklinik, Filderstadt 1992.

8   Sommer, M. Zur praktischen Anwendung des Ingwerwickels. *Der Merkurstab* 2006; 59 (6), pp. 538–540.

9   Eichler, E. *Wickel und Auflagen.* Gesundheit Aktiv – Anthroposophische Heilkunst, Bad Liebenzell 1991, p. 15 f.

10 Fingado, M. *Compresses and Other Therapeutic Applications.* Floris, Edinburgh 2012.

11 Pelikan, W. *Healing Plants.* Mercury Press, Spring Valley 1997.

12 Weckenmann, M. Die offiziellen Lamiaceen (Labiaten). *Beiträge zu einer Erweiterung der Heilkunst* 1978; 31 (4), pp. 122–134.

13 ibid.

14 Weckenmann, M. et al. *Verlaufsbeobachtungen während einer Lokalbehandlung bei Patienten mit varikösem Symptomkomplex.* Erfahrungsheilkunde 1987; 36 (4), pp. 201–210.

CHAPTER XII

Rhythmical Einreibung According to Wegman/Hauschka

URSULA VON DER HEIDE · REVISED BY MONIKA LAYER

Rhythmical oil applications, known as Rhythmical Einreibung according to Wegman/ Hauschka, are widespread in anthroposophic nursing care (Translator's note: The German word *Einreibung* means "inunction" and is used internationally to show that a specific, well-defined form of treatment is meant.) This chapter will introduce the basic circle, straight line, and figure-eight application forms and give examples of their implementation. It will close with indications and effects and discuss ways of learning these techniques.

→   Learning objectives, see end of chapter

1.   Touch in nursing care

Hardly any encounter between a nurse and her patient happens without physical contact. It is not for nothing that we speak of "treating" the patient and this includes not only rhythmical oil applications themselves, but also washing, positioning, and mobilization. Other actions such as measuring pulse, temperature, and blood pressure are also associated with physical contact between the people involved. This already applies to the mobile and awake person who stretches out his arm towards the nurse so that she can put the blood pressure cuff on, and even more so to the seriously ill person with clouded consciousness, whose arm must be carefully lifted and supported in order to secure the cuff.

1.1   Closeness and distance

People who are dependent on nursing assistance find themselves isolated per se: they are torn out of their accustomed environment, unknown specialists are taking care of them, their whole everyday life is turned upside down, etc. Whether the help needed is expressed in physical touch or in conversation depends on the situation. The need for physical closeness is hardly verbalized, often only when the patient requests help with washing his back, or when he asks for an oil application. The writer Vilma Sturm (1912–1995) impressively described how intense the desire for touch and closeness really can be, especially in a strange, sober environment: " . . . between all the hands that carry syringes and tubes and fever gauges and tables and pens, I see a few empty hands. What a desire to be touched by hands! [The nurse] really takes my outstretched hands into hers. I content myself with this, although I strongly wish she would sit on the edge of my bed and put her arm around my shoulders!"[1]

It is not uncommon for the nursing situation to create a proximity between the nurse and the patient that otherwise only exists between people close to one another in a family. This physical closeness alone, which in almost all nursing activities is well within the usual social distance of one to four meters and may even intrude on the genital area[2], makes for unusually direct contact between strangers.

How do nurses deal with this proximity? Do they come up against their own limits? One might suspect that nurses would be overwhelmed by this closeness. In fact, this does happen, and it is then felt intensely. Professional nurses, as well as other body therapists, prepare for this situation during training and learn a targeted approach to closeness and distance. It can therefore be assumed that such situations of feeling overwhelmed only occur when other factors, such as high work pressure, lack of time, etc., play a role. As a defensive mechanism—regarded as a counter-movement—efforts to create distance can occur, which may be seen, for example, in excessive bustling, with a subjective experience of being constantly short of time. Closeness and distance are equally important in nursing care, as long as they are in balance. Distance enables more impartial observation and thus possibly more precise perception of the patient's situation, but it often prevents a relationship with the patient through strong insistence on boundaries. A high degree of closeness, on the other hand, favors an empathetic and understanding relationship and a comprehensive perspective, but makes it difficult for the nurse to assess situations realistically and in extreme cases can lead to an inability to act. As nurses attend to patients in a very concentrated manner, it can be a healthy counter process to distance oneself from the situation, to detach oneself inwardly and view the situation as if from outside.

1.2 Qualities of touch

Closeness and distance also play into the type of touch used. It is a sign of initial shyness or uncertainty when nurses only touch patients with their fingertips. Ashley Montagu (1905–1999) described this analogously for mothers who initially touch their newborn children only timidly with their fingertips before gradually losing their shyness and daring to touch them with the whole palm of their hand.[3] The quality of the touch thus changes fundamentally and acquires a secure and committed character. The rather spotty and local feeling that the fingers evoke gains an extensive, enveloping and warming quality when touched with the entire hand. This fact, which can be experienced by everyone, is especially cultivated when giving Rhythmical Einreibung treatments.

Other qualities of touch are related to the treating hand itself. If the skin is cracked and brittle, this has an effect on the quality of the touch and thus also on the quality of the treatment. The same applies to long nails and cold hands. The latter are felt to be unpleasant on almost all parts of the body, except for a few exceptions, such as a cool hand on a fever-hot forehead.

Perceptible qualities of touching as well as being touched are:

- Warmth or cold
- Dryness or moistness
- Tension or flaccidity
- Smoothness or roughness
- Quantity and quality of body hair

The intensity of the touch is another quality feature. It offers a spectrum from slight tickling to painful pressure, with the aim being to find the middle between these poles.

The nurse's intentions are strongly perceived by the other person. Am I placing my hand to perceive the skin temperature superficially, to feel any muscular tension, or to signal: "I'm here, you're not alone!" These are variations that are communicated directly to the person being treated, as experience shows.[4]

During a Rhythmical Einreibung treatment, a non-verbal conversation often develops, in which the treated person reacts as a matter of course to clear requests from the hands, for example by raising a leg without talking about it. In the sense of this dialogue, it is important that nurses notice when a patient is tense and cannot or will not allow a certain type of touch.

Digression: Skin function

With a surface area of two square meters, the skin is the largest of our sensory organs. In addition to the perceptual ability generally described as the sense of touch, it carries sensory cells for the differentiated perception of touch, pressure, tickling, itching and burning, as well as vibrations, heat, cold and pain. The skin acts as an organ for storage, excretion and absorption. The latter is important for the effect of any substances that may be applied.

As an organ of expression, skin allows emotions such as shame, fear and excitement to appear externally, e.g., through flushing, becoming pale, or sweating. That's why we speak of the skin as the "mirror of the soul."[5]

Another important function is protection against mechanical and chemical damage. The skin has immunological functions and it forms a border, a barrier between the 'I' and the 'you.'

At the same time, skin acts as a contact organ for the environment and facilitates exchange with it. A person with so-called "thick" skin appears less sensitive and more robust than "thin-skinned" fellow human beings, for whom the same attacks immediately get "under their skin."

The fact that the sense of touch develops very early in the embryonic state indicates the central role of physical contact in human life. As the primary sensory organ, the skin is the infant's first communication medium, and tactile stimulation is an essential element in its development.[6]

The skin as a boundary to the environment enables us to experience our separate existence. By defining ourselves or pushing against our outer boundaries, we become aware of our own identity, both directly and figuratively. This applies to childcare, where attention is paid to wrapping firmly and making sure that the bed is not too large, as well as to adult care. In experiments in which test persons were wrapped in cotton wool in dark test chambers without anyone addressing them, they experienced sensory illusions ranging to hallucinations, which were attributed to their lack of awareness of their body's limits.[7]

Parallels for nursing care are obvious. Patients who are bedridden for a long time often describe that they no longer have any feeling for their legs. Especially in elderly people we can often notice that they have a reduced feeling for their body. In addition to the age-related loss of sensory functions, missing stimuli are a problem. Old people often lie motionless in bed for long periods of time without noticing their numbness, let alone being able to remedy it. Many problems of depressively disgruntled, apathetic and confused patients can be traced back to a lack of sensory stimulation and a lack of being consciously addressed.[8] In such cases, a Rhythmical Einreibung treatment helps them to become aware of the respective part of their body.

The hands are communicating organs through which the patient feels the condition and mood of the nurse.[9] And since nursing care is an occupation of contact, nurses should be "touch professionals."[10] Reasons and situations which favor the avoidance of contact are, e.g., feelings of shame on the part of the patient, or shame or a wish to be distant on the part of the nurse. Personal aversion, fear of sexual reinterpretation of a rhythmical oil application, feelings of disgust and rationalizing them as hygiene regulations often make it seem imperative to wear gloves when administering an oil application. This unfortunately results in a loss of a large part of the quality, which is why gloves should only be worn in exceptional cases, such as when there is a risk of infection or when the nurse is allergic to substances used in the treatment.

All in all, touch is to be regarded as an opportunity to convey humanity and to reach not only the physical but also the patient's soul and spirit.[11] By creating nurturing physical contact, warmth, presence and calming, we take into account elementary human needs, the fulfillment of which promotes the healing process.

In addition to the ability to perceive and communicate, this hands-on treatment of patients is a necessary part of nursing care. The hand as a universal instrument is of great importance. It is an organ of perception, and at the same time also a recognizing organ which can "grasp" what needs to be understood. Moreover, hands can transform things—our whole culture is ultimately created by their actions.

As a tool of nursing care, the relaxed hand adapts to the body's shape. This suppleness creates a soft, comprehending touch instead of a cramped or hard one. If it is possible to achieve this quality of touch in the respective care situation, then we accomplish more than just cleaning the body during whole-body washing, more than just applying the ointment during thrombosis prophylaxis, more than just gripping the lower arms during mobilization. Through such touching that is in line with humanness, the patient feels comprehended in his being, and this gives him a feeling of security, comfort and being understood. This in turn enables him to develop trust, which forms the basis for every relationship.

2. What is Rhythmical Einreibung?

A complex manual activity such as Rhythmical Einreibung can naturally only be inadequately explained in words. Direct instruction by trained nurses *plus* independent practice are indispensable prerequisites for learning to apply the technique competently. The following description must therefore be limited to describing experiences and working out fundamental aspects that may arouse interest for further study.

What, then, is Rhythmical Einreibung? First of all, substances are applied to the surface of the body during treatment, and they have an effect on the organism via the skin. These are oils, ointments, and lotions which, in addition to the general nursing effect, have specific effects through the addition of certain medicinal plants or metals. The adjective "rhythmical" also means that the method for applying the substance is not arbitrary, it is based on the laws of rhythm [→ Chapter "Rhythm"]. This rhythmical application of substances occurs in basic figures derived from the human form.

Rhythmical Einreibung treatments are carried out directly on the body, but with the intention of affecting the entire human being, i.e., the person's etheric and soul body, as well as their I-organization. In anthroposophically extended nursing care, Rhythmical Einreibung is used both prophylactically and therapeutically.

The roots of Rhythmical Einreibung lie in the rhythmical massage developed by Ita Wegman (1876–1943). This doctor, who worked closely with Rudolf Steiner, had learned Swedish massage before studying medicine and thus had a special connection to manual therapies. She herself carried out many such treatments during her medical work, often as part of her rounds. One of her special focuses was in the field of rhythmical organ embrocations. According to the descriptions of the nursing staff working with her, Ita Wegman had the ability to vary the treatment individually according to the patient's personality and situation. In subsequent years, Wegman's assisting physician Margarethe Hauschka (1896–1980) took over the teaching of rhythmical massage therapy and set up courses for doctors and nurses. A school for art therapy and rhythmical massage therapy was established in Bad Boll, Germany, in 1962. Margarethe Hauschka further developed the basic forms of rhythmical massage therapy in collaboration with Irmgard Marbach (1921–2008). In the following years, nurses worked intensively with rhythmical oil embrocations and worked out aspects of technique and application. As a result, various publications are available that describe the entire spectrum of rhythmical oil applications.[12, 13, 14] Mathias Bertram researched and described the effects of Rhythmical Einreibung on a physical, mental and spiritual level as part of his doctoral thesis.[15] In 2011, the International Forum for Anthroposophic Nursing (IFAP) published a "Handbook for the Certification of Experts in Rhythmical Einreibung according to Wegman/Hauschka," which explains the path to qualification, among other things.[16]

The spectrum of Rhythmical Einreibung includes organ embrocations, partial-body treatments, whole-body treatments, and the pentagram or five-pointed-star treatment. Rhythmical Einreibung treatments of the spleen, liver, kidneys, heart and bladder are usually performed with metal ointments in forms corresponding to the respective organ.[17]

In Rhythmical Einreibung treatments of the whole body, as the name suggests, the whole body of the patient is treated, except for the head. There are different indications for this, which are specified by a corresponding selection of substances. If you want the treatment to be soothing, use lavender oil.

- *Lavandula, Oleum aethereum 10%* (WALA)

- *Lavender 10% oil* (Weleda)

If a warming effect is to be achieved, St. John's wort oil or Solum oil are suitable:

- *Hypericum ex herba 5%, Oleum* (WALA)

- *Hypericum, Flos 25% oil* (Weleda)

- *Solum oil* (WALA)

If the whole-body Rhythmical Einreibung is to have an upbuilding and invigorating effect, use sloe oil or mallow oil, for example:

- *Prunus spinosa e floribus W 5%, Oleum* (WALA)

- *Mallow oil* (WALA)

Careful handling of warmth must be ensured during the treatment. Often it seems advisable to start with partial treatments to avoid overwhelming the patient with 15 to 20 minutes of very intensive whole-body Rhythmical Einreibung.

Partial-body Rhythmical Einreibung includes:

- Rhythmical Einreibung of the arm
- Rhythmical Einreibung of the chest
- Rhythmical Einreibung of the abdomen
- Rhythmical Einreibung of the leg and foot
- Rhythmical Einreibung of the back

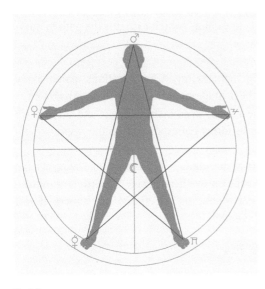

Fig. 1: Pentagram

Each of these partial-body treatments can be performed independently for itself or combined in a whole-body Einreibung. Indications are functional disorders such as digestive problems, sleep/wake rhythm disorders, pain/tension, respiratory problems, etc. The substances are selected according to the indication. A distinction is made between nursing orders and medical prescriptions by physicians. The boundary is a simple one formally, but difficult to draw in terms of content. For example, prophylaxis is the primary indication for nursing care, while therapy is the primary indication for the work of doctors.[18]

The pentagram Einreibung is a treatment based on the human form as a five-pointed star. Treatment is done on the forehead, forearms, and lower legs. It can be used for conditions of physical or mental numbness or dissolution, to support convalescence and to strengthen the heart.[19]

2.1 Basic forms

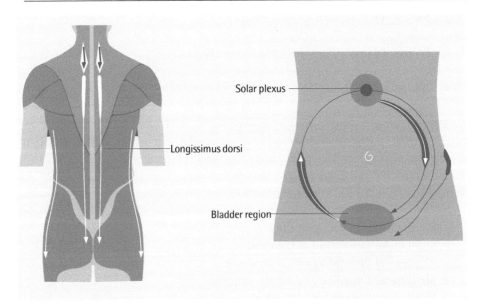

Solar plexus

Longissimus dorsi

Bladder region

Fig. 2: Straight back strokes[20] (left) and circle for Rhythmical Einreibung of the abdomen[21] (right)

ELEMENTS OF PRACTICAL NURSING

All Rhythmical Einreibung treatments are composed of the basic forms "circle" and "straight line" in different variations and combinations. The straight line can occur alone, e.g., in the form of strokes along the back, or we can use only a circle, e.g., in two-handed abdominal treatments.

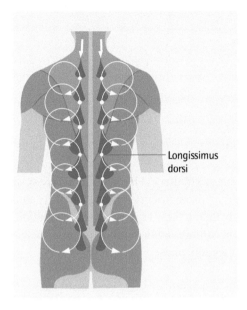

Longissimus dorsi

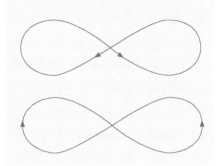

Fig. 4: Figure eight

Fig. 3: Combination of circles and straight lines; one-handed Rhythmical Einreibung of the back[22]

When circles and straight lines are combined, there is a variety of forms via which the Rhythmical Einreibung treatments "sculpt" the body. [Example: Figure eight, one-handed Rhythmical Einreibung of the back].

The forms that must be learned are determined by the individual.[23] An example is when the rhythmical application of oil follows the course and shape of the muscles, ribs or intestines.

2.2 The importance of rhythm

Differentiating the quality of touch creates the *rhythmic quality* that forms the central element of this treatment. According to Wilhelm Hoerner (1913–2013), rhythmical processes are characterized by the following properties:[24]

- Polarity and mediation
- Continuous renewal
- Flexible adaptation

In the human organism, the lungs and heart represent the rhythmic system. Breathing and the heartbeat appear as archetypes. Both take place between the polarities of narrowness, contraction, and being pressed versus expansiveness, loosening and letting go. Thus, rhythm requires two opposites to occur, such as stillness and movement. Goethe (1749–1832) described this process in a wonderfully poetic way using the example of breathing:

> *In breathing grace may twofold be:*
> *We breathe air in, and set it free;*
> *The inbreath binds, the out unwinds;*
> *And thus in marvels life entwines.*
> *Thanks be to God when we are pressed,*
> *Thanks be again when he grants us rest.*

Applied to the quality of touch and movement of Rhythmical Einreibung, we speak of the polarities of expansion and contraction or (isometric) increasing intensity and relaxation. A breathing quality is achieved by taking these aspects into consideration. Each individual stroke and each circular form contains an increasing (rising, crescendo) phase and a decreasing (subsiding, decrescendo) phase.

Edelgard Große-Brauckmann has worked out and described these interrelationships.[25] She particularly emphasizes the turning moments, which are among the most important in rhythmic activity.

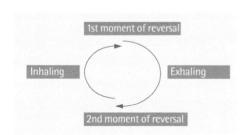

Fig. 5: First and second turning moments

In respiration, a turning moment can be found between inhalation and exhalation, as well as between exhalation and inhalation: this is a brief pause that allows the reversal of the flow of breath. In Rhythmical Einreibung, there is a turning moment after the contraction phase, with an isometric relaxation of the hand initiating the relaxation phase; the other reversal occurs as a pause after the loosening phase, when the binding action is resumed. Already Hippocrates (460–370 B.C.) said that everything is based on binding and loosening.[26]

Rudolf Steiner described rhythm as the carrier of health, from which the actual healing powers emanate. In a conversation he pointed this out to Rudolf Hauschka (1891–1969): "Study rhythm; rhythm carries life."[27] In addition, there is the experience that rhythm, in contrast to beat, has an invigorating and transforming effect. "Beat repeats, rhythm renews."[28]

In particular, it is the effort to achieve a rhythmic quality that has an invigorating, ordering and harmonizing effect, also on the person providing the treatment. Experienced practitioners often describe that they can "unwind" well during a Rhythmical Einreibung treatment, despite time pressures and other urgent tasks. They get into a kind of state of calm themselves and thus experience the balancing effect that rhythm has.

2.3   Other characteristics of quality

The possibility of transformation as a basic principle of life finds expression in the constant renewal in which a rhythmic process is always similar, but never identical. Just think of waves on a beach and of Rhythmical Einreibung, where each form is shaped somewhat differently.

Flexible adaptation occurs in waves, for example, in response to a change on the beach or the turn from low to high tide. Changes in Rhythmical Einreibung succeed effortlessly as the hand adapts to the respective body shapes.

Another essential feature of Rhythmical Einreibung is the principle of working "from lightness for lightness." Certain principles are to be considered in the technique for treatment, since our aim is particularly to address the living forces in the human organism: rather than following the physical laws of gravity, Rhythmical Einreibung works with forces of buoyancy or lightness, as in qualities of water. In practical terms, this means giving lightness to the quality of touch and movement rather than working with pressure and force. Close but light contact leads to a sucking effect through which the body tissue "comes along" without being pulled or pressed. In this way, the organism can reorganize itself without any compelling foreign influence.

3.   Administering a Rhythmical Einreibung treatment

Example

Mrs. L. is still very exhausted and weak during convalescence after pneumonia. Her physician has prescribed arm treatments with sloe oil (*Prunus spinosa e floribus W 5%, Oleum* (WALA)) to strengthen and fortify her, which she will receive today for the first time.

Preparation:

I inform Mrs. L. before breakfast and agree on a time for her Rhythmical Einreibung treatment. It is important to eliminate as many factors as possible in advance that might interfere with a smooth course of treatment. This includes the planned activities of the patient as well as any pending therapies and examinations. We talk about the procedure and about how important it is that she come rested and not in a rush. The post-treatment rest is an important part of it, as the Rhythmical Einreibung only unfolds its full effect during the rest. Therefore, careful planning includes ensuring that enough time and (inner) space are available.

To prevent the danger that other therapists might want to work parallel to the planned treatment, I suggest that she keep a timetable, which can be viewed by all involved and where she can note down any fixed appointments. Then the regular therapies and other activities can be carried out at the same time each day. Such a timetable allows for a rhythmical day.

Mrs. L. asks if she will have to take off her nightgown, which I confirm. I estimate the duration of the arm treatment with preparation and rest to be about half an hour.

Before I enter the room, I prepare the material by preheating two towels with hot-water bottles. I warm the prunus oil (*Prunus spinosa e floribus W 5%, Oleum* (WALA) in my hand directly before I apply it.

For longer treatments I sign off with my colleagues so as not to be interrupted by visitors or staff. During the treatment and rest, it has proved successful to affix a "Please do not disturb" sign to the door of the patient's room. I ask Mrs L. to get up briefly and go to the toilet, if necessary, so that she can relax better. I disconnect the telephone to avoid interference.

One fellow patient is not in the room right now, the other is bedridden. Since the air seems to be quite used up, I air the room and ask the other patient if she needs anything, because I will be concentrating on the Rhythmical Einreibung afterwards. A screen serves to block the view between the beds.

I like to close the curtains to create an enveloping atmosphere. This is especially important when the light from the window is blinding. I also deal with the bedside lamp and other light sources that need to be altered or dimmed so that the patient does not have to look directly into the light.

Now I help Mrs. L. to take off her nightgown, then I cover her arms and chest separately with towels and with the blanket.

Since cold feet impair the effectiveness of the treatment, I check whether her feet are warm and, if necessary, apply a hot-water bottle or administer a foot treatment beforehand.

When everything is ready, I take off my watch and pin my hair so that it doesn't hinder me during the treatment. The same applies to long, wide sleeves, which disturb and distract from the Rhythmical Einreibung when they brush over other parts of the body. If necessary, I warm up my cool hands when washing them or use a hot-water bottle. I am already concentrating on the patient, the reason for administering the Rhythmical Einreibung and the goal that I want to achieve with it.

The treatment

The procedure includes preparing the bed, such as raising the head end, as well as giving any assistance that may be necessary when undressing. The prepared, warmed cloths serve on the one hand to protect the bed from oil or ointment, and on the other to cover the patient, to better maintain her warmth. After the clothing over the area to be treated has been removed, I cover it with cloths that can be quickly removed and replaced, and position the patient safely and comfortably.

At this point I would like to remind the reader of the rhythmical quality and the lightness that are central to Rhythmical Einreibung treatments. To ensure that warmth is not lost, I uncover the area to be treated only immediately before I am ready to start on it. It works well to pull back the duvet first but remove the cloths only after the oil is in my hand warming up. Experience has shown that planning and consideration are required to organize the covering and uncovering in such a way that the patient does not get too cold, the process is calm and fluid and my concentration on the Rhythmical Einreibung itself is maintained.

Clear, targeted and well-considered movements play an important role in uncovering and covering, and they also determine the treatment itself. The important thing is to avoid overdoing anything: your forms should be simple, plain and without "frills." If you feel that you must do a lot, "frills" can easily develop. You should therefore imagine a movement impulse that flows as if radiating from behind through your arm into your hand, following its motion. This picture helps us to perform deliberate movements instead of "flailing about" with our elbows or wrists.

Attention must be paid to the flowing transitions between the different forms. They contribute to the harmonious whole. This also includes a clear, consciously formed beginning and end.

As a practitioner, I stand at the side of the patient's bed with one foot slightly in front of the other, looking in the direction of Mrs. L.'s face. The placement of my feet enables me to change my position by shifting my weight in such a way that I can reach more distant parts of her body, such as her shoulder, without falling out of the sequence of movements. I do not lean against the edge of the bed, because this makes working "from levity towards levity" more difficult. My attitude of attention to what I am doing finds expression in my rounded back and inclined head.

I apply the substance to the arm in a generously executed basic form before I start the actual Rhythmical Einreibung. The amount of oil directly influences the quality of the treatment: if I take too little, I easily get "caught" and "bogged down"; if I take too much, I just "slide" over the skin and cannot "suck" any body tissue.

The treatment requires concentration, which is why conversation should be avoided if possible. If you talk during the treatment, the patient may feel that too much is being demanded of her at once. So that Mrs. L. would not be unsettled by my resolute silence, I pointed out to her in the preliminary conversation that I did not intend to speak during the treatment.

A danger of this concentrated work is to bend too close to the patient and thus not keep the necessary distance. Such lack of distance is often experienced as being personally oppressive. Therefore, I try to observe myself as I work to the extent that I can correct my distance if necessary.

Finally, we need to look at the duration of the Rhythmical Einreibung. It is relatively short, but from the point of view of the person being treated, it could be extended for a long time because of its beneficial effect. However, it has proved far more effective to give an impulse with a short treatment. The guideline values for a whole-body Rhythmical Einreibung are approximately 20 to 30 minutes, for treatments of the leg or arm 15 to 20 minutes (including preparation and follow-up), and correspondingly shorter times for other partial treatments.

Follow-up

Now I inform Mrs. L. that she is welcome to fall asleep during her rest and that I will look in on her in thirty minutes. After she is well covered and is lying comfortably, I prepare the bell for her in case she needs anything. During the rest I try to protect her from disturbances. If she wishes, I close the curtains completely.

After washing my hands and disposing of the materials, I reflect on the treatment process:

Was the duration good? Was the patient relaxed? How did her skin feel? Did she need little or a lot of oil? What was the temperature of the different areas of her skin? How did the patient appear after the treatment?

I try to rethink the process and to plan improvements for the next treatment, depending on her respective reactions.

4.   The effects of Rhythmical Einreibung

The effectiveness of a Rhythmical Einreibung treatment can be observed directly from observation of the patient on the one hand and from the patient's own experience on the other.

Example

Mrs. B., who has had her first Rhythmical Einreibung treatment during an acute migraine attack, describes her experience of a calf and foot treatment so vividly that I ask her to write down her report. Mrs. B. suffered from a severe migraine headache, nausea and ice-cold feet at the time of the treatment.

"May I come? Are you ready? Are you coming with me?—the hands ask. They glide down asking, a few times, until I'm ready. Below, they answer me that they will stay. But not in one place, no, other places are also greeted by them. They no longer approach me with questions, they are more familiar with me, I am more familiar with them. The question stays in the background. Like soft water they surround me, gliding forward, forming a vortex at an obstacle, in constant motion, calm, stagnating nowhere.

Gradually I can approach the hands more, move fluently with them, expand myself, warm myself, round myself. Much too soon the hands say goodbye to me, with a soft but decisive movement. But what joy—the living flow, the warm stream, the calm expansiveness remain, even without the hands. They didn't take it with them, they left it with me."

The above report contains some essential effects of Rhythmical Einreibung: living flowing, warm streaming and a calm expansiveness.

In order for these effects to occur, it is important to first approach the patient carefully and cautiously, and thus with the caregiver's unspoken question: "May I come? Is it all right with you?" This first cautious inquiry leaves the treated person free to decide whether he is able and willing to follow along. If this is not possible, depending on the area to be treated and the indication, we seek other ways to achieve the desired effect or to apply the prescribed substance. For example, instead of rhythmically applying caraway oil on the patient's stomach, we can apply an oil compress. It is important to keep a constant eye on whether the treatment is desired or not, because rejection of Rhythmical Einreibung is often an initial reaction that no longer occurs after a few treatments and after a trusting relationship has been established.

Every external application addresses a question to the organism, which the organism answers with a reaction. Such a question can of course be heard or not. If it is asked too timidly or too quietly, it may be easier to overhear it; if the necessary rest is lacking afterwards, it will be difficult to formulate an answer. If, however, it is possible to find the right quality of treatment, the person will feel personally addressed and recognized.

Example

An elderly lady who has been prescribed bed rest because of a pelvic fracture appears increasingly impatient and complains about massive sleep disorders. In a conversation she reports that she cannot bear this kind of immobility, especially since she is a person who must move a lot in order to feel comfortable. She usually goes for long walks, then feels comfortably tired and can sleep well. She confirms my assumption that she cannot perceive her legs and feet at all now.

I offer her a foot treatment, which I administer with stimulating, invigorating qualities of touch and movement. I pay particular attention to the rhythmic quality, on the one hand, and strong down-strokes on the soles of the feet on the other, in which I lift her foot from its relaxed extension to the equivalent of a right angle when standing. The effect is astonishing: The patient feels revitalization and later pleasant tiredness in her legs and feet—like after a long walk. She falls asleep during her post-treatment rest.

Her organism reacts to the desired stimulation given by Rhythmical Einreibung and sole strokes with relaxation, enabling her to fall asleep.

If we pay special attention to the described quality of Rhythmical Einreibung when teaching, practicing and administering, it is possible to have a direct effect on the life currents in the organism. When we stimulate the etheric body, we can observe qualities of invigoration and expansion. Patients often describe that their treated leg or arm feels much lighter and seems to lie up to 20 centimeters higher than their untreated extremity.

The feeling of lightness is directly connected with the alleviation of discomfort. For example, a patient with posture-induced tension in her back requested in her Swabian dialect: "Make me wings again, please!" At first it may seem unusual not to press and knead a hard shoulder area, but on the contrary to work it with gently sucking hand movements. In cases of tension the soul is expressing itself too strongly locally; we can bring it back into flow with stimulating and invigorating movements, following etheric laws. The rhythmic stimulation of parts of the body other than those affected locally has also proven to be effective: in the case of a tense neck, for example, we treat the sides and back.

Many patients with painful conditions express immense relief after a Rhythmical Einreibung treatment, especially if they have pain caused by tension and cramps or prolonged lying in bed. Often, we do not treat such conditions locally, since already too much consciousness prevails at the painful place. We remedy the situation by bringing consciousness to other areas. For example, a migraine headache can be alleviated with an efferent Rhythmical Einreibung treatment of the calves.

People with asthma or respiratory problems often describe recovering a sense of expansiveness after a rhythmical Einreibung treatment of their back or chest. In contrast to the oppressive constriction of being short of breath, this is perceived as relieving to the highest degree.

We can see from the ice-cold feet of the young woman described above how closely stagnation in the warmth organism is connected with many pathological phenomena. If it is possible to guide the warmth back into the cold feet via Rhythmical Einreibung, excessive metabolic processes present in the neurosensory system during migraine are diverted to the limbs. The treatment follows the same direction of action as a mustard footbath.

Rhythmical Einreibung stimulates the patient's own activity and self-healing powers through the flowing activity of their etheric body.

Rhythmical Einreibung also speaks to the soul. The feeling of being understood develops into trust between the practitioner and the patient.

Example

During the first days of his stay in the hospital, Mr. M. appears to be very tense and stiff. After a Rhythmical Einreibung treatment of his back, his rigid posture is released; there is room for grief and tears. He tells me that he can feel himself again, with all his feelings from fear to hope. In our subsequent conversations Mr. M. often expresses his worries and his changing attitude towards life.

Last but not least, Rhythmical Einreibung has an effect on the human 'I', which becomes increasingly involved in the organism through the flow of warmth.

A safe, clear and loving touch often means more than many words. Withdrawn or "difficult" patients in particular react by opening up, usually surprisingly, and by asking central questions. The following information comes from Margarethe Hauschka: "The feeling of compassion and helpfulness, even love itself, as Rudolf Steiner once described it, should be transformed into careful technique. Then the patient feels immediately taken care of and understood, even much better than when unnecessary and above all unsolicited advice is brought to him. One will experience that such an attitude can only promote a normal, warm, human relationship between the patient and the masseur [nurse]."[29]

Such an attitude brings with it a loving orientation towards the patient. If the patient feels our desire to achieve "careful technique" and notices that the encounter is free of personal inclinations and desires, he can allow the treatment without too much personal sympathy. The physical gesture of the nurse during the treatment, i.e., her slight bending and turning towards the patient, thus becomes an inner posture in the figurative sense.

The quality of a Rhythmical Einreibung treatment results not only from the technique, but also from the motivation of the practitioner.

5. Touching must be learned

In most nursing situations, we encounter strangers with whom we must first familiarize ourselves. Since we are not in the role of a mother who has a deep relationship with her child, finding an unbiased way of touching is much more difficult for us as nurses. The quality of touch must be learnt anew, the art of following the body's forms in a simple and unbiased way and adapting our hand smoothly.

Art is related to skill and refers to a skill acquired through practice. Craftsmanship is closely related to art; it is, so to speak, the wet nurse of art, for art draws its nourishment from craftsmanship. Mastery of the skill, together with constant practice, knowledge, and experience, are the basic prerequisites for qualified practice. The psychoanalyst Erich Fromm (1900–1980) emphasized that an artist must have an interest in his profession in addition to skill and knowledge; his cause must be more important to him than anything else.[30]

This interest, as the third prerequisite for learning an art, plays a key role in nursing care and especially in Rhythmical Einreibung. It concerns interest in people as well as interest in the treatment and its optimal effectiveness.

Our descriptions so far have illustrated how complex and technically demanding the practice of Rhythmical Einreibung is. The necessary training involves a long process that includes both theoretical and practical elements. An essential part of the learning process is to experience Rhythmical Einreibung treatments on one's own body. Anyone who has personally experienced an abdominal embrocation given by icy cold hands is unlikely to be indifferent to the detail of hand temperature. Anyone who got nauseous from too much pressure or who had to go to the toilet immediately afterwards has also had experiences that let him take seriously the (side) effects of unprofessional treatment. Self-experience rounds off the theoretical knowledge and practical exercises.

The following exercise gives a better idea of the necessary quality of skin contact in Rhythmical Einreibung:

> Try to place your hand on a smooth surface of water and move it in circles with so little pressure that you do not immerse your hand or "break through" and yet are still fully at the water level. You can feel that when you carefully lift off your hand, the surface of the water goes along with it, remains "stuck," so to speak, or is "sucked" upwards.

It is precisely this experience that is meant by the sucking quality of touch, by "working with the body tissue." It shows that Rhythmical Einreibung is in fact a dialogue in which the tissue of the treated person always approaches the nurse to a certain extent.

6. Final considerations

The combination of substance (remedy) and its rhythmical application results in increased effectiveness. Compared to the simple application of ointment or an oil compress, or "applying the stuff somehow," a Rhythmical Einreibung enhances the effect of the substance.

Accordingly, not only is the substance decisive, but also the quality of the treatment achieved by "careful technique."
The effects of Rhythmical Einreibung support life processes in the human body. This, in turn:

- Calms/deepens respiration
- Relaxes in cases of agitation/anxiety
- Relieves cramping
- Promotes the rhythm of sleeping and waking
- Improves blood circulation
- Promotes warming through
- Stimulates digestion
- Awakens a new awareness of the person's body, so that a paralyzed part of it, for example, can be experienced as being part of it again[31]

It seems to be due to the quality of rhythm that the organism "responds" to the impulse of Rhythmical Einreibung in a way that corresponds to the body's current condition. This means that, to achieve self-regulation, the body reacts to the same treatment one time with relaxation and another time with activity.

The touch quality developed in Rhythmical Einreibung can be transferred to many other nursing activities, e.g., to whole-body washing, which is carried out according to similar principles and basic forms. The extent to which "humanizing" touch is experienced and the direct effects that it has on the well-being of patients is shown by the example of a young woman who, after a case of sepsis, retrospectively described her memory of her first whole-body wash as something that made her "human again at that moment."

Rhythmical Einreibung is therefore more than a technique used in specific nursing care situations; it is also an attitude that inspires our daily work in many respects. Especially its rhythmical element can become a prototype for the polarities of nearness and distance in social interaction, yet also for dealing with engagement/relaxation, thinking/doing and perception/reflection in our personal life or in our daily routine on the hospital ward. Rhythmical Einreibung contributes to the shaping of nursing care, especially as it gives every nurse access to professional independence. This chapter was intended to encourage you to learn and develop the art of Rhythmical Einreibung.

Category	Example learning objectives	Recommended learning path
Skills	You are developing quality awareness for touch in nursing care.	A
Your own learning objective		
Relationships	You understand nursing as a profession of contact.	B
Your own learning objective		
Knowledge	You know the effects and indications of Rhythmical Einreibung according to Wegman/Hauschka, as well as the importance of rhythmical movement and touch qualities for well-being.	C
Your own learning objective		

References

1 Sturm, V. *Krankenbett*. Herder Verlag, Freiburg im Breisgau 1988, p. 9.

2 Büschel, M-M. Pflegende müssen ihre Hände mögen. Der Stellenwert der Berührung im Pflegealltag. *Pflegezeitschrift* 1994; 47 (6), p. 367.

3 Montagu, A. *Körperkontakt*. Klett-Cotta Verlag, Stuttgart 2012, p. 88.

4 Helmbold, A. *Berühren in der Pflegesituation. Intentionen, Botschaften und Bedeutung*. Verlag Hans Huber, Bern 2007.

5 Condrau, G.; Schipperges H. *Unsere Haut. Spiegel der Seele, Verbindung zur Welt*. Kreuz Verlag, Freiburg im Breisgau 1993.

6 Montagu, A. *Körperkontakt*. Klett-Cotta Verlag, Stuttgart 2012.

7 ibid.

8 Inheste,r O.; Zimmermann, I. *Ganzkörperwaschung in der Pflege. Anleitung und Hilfen für Pflege-personal und pflegende Angehörige*. Schlütersche Verlagsgesellschaft, Hannover 1990.

9 Inhester O. *Ganzkörperwaschung. Analyse einer komplexen Situation als Beitrag zur Förderung pflegerischen Denkens*. Die Schwester/Der Pfleger 1992; 31 (8), p. 712.

10 Hug, M; Reiner, S.; Surina, G. Routinierte Berührungen. *Die Schwester/Der Pfleger* 1988; 27 (10), p. 770.

11 ibid.

12 Batschko, E-M. *Einführung in die Rhythmischen Einreibungen*. Mayer Verlag, Stuttgart 2010.

13 Fingado, M. *Rhythmic Einreibung. A handbook from the Ita Wegman Klinik*. Floris Books, Edinburgh 2011.

14 Layer, M. (ed.). *Handbook for Rhythmical Einreibungen according to Wegman/Hauschka*. Temple Lodge, Forest Row 2006.

15 Bertram, M. *Der therapeutische Prozess als Dialog – eine strukturphänomenologische Untersuchung der Rhythmischen Einreibungen nach Wegman/Hauschka*. Witten/Herdecke University 2005.

16 International Forum for Anthroposophic Nursing (IFAP) in the Medical Section of the School of Spiritual Science at the Goetheanum (ed.): *Handbuch zur Zertifizierung von Expertinnen/Experten für Rhythmische Einreibungen nach Wegman/Hauschka* (IFAP), Dornach 2011.

17 Layer, M. (ed.). *Handbook for Rhythmical Einreibungen according to Wegman/Hauschka*. Temple Lodge, Forest Row 2006.

18 Große-Brauckmann, E., in Layer, M. *Handbook for Rhythmical Einreibungen according to Wegman/Hauschka*. Temple Lodge, Forest Row 2006.

19 Heine, R., in Layer M. *Handbook for Rhythmical Einreibungen according to Wegman/Hauschka*. Temple Lodge, Forest Row 2006.

20 Layer, M. *Handbook for Rhythmical Einreibungen according to Wegman/Hauschka*. Temple Lodge, Forest Row 2006.

21 ibid.

22 ibid.

23 Hauschka, M. *Rhythmical Massage as indicated by Ita Wegman*. Mercury Press, Spring Valley 1991.

24 Hoerner W. *Zeit und Rhythmus. Die Ordnungsgesetze der Erde und des Menschen*. Verlag Urachhaus, Stuttgart 2006, p. 24.

25 Große-Brauckmann, E., in Layer M. *Handbook for Rhythmical Einreibungen according to Wegman/Hauschka*. Temple Lodge, Forest Row 2006.

26 Hauschka, M. *Rhythmical Massage as indicated by Ita Wegman*. Mercury Press, Spring Valley 1991.

27 Hauschka, R. *Wetterleuchten einer Zeitenwende*. Salumed Verlag, Berlin 2012, p. 85 ff.

28 Husemann F.; Wolff, O. (ed.). *The anthroposophic approach to medicine*, vol. III. Mercury Press, Spring Valley 1980.

29 Hauschka, M. *Rhythmical Massage as indicated by Ita Wegman*. Mercury Press, Spring Valley 1991.

30 Fromm, E. *The art of loving*. Harper, New York 2006.

31 Große-Brauckmann, E., in Layer M. *Handbook for Rhythmical Einreibungen according to Wegman/Hauschka*. Temple Lodge, Forest Row 2006.

CHAPTER XIII

Compresses in Anthroposophically Extended Nursing Care

GABRIELE WEBER

Compresses have been part of the treasure trove of healing remedies in all cultures for thousands of years. In Anthroposophic Medicine, they are used to bring healing to the organism via the neurosensory system. Decisive for the effectiveness of an application is its correct implementation, not just the selection of the right substance. This chapter will present aspects to consider when finding indications, as well as give practical examples.

1. Introduction

Compresses are external applications. They initially act on the patient via the skin, which is an organ of the neurosensory system. From there, a range of effects unfolds over the entire organism, including the patient's rhythmic and motor-metabolic systems.

The effects of external applications range from calming, ordering and channeling away to stimulating a variety of metabolic processes. In addition, patients experience these treatments as beneficial, as a special form of therapy and nursing care that reaches them mentally and spiritually.

The external applications discussed here include:

- Compresses that wrap completely around a part of the body.
- Compresses and ointment cloths that usually cover one area of the body.
- Oil cloths, which represent a milder form of heat application and usually stay on longer.
- Poultices: moist packs with farmer's cheese, mustard powder, or mashed potatoes, for instance.

Other external applications are rhythmical oil applications (Rhythmical Einreibung), washes and baths.

1.1   Historical origins

Compresses have been known as remedies for thousands of years. In recent times, therapists such as Sebastian Kneipp (1821–1897, Kneipp hydrotherapy), Vinzenz Priessnitz (1799–1851, Priessnitz compresses) and Leopold Emanuel Felke (1856–1926, Felke clay packs) became known for natural healing methods of this type.

As external applications, compresses are a form of hydrotherapy and thermo-therapy. Anthroposophically extended medicine uses substances from the mineral kingdom (e.g., copper or potentized gold in an ointment base), the plant world (e.g., calendula and chamomile as essences or teas) and the animal kingdom (e.g., farmer's cheese or honey). By now we can speak of a renaissance of external applications in therapy and nursing care.

An interesting study was done on the results obtained from compresses that are wrapped entirely around part of the body. Of the 221 patients who were treated as in-patients in a wide variety of specialist fields, 70% of those surveyed noticed a clear or very clear improvement in their condition, which they attributed to the compress-es. The majority of patients were able to recover through the application. Overall, more than 70% of the patients rated the success of the application as very high to significant.[1]

1.2   Compresses as part of anthroposophically extended nursing care

Nursing care extended by an anthroposophic understanding of the human being be-gan with the opening of two clinical therapeutic institutes established by Rudolf Steiner in Arlesheim (Switzerland) and Stuttgart (Germany) in 1920. Many new as-pects for nursing work resulted from Steiner's concept of the four subtle members constituting the human being, as well as from knowledge of the threefold functioning of the human organism.

From the very beginning, external applications were part of the nursing staff's field of activity and the treatments still play an important role in therapy today. We draw on many years of experience for our practical work, which is increasingly being researched in a targeted manner. In this context, reference should be made to studies that were done on the effects of ginger.[2, 3, 4]

Even outside of anthroposophic nursing care, the subject of compresses is increas-ingly attracting attention. This can be seen in publications in the relevant nursing literature, as well as in small research projects reported in the trade press.[5]

An anthroposophically expanded view of the human being enables us to deter-mine the indication and effect of the corresponding measures in a targeted manner. In particular, it is the threefold functioning of the human organism that serves as a basis for understanding this aspect of treatment.

Various publications on the subject can be found in the bibliography at the end of this chapter. In addition, it is highly recommended that you attend an advanced training course.

2. Understanding the effects of external applications

If we look at the origin of the word "therapy," we find the Greek word stem "therapon," which means "servant, companion." Nurses are companions of sick and old people. Nurses are there for the patient around the clock. They know the person's needs, worries and sufferings, they know what needs to be done.[6]

External applications are to be regarded as healing remedies, i.e., as part of medical treatment, and they are therefore prescribed by doctors. Practice shows, however, that their prescription is often suggested by experienced nurses. A simple ICD diagnosis (International Statistical Classification of Diseases and Related Health Problems) is often not enough to arrive at a correct indication; we also require meticulous observation of the patient's symptoms and well-being.

2.1 The relationship between the threefold human being and medicinal plants

As shown in the chapter on functional threefolding [→ Chapter "The Anthropological Foundations"], we find a threefold structure in the human body.

Our neurosensory system, which enables us to have a relationship with the outside world through our absorption of sensory impressions, needs stillness for this activity. Coldness tends to prevail. "You must keep a cool head to think clearly." This folk saying characterizes an essential aspect of our neurosensory system. People are quickly tired by thought activity and constant absorption of sensory stimuli. These activities have a degenerating effect and they need to be balanced through upbuilding forces found in our metabolism.

The human motor-metabolic system creates life. Movement and warmth predominate when metabolic processes occur in the abdominal organs or muscles.

When stillness and cold predominate in the neurosensory system, this can lead to hardening, such as in cerebral sclerosis. When movement and warmth in the motor-metabolic system become excessive, this is followed by inflammation and processes of dissolution, such as diarrhea.

A mediating element, the rhythmic system, harmonizes between the neurosensory and motor-metabolic systems. The rhythmic system pulsates through the entire body and lives between the neurosensory activity that prevails in the head, i.e., in the upper part of the body, and the metabolic activity that prevails in the lower part of the body.

Similar processes can also be found in the plant world. This enables us to apply medicinal plants to treat specific corresponding disease processes.

In plants, three systems can be distinguished:

- The root area, which grows in the cool soil and ensures the absorption of nutrients and water.
- The stem and leaf area that causes nutrients and juices to rise and fall.
- The flower that emits its unique scent in the warmth of the sun, attracting insects and—after pollination—forms fruit and seeds.

Human being		(Medicinal) plant
Upper human being, neurosensory system	Head	Root
	Receives sensory impressions	Receives nutrients
	Stillness	Stillness (through being rooted in the ground)
	Cold	Cold
Middle human being, rhythmic system	Heart/lung	Leaf
	Balancing/compensating	Rise and fall of juices (spring-summer/autumn-winter)
	Mediation between the upper and lower human being	Mediation between the upper and lower plant
	Harmony	—
Lower human being, motor-metabolic system	Metabolic organs, muscles	Flower, fruit and seeds
	Release of digestive secretions	Release of scents (essential oils) and pollen
	Movement	Moving pollinator in the flower
	Warmth	Warmth

Chart: Relationships between human beings and plants

2.2 Health and illness

Human life processes are subject to certain fluctuations. We are never dealing with a straight progression; life always oscillates between two poles. This applies to body, soul and spirit. There is constant fluctuation between upbuilding and degenerating processes, and this is linked to certain rhythms. During the day, processes of consciousness predominate in our neurosensory system. At night, when we are "unconscious," a healthy balance is restored. We therefore find that the motor-metabolic system has its main activity at night, when the body regenerates itself. But metabolic activity outweighs conscious activity after a sumptuous lunch, as well. This is succinctly expressed in a popular saying: "A full belly doesn't like to study."

So, the human being strives to keep the two poles in balance or to regain balance again and again. We call this activity "health." Disease happens when there is a loss of balance or balancing forces.

Such processes have their place not only spatially, i.e., in a person's physical body, but also temporally, in their biography. Whereas in childhood the building up of physicality predominates, in old age the body is predominantly in decline.

The incidence of disease is very different from individual to individual. Therefore, each person's recovery of lost equilibrium is different.

2.3 Stimulating and supporting self-healing powers

We have thus seen that the human organism strives to keep all processes in balance. When it does not succeed, diseases develop. A possible basic tendency that can occur is hardening (sclerosis). We find hardening in almost all regions of the body, and it always causes a restriction or loss of function in the affected organ. Sclerosis is irreversible, but the speed at which it progresses can be influenced.

The opposite pole to sclerosis is found in diseases which are inflammatory or feverish. The classical course of such diseases can be observed in childhood illnesses. The child's temperature rises very rapidly, and the symptoms worsen until a crisis is reached. This can also be seen as a turning point. Soon the crisis is over, the child's temperature drops, and recovery and healing begin. The fever is a reaction of the immune system, it increases metabolism. Unfortunately, we have fewer opportunities to observe such typical disease progressions today, as fever is often mistakenly fought against.

It is helpful to recall these polar disease tendencies again and again when we aim to stimulate self-healing processes with the help of external applications. It is important to know, for example, that osteoarthritis initially leads to deposits in the joints, which are associated with a loss of mobility. When this becomes chronic, it results in stiffening and deformation. In this phase, patients usually try to keep warm. This hardening is interrupted again and again by acutely inflammatory phases. Now the patient suddenly develops a fever, and his joints are overheated and feel hot. Then the person is often grateful for local cooling. This shows that the organism is trying to overcome the hardening process through inflammation.

This is where therapy and nursing care can help. We begin by observing the patient's warmth organism and this enables us to find the specific treatment that is needed. We must keep the aim of the treatment always in mind. Should warmth be generated, or should it be dissipated or even eliminated? By the way, a good guide for healthy warmth distribution in the organism is wonderfully summarized by a German proverb: "Head cold, feet warm, this makes the best doctor poor."

3. Lemon

There are three main applications for lemons. All are based on the affinity between citrus fruit and metabolic processes in the human body.

To understand this, we must consider the plant as a remedy. If we were to limit our considerations to an analysis of the fruit's ingredients, we would find only limited indications for understanding lemon as a remedy. Where should we direct our attention?

Any substances found by chemical analysis represent an end product of the plant's developmental process. It is looking at this process and seeing it in relation to the disease process that puts us on the right track. The lemon tree grows in the warm, sun-drenched south. The small, evergreen tree can flower and produce fruit at the same time, which is unusual, and it yields up to two thousand lemons per year. This is a sign of very lush growth and metabolic activity. For external use we select the fruit of the lemon plant. In it—mainly in the skin—we find a characteristic essential oil.

Our mouth waters when we imagine a lemon or see, smell or taste one. Soon we feel a clear tightening and contraction. We attribute this effect to the lemon's acidity. However, it is not only the acidity of the final product that is important, it is the way in which the lemon manages the acidity. The fruit retains its acidity despite increasing maturation in sunlight and, unlike most other citrus fruits, such as oranges, does not become sweet. This shows the strong enclosing and delimiting power of lemon. It successfully shields itself from heat and light and maintains its juiciness against the hardening, drying influences of the world around it. This demarcation increases in wrinkly old fruit. Old lemons are often rock-hard, and their skin is thin, yet they are still full of juice inside.

Lemon is used to treat the following disease processes:

- As a *throat compress*, moderately tempered: for incipient painful sore throat inflammations and flu-like infections.
- As a *chest compress* for pneumonia and bronchopneumonia accompanied by fever.
- As an *addition to calf compresses* to counteract fever in childhood illnesses and febrile illnesses in general.

If we look for a common characteristic of all the mentioned indications, we can see that these are cases in which metabolic processes have taken over in body regions in which they are not normally found. A sign of this increased metabolic activity is increased production of secretions. The forces in the lemon are used to return the derailed metabolism to its normal level. Even the addition of half a lemon to a hot foot bath, or the application of a slice of lemon to the soles of the feet overnight, can have an impressive effect on the onset of flu infections. The lemon presents the body with something like an image of structured metabolic processes which it can use as a guide.

The lemon's structuring metabolic forces redirect the outflowing (mucus production) and dissolving processes (fever fantasies and agitation) back into healthy channels. This immediately improves the symptoms.

Part of plant used	Fruit, mainly peel
Characteristics	Control of metabolic processes, Boundary against heat and light
Indications	Displaced, increased metabolic processes with secretions
Kind of application	Moderately tempered compress
	Hot compress
Location	Throat, chest, calf

Chart: Lemon compresses

3.1 Practical implementation using the example of a lemon chest compress

Administering a lemon chest compress requires a certain amount of skill. It is best to work in pairs, because the compress must be prepared quickly so that the inner cloth soaked with lemon does not get cool.

INDICATIONS: Pneumonia or bronchitis associated with high temperatures and mucus production.

CONTRAINDICATIONS: Skin damage and citrus fruit allergies.

MATERIALS: 1 lemon, 500 ml of very hot water (75 to 80°C, or 167°F to 176°F), a shallow bowl, sharp knife, fork, glass, cloth for the compress (large enough to wrap around the whole chest), flannel or wool as an outer cloth all around, a wringing-out cloth.

INSTRUCTIONS: The compress cloth must completely enclose the patient's chest. Roll it up from both ends to the middle and then place it in the wringing-out cloth so that two free ends remain. Pour the hot water into the bowl. Halve, then press lemon into the water with its cut surface downwards, spear it with a fork and carve it into a star shape with a knife. Then vigorously squeeze out both lemon halves under water (using the glass). Small bubbles will rise, and the typical fresh scent of lemon will emerge. Now you dip the compress cloth (in the wringing-out cloth) into the hot lemon water, keeping the free ends dry, which you then use to very firmly wring out the cloth afterwards. Next you wrap the hot cloth from both sides—starting at the back—very quickly around the chest of the patient and then fix the outer cloth firmly around it. It is important that the damp cloth be completely sealed in. Now cover the patient well so that he neither sweats nor freezes.

DURATION: Between 30 and 45 minutes, then rest for at least 15 minutes. This application can be repeated once a day until the symptoms diminish and the fever subsides.

4.   Cabbage leaves

External applications with savoy cabbage or white cabbage leaves are not well known, but cabbage leaves are used in nursing care by placing them directly on the affected body region and fixing them in place—washed, freed from thick leaf veins, crushed and possibly warmed up slightly. The indications are manifold, and the range of effects is impressive.

First, let us look at the plant. Cabbage plants belong to the cruciferous family. These grow primarily on scarcely fertile, barren soils. We find a particularly large number of "weeds" in this family, as the plant can wrest life from poor soil conditions. All processes, from germination to rooting, leafing, flowering and fruiting, follow each other quickly and start very early in the year.[7] The plant absorbs sulfur from the soil and binds it in mustard oil glycosides. These determine the characteristic taste of the raw leaf, which can be described as intense, pungent, biting and peppery and which sometimes also has something cool about it. You can smell the sulfur only when the leaf is damaged. Everyone knows the biting and sometimes tear-eliciting smell that cabbage gives off when being cut. When cabbage leaves are boiled, the heating process makes the taste milder and a sulfuric smell is generated.

External applications use the leaves. The cabbage plant's juicy, fleshy leaves grow so tightly around each other that it is difficult to gradually remove them. So, we are dealing with a tightly closed, outwardly rounded growth in which the stem is compressed to almost nothing. This compact structure also makes it difficult for people to digest cabbage dishes.

Proven *indications* for which cabbage leaves are used in external applications are lymph congestion, thrombosis, ulcus cruris, decubitus ulcers, abscesses, rheumatic diseases, menstrual complaints and metastatic pain (soft tissue and bone metastases).

At first glance, these diseases appear to be very different. However, they have common characteristics: they are chronic, progressive diseases. One gets the impression that the person's life processes have pulled themselves out of the organs and thus, for example, liquids and substances remain lying as if "dead" and are no longer integrated into the organism as a whole. Dying processes can be the direct result in case of venous ulcers and bedsores. Life escapes bit by bit. This also applies to rheumatism, in which inflammatory and hardening processes alternate.

Cabbage leaves can bring relief in such cases. Accumulated liquids start to shift, the liquid is lifted out of heaviness and reintegrated into the metabolism. Abscesses can mature and open up, wounds can be cleansed and revitalized. Where stagnation prevailed, movement now occurs. It is therefore understandable that the patient may experience an increase in pain at the start of treatment. The pain-relieving effect of cabbage compresses on metastases is particularly impressive.

The strong vitality of the cabbage plant makes it possible to reintegrate disease processes back into life.

Part of plant used	Savoy and/or white cabbage leaves
Characteristics	Revitalization of unfavorable soil conditions
Indications	Metabolic decline Death processes
Kind of application	Cabbage leaf compress (cool to tempered)
Location	Locally, on the affected area

Chart: Cabbage compresses

4.1 Practical implementation using the example of a joint compress

The first step is to determine the stage of the joint disease. In the case of an overheated, swollen and very painful joint, such as in the acute relapse of rheumatic disease, it is preferable to use a cool application. Cold reduces metabolism and has an antiphlogistic and analgesic effect. In the long run, however, the symptoms worsen. When used over a longer period of time, the cabbage leaves should therefore be applied at room temperature.

When treating osteoarthritis accompanied by painful movement, we lightly heat the cabbage leaf between two hot-water bottles. The heat reduces the viscosity of the synovial fluid and has a positive effect on morning pain and mobility.

It is recommended to use cabbage leaves from controlled organic cultivation. A certain odor that "fine noses" find unpleasant cannot be avoided when a cabbage application is kept on for several hours.

INDICATIONS: Painful, swollen joints as part of rheumatic disease or during the inflammatory stage of osteoarthritis.

CONTRAINDICATIONS: None.

MATERIALS: White cabbage or savoy cabbage, a sharp knife, rolling pin or bottle, a tea towel, duvetyn fabric or an elastic compress wrap, possibly two hot-water bottles.

INSTRUCTIONS: Remove as many cabbage leaves from the cabbage as are needed to well cover the affected part of the body. Discard withered and damaged leaves. Wash the leaves in lukewarm water, cut out the thick middle ribs and place the rest in a drying cloth. Next, vigorously roll across the leaves with a rolling pin, so that juice escapes and the structure becomes softer. Then warm the leaves slightly between the hot-water bottles or place them directly on the respective part of the body and fix them in place with the duvetyn fabric or elastic compress wrap, in a way that mobility is not restricted.

DURATION: If the skin is intact, the compress can be used for hours or even overnight. A post-treatment rest is not necessary.

5.   Chamomile

Chamomile is one of the best-known medicinal plants to this very day. Who hasn't experienced the soothing effect of chamomile tea in cases of indisposition, stomach ailments or cramping abdominal pain? Chamomile is also used to treat badly healing and infected wounds. For some of us, chamomile is the epitome of an herbal remedy and evokes pertinent memories. Heinrich Waggerl (1897–1973) wrote:

Chamomile
The Creator bestowed on chamomile
the power to quench the body's pain.
It flowers and waits undaunted
for someone with a stomachache.
People, however, in their torment,
don't believe in what's available
They shout for pills.
Spare me chamomile, they cry,
for God's sake.[8]

Fortunately, chamomile has been preserved as a remedy. Externally, it is used as a hot abdominal compress for the indications mentioned, since as a flower it has a special relationship to the metabolic pole in the human body.

Botanically speaking, chamomile belongs to the family of composite flowers. This plant family can be found in almost all zones of the earth where it is warm and bright. It loves light and warmth and needs them to form its flower heads. It grows relatively rarely in the wild and is often confused with similar composite flowers. It can be clearly identified by its hollow, air-filled flower receptacle.

Already in autumn, first small leaf rosettes develop from the seeds, which become strong in winter under ice and snow and from which juicy green shoots with many leaves develop as warmth increases. When the plant starts to flower, its leaf and stem growth are pushed apart by strong branching, making the plant appear sparse and translucent. The more flowers there are, the more the growth in leaves diminishes. The leaves turn yellow and finally dry up completely. The delicate yellow flowers give off a sweet, aromatic, typical chamomile scent when touched lightly.[9]

The plant forms its characteristic essential oil in the flower with the help of the sun's warmth. We obtain this by distillation; it is also contained in tea. Treatment with chamomile releases light and warmth. We can bring this all-pervading golden warmth to a patient's body by means of an abdominal compress, for example.

In the disease processes mentioned, warmth—as a typical quality of the metabolic system—is reduced. This is often accompanied by frozenness. Instead of movement, we find inertia and cramping tendencies, which manifest in flatulence and constipation, for instance. In cases of agitation and nervousness the soul lacks shielding [→ Chapter "The Human Warmth Organism and Its Care"]. Chamomile applications quickly alleviate the person's discomfort, providing pleasant warming and relaxation.

However, hot compresses are contraindicated for all forms of unclear and acute abdominal complaints, i.e., any that are not reliably diagnosed!

Part of plant used	Flower
Characteristics	Intensive connection to light and warmth
Indications	Stagnant, convulsive processes in the motor-metabolic system
Kind of application	Hot compresses
Location	Abdomen

Chart: Chamomile abdominal compresses

5.1 Practical implementation using the example of a hot abdominal compress

Hot chamomile abdominal compresses require good guidance and skill. It is important for the patient to know beforehand that this compress must be quite hot to begin with, otherwise too much heat would be lost. After three or four breaths the temperature becomes pleasant.

INDICATIONS: Wherever there is a lack of warmth and relaxation, such as painful cramps in the gastrointestinal tract, menstrual cramps, a feeling of fullness, nervous restlessness, insomnia.

CONTRAINDICATIONS: Acute, unclear abdomen, heavy menstrual bleeding, fever, cold feet, skin injuries in the area of the compress.

MATERIALS: 500 ml of hot, fresh chamomile tea in a thermos flask, duvetyn fabric or wool cloth as an outer cloth all around, a compress cloth, a wringing-out cloth, a bowl, a hot water bottle with a cover.

INSTRUCTIONS: The flannel fabric or wool cloth serves as an outer cloth and is applied all around the body. Fold the compress cloth to the right size, roll it up and place it in the wringing-out cloth. The rest of the steps are similar to those of the lemon chest compress. Finally, place the hot-water bottle on the patient's stomach.

DURATION: About 30 to 45 minutes, then at least 30 minutes for the post-treatment rest.

6.   Mustard

Special attention should be paid to this application. Mustard is an effective remedy that must be handled responsibly, as burns can occur if administered improperly.

How is this enormous generation of heat to be understood, when the mustard powder is dissolved in water at a maximum temperature of 40°C (104°F) and applied as a foot bath or poultice?

Like cabbage, the mustard plant belongs to the cruciferous family. Plants of this family grow all over Central Europe, partly wild. With regard to soil conditions, mustard is undemanding and, like the cabbage plant, exhibits a high level of vitality.

However, the mustard plant's sulfur processes are not located in its leaves, they are in the seeds. This is where we find the connection to warmth processes. These warmth processes appear when mustard oil glycosides dissolve in water to form volatile mustard oil. As mustard irritates the skin and mucous membranes, it fires up metabolic processes.

Important *applications and indications* for mustard powder:

- Chest compress: for pneumonia and bronchopneumonia.
- Footbath: for the onset of influenza with headaches, or migraine attacks and chronic asthmatic complaints.

To arrive at a differentiated indication for the use of mustard powder, it is necessary to consider the course of a disease. In cases of pneumonia we begin by asking:

- Is it chronic or acute?
- Is the phlegm blocked and can't be coughed up?
- What about body temperature—does the patient have a high fever or a moderate one?
- Does the patient appear to be very weak or does she still have the strength to overcome the disease?

When pneumonia takes the classical acute, febrile course and the patient can survive the high fever without serious physical or psychological impairment, mustard powder chest compresses support the healing process. When the fever impairs the patient's general condition through headaches, circulatory weakness or excessive somnolence, lemon compresses to the chest or calves provide relief.

If it is a protracted illness with a low fever (below 38.5°C, or 101.3°F) or pneumonia treated with antibiotics, where the fever usually drops quickly, a ginger chest compress is recommended.[10]

In cases of migraine and head colds, excessive metabolic processes manifest in the form of pressure and pulsation in the head, as well as hotness and increased secretion. These phenomena occur frequently and massively in places where they do not belong.

These shifted metabolic processes must be brought back to their natural place with a foot bath, i.e., with an application to the lower limb system.

In chronic asthma, stimulation of the metabolic limb pole often results in a release in the rhythmic system, which has a positive effect on spasticity. Note how sluggish and solidified the entire digestive system of asthma patients often is. Stimulation therefore has a liberating effect on their rhythmic system.

Mustard helps to bring the wrongly localized metabolic processes back to where they belong, or to ignite sluggish inflammatory processes, enabling a turn for the better.

Thus, mustard's effect differs substantially from that of lemon or cabbage, which do not have such rapid stimulating effects. Consequently, a mustard application at the beginning of treatment is given for a maximum of two to five minutes, or up to ten to fifteen minutes for patients who are used to it, while cabbage leaves can be applied for several hours.

Part of plant used	Seeds	
Characteristics	High vitality, sulfuric processes	
Indications	Increased metabolic processes:	Displaced metabolic processes:
	Pneumonia, broncho-pneumonia	Beginning influenza, headaches, migraines, chronic asthma
Kind of application	Mash poultice	Partial bath
Location	Chest	Feet and lower legs

Chart: Mustard powder chest compresses, mustard powder footbaths

6.1 Practical implementation using the example of a mustard powder foot bath

The use of mustard powder can lead to burns if carried out improperly. Compared to a mustard compress, the footbath develops its effect more slowly and gently. The water temperature should not exceed 40°C (104°F), otherwise proteins will coagulate, and the mustard oil will not be released.

INDICATIONS: To draw off in cases of rhinitis, colds, flu infections, severe headaches, migraines.

CONTRAINDICATIONS: Vascular diseases, sensory disorders, skin irritations, allergies.

MATERIALS: Two hands full of black mustard powder, a foot-bath tub (preferably up to the knees), a bath towel and bath mat, lukewarm water for rinsing off mustard residues (a shower head or jug), olive oil or skin protection oil (e.g., *Calendula oil* (Weleda)), warm socks.

INSTRUCTIONS: First fill the tub with lukewarm water, then have the patient put their legs in it. Add the mustard powder and have the patient spread it around with their feet.

DURATION: The duration is initially 5 minutes and increases to up to 15 minutes for patients who are familiar with it. The decisive factor is whether the patient is still able to withstand the tingling or burning sensation. At the end, any mustard residues are removed with lukewarm water and the legs are dried well. A thin layer of skin oil is then applied to the areas treated. Socks protect against renewed cooling. The application is very suitable when there are signs of a beginning cold, preferably before going to bed. Having warm feet leads to restful sleep.

7. Observing and influencing metabolic activity and warmth processes

The effectiveness of all external applications depends on the specific indication. This in turn requires precise observation and assessment of the metabolic processes in disease processes.

As nurses, we must ask ourselves the following questions before we carry out the prescribed application: in which direction should the stimulation or support of the person's self-healing powers go? Does their metabolism need to be stimulated, pushed back or ordered in a targeted way?

An important reference point for finding and evaluating the indication is our observation of the patient's body temperature. We have to consider that people feel warmth very individually and therefore subjectively [→ Chapter, "The Human Warmth Organism and Its Care"]. It is also necessary to detect the flow and radiation of warmth during treatment. During hot applications, the patient's warmth organism expands; during cold applications it contracts.

Some basic rules must be observed, which are presented in the following paragraphs.

8. Basic rules for administering compresses

8.1 Substances

The selected examples show that we use a wide variety of substances. As with the administration of medications, we require precise knowledge of the substance's effects, side effects, indications and methods of application.

For external applications we usually work with plant extracts. Wherever possible, we use products from controlled organic cultivation.

When using teas, great care must be taken with quality. The plant substance should be fresh, for example, and thus contain a certain quantity of essential oils.

The preparation of tea depends on the part of the plant used (flower, leaf or root). The rule of thumb is: the more solid the component, such as a stem, the more intensive the form of preparation, e.g., we boil it.

When preparing delicate chamomile flowers for a hot abdominal compress, a short infusion (two minutes) is enough to extract the essential oils from the flower. If the chamomile tea is left to steep for longer, it quickly tastes bitter because, in addition to essential oils, bitter substances have also been extracted. These are important for wound irrigations because of their anti-inflammatory and anti-irritant effect. The type of preparation can be looked up in the literature mentioned at the end of this chapter. Especially recommended are the publications of Monika Fingado and Els Eichler.[11, 12]

8.2 Materials

In addition to teas, oils, aqueous-alcoholic extracts and ointments, we also need textiles to administer compresses: cloths—soaked with substance—which we can place directly on the skin, and cloths which we place on top of the substance cloth to create a warm enclosure. These cloths must also meet certain requirements.

The *inner cloth*, the actual compress, must absorb the substance well, be skin-friendly and permeable to air. The latter is important so that the compress does not become a sweat pack. Thus, only cotton, linen, and silk can be considered. Since hospital laundry must be boil-proof, silk is omitted here. The final *outer cloth* must above all hold heat well, be soft to the touch and also be permeable to air. Pure wool best meets these requirements, e.g., in the form of natural wool fleece, but flannel and terrycloth are also suitable materials.

An additional cloth between the inner and outer cloth is sometimes required, such as to protect the woolen cloth from soiling and felting. This intermediate cloth is made of cotton or linen.

Unfortunately, it is quite difficult to get pure cotton linens in hospitals. If used regularly, it is a good idea to have your own assortment of different sizes available at the nursing station.

8.3 Special preparations for compresses

When the decision to administer an external application has been made, you should consider the criteria for appropriate implementation before starting your work.

First, remember to inform the patient. Since we require his cooperation, he must be informed about the sense and purpose and also about the process, as well as possible reactions. If it is difficult for the patient to cooperate, we select "milder" applications, such as an oil cloth or ointment cloth compress, e.g., for children and disoriented people. The reaction is not always as spectacular as it is when mustard is used. It is therefore all the more important that the patient observe himself and inform us of any slight changes.

Some applications have a stimulating effect on excretion processes. It is therefore recommended that the patient go to the toilet beforehand. When administering mustard powder chest compresses, have enough tissues or a cup ready for the mucus. Since many compresses stimulate breathing, it is necessary to provide for fresh air in the room beforehand. Nevertheless, the room should be warm during the application. Often there is a great need for rest during a compress, or the patient falls asleep during or after the application:

- Is she lying comfortably?
- Is a bright ceiling light or the sun blinding her?
- Can she sleep in peace, or is she due for another examination?
- Will visiting time soon begin, with unrest in the room?

All these questions have to be clarified in advance, because it is not only the time required for the application that is important, we also need to ensure time for the rest and relaxation phase afterwards.

To create good framework conditions, external applications must be integrated into the daily routine of the patient and the workflow of the nursing staff. It may require some time changes or the creation of a timetable for the patient. In addition, the application should be regular and always at the same time of day.

The final steps of the preparation phase, such as soaking and wringing out the cloths, take place directly at the patient's bed. In this way he already participates in the implementation and possibly already helps with the preparation.

The greater care the nurse takes, the greater the patient's attention and inner involvement will be; this can convince even skeptical patients.

8.4 Priorities for monitoring

Intensive observation is essential. This applies both to identifying the correct indication and to supporting the patient during the application.

An interplay of questions and answers contributes to a better understanding. How often do we ask a person questions without really waiting for an answer? Such an attitude may indicate a lack of attention or, worse still, a lack of interest. However, interest in the answers is essential to develop oneself as a questioner and to learn new things. When applied to external applications this means: the application is a question that we ask of the organism. The response to this question is the reaction of the patient—on a physical level as well as on a soul level.

Initially, we turn our attention to the patient's warmth organism. A person's own sensation of warmth represents a completely subjective perception and it is often highly disturbed in ill people.

Compresses emphatically appeal to the warmth organism.

Criteria for observing the warmth organism:
- Rectal temperature before and after application
- Temperature curve during the day
- Temperature at the extremities
- Warm and cold zones on the body
- Changes in the patient's perception of warmth

All observations have their significance for treatment.

Other monitoring tasks:
- Improvement/worsening of complaints due to heat/cold
- Changes in excretion processes (sweat, sputum, urine, stool)
- Influence on the person's consciousness
- Quality of sleep (sleeps better/worse, falling asleep/sleeping through, dreams more/less)
- Changes in the need for rest and withdrawal
- Changes in the cardiovascular situation (blood pressure, pulse)

Our observations allow us to assess the effectiveness of the application. This depends on the proper implementation and the correct indication. Here lies a great responsibility for nurses. The doctor depends on our skills and experience. In addition, our observations allow us to make any possibly necessary modifications or corrections in the way we administer the compress.

In addition, the following notes are important:
- Small steps often lead more gently to the goal of healing.
- Never wrap a patient's calves with ice water.
- According to the motto "less is more," it is sometimes necessary to gradually acclimate the patient to the temperature of a compress, e.g., to warm up an abdominal compress a little more from day to day or to increase the duration of a mustard powder compress by one minute per day.

8.5   New qualities in the therapeutic process

Even though compresses have long had a firm place in anthroposophically extended medicine, this is still an area that has potential for development. It is waiting to be explored with researching awareness, in order to cultivate an even more conscious handling of these wonderful therapeutic possibilities.

8.6   The nurse's inner attitude

The inner attitude of the nurse essentially determines the quality of an external application. The right attitude towards the matter in hand promotes therapeutic effectiveness. Our attitude is reflected in our learning to understand the medicinal plant, it makes us awake to our observations and allows us to be careful and loving in the way we prepare and administer the application. The world opens up to us when we ask questions, and we can arrive at new insights. If the patient notices that the nurse is approaching him with warm interest, he is also more inclined to open up and express personal feelings.

Such a questioning and interested attitude is inextricably linked with the therapeutic process. It increases the healing effect of the plant.

Questions arouse interest, you draw attention to what is being done. This is the only way to overcome the stage of pure trial and error and gather detailed perceptions about the effect of an application. This keeps our senses awake and preserves us from falling into an unthinking "daily grind." We aim for a routine of learned, practiced, and ultimately professional action. This is what this chapter aims to convey.

References

1   Simoes-Wüst, A.P., et al. Wie Patienten Wickelanwendungen (ein) schätzen: Ergebnisse einer Umfrage in einem anthroposophischen Akutspital. *Der Merkurstab* 2014; 67 (2), pp. 92–97.

2   Heine, R., et al. *Praxisintegrierte Studie zur Darstellung der Frühwirkungen von Ingwer (Zingiberis officinalis) als äußere Anwendung.* Selbstverlag Filderklinik, Filderstadt 1992.

3   Therkleson, T. Topical ginger for the chronic inflammatory condition of osteoarthritis. *Der Merkurstab* 2013; 66 (2), pp. 145–149.

4   Sommer, M. Zur praktischen Anwendung des Ingwerwickels. *Der Merkurstab* 2006; 59 (6), p. 538–540.

5   Faschingbaue,r C. Schonendere Fiebersenkung durch Zitronenwickel. *Pflegezeitschrift* 1995 (6).

6   van Benthem-van Beek, Vollenhoven, A., et al. *Krankenpflege zu Hause auf der Grundlage der anthroposophisch orientierten Medizin.* Verlag Freies Geistesleben, Stuttgart 1996.

7   Pelikan, W. *Heilpflanzenkunde.* Band 1. Verlag am Goetheanum, Dornach 2012, p. 133 ff.

8   Waggerl, K.H. *Heiteres Herbarium.* Otto Müller Verlag, Salzburg 1950, p. 20.

9   ibid.

10 Sommer, M. Zur praktischen Anwendung des Ingwerwickels. *Der Merkurstab* 2006; 59 (6), pp. 538–540.

11 Fingado, M. *Compresses and other therapeutic applications: A handbook from Ita Wegman Klinik.* Floris Books, Edinburgh 2011.

12 Eichler E. *Wickel und Auflagen.* Verein für Anthroposophisches Heilwesen, Bad Liebenzell 2000.

CHAPTER XIV

Active Principles in External Applications

The Nature of External Applications—How They Differ from Other Medical and Nursing Interventions

ROLF HEINE

The term "external applications" is an undefined collective term for a wide range of therapeutic and nursing measures such as baths, rhythmical oil applications (known as Rhythmical Einreibung), and compresses. In addition to their use in professional settings, external applications have traditionally played an important role in self-treatment. There is now comprehensive self-help literature and online information available to explain and train these methods, which previously were mostly passed on within family traditions. Based on extensive analysis of the literature, André Fringer and his working group first proposed the following definition of external applications in nursing in 2015.[1] This definition includes the character of external applications, how they work, their types and possible variations. It is a starting point for scientific investigation of external applications. In particular, this definition makes it clear that the impact of external applications is not limited to the effect of substances. Rather, other dimensions of efficacy must be taken into account to provide appropriate indications and develop suitable study designs.

→   Learning objectives, see end of chapter

What external applications are: "External applications in nursing care are therapeutic interventions based on salutogenetic principles, in which direct or indirect forms of contact with the sensory organ skin and/or the neurosensory system are used to stimulate processes designed to alleviate complaints, heal illnesses, and increase well-being, and whose foundations are based on complementary nursing and medical systems, encompassing structural, functional, and therapeutic interventions, as well as knowledge, techniques, and expertise, and which must be learned to be able to administer them professionally."

How external applications work: "External applications act systemically (mechanically, physiologically, psychologically, spiritually and socially), primarily reciprocally between the therapist and the person being treated, as well as secondarily affecting the person's relatives and others around them."

Kinds of external applications: "The aim and purpose of the therapeutic intervention determines the type of 'external application', whose stimuli can be physical (e.g., warmth, cold), rhythmical (e.g., tempo, intervals, pauses), chemical (e.g., active substances) and tactile (e.g., types of contact), whereby the intensity, location, duration and frequency of the measure vary according to the diagnosis and the physical and mental condition of the patient."

	Substances and mediums	Comment
Baths and partial baths	water, warmth, emulsified essential oils, emulsified fatty oils, water-soluble substances	oil dispersion bath brushing resembles massage. In flow baths the water is moved around
Washes and partial washes	water, warmth, emulsified essential oils, water-soluble substances, movement	elements of rhythmical oil applications are incorporated into bed baths
Compresses	water, warmth, essential and fatty oils, water-soluble substances	absorption of substances via the skin during occlusion is especially intensive
Oil embrocations, massages	essential and fatty oils, touch	intensive interaction between patient and practitioner

Chart: Kinds of external applications

1. Effect factors

Different factors determine the effect of any external application:
1. The substance used (e.g., lavender, lemon, copper)
2. The medium that conveys the substance (e.g., water, oil, temperature)
3. The rhythm (e.g., time of day, frequency, dosage)
4. The setting (e.g., attention, touch, quiet)

Each of these factors also has an effect when isolated from the others. When a nicotine patch is applied, the only effective factor is presumably the substance, according to the dosage. Simply cooling a sprained joint has an analgesic and decongestant effect even without an added substance. Rhythm created by pauses, for example, has its own therapeutic benefit. Attentive interest shown to a suffering patient has effects that also occur without the use of a physical substance or therapeutic medium.

These factors are also important for other routes of administration, but their relevance for external applications is polar opposite to that of oral administration. Substance is the most important factor in oral administration, yet it can be completely missing from an external application. A hot water bottle warms without any 'substance', it has an antispasmodic and relaxing effect, but can cause burning when overdone. The setting, on the other hand, such as undisturbed post-treatment rest, is of the utmost importance for external applications, while it is of no obvious importance for oral administration, beyond the placebo effect (exceptions confirm the rule, as with the substance-dependent effect of a mustard compress and the setting-dependent effect of mind-altering drugs).

The factor "rhythm" (frequency, dosage and time of day) is relevant for all forms of application. The following table compares the different application forms.

	External application	Inhalation	Injection	Enteral medication
Approach or organ	Skin, neuro-sensory system	lungs, rhyth-mic system	blood, rhyth-mic system	mouth, stomach, bowels, metabolic system
Primary sense impression	warmth, smell, touch	smell	pain as a side effect	taste as a side effect
Dependence of the primary effect on the setting	++++ strong	+++ weaker	++ minimal	+ very minimal
Dependence of the primary effect on the substance	++ minimal (with the exception of skin irri-tants)	++++ strong	++++ strong	++++ strong
Dependence of the primary effect on the medium	++++ strong	+ very minimal (only aerosols are applied)	+ very minimal (only liquid substances are applied)	+ very minimal (with suitable galenicals)
Dependence of the primary effect on rhythm	++++ strong	++++ strong	++++ strong	++++ strong

Chart: Comparison of different forms of application

2. Substances in external applications

The chapter "Compresses in Anthroposophically Extended Nursing Care" presents examples of various substances: lemon, chamomile, mustard, and white cabbage. The first three come from fruit, flowers and seeds. They have an effect especially on human metabolic processes and limbs. White cabbage leaves balance processes of degeneration and upbuilding, as in wound cleansing and wound healing, thus supporting the rhythmic system.

Rudolf Steiner, following the alchemical tradition, described warmth-related substances and those that tend to dissolve, smell and spread out into the space around them as "sulfuric substances." Sulfur is the mineral archetype of a strongly smelling, easily flammable and chemically readily transforming substance. In plants, sulfuric processes are mainly seen in flowers and fruit.

Rudolf Steiner called substances that easily crystallize, form shapes, and transparently absorb light but only little heat, "sal-like substances."[2] In plants it is especially the roots and seeds that have this tendency to become firm and durable. Table salt is the archetype for saline-like hardening and clarification processes.

Between sulfur and salt processes we find a mediating, balancing "mercury process." Substances that support this process can act in the direction of both dissolution and hardening. These include, for example, white cabbage, honey, and farmer's cheese.[3]

The following table assigns some substances to these principles and gives indications and contraindications.

Sulfuric substances	Principle	Used externally as	Indication
Chamomile flower	strengthens metabolic activity; counters forming, nervous, cramping processes; dissolves indurations in the gastrointestinal system	moist-warm abdominal compress	irritable stomach; examination anxiety, nausea with vomiting; abdominal cramps with acute gastroenteritis or for chronic inflammatory bowel syndrome CAUTION: Not for acute inflammations such as appendicitis!
Mallow flower	gentle warming through and lightening up; relieves tension; strengthens vitality (summer ripe)	warm thorax oil compress or Rhythmical Einreibung of the chest	convalescence, exhaustion
Blackthorn flower	gently warms through and lightens up; relief of tension; strengthening vitality (spring forces)	Rhythmical Einreibung of arms or thorax	convalescence, exhaustion

Lavender flower	loosens, relaxes	warm thorax oil compress or Rhythmical Einreibung	asthma, difficulty falling asleep
Rose flower	strong mental/emotional effect, harmonizing and strengthening	Rhythmical Einreibung of the limbs or thorax	exhaustion, despondency, vulnerability
St. John's wort (leaf and flower)	lightens up; repels pressing environmental influences by strengthening one's own metabolic forces	Rhythmical Einreibung of the limbs or thorax	depressive moods, emotional over-excitedness; burning pain
Mustard powder (seeds)	strengthens metabolic activity; hyperemia; repels overly formative forces; strong centrifugal spread of warmth	thorax compress shoulder-neck compress foot bath	acute febrile infections of the respiratory tract; muscle tension hypotension, depression, migraines
Fennel, Anise, Caraway (seed-like fruits)	gentle, inward pressing warmth; mild stimulation of digestive activity eliminating gas	abdominal oil compress or abdominal tea compress	obstipation, full feeling, bloating
Sulfuric leaves	Principle	Used externally as	Indication
Yarrow	dissolving substances like etheric yarrow oil (with azulene) penetrate the strictly articulated, finely chiseled leaf dissolving and forming forces work together harmoniously	yarrow liver compress	to stimulate liver activity in case of depression; detoxification after chemotherapeutics
Rosemary	the flowers reach deeply into the leaf area very aromatic leaves sulfuric forces work in the rhythmic system	rosemary oil application to the legs, rosemary foot bath	hypotension, circulatory weakness, chronic fatigue, depression

Sulfuric roots	Principle	Used externally as	Indication
Ginger powder (rhizome)	strengthens metabolic activity in neurosensory system repels overly formative forces a strong pervasion of warmth spreading inward, also reaching the soul	kidney compress	chronic inflammation, convalescence, exhaustion
Onion	strengthens releasing processes in the neurosensory system	ear bags	middle ear infection
Horseradish	strong warmth development and secretolysis in neurosensory system	compress on forehead, cheek bone or neck	sinus inflammation
Mercurial substances	Principle	Used externally as	Indication
White cabbage	enlivens hardened, edematic tissue support of the exudation phase in wound healing	compress on wounds and limbs	ulcus cruris, mastitis, congestive dermatosis, lymphedema
Farmer's cheese (quark)	cools and relieves inflamed congested tissue	compress on chest, veins, thorax	mastitis, thrombophlebitis, pleuritis with effusion
Honey	promotion of wound secretion (dissolving) and epithelialization (forming)	wounds	wound treatment
Saline substances	Principle	Used externally as	Indication
Oak bark	forms and tans	washing, dabbing with alcoholic or aqueous extract	eczema, hemorrhoids
Quartz sand	forms	sand bath	rheumatism, arthritis

Medicinal clay	forms, dries	poultice	eczema, arthritis
Equisetum	forms	chest compress, kidney oil cloth	pneumonia with abscess tendency, nephritis

Chart: Assignment of substances according to the Tria Principia (sal–sulfur–mercury)

2.1 Active principles in sulfuric substances

a) Supporting inflammatory processes
Inflammation is a primarily healthy reaction to a foreign body, whether it is a splinter in the hand or a bacterium in the lungs. If we want to promote this "good" intention of inflammation, we can do this with warmth and with sulfuric acting substances. Examples of this are the maturation of a furuncle with the support of St. John's wort oil, and mustard compresses for pneumonia. The latter forces the heat of an inflammation from the inside of the organism outwards towards the body's surface, leading to relief from shortness of breath and dissolving mucus.

b) Warming cold, lifeless, sclerotic organs
Where metabolic activity has withdrawn from the organism, sulfuric substances stimulate blood flow in the affected region. An example of this would be cramped, cold shoulder muscles, which are warmed and revitalized by essential oils or mustard powder compresses. This principle of action requires an intact capacity to react within the organism. A cachectic elderly person does not develop warmth from the stimulus of a mustard compress but is rather left with local skin damage. Scars do not dissolve even if they are lovingly rubbed with essential oils. Nevertheless, the vitality of the surrounding tissue can be maintained by regular treatment with blackthorn blossom or almond oil.

2.2 Active principles in mercurial substances

a) Transferring the sulfur principle to the rhythmic system
Representatives of the Labiatae family, such as lavender, rosemary, thyme, sage, peppermint and Melissa, produce sulfuric substances, i.e., fragrant, slightly volatile essential oils, mainly in the leaf area. During treatment the sulfur pole of these plants fills the patient's rhythmic system, which is related to the leaf region. [→ Chapter "Compresses in Anthroposophically Extended Nursing Care"]. Warmth is carried into the patient's respiration and blood circulation in a revitalizing way. It dissolves deposits such as mucus (e.g., in the case of colds), supports inflammation as a self-healing process (e.g., in the case of bronchitis), or stimulates sluggish blood circulation (rosemary, sage).

b) Transferring the sal principle to the rhythmic system

Plants such as field horsetail carry the hardening sal principle into the leaf area of the plant (silicification). This is taken advantage of when inflammatory processes get out of control, for example by using horsetail chest compresses to treat pneumonia with empyema formation.

c) Transferring the sulfur principle to the neurosensory system

In the case of "sulfuric roots" (correctly called rhizomes in many cases, i.e., stalks growing underground), such as ginger or onions, the sulfuric-flowering quality is drawn down into the region of the plant's hardening pole (the sal-root pole). When used to treat the human being, sulfur unfolds its effect in the neurosensory system. The use of horseradish for sinusitis or onions for inflammation of the middle ear are excellent examples of this principle. So, too, does the effect of ginger rhizomes on chronic states of mental hardening—when someone lives too much "in their head"—illustrate the shift of the sulfur principle to the sal-neurosensory pole in the human being.

d) Mercurial moderation to facilitate dissolving processes

White cabbage is a typical mercurial plant. It is predominantly a leaf structure with marginal roots and inconspicuous flowers. As a wound dressing for poorly healing wounds, such as ulcer cruris or bedsores, it stimulates wound secretion and contributes to wound cleansing and vitalization.

Honey works in a similar way. In a wound it quickly dissolves its mercurial gel-like consistency and strongly promotes exudation.

e) Mercurial moderation to facilitate formative processes

When a farmer's cheese (quark) compress is applied to an inflamed vein or an engorged, inflamed breast, it cools the inflamed organ. The gel consistency of the farmer's cheese dries, hardens and absorbs moisture from the tissue. The tissue is firmed up and the accumulated fluid is set in motion.

Honey and cabbage leaf have a similar effect if they are not used in the exudation phase but in the epithelialization phase of wound healing. The honey now crystallizes and forms, while the cabbage leaf dries and protects the delicate epithelium.

2.3   Active principles in saline substances

a) Forming

Even mere cooling reduces acute inflammations, such as those caused by sprains, burns or eczema. In case of sprains, the addition of table salt to a moist and cool compress supports this formative process. Arnica essence has a soothing effect on hematoma and pain, especially with blunt injuries.

In eczema, any substance applied externally may cause further irritation. In this case, simply covering with gauze bandages can provide the required formative influence.

In the case of abrasions, dabbing with an oak bark decoction limits exudation, alleviates pain and supports the epithelialization process.

b) Dissolving

A resilient organism tends to resist excessive forming by external influences. Rhythmical Einreibung with table salt stimulates perspiration and blood circulation in the skin.

Rudolf Steiner gave the following meditation on the three working principles sal, mercury and sulfur in January 1924 in Dornach:[4]

You healing Spirits,
You unite
With Sulfur's blessing
Of the ethereal fragrance;

I will unite my soul's knowing
To the fire
Of the blossom's aroma;

You come to life
In upward springing Mercury
Dewdrop
Of growing
And becoming.

I will arouse my soul's life
With the glistening drops
On the morning leaves;

You make your halting place
In the Earth Salt
Which nourishes the root
In the soil.

I will strengthen my soul's being
On the hardening salt
With which the Earth
Attentively cares for the roots.

3. The medium through which a substance is conveyed

External applications already have an effect on body and soul through heat or cold. Moderate heat relaxes, moderate cold contracts. Very strong heat and cold have destructive effects.

In baths and washing, it is primarily the element of water that has an effect, at a certain temperature and, if necessary, with an added substance. Warmth or cold can be considered for poultices and compresses, and moisture or dryness are also important. Last but not least, there are applications in which the carrier element has hardly any effect of its own. This is the case with ointment cloths (compresses). Even a gel is no longer neutral as a medium and is deliberately used for cooling.

We differentiate between warm, cold, dry, moist and neutral applications. Two qualities always appear together.

Medium	Examples	Used for
Dry-warm applications	hot water bottle cherry pit bag oil cloth*	cold, freezing, weakness, exhaustion for disturbances in the warmth organism
Moist-warm applications	mustard chest compress ginger chest compress tea compress†	obstruction, full feeling, tension, cramps, shortness of breath, flatulence for disturbances in the air organism
Moist-cold‡ applications	farmer's cheese (quark) compress arnica essence compress lemon calf compress	inflammation with strong edema formation, warmth congestion, contusions for disturbances in the fluid organism
Dry-cold applications	cool pack	fractures for disturbances in the physical organization

Chart: The medium used for compresses and poultices

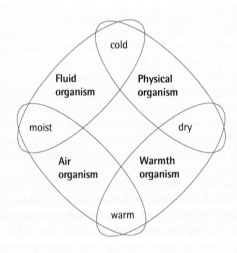

Fig. 1: The four qualities and the medium used in external applications

---

*   Oil is fluid but does not appear moist.

†   Such as with chamomile or yarrow tea

‡   The applications are generally 2–10°C (3.6–18°F) below body temperature. They are felt to be cool, but not cold.

In the Hippocratic and alchemical traditions, 'wet' – 'dry' – 'warm' – 'cold' are referred to as the 'secondary qualities' of the four elements. Warm-dry corresponds to the element fire, warm-moist to the element air, cold-moist to the element water, cold-dry to the element earth. Disturbances in the interaction between the elements fire (warmth), air, water (liquid) and earth (physis) are thus indications for the use of compresses and poultices [→ Chapter "The Anthropological Foundations of Nursing Extended by Anthroposophy"].

It should be noted that dry-warm applications may only be used if the fluid organism opposite the warmth organism in Figure 1 is intact. Cold edemas should not be treated with dry heat, as this increases fluid retention. Warm-moist applications are contraindicated if the physical organism is destroyed or endangered. Acute appendicitis with risk of perforation is an absolute contraindication for moist-warm applications!

In nature we find dry heat in desert areas, humid heat in the tropics and wet cold in cold ocean areas such as the North Sea. Dry cold governs northeastern continental climates, such as in the Russian taiga. External applications are essentially climate therapy brought to the treatment room and the patient's body.*

3.1   The importance of warmth

Heat and cold play decisive roles in all the qualities mentioned above. They are polar phenomena. External warmth and cold are perceived in relation to one's own body temperature. Objects and the environment appear cold when our hand is warmer than they are; warm when their temperature is higher.

Moisture increases the effects of cold and heat. A temperature of 8 degrees Celsius (46.4°F) seems colder on a foggy November day than on a dry January day with temperatures below freezing. The perceived heat in a sauna at 90 degrees Celsius (194°F) increases dramatically when water is poured on the rocks, which causes the humidity to rise. The physical phenomena affecting the organism in these cases are heat conduction, heat convection (heat exchange), evaporation and heat radiation.

"The 'I' lives in warmth." Rudolf Steiner described the warmth organism as the place through which the 'I' expresses itself in the body. [→ Chapter "The Human Warmth Organism and Its Care"]. Stimulation and regulation of warmth via external applications is thus always also a stimulation of the 'I'-organization. In cases of physical hypothermia, the 'I' is completely fixed on its own body. Uncontrollable shivering overlays voluntary movement. In cases of hyperthermia and fever, consciousness is dulled. Concentration is difficult. Body and soul tend towards disintegration. A "human" body temperature of 37 degrees Celsius (98.6°F) is the basis for free, responsible decision-making. It is therefore fundamental to provide cooling, immobilization and "forming" in case of acute inflammation, and to administer heat stimulation from

---

* Rudolf Steiner described in his lecture cycle *Mystery Knowledge and Mystery Centers* how Aristotle (384–322 BC) gave his pupil Alexander (356–323 BC) a lesson in which he taught him about the climatic qualities of landscapes. Starting from Macedonia, Alexander's home country, he described the qualities of the northeast as humid-cold, related to the element water (North Sea), the southeast, related to the element fire (Arab desert), the southwest, related to the element air (Central Africa) and the northeast, related to the element earth (Asia's steppes).

the outside in case of "cold," sclerotic diseases. This is not contradicted by the fact that warmth therapies are also used for acute inflammations. A mustard compress for pneumonia or a thyme oil compress for bronchitis support the fever gesture of the organism, because the fever itself is "warmth therapy" to counteract a foreign body (microorganism). The microorganism itself finds optimal conditions for reproduction if the patient is weakened or has a cold.

4. Rhythm (time of day, frequency, dosage)

Morning and evening

A mustard foot bath in the morning has a different effect than one in the evening. In the morning it refreshes and stimulates, in the evening it loosens and leads to sleep. This phenomenon can be observed in many applications, such as rosemary skin applications.

Above and below

The location of a treatment can show effects that are not restricted to the area of skin that has been treated. A Rhythmical Einreibung treatment of the feet and legs stimulates excretion more and thereby has a rousing effect, while a Rhythmical Einreibung treatment of the hands and arms promotes metabolism and thereby calms the person. Treatment of the lower extremities (normally more involved in will activities) makes them more sensitive to perception of the outer world. Treatment of the hands and arms (normally more involved in perception) emphasizes the will aspect, resulting in tiredness and introversion.[5]

Dosage

As with all treatments, dosage plays an important role:
- Weak stimuli stimulate (a short, cool rinse stimulates the skin's circulation and warmth generation)
- Strong stimuli obstruct (a strong cold application reduces circulation and the treated person stays cold)
- Very strong stimuli destroy (long-lasting, severe cold leads to freezing)

The examples above illustrate that rhythmical aspects have to be considered when determining the effect of an external application. The organism responds to the external stimulus according to its own capacity to react. A weakened organism can only react to the stimulus with a weak response. A cachectic, exhausted patient is unable to respond with warmth generation to a mustard compress. The response will not go beyond local skin irritation or even skin damage. On the other hand, a patient with a sensitivity or allergy to composites can respond to very small doses with a severe localized or generalized inflammatory reaction.

The phenomenon that an application works differently in the morning than in the evening can be explained by human biorhythms: stimulation in the morning supports the person's natural and healthy tendency to incarnate, even when they may have little inclination to adjust to the day because of hypotension or depression. On the other hand, stimulation such as with mustard or rosemary, used in the evening, is a very suitable remedy for patients who have done too little physically during the day, due to being confined to their bed or because of one-sided intellectual work. Here, metabolically stimulating substances incarnate, especially in the rhythmic and motor-metabolic systems, and provide the impetus for letting go or excarnating.

The importance of post-treatment rest
The interplay of external stimulus and internal response reveals the important role of rest in any external application. Rest enables rhythmical switching from an emphasis on neurosensory stimulation to a warming phase with emphasis on the metabolism. If the metabolism's response occurs already during the application, as is often the case with yarrow chest and abdominal compresses, then the post-treatment rest serves to gradually adapt the spreading warmth to the conditions that will be there once the compress and hot water bottle have been removed.

Helping oneself
External applications match the need of many patients to assume an active role in healing, rather than merely passively indulging in therapy. This applies in three respects:
- External applications are available without a doctor's prescription, often with substances available at home.
- The reaction of the body (warmth, blood circulation, respiration, digestion, well-being) immediately after the application shows the activation of the person's self-healing powers.
- Actively giving rhythm to everyday life through arranging for the setting (planning the treatment, allowing for intervals and post-treatment rest) has a positive effect on the person's lifestyle.

This raises the question of whether external applications should always be administered by a nurse (or family member, doctor, therapist) or whether self-therapy plays an equally important role in self-healing from the point of view of empowerment. The answer is that both are true. The first application should always be performed by a nurse. This is the only way to ensure that the desired effect is achieved—through correct application. This will encourage the patient to carry out the application themselves if necessary in the future. With severely ill and exhausted patients, nurses should always administer the treatment.

Psychosomatic patients would usually be able to put on a compress themselves, in terms of their physical strength. Nevertheless, there is a place for a kind of therapeutic regression in which the patient can surrender herself to ministration and care. In this case, it remains advisable to relieve the patient of the task of performing the application. In cases where an assumption of responsibility for the daily rhythm and self-treatment is indicated, the external application is transferred to the patient early on. This is the case with many chronically ill patients!

Frequency and duration of external applications

The subtle members of the human fourfold nature (physical body, etheric body, soul body and 'I'-organization) each have their own specific rhythms:

- 'I'-organization: 24 hours (one day and one night)
- Soul body: 1 week (the week marks a social rhythm. Sundays are free and are followed by work on Monday, etc. Physical processes, such as wound healing, are also subject to the 7-day rhythm.)
- Etheric body: 1 month (the menstrual cycle and the maturation of skin epithelia are subject to this rhythm. A holiday or cure can reach a more profound level of regeneration after 4 weeks.)
- Physical body: 1 year (bone healing after a fracture is completed after one year. Pregnancy, during which a human child matures, lasts 9–10 months– a little less than 1 year, depending on how it is calculated.)

External applications often work after a single application. Arnica, mustard, a bath, a massage have a direct effect on a person's 'I'-organization via their senses and warmth. In many cases these can be genuine emergency measures.

Acute inflammatory illnesses such as colds, flu or pneumonia last about one week. Here a daily application, such as a thorax compress, is indicated for one week. Afterwards, the application can be reduced to two or three times a week, if the course of the illness requires it in severe cases. In convalescence, it is enough to use it once or twice a week for a period of four weeks. The same applies to chronic diseases. In periods of relapse, daily treatment for a week is recommended, followed by a continuation for about one month. Many patients with chronic diseases benefit from treatment in the spring, summer, autumn and winter, with four to eight treatments per series (e.g., in conjunction with a fasting cure or holiday).

5.   Attention–giving, setting, and touch

Most patients remember an external application due to its specific setting. Initial uncertainty about the primary effect of warmth, cold or substance on the skin is accompanied by the proximity to the caregiver, who usually applies the treatment to the chest, back or abdomen, i.e., to relatively intimate areas of the body. The patient can feel secure when she trusts in the safety of the application and the protection provided by the setting. Relaxation occurs, warmth penetrates her entire organism.

Each external application is connected with specific sensory impressions, with pleasant warmth ("like being next to a masonry heater") or refreshing cold ("like on a clear winter morning"), exotic or familiar smells (e.g., ginger or rose) and mindful touching [→ Chapter "From the Question of Meaning in Cancer to the Cultivation of the Senses"]. Sensory impressions alone would not be effective if they were not followed by a balancing response of the metabolism. The sensory impression leads to awareness of the perceived substance, the metabolic response compensates for the degrading effect of the sensory impression. The sensory impression is connected to waking consciousness; the metabolic response happens unconsciously. A rich spectrum of—usually pleasant—sensations develops between the sensory impression and the metabolic response.

When the patient connects positively with sensations, he enters a period of daydreaming, where inner images and memories appear. Thoughts pass by, the breathing deepens, and inner warmth develops. This phase only occurs when the patient can relax, when he does not have to keep alert or maintain anxious control of the application but can surrender to the surge of inner images. With many applications, daydreaming may transition into a short phase of real dreaming.

The phase of daydreaming and dreaming leads to a short, dreamless sleep, often a momentary sleep. From this sleep the patient awakens refreshed and strengthened. The entire external application first prompts an excarnation process in which the soul body and 'I' separate from the etheric and physical bodies (falling sleep). Then follows an incarnation process, a renewed binding of the soul body and 'I' with the etheric and physical bodies.

	Waking	Dreaming	Sleeping
Body	sense impressions (external warmth, cold, aroma, touch)	circulation (blood, breathing)	metabolic response (inner warmth)
Soul	feeling (pleasant, unpleasant)	inner pictures (imaginary journeys, memories)	dreams (images are no longer steerable)
Spirit	assessment ("that smells like chamomile")	Imagination (true image, e.g., chamomile as a healing substance)	Inspiration (unconscious relaxation and awakening with new ideas)

Chart: The transition from waking to sleeping in body, soul and spirit during external applications

A) GINGER KIDNEY COMPRESS

MATERIALS:
- 1 tablespoon of ginger powder (Rhizoma zingiberis)
- Olive oil (or any other oil without fragrant additives)
- 1 gauze diaper (folded four times—size approx. 25 x 15 cm)
- 1 cloth to hold it in place (flannel or terry-cloth towel)
- 1 post-treatment rest cloth (flannel or wool, e.g., a wide woolen scarf)
- 300 ml hot water (approx. 70°C, or 158°F)

TIME OF DAY / DURATION:
- Time of day: in the morning
- Duration: 30 minutes, post-treatment rest about 10 minutes

INSTRUCTIONS:
The patient should empty her bladder and take a comfortable position in the bed before the application. A knee roll can be placed under the knees to relax the abdominal muscles and lumbar spine, as needed. The feet should be warm before the application (put a hot water bottle on them, if necessary).

Let the ginger powder soak in hot water. Grasp the folded gauze diaper at its narrow ends and immerse it in the hot water so that it soaks up the ginger brew and the ginger powder spreads evenly over its surface. Firmly wring out the gauze diaper.

Place the gauze diaper on the kidney region and the fastening cloth over it around the hips. Fix the cloth in place tightly, but without constricting, and tuck the bedcovers in around the patient's hips. If a hot water bottle was used to warm the feet, remove it now.

The room should be slightly darkened. Switch the phone off and tell the patient that the application will last for 30 minutes.

After 30 minutes, remove the compress, dab any leftover ginger powder off the skin, apply olive oil lightly and quickly to the skin and cover it with the post-treatment rest cloth.

End the rest after 10 minutes at the latest and remove the cloth.

TYPICAL EFFECTS OF A GINGER KIDNEY COMPRESS:
- **Warmth:** The patient initially perceives the compress as being hot. After a very short time, the temperature drops, and the compress seems cool. It now takes almost 10 to 15 minutes until the region under the compress slowly warms up. The subjective temperature oscillates between cool and hot, until it stabilizes at a high level after 15 minutes.

- The warmth moves from the application area towards the thorax and head, as well as towards the hips, knees, lower legs, and feet. Many patients report a peculiar spreading of warmth. They do not perceive the heat as being centered on their skin, but rather as being located outside the body or beneath the surface of their skin. This warmth now "washes around" the inner organs in rhythmic waves. Some people experience it vividly, as if it were a "heat scan." As rhythmically flowing warmth, the current reaches the abdominal wall and excites a special heat sensation in the area of the solar plexus in some patients. These or similarly detailed descriptions of the flow of warmth during ginger kidney compresses occurred in several hundred subjects over the last 40 years. A systematic observational study on the typical effects of ginger applications was carried out on patients at the Filderklinik in the 1990s.[6]

- **Breathing:** The patient's breathing deepens and slows down during the application. This is to be expected due to the setting (the patient is lying in bed, not doing anything) and is not ginger-specific. However, many patients report an emphasis on the inhalation phase, especially towards the end of the compress time. Asthmatics find that obstructions relax and mucus is loosened.

- **Excretion:** Increased saliva flow, occasionally stimulation of digestive activity and appetite occur during the treatment. Some patients experience increased urination after the kidney application.

- **Circulation:** Pulse acceleration is more frequent, small increases or decreases in blood pressure occur less often.

- **Mood:** The effects on the patient's mood during and after the application are particularly pronounced. After an initial alertness and attention to the activity of warmth and cold in the body, and a certain irritability toward sounds and light coming from the surroundings, inner images begin to shape the person's mood. Patients report distant past memories of peculiar intensity, waking dreams, and even "dream journeys" through imaginary landscapes (see the pictorial description of spreading warmth). Their feelings are mostly "in a minor key," contemplative, internalized, sometimes full of longing or sadness. If patients are asked about these feelings after the treatment, some are moved to tears.

- **Consciousness:** The first phase of the application is characterized by alertness and attention to the warmth activity. When the heat generation begins, this phase changes into a very contemplative stage (as described above). Daydreams can pass into sleep, which often lasts for only a moment. Patients awaken from this sleep phase with vigor and a desire to do something. Sometimes a new cycle begins of increased alertness—daydreaming—momentary sleep—refreshed alertness.

- **Post-treatment rest:** During the post-treatment rest, the spread of warmth may increase. Some patients report that their body has only now completely warmed up. The rest period is to be ended after about 10 minutes. If the patient stays in bed longer, it may occasionally happen that she gets a feeling of "standing beside herself," of not waking up properly.

Indications for ginger kidney compresses	
Principle	**Examples**
generation and internalization of warmth in an exhausted warmth organism	chronic inflammatory diseases such as Crohn's disease, chronic bronchitis, Pink Buffer-type COPD
	acute inflammation without fever, e.g., antibiotically treated pneumonia, viral pneumonia
loosening up a rigid soul body	asthma (when obstruction is the main thing), irritable bowel syndrome
releasing entrenched images and thoughts	depression in a neurasthenic constitution, compulsions
Contraindications	
Principle	**Examples**
kidney damage	acute kidney inflammation
mental illness	untreated traumas, delusional psychoses

Chart: Indications and contraindications for ginger kidney compresses

B) MUSTARD CHEST COMPRESS

MATERIALS:
- 3 heaped tablespoons of black mustard powder (Semen sinapis niger)
- Olive oil (or any other oil without fragrant additives)
- bed protection (e.g., incontinence pad)
- 1 gauze diaper
- Cellulose or paper towels (30 x 40 cm)
- 1 cloth to hold it in place (flannel or terry-cloth towel)
- 1 post-treatment rest cloth (flannel or wool, e.g., a wide woolen scarf)
- 300 ml warm water (below 60°C or 140°F!)

TIME OF DAY / DURATION:
- Time of day: afternoon, evening
- Duration: 2–15 minutes (depending on skin tolerance!), 30 minutes of post-treatment rest

INSTRUCTIONS:

The patient should empty his bladder and take a comfortable position in the bed before the application. A knee roll can be placed under his knees to relax the abdominal muscles and lumbar spine, as needed. His feet should be warm before the application (put a hot-water bottle on them if necessary). Place the bed protection at chest height on the bed.

Spread out a layer of cellulose on the middle of the gauze diaper. Spread the mustard powder evenly with a spoon on top of the cellulose over the area that will cover the back (approx. 35 x 25 cm). The mustard powder should cover this surface with a continuous yellow layer. Apply a second layer of cellulose and turn over the edges of the cellulose to the boundary of the surface covered by mustard powder. Similarly fold the gauze diaper. Loosely roll in the two narrower ends of the resulting pack.

Soak the pack in the warm water. A yellowish liquid will seep out. Make sure that the core of the pack is also moistened. Mustard only unfolds its effect if it has absorbed water and has not been heated above 60°C (140°F)! Now carefully squeeze out the soaked pack, so that no excess fluid escapes.

Place the pack on the thorax from the shoulder blades to the lower ribs and fix it in place with the fastening cloth. The patient lies down on the bed protection and you wrap the fastening sheet loosely around his chest.

Heat is generated as soon as the pack is placed on the skin. This requires the presence of the nurse during the first application. The pack should be tolerated for at least two minutes during the first application. If the burning sensation seems unbearable, remove the pack and assess the condition of the skin. The first application must not exceed five minutes! If the patient's skin tolerance allows it, i.e., if the redness has completely disappeared after 24 hours, then the duration of the application can be increased gradually up to 15 minutes.

After removing the pack, immediately apply olive oil to the reddened areas of the skin. Loosely place the post-treatment rest cloth around the thorax and cover the patient well. The post-treatment rest period is at least 30 minutes. If the patient has not fallen asleep after the treatment, remove the post-treatment rest cloth.

TYPICAL EFFECTS OF A MUSTARD THORAX COMPRESS:

- **Warmth:** Immediately after the application of the compress, the patient feels a strong burning sensation which can increase almost to intolerance. After about two minutes, the patient gets somewhat used to or adapts to the skin irritation. Nevertheless, the heat increases continuously until the pack is no longer accepted. In indolent or "performance-oriented" patients, or those with impaired perception, such self-protecting perception may not occur, which will lead to first and second degree burns if the nurse does not terminate the application in time.

- The skin irritation intensifies again immediately after the pack is removed and until oil is applied. The local burning often only turns into a sensation of warmth after the compress has been removed. Heat radiates noticeably from the strongly reddened skin area. In patients without fever, this can lead to cooling (especially of the extremities) and even to chills. Care must therefore be taken to ensure that suitable clothing or warm blankets are used.
- **Breathing:** The patient's breathing remains very superficial at first, once the pack is in place. Only after the compress has been removed does their breathing deepen, usually with an emphasis on exhalation. The now beginning loosening of mucus and secretions noticeably facilitates breathing in patients with asthma, bronchitis, pneumonia or COPD.
- **Excretion:** Increased saliva flow, stimulation of digestive activity and appetite sometimes occur during the treatment. Secretion in the airways is loosened.
- **Circulation:** There is often an accelerated pulse.

- **Mood:** Impressive is the patient's exuberant, sometimes anxious mood during the strong burning phase, which gives way to great relief once the compress is removed. Most patients fall asleep dreamlessly during the post-treatment rest.
- **Consciousness:** The first phase of the application is characterized by alertness and attention to the pressing skin irritation. Most patients want to sleep after the pack is removed. They wake up as after a restful sleep, but feel less of a desire for action, rather a sense of quiet power within themselves.
- **Post-treatment rest:** Usually the burning sensation does not give way to the spread of warmth until the post-treatment rest. Only now does the body seem completely warmed up. The post-treatment rest should always last at least 30 minutes and should not be interrupted if the treatment marks the start of a prolonged sleep.

Indications for mustard thorax compresses	
Principle	Examples
support for the body's inflammatory reaction	acute feverish diseases such as bronchitis or pneumonia
guidance of warmth processes to the outside	asthma (when congestion is the main thing), COPD (blue-bloater type), hypotension
stimulation of a sluggish soul body	depression (hysterical constitution)

Contraindications	
Principle	Examples
damaged skin	thin skin, burns, skin irritation, neuro-dermatitis, hypersensitivity
overstraining the circulatory system	decompensated heart failure

Chart: Indications and contraindications for mustard thorax compresses

Caring attention and the setting as independent principles

The foregoing description clearly shows that external applications are associated with specific states of consciousness (sense impressions, sensations, moods, dreams, sleep). To readers without personal experience, these descriptions may seem exaggerated or even fantastic. They are not, as has been shown by hundreds of examples with healthy volunteers and patients with different diagnoses. However, patients who only remain in the first phase of sensory sensations do not arrive at relaxation or sleep. They will not be able to report anything about the deeper dimensions of the application. This changes if it is possible to give the patient a way through these levels of consciousness by taking suitable care of the environment (quiet, security, warmth). Now there will be signs of substance-specific patterns, as demonstrated by the impressive examples above. Only the appropriate setting (attentive care, atmosphere, post-treatment rest) enables a deeper dimension to take effect. The post-treatment rest is the period of time in which the application "switches" from stimulation of the senses to a metabolic response. Enabling relaxation and sleep are therefore part of the therapy and they are as important as the substance and medium.*

5.2 Touch

Physical contact is unavoidable with external applications. Rhythmical oil applications (Rhythmical Einreibung) and massage cultivate the art of touching in a special way [→ Chapter "Rhythmical Einreibung According to Wegman/Hauschka"]. The rhythm of delving down into the skin tissue, the reversal point before releasing the hand and reconnecting again after a pause is like a small-scale version of the above-mentioned larger rhythm experienced over the course of an external application. Mathias Bertram also describes a three-stage effect of Rhythmical Einreibung. Patients and experts refer to the stages as "Letting go—Being at one again—New ability."[7] "Letting go" corresponds to exhalation or excarnation, "being at one again" to differentiated self-perception, and "new ability" to awakening from restful sleep feeling refreshed and energized. Rhythmical Einreibung is thus a model for health training.

---

* In ancient mystery medicine, "healing sleep" was a method of dreaming one's own healing path. After purifying preparation (catharsis) the priest-doctor put the patient into a sleep similar to death, from which he awakened to become aware of healing substances, necessary behavioral changes and moral insights. The healer-priest interpreted these experiences and they inspired the therapy.

This also applies to the nurse himself when he provides Rhythmical Einreibung or other external applications. Immersing oneself in the rhythm of Rhythmical Einreibung, in the calm of a treatment or the nourishing atmosphere of a body compress has an immediate effect on the person providing the treatment. Especially in the case of Rhythmical Einreibung, one can observe how it is not only the patient who benefits from the treatment, but also, for example, a neighboring patient, affected by the mood, may relax and fall asleep.

This creation of a healing atmosphere is therefore not something external, it is rather a joint formation of "healing substance" by the nurse, the patient and the application.

The very close, gentle touch of a treatment with Rhythmical Einreibung can awaken sympathy, but also antipathy in both the patient and the practitioner. On both sides, the emergence of sympathy and antipathy is an expression of the fact that a rhythmic, middle, mindful—what used to be called "chaste"—quality was not achieved. In sympathy, the practitioner and the patient go out of themselves; the practitioner typically when his or her hand connects with the tissue, the patient when the hand lets go again. In antipathy the patient and the practitioner isolate themselves from each other; the practitioner when he pulls back his hand, the patient when the practitioner's hand connects with the patient's body. Too much sympathy and too much antipathy are ultimately expressions of an imbalance and a lack of rhythmic balancing between the forces. It is only in a state of balance that people meet from 'I' to 'I'.*

6.   Evaluating external applications

This chapter describes the active factors in external applications. External stimuli are regarded as the causes of changes in the condition of the organism. These we differentiated into chemical stimuli (substances) and contact or temperature stimuli (medium). Such stimuli have a "place" on the body and are set in a specific temporal context that has a decisive influence on the direction of action (rhythm). The organism interacts with itself and the environment. For example, a chamomile steam bath relaxes the muscles of the pelvic base and bladder. The patient's breathing deepens and her cheeks turn rosy. A space of consciousness can unfold in our attentiveness to this interaction that cannot be satisfactorily explained by a mere stimulus-reaction or cause-effect scheme. Comfortable coziness, trust and joy shine in the mirror of the soul, or dark spaces of sorrow and pain open up. These experiences influence the patient's further actions. She can now feel motivated to get involved in the treatment and actively take care of rest and relaxation. In her pelvic floor, the warmth increases awareness and circulation. These are good prerequisites for overcoming a bladder infection with one's own forces and building up long-term resistance to germs. The external application has become an act of self-care.

---

*   Rudolf Steiner described "being pressured by the other" and "dissociating oneself from being pressured" as the way that sensing the 'I' of the other person works [→ Chapter "From the Question of Meaning in Cancer to the Cultivation of the Senses"].

A scientific study of external applications and the factors postulated above looked at the following questions:

- Substance: How are substances absorbed via the skin? How do they affect the organism?
- Medium: How do warmth and cold, pressure and suction affect the organism?
- Rhythm: At what point in time do which stimuli have an effect in what strength (dosage, duration) and at which place in the body?
- Caring attention and the setting: What paths does consciousness take with different applications? How does consciousness affect the body and how does the body affect consciousness? What influence do attention and setting have on these processes?

Mathias Bertram and Harald Kolbe presented an 'ecological model' for the scientific investigation of the effectiveness of therapeutic interventions.[8] In this paper they distinguish between the following perspectives:

- Mind-body perspective (interaction between a person's mental state and their physical condition)
- Body-mind perspective or embodiment (changing the mental condition via physical imprints)
- Phenomenological-physical perspective (examination from the subject's perspective, from the empathic perception of the viewer and from objective observation or measurement of processes)

The "ecological model" focuses on the systemic relationship between body and consciousness. This complements the scientific approach that is still favored in medicine today. It makes it possible to draw complex correlations between the subjective well-being of the patient (e.g., feeling of lightness, refreshment, pain relief) and objective measurements on the body (e.g., breathing, pulse, blood pressure), put them into a context and describe the effects holistically. The "ecological model" is particularly suitable for demonstrating the principles of "attention" and "setting."

Example:

Typical effects of a "sounding bath"[*]

First, there is a description of the setting in which the effects were found:

"As part of the care process, patients were questioned about their condition after treatment. The effects described below are based on spontaneous oral descriptions of the people treated (both patients and healthy volunteers). These effects occur in almost all patients and experimentees. The communications from patients and test persons are differentiated in different ways."[9]

The effects observed by the patients and test persons are then presented. They constitute the "first-person perspective" of the ecological model. The described effects *"range from purely vegetative expressions of a somnolent or unconscious patient (such as reddening of the skin, respiration) to general verbalizations ('was*

---

[*] [→ Chapter "Variations in Whole-Body Washing," Section "Sounding bath"]

pleasant') to detailed descriptions of physical, bodily and psychological experiences."[10] When collecting the reports, it should be noted that, in addition to the individual diversity of the experiences, there is often also a large variance in linguistic expression. *"For example, terms such as refreshing, invigorating or flowing through were used to describe a 'vitalizing' effect on the person's experience of their body. These words are by no means synonymous or interchangeable. They describe a specific state of mind, the understanding and interpretation of which, however, are equally elusive to an exact definition of meaning. The choice of words and interpretation is not only determined by the actual perception of the body, but also by the vocabulary and the conceptual differentiation of the patient and interpreter of each situation of illness and communication."[11]*

This is followed by an interpretation of the linguistic utterances of the test persons and patients. This is necessary to broaden the concept of the effect of an application and not to confine it to standardized expressions. *"The effects mentioned here are therefore not defined or calibrated consequences of the treatment, rather they represent an effect figure or pattern of effects. This is the pattern that is meant when we speak of 'effects' below. The division into physical, bodily, psychological and interactive effects classifies these into the experiential dimensions of the model created here. The term 'mental effects' refers to effects that occur without a conceptual reference to the body and describe 'interactive effects' in relation to the environment (meaning the practitioner and the person's own biography in this case)."[12]*

Here is a list of physical, bodily, mental, and spiritual effects by way of example:

Physical effects:
- *slight reddening of the face as an expression of increased blood circulation in the skin*
- *warming of the hands and feet*
- *reduction of the respiratory rate*
- *relaxation of muscle tone*

Bodily effects (experienced on the body or effects expressed in terms of physicality):
- *feeling relaxed*
- *feeling secure, folded in, protected, warmed up*
- *feeling refreshed, invigorated, stimulated, permeated by flow*
- *feeling light or heavy, feeling round, erect or even 'whole'*
- *experiencing (pain) relief*
- *wholly present in oneself*

Mental effects (perceptions that are detached from conceptions of physicality):
- *serenity*
- *joy, confidence*

- *relief from fears, worries*
- *mindfulness of sensory impressions*

Spiritual effects (intersubjective and trans-subjective effects regarding the relation to the environment or the value horizon of the treated person):
- *trust (in the practitioner, the situation, fate, oneself)*
- *dignity, respect (feeling respected, experiencing the dignity of the setting)*
- *blessing (feeling blessed, experiencing the presence of a "higher" being)*
- *gratitude (towards the practitioner, "to be able to experience something like this," towards existence)*
- *superpersonal love*[13]

Finally, the effects are weighted. This avoids premature expectations and invites the observer to add his own perceptions to the observations mentioned above. *"The effects of a 'sounding bath' are manifold. Not every treated person experiences all of the effects (such as warming of the hands). Some effects also appear to be almost opposites (e.g., a heavy feeling in the legs after treatment versus a light feeling in the legs after treatment). Some effects can be dominant in a treatment, but later they take a back seat (i.e., 'refreshment') when the same patient is treated again."*[14]

The assessment by the therapist is supported by the patient or test person's own assessment: *"In this context, it is relevant to know how the patient himself assesses the effects and therapeutic benefits, or what significance he attaches to the effect and benefits. In the case of a 'sounding bath,' for example, the purely physical effects (such as facial reddening, reduction of the respiratory rate) are generally irrelevant to the patient, if they are noticed at all. The bodily effects (how relaxed or enveloped the person feels) on the other hand, have a greater meaning, since they are by definition related to the person's own body perception and physical being. Even more relevant to the patient are psychological effects (like serenity, joy and others). These are no longer closely tied to the body and they have the greatest experience value. They impress the patient particularly by relieving suffering for a moment and improving his mood. But it is the spiritual effects (e.g., trust or respect) that are of utmost importance for the patient. These are perceived as transcending the body. They can therefore also be remembered by the patient, even if the patient's physical condition deteriorates. Remembering a state of trust, respect or gratitude, for example, can bring it to mind and renew it, even if the triggering treatment (a 'sounding bath' in this case) occurred some time ago. When this active renewal of the experience in the patient's memory succeeds, the intervention will have a lasting effect. Ultimately, 'sounding baths' could even revive experiences that the patient had in the past, for example in his childhood, as feelings of security, joy and respect, now recalled to the present. In fact, both patients and test subjects describe their experiences using terms, images and comparisons from childhood or their spiritual life ('I last experienced this feeling of security as a child' or 'The respect that I experienced in the treatment reminds me of Christ's washing of the feet').*"[15] This perspective is so remarkable because it extends originally expected outcomes, such as alleviating symptoms, through parameters that the patient did not perceive until the treatment. This leads to new conclusions regarding the mode of action and thus also the indication for any application.

"The ability of the patient to call up elementary positive (body-free) experiences of soul and spirit out of his or her own strength is an important salutogenetic competence. It is the basis for mental resilience and resistance.* By conveying elementary experiences through water, warmth, touch and an attitude of devotion, respect and attentiveness, 'sounding baths' can lead the patient back to layers of deep trust, being one with oneself, comfort and security. The reconnection with this 'primordial ground' evokes associations with the Latin term' 'religere' ('reconnect'), i.e., the etymological origin of the word 'religion.' Many patients then also characterize 'sounding baths' as 'holy deeds' or believe them to be ritual acts."[16]

This observation and description of the effects of an external application in the sense of the ecological model does not provide proof of efficacy in the scientific sense. It does serve as a good description of the character and type of an external application. It provides more valuable assistance for the indication, implementation and modification of an application than any statistical determination that a particular application in the case of indication "X" leads to a reduction of symptoms in a certain percentage of patients.

7. Cognition–Based Medicine (single case studies)

The current gold standard of scientific studies in medicine is the Randomized Controlled Trial (RCT). A group of patients to be tested is randomly assigned to a treatment, called randomization. Another group, also randomly selected, receives either a placebo or a treatment with a method that is deemed to be effective. The RCT is considered to be the highest level of evidence-based medicine (EBM). Good RCT study designs are extremely time-consuming and costly, and have rarely been used for research into external applications. In nursing science, other methods are therefore being sought to obtain evidence of efficacy for external applications. In most cases, descriptive, qualitative research methods are used. In recent years, special attention has been paid to a procedure that enables a high degree of evidence for medical procedures to be generated from individual case descriptions, known as cognition-based medicine (CBM):

"Cognition-based medicine is a newly developed methodological system of scientific medicine. The starting point is criterion-supported, valid and reliable efficacy assessment of individual patients. These principles and various criteria have been an-

---

* Resilience is the ability to deal with life-cycle crises by relying on personal and socially mediated resources in most cases and using them as an opportunity for one's own development. [→ Welter-Enderlin R, Hildenbrandt B (ed.). Resilienz. Gedeihen trotz widriger Umstände. Carl-Auer Verlag Heidelberg 2006] *alyzed and explained. CBM enables a methodological professionalization of medical judgment as well as an explication of medical experience and medical expertise. CBM study designs extend the spectrum of clinical research; they range from criteria-based therapeutic causal recognition to new forms of evaluation in cohort studies."*[17]

Individual case studies, carefully researched and documented according to the observation criteria of CBM, are also suitable as a method for scientifically examining external applications (for which no uniform implementation descriptions exist so far). Particularly issues with well definable and measurable outcomes, such as pain or exhaustion, could be proven with comparatively little effort in individual cases.

7.1 Evaluation of external applications in practice

Anyone who administers external applications is required to evaluate and document the results. The following fields of observation have proven helpful for the collection and presentation of the characteristic effects:
  • Current pain and discomfort
  • Warmth (warm and cold zones on the body)
  • Breathing (deep, superficial, chest or abdominal breathing)
  • Skin (dry, moist, cracked, brittle, reddened, inflamed, edematous, ...)
  • Excretions (sweat, saliva flow, urination, stool urgency)
  • Body tension (balanced, flaccid, weak, wiry, tense)
  • Mood and consciousness (balanced, 'major', 'minor', cheerful, exuberant, sad, downcast, depressed, dreamy, sleepy, tired, sleeping, awake, irritated)

Depending on the application, other observations such as pulse or blood pressure may be required, or there may be unexpected reactions expressed by the patient or observed by the practitioner.

Here below is an example of a form that is used for treatment with Rhythmical Einreibung that serves to document the course of treatment, and an evaluation form for such treatments. The collection and evaluation of many treatment reports enables conclusions to be drawn about the effectiveness of a method. A modified observation sheet can be used for treatment with other external applications.

Patient Name, Date of Birth	Diagnosis
Treatment no.	

Application / Substance

Indication / Wish / Aim of the Treatment

	Before the treatment	During / After the treatment
Warmth		
Pain		
Breathing		
Skin		
Excretion		
Tension		
Mood		
Special		

Anthroposophic–anthropological nursing assessment

Date, Signature

Fig. 2: Treatment report for Rhythmical Einreibung, developed by Monika Layer

Patient Name, Date of Birth	
1 **Location of Rhythmical Einreibung** e.g., shoulder	
2 **Substance used** e.g., *Cuprum met. praep. 0.4%* ointment	
3 **Type of Rhythmical Einreibung** e.g., five-pointed star	
4 **Reason for the treatment** Multiple answers possible, under-line each symptom	o cold, fear, not feeling oneself in the body o rigidity, pain, irritation o congestion, lifeless tissue, feeling of heaviness o perceptual disorders, sensory disorders o other reason:
5 **Purpose of the treatment** Multiple answers possible	o to warm through o to "lighten up," bring into lightness o to invigorate, bring flow o to envelope, promote a feeling for the body o other reason:
6 **Condition 5 minutes after the treatment** Change compared to 4	o worse o the same o slightly improved o markedly improved o no complaints anymore o other reactions:
7 **Condition 2 or more hours after the treatment** Change compared to 4	Time after the treatment: Reactions: o worse o the same o slightly improved o markedly improved o no complaints anymore o other reactions:
Date, Signature	

Fig. 3: Form for evaluating Rhythmical Einreibung treatments

The attached evaluation sheet does not primarily refer to medical diagnoses or symptoms. It is also not designed to treat them, but rather assigns certain phenomena to the human fourfold nature and relates the effect of the treatment to changes in the fourfold nature.

Subtle body / Element	Reason for treatment	Purpose of treatment
'I' 'Fire'	cold, fear, not feeling oneself in the body	to warm through
Soul body 'Air'	rigidity, pain, irritation	to lighten up, make more airy, convey sense of lightness
Etheric body 'Water'	congestion, lifeless tissue, feeling of heaviness	to invigorate, bring flow
Physical body 'Earth'	perceptual disorders, sensory disorders	to envelop, promote a feeling for the body's form

Chart: Observation areas according to the human fourfold nature

7.2 Vademecum of External Applications

A collection of reports on experiences with external applications is available in the "Vademecum of External Applications," which has been published online by the *International Forum for Anthroposophic Nursing*.* It contains numerous external applications that are used in anthroposophic nursing care and medicine, searchable by substance, indication and type of application. Some detailed descriptions and case reports are also available there.

The Vademecum lives from the experience reports that nurses, therapists and doctors send to the editors.

The publication process is as follows:
- The user enters his or her experience in an online documentation sheet
- The editors edit the field report and check the plausibility of the information
- If necessary, they contact the author
- The report appears online

The Vademecum is not only a source of information for finding indications and implementing external applications. It should also become a lively forum for exchanging experiences and, in the long term, a quality assurance instrument for external applications. Experts in administering external applications are cordially invited to share their experiences.

---

* www.pflege-vademecum.de (Checked May 2020)

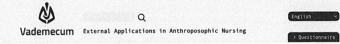

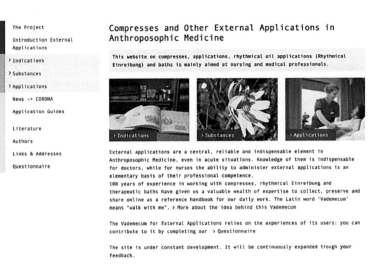

Fig. 4: Nursing Vademecum homepage www.pflege-vademecum.de

YARROW LIVER COMPRESS

SUBSTANCE:

Yarrow tea

MAIN IDEA:

Moist-hot liver compresses support liver function in a way that positively influences the unpleasant effects of a stressed liver, such as sleep disorders, depressive moods, lack of drive and liver capsule pain.

INDICATIONS:

- Digestive problems and weak digestion
- Support of anabolic liver metabolism
- To stimulate detoxification, e.g., during fasting, after antibiosis, chemotherapy
- General exhaustion
- Alcohol withdrawal

- Depression
- Liver capsule pain
- Sleep disorders: Day-night rhythm reversal, difficulty in falling asleep or sleeping through the night, especially when waking up nightly at the "liver hour" (about 3 o'clock in the morning)
- Chronic hepatitis
- Hepatic cirrhosis
- Hepatocellular carcinoma
- Liver metastases
- Irritable bowel syndrome

MATERIALS:
- Prepare the tea: Pour ½ liter of boiling water over 3 teaspoonfuls of yarrow (including the flowers), cover and let steep for 3 to 5 minutes
- Fold the double woven cotton cloth to the required size (approx. 12 x 20 cm), then roll up
- Fold a covering cloth (e.g., flannel or terry-cloth towel) so that it is slightly larger than the compress cloth to be covered
- Long wool cloth, flannel, or bath towel
- Bowl
- Make sure the patient's feet are warm before applying the compress
- Rubber gloves for wringing out the compress, if needed

INSTRUCTIONS:
- Prepare the materials
- Prepare the patient
- Place the wool cloth and flannel layer under the patient's back
- Lay the prepared double woven cotton cloth in the bowl
- The more thoroughly you wring out the hot cloth, the hotter the compress can be applied!

From now on, work quickly so that the moist compress does not cool down prematurely. Fan* the liver area as hotly as possible, until the patient tolerates the heat (the right rib covers the liver by two thirds)

- Lay it on as hot as possible without burning the skin. The temperature varies greatly from patient to patient
- Firmly wrap the wool and flannel cloth around the patient's upper abdomen, free of folds

---

* To "fan" means to move the hot compress several times towards and away from the body's surface using rapid, rhythmic movements, before touching the skin. The compress meanwhile cools down to a tolerable temperature and the skin simultaneously becomes accustomed to the heat.

DURATION:
- 30 minutes

Caution: The compress should be removed as soon as the patient feels cold or experiences the compress as being too cold.
- Pull out the moist compress materials without opening the wool cloth.
- Work quietly and gently, in order to not disturb the compress rest.

POST-TREATMENT REST:
20–30 minutes, or as long as the patient finds it pleasant

FOLLOW-UP:
Rinse, wring out, and hang up all of the cloths to dry.

Reliability	Well-proven in many patients
Dosage	Once a day to twice a week • Afternoon application: for digestive complaints and Nausea, "detoxification" • Evening application: for exhaustion, sleep disorders, to stimulate anabolic liver metabolism
Onset of effect	• Immediately after/during the first application: pain reduction for liver capsule pain, elimination of gas • For detoxification, sleep disorders and general weakness: after several days to several weeks
Duration of therapy	At least 4 weeks, longer according to need
Other options	Yarrow oil compresses can be applied as an alternative.
Warnings	Do not use in cases of: • Acute inflammation • Sudden abdominal pain of unknown origin • Fever • Suspicion of internal bleeding • Acute abdomenal pain

Fig. 5: How to apply a yarrow liver compress, as described in the "Vademecum of External Applications"[18]

Category	Example learning objectives	Recommended learning path
Skills	You are able to administer ginger and mustard applications in such a way that the typical bodily and mental effects occur.	A
Your own learning objective		
Relationships	You can bring yourself to a state of inner quiet while administering an external application.	B
Your own learning objective		
Knowledge	You understand the principles of external applications	C
Your own learning objective		

References

1 Fringer, A.; Layer, M.; Widmer, C., et al. Äussere Anwendungen in der Pflege. *Eine Review gestützte Definitionsentwicklung.* Konferenzpapier der FHS St. Gallen, University of Applied Sciences, St. Gallen 2015. Download from www.researchgate.net/publication/283341981_Aussere_Anwendungen_in_der_Pflege_Eine_Review_gestutzte_Definitionsentwicklung.

2 Rozumek, M. Tria Principia. In: Meyer, U.; Pedersen P. (eds.). *Anthroposophische Pharmazie.* Grundlagen, Herstellprozesse, Arzneimittel. Salumed Verlag, Berlin 2016, pp. 66–69.

3 ibid.

4 Steiner, R. *Meditative Betrachtungen und Anleitungen zur Vertiefung der Heilkunst* (GA 316). Rudolf Steiner Verlag. Dornach 2008. Lecture of Jan. 5, 1924. "You healing spirits": translator unknown. "I will unite my soul's knowing": translated by Dana L. Fleming and Christopher Bamford, in: Steiner R. *Mantric sayings 1903–1925.* SteinerBooks, Great Barrington 2015, p. 289.

5 Steiner, R. Lecture of April 5, 1920, in *Introducing anthroposophical medicine.* SteinerBooks, Great Barrington 2011.

6 Glaser, H.; Heine, R.; Sauer, M. et al. *Praxisintegrierte Studie zur Darstellung der Frühwirkungen von Ingwer als Äußere Anwendung.* Verband für Anthroposophische Pflege 2001. Request information leaflet (in German) from mail@vfap.de.

7 Bertram, M. *Der Therapeutische Prozess als Dialog. Strukturphänomenologische Untersuchung der Rhythmischen Einreibungen nach Wegman/Hauschka.* Dissertation, Witten-Herdecke 2005. Pro Business Verlag, Berlin 2005.

8 Bertram, M.; Kolbe, H.J. Entwurf eines ökologischen Modells therapeutischer Prozesse. In: Bertram K, Kolbe H.J. (ed.). *Dimensionen therapeutischer Prozesse in der Integrativen Medizin.* Springer Verlag, Wiesbaden 2016.

9 Heine, R. Die Klingende Waschung. In: ibid., pp. 126–129.

10 ibid.

11 ibid., p. 127.

12 ibid.

13 ibid., p. 127 f.

14 ibid., p. 128.

15 ibid., p. 128 f.

16 ibid., p. 129.

17 Kiene, H. Was ist Cognition-based Medicine? In: *Zeitschrift für ärztliche Fortbildung und Qualität im Gesundheitswesen* 2005;99, pp. 301–306.

18 www.pflege-vademecum.de/schafgarben_leberwickel.php (Checked May 2020).

Specializations in Nursing Care

CHAPTER XV

Pregnancy, Childbirth, and Puerperium as Stages of Human Becoming

ANNA WILDE · REGULA MARKWALDER

This chapter will present pregnancy, childbirth and puerperium from an anthroposophic understanding of the human being and describe nursing assistance for pregnant women.

→   Learning objectives, see end of chapter

1.   When does human life actually begin?

This is a question that has always occupied mothers and fathers, theologians, scientists, gynecologists, writers, and philosophers. It has stirred hearts, heated spirits, given rise to discussions and controversies, and still does. This is a question that has been shaped by social, religious and economic transitions throughout history. Is there a moment that could be called the beginning of life? This is closely linked to the question of human becoming, which encompasses life and death and can lead beyond them. "Human becoming" is generally understood to occur in the womb during embryonic development, yet anyone who allows themselves to be touched inwardly by the sight, the sounds, the scent, and the radiance of a newborn baby can confirm that this child is not a blank page. This being is not exclusively the product of a biological process that has resulted from the inheritance stream of its parents, ancestors, and folk, it is a being that already has a journey behind it. Much is spoken and written today about the immortality of the human soul. When thinking about the beginning of human life, we naturally arrive at the question of pre-existence, of a time before birth. What is the origin of the human being? The words "human becoming" contain one of the essential aspects: the becoming, the development, the transformation, the journey. We have all experienced more or less closely how everything changes fundamentally with the birth of a child. Do we notice the first, tender announcements of the arriving human being?

Birth and death cannot actually be beginnings or ends, rather they are transitions, or gates from one state to another, moments of transfer between two different forms of existence. The actual moment of birth or death is a fleeting one, often lasting only fractions of a second, in the intensity of which past and future meet in the present. It is a moment in which we look back at what has been, and at the same time look ahead to what is to come.

What is being transformed? When people are sick and dying, we observe that their bodies are inclined more and more towards the earthly. At the moment of death, the physical body becomes a corpse and begins to decay. But the etheric body, soul and spirit do not decay. Rudolf Steiner described how these three higher members of the human being continue to develop even after physical death, which is an idea having to do with reincarnation and karma.

Patients who have clinically died and returned to life tell of moments in which they saw memory pictures of their life spread out before them. Their past appeared before them as a retrospective of their life, as an objective tableau. Such experiences are connected with the etheric body letting go of the physical body. Just as the physical body returns to earth after death, so the human etheric body is absorbed by the cosmos. The acquired abilities of this etheric body do not dissolve, they persist.

At the next higher level, the soul body frees itself from its physical bond and the deceased person experiences the happiness and suffering that he has inflicted on others during his life. Consistently and exactly, the person reexperiences his or her life in this way, starting from the moment of death and going backwards to the moment of birth.

Experiences of this kind gradually arouse and reinforce an increasing need to create possibilities for compensation through a renewed life on earth. This need changes into a longing, an urge; the 'I' wants to return to earth to balance what has happened, to follow its impulses.

The 'I' creates a connection from one life to the next by experiencing the past and working to shape a future body with the help of spiritual beings, i.e., with angels. In the new life, a new body will be available to him as a suitable tool for the tasks to be accomplished. On its way to the new birth, the spiritual archetype of this human being also takes with it the abilities that had been acquired in previous lives on earth.

By means of conception, the physical body provided by the parents becomes a vessel for the descending being. The incarnating individuality connects itself with the germinating physical body from the moment of fertilization and thus enters into a connection with the inheritance stream of a folk and family. From about the third week onwards, this individuality increasingly influences the physical development of the embryo. A multitude of forces contribute to this mysterious process of becoming, which is hardly comprehensible to our thinking.

Similar to the life review immediately after death, before birth there is a prenatal preview of the coming life's future possibilities. This knowledge is usually forgotten. We shall let these considerations resonate in the background when we now look at pregnancy, childbirth and puerperium.

2. Pregnancy

In no other situation in life can we find such a connection between two beings as the one between a mother and her baby during the time of pregnancy.

This does not only concern physical connections. There is, as it were, a sensitive interplay between the mother-to-be and the growing child at the level of soul and spirit.

Maybe the woman doesn't yet know about her pregnancy. The changes she is undergoing in her organism soon make her aware of it. She often remembers less obvious indications only in retrospect.

Pregnancy can be divided into three main stages:

The first three months
During the first three months there are sometimes unpleasant physical and psychological symptoms. This "nesting time" can bring the woman into unbalanced, vulnerable, unstable and moody states. The conflict between the two beings can be expressed in the mother's discomfort and nausea. In this first period, a "quiet struggle" takes place between the woman who was accustomed to exist as an individual, as someone who sought to be independent, and this other being who wants to develop within her. The woman is, so to speak, pushed somewhat out of her corporeality; the child, on the other hand, descends from supersensible realms and develops its earthly body more and more. Both beings are moving towards each other, are getting to know each other.

This experience of being lifted above herself is perhaps one of the reasons for the great changes the pregnant woman is experiencing. These changes call for understanding, for loving participation. A little humor often works wonders. There is creative activity in the woman's abdomen which also has a stimulating effect on her neurosensory system: extreme tastes, smells and fantasies can occur. Who doesn't know these highly acute desires for sauerkraut or strawberry ice cream, for herring or Sacher cake, for pickled gherkins or cream slices? A father-to-be can make this area a personal concern and in this way positively influence the well-being of the woman and the developing baby.

The middle trimester
The middle stage of pregnancy often turns out to be a more balanced, healthy time for the woman and her loved ones. Her thoughts become more concrete, the physical inconveniences of the early days have mostly subsided. A quiet, inner joy grows. The search for a suitable place for the birth also falls into this time. The practical preparations begin. Questions, wishes, ideas, perhaps also fears concerning the birth event are grateful for open, receptive ears.

The last three months of pregnancy

The woman's experience changes again towards the end of the pregnancy, when the baby has already completed a considerable part of its physical development; as her baby becomes more earthly, increasing in corporeality, she feels her own heaviness more strongly. Her legs are hot and swollen in the evenings, her back hurts, her movements become more difficult. A new balance must be found by shifting her body weight. Disturbances and pathological changes therefore occur more frequently in the first and last third of pregnancy.

Expectant parents are more and more concerned with the question of caring for the pregnancy and preparing for a suitable birth. A large, varied range of possibilities is available to them. The woman experiences her pregnancy both as a physical process, and as one of soul and spirit. Accordingly, she and the father increasingly seek access to all these levels. Thus, regardless of any special methods, the basic attitude behind all efforts to accompany a pregnancy should be to create space for the expectant mother's healthy, genuine feelings and sensations towards her baby and herself. Birth preparation encourages expectant parents to understand and share these processes and empowers them to express their questions, fears and uncertainties.

The practical part gives suggestions for dealing with the inconveniences of pregnancy and offers exercises that promote the progress of the birth through active co-operation. Often such courses are a time—especially for a working woman—in which she can give her undivided attention to herself and her baby—a very valuable aspect in birth preparation.

It is also a time to cultivate her inner world, the intimate sense of connection, the quiet conversation between the mother, between the parents and the baby.

> What a pregnant woman carries in her thoughts, her feelings, her actions has just as much influence on the well-being of the baby as nutrition via the placenta.

Every woman will feel how she can be close to her baby. It can often be observed that new areas of perception open up through the time of pregnancy: the woman notices things and people she had previously overlooked; pregnancy as a time in which the expectant mother can see more, hear more, read more between the lines. What is being revealed to the mother here—can it be understood as a message from her baby?

Madonna paintings can offer a suggestion for encountering a baby inwardly. The "Sistine Madonna" by the painter Raphael (1483–1520) holds a special intimacy. The original can be found in Dresden, Germany, in the Gallery of Old Masters.

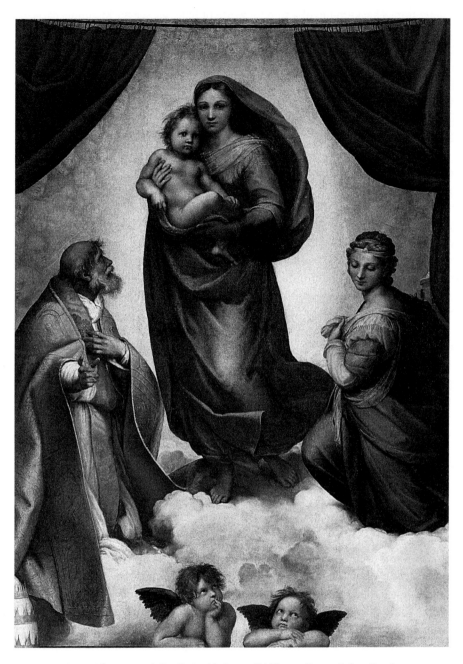

Illustration: Raphael (1483–1520): The Sistine Madonna, Old Masters Picture Gallery, Dresden

Coming from a background of a shining world of light, we see the Madonna carrying the child to earth. The child detaches itself from the community of heavenly beings depicted as angelic heads: they say goodbye and gaze after the child of light on his way to the human community. The Madonna holds him on one side next to her warm, red glowing heart, supported by her hand and wrapped in her robes; on the other side the child is directly connected to the world of light. One knee pointing towards the earth indicates his future, his earthly life. As he descends, he encounters two figures. The male figure looks back: "Where have you come from?" The female figure asks, with her gaze turned towards the earth: "Where are you going?" The dynamics of this perspective are an important element. The Madonna is carrying her child unerringly towards us. The wind is blowing her robes. She and her child are still borne by cloud formations. However, down below, a wood-like beam completes the picture, on which the putto angels rest as a sign of our human idea of the heavenly world. We as observers would have had to stop at this earthly threshold if the green curtain to the sky had not been slightly opened. The miracle of incarnation does not pass by the Madonna without a sign: the splendor of the starry world shines through the light in her face. Her dignified appearance shows the enveloping, protective, supporting role of a loving mother in an upright, free posture.

Every pregnancy is a mystery for the world of the senses. Changes are visible and can be experienced, but the actual happening takes place hidden behind the curtain. Birth, the transition from pre-earthly to earthly life, is the moment when the curtain opens momentarily so that the mystery that grew during pregnancy can come to light. The "Sistine Madonna" represents a special birth, the birth of Christ. But heaven flashes open for a moment at every earthly birth. Contemplating paintings like this can contribute to a healing care of pregnancy—as well as provide support and a source of strength for the birth.

3.   Birth

What actually happens during the physical birth of a human being? It is not about describing what happens—no mother will experience the births of her children as being the same every time, no midwife can rely on things being consistently the same. Each birth will be as unique as each human being, each person's life, each person's dying. It is a highly mysterious, complex and multi-layered process between mother and child—also between mother, father and child, and in the broadest sense between human beings and the spiritual world. It can be looked at from different perspectives, from the mother's or child's point of view. It presents itself as a religious, social, socio-cultural, medical, hormonal, biological and sexual act.

Hidden from the outside world, the embryo rested, grew and moved, surrounded by various enveloping layers. The amniotic fluid, which protects the embryo from vibration, has an enveloping quality that allows the baby to live in weightlessness. Surrounded by the two inner amniotic membranes, the amnion and chorion, the baby lives in this fluid. Enveloping layers are boundaries, but they also enable connections.

The umbilical cord connects the unborn baby with the placenta, the marvelous organ of nutrition and respiration. The uterus forms another layer around the life in progress, and all of this is enclosed by the maternal abdominal wall.

The baby pushes all these covers off at birth. What meets him? What is he expecting? First, he is received by human hands. The newborn unreservedly entrusts himself to these hands. It is to these people—to these parents' hands—that the baby wants to come. Newly born he lies on his mother's breast. Gradually, a feeling of well-being, of contentment, arises when, after the great moment of seeing the light, he is embraced, touched, comforted and kept warm by the hands of his parents. Maybe the baby starts to quietly look around with interest. For the future of the young family it is of great value when the eyes of the baby and parents can meet during this amazing wakefulness of the first minutes. Before the birth, the mother's inner life of soul and spirit, her joy, her worries, her love and her interest, reached the baby through the protective layers mentioned above. Now that these have been thrown off, the parents bestow their inner attention through the active love of their hands, among other things. Their greeting affirms the will that has led this baby to earth. The baby feels encouraged and confirmed by this step, so that he feels right into his body: "It's all right. I'll stay here." The first moments of life are among the most formative of a person's whole life. These have been some thoughts about birth as an "experience of revelation."

Let us now look at birth from another angle. In the womb, the growing baby is completely surrounded by fluid. Its cardiovascular system began to develop and function early on.

What about breathing? The placenta is responsible for the exchange of gases, i.e., it supplies the baby's organism with oxygen and removes waste products. Within the womb, the baby's lungs have not yet unfolded, they literally stick together. No air has touched them yet. Liquid moves inside them too. This changes abruptly at the moment of birth. The narrowness of the birth canal forces the fluid out of the lungs, making room for another element. In this moment the human being becomes an earth being, because he has taken the step from water to land through his first breath, through regular inhalation and exhalation. The fact that this elementary change in life takes place does not just have physiological significance. The biblical creation story indicates that air is the bearer of the human soul.

> *"And the Lord God formed man of the dust of the ground, and breathed into his nostrils the breath of life; and man became a living soul."*
> Genesis 2:7

Another aspect of birth must not go unmentioned in the context of these remarks. Obstetrics has undergone tremendous changes in recent decades. From an invasive medical discipline, in which the possibilities of technology exerted great fascination, the pendulum has swung back to the opposite side. This was demanded by the affected women themselves. The French obstetrician Frédérick Leboyer took a first step in this direction with his important suggestions and encouragements for "gentle birthing."

Is it only the mother who suffers the pain of childbirth? Let us remember the picture of the "Sistine Madonna": the child detaches himself from the vastness of the cosmos, passes through the eye of the needle of birth and, as a newborn, perhaps lies somewhat exhausted on his mother's breast. It is a long journey, where a lot has happened! The vast expanse of heaven must be born into a limited body. Is there such a thing as "incarnation pain"? The descending human soul wants and must follow this condensation process into earthly existence. The baby's parents can develop an understanding for this and support this process. This is especially true for the mother, because she is the only one who consciously meets the child in its pain through her own pain, through her contractions. Thus, the mysterious, probably meaningful connection between the mother's pain and that of the child can become more tangible and understandable in its significance. For midwives and obstetricians, it becomes a constant challenge, a constant concern, to accompany the woman through this experience, if possible.

The four elements earth, water, air and fire (warmth) offer a variety of aids to assist women with labor pains. We apply the element of earth, of solidity, of form by massaging with our hands, exerting counter-pressure at the place of the greatest pain and thereby relieving it. The father-to-be can be involved in this. The various positions that the woman can take, especially shifting from one to the next, are part of this.

Warm water can often relieve and relax pain in a wonderful way; it sometimes contributes amazingly to positive birth progress. We can use full baths or footbaths.

> Birth can be described as a major exhalation. The received being has been released, exhaled.

For the woman who is giving birth, breathing is a valuable instrument for working with and actively countering contractions. Guided breathing using tones is also helpful.[1] The woman often finds her own rhythm herself, sometimes she needs guidance, so that the father and midwife together with the woman "breathe along" with one contraction after another.

And last but not least: it is difficult to give birth with cold feet, just as it is difficult to fall asleep when you are cold. When you're cold, you always hold on a little bit, you can't let go. But relaxation is the Alpha and Omega of childbirth. Often a pair of wool socks, a hot-water bottle on the back, a warming hand on the shoulder can help. And it is not only heat measured in degrees Celsius that plays a role. Soul warmth—the mood, the inner attitude of those present—is of inestimable, decisive value for the birth event.

4. The puerperium

One part has been completed, a great deal of work has been done and survived, the pain is already largely forgotten. The joy of welcome is usually great, the long-awaited guest has arrived and from one moment to the next life changes completely for the mother, the parents: not only a baby was born, a *family* was born.

> "Not only does the mother give birth to the baby,
> the baby also gives birth to the mother."
> Gertrud von Le Fort (1876–1971)

The puerperium is a time of getting to know one another. Mother and baby were inseparably connected until the moment of birth. The cutting of the umbilical cord separates them into two physically independent organisms, yet they belong directly to each other. They should be close, physically close, able to see, hear, feel, taste, smell, breathe the same air—during the day and especially at night. Thus, the mother and with her also the father can grow naturally into their new tasks, learn to recognize what their baby needs, what he wants to express, how they can meet him, how they can respond to him. Not only the parents get to know their baby. The baby gets to know his parents and thus the world with its laws, because he comes from a world with different laws. No one is ever more open, receptive, influenceable and impressionable than a newborn baby. Every impression made on the baby (in every respect!) shapes him and is accepted by him. Everything in the baby's environment is important, especially the mood of the people surrounding him. He needs rest from unnecessary disturbances, so that these subtle processes can occur as undisturbed as possible.

Already during pregnancy, often also during childbirth, the woman is in conversation with her baby, often without audible language.

In the puerperium, this dialogue is to be transformed and continued. One form of conversation with each other happens during nurturing, breastfeeding.

At birth, the skin of the newborn baby has a more or less thick layer of Vernix caseosa, a greasy-white, ointment-like substance that contains important nutrients. It is supposed to protect the skin in a moist environment. Within a very short time it penetrates into the skin and thus forms a kind of initial nutrition as well as a warm enveloping layer. We have already mentioned the great, attentive vigilance and openness of the newborn in the first hour of life, often followed by a deep sleep. When awake, the baby often makes his first seeking and sucking movements. If you put the baby on his mother's breast, in many cases he will already know exactly what to do. If mother and baby remain close in the following days and nights, breastfeeding can become an encouraging give-and-take, a deep experience for mother and baby. Nowadays it will not be necessary to inform people about the advantages of breast milk nutrition or to prove that breast milk is the best nutrition in the first months. Milk production comes from the upper part of the human being, from the chest and arm area. It is very sensitive to temperature fluctuations. It is therefore advisable for every breastfeeding mother to protect herself from drafts and to keep her upper body warm. It is not just for the mother that warmth plays an important role; the baby also needs the element of warmth so that he can move undisturbed into his "earthly dwelling."

Clothing as a "memory," as a continuation, as a detachment from the noble enveloping layers of the prenatal period should keep the baby warm at a constant temperature. In warmth she thrives best. Natural fibers allow the skin to breathe and are able to create a balance to the outside world.

The warm, loving touch of her parents' hands happens during body care among other things. Through the comfort that the baby experiences unconsciously, she connects more strongly with her corporeality. This connection is the basis for strong, healthy, physical, mental and spiritual development. The younger the child, the more vigilant, careful and unobtrusive we will be in caring for him or her.

5. Lily and rose

The arts can express the essence of things in a way that cannot be said with words. You may have perhaps felt this in our contemplation of the "Sistine Madonna."

Painters have repeatedly associated the white lily and the red rose with conception and birth, thus highlighting them in a special way.

In pictures of the Annunciation, the angel Gabriel approaches Mary with a lily in his hand. The white, pure, innocent lily acts as a messenger for the spiritual world. It is a plant with a beguilingly heavy scent. The announcement of a child through the lily appears as an image for the descent of the soul from the spiritual into the earthly world.

The red rose, which can often be found in birth depictions (e.g., "Madonna in the Rose Garden," Martin Schongauer, Colmar), gives us a completely different impression. The harmonious rose symbolizes love that connects with the earth. The rose reveals an enhancement of its earthly qualities in its formation of thorns and wooden branches.

While the radiant lily remains dreaming in fragrance, the rose shows an awake, individual will to live.

The lily transforms into a rose igniting its own spark of life through the gate of birth: the transformation of the lily into a rose is an image of the earthly task that the child loves and has chosen to take hold of during its process of incarnation.

Category	Example learning objectives	Recommended learning path
Skills	You create an appropriate atmosphere for mother and child before, during and after birth.	A
Your own learning objective		
Relationships	You accompany pregnancy, childbirth and puerperium out of your understanding for the special situation of the (expectant) mother.	B
Your own learning objective		
Knowledge	You understand birth and death as threshold events between the spiritual and the earthly world.	C
Your own learning objective		

References

1   Hemmerich, F.H. *Geführtes Tönen zur Geburtshilfe.* Hygias Verlag, Westheim 1997.

Further reading

- Steiner, R. *The principle of spiritual economy.* Anthroposophic Press, Hudson 1986.
- Steiner, R. *Prayers for parents and children.* 4th ed. Rudolf Steiner Press, Forest Row 2012.
- Steiner, R. Lecture of Dec. 30, 1922, in *From comets to cocaine: 18 lectures to workers 1922–23.* Rudolf Steiner Press, London 2000.

CHAPTER XVI

Neonatal Nursing Care
Care Is Education—Education Is Care

INGE HEINE · ROLF HEINE

This chapter will provide information on the practical care of healthy newborns. It will show how the infant's transition from the womb to our world can happen in a child-friendly way through shaping the environment, initial care, diaper changing and dressing, breastfeeding and skin care. Care is the first step in educating to freedom.

→   Learning objectives, see end of chapter

1.   Parental counselling as a focus of postpartum care

The wish of parents to leave the hospital as soon as possible after childbirth, as well as case-based lump-sum insurance plans, place special demands on the care of newborns and mothers who have recently given birth. Since parents can hardly be given a satisfactory introduction to the care of their child within a few hours or days, decisive importance must be assigned to early accompaniment of expectant parents during pregnancy and after childbirth. Midwives, doctors and nurses complement each other in the respective counseling and support services that they offer.

Since today's expectant parents can only rarely look back on experience in caring for newborns, infants or small children, they lack assurance and often also healthy self-confidence for correct handling of their child's everyday expressions and needs. The questions of expectant parents are shaped by the belief that there is "a scientifically proven truth" of what is good for children and what harms them. Medical science is the authority to trust—not social traditions any longer. This widespread attitude undermines the parents' ability to make judgments based on their own perceptions. This is where every consultation must begin. The aim is to train the mother and father's perceptive faculties and powers of judgment, to give them self-confidence and the courage to develop their own competence. The counseling services offered by midwives, professional nurses and self-help groups also create social networks which must replace the traditional relationship structures of extended families in a modern way.

2.   The didactics of parent counseling

Basically, we can distinguish between four different counseling situations:

- Before the birth: birth preparation courses, parenthood preparation courses (caregiving, breastfeeding and education)
- During the first phase of life: breastfeeding counseling, demonstration and practice of body care, diaper changing, postnatal exercise courses
- After the puerperium: individual parent counseling, parent-child groups, rhythmical embrocations for babies, breastfeeding groups
- Crisis intervention: for problems of all kinds

Before the birth
Before the birth it is important to reduce fears and uncertainties. This is usually achieved by providing information about the "normal" course of pregnancy, birth and puerperium. Possible complications should usually be discussed upon request or when there is direct cause. Vividly described examples often have more to offer than comprehensive theoretical explanations. The inclusion of images, dreams and fairy tales can create a connection between abstract knowledge and the parents' often-unconscious fears and hopes.

During the puerperium
In the postpartum period parents can hardly be reached via their intellects. They are still too much under the impression of the birth and the new human being who has placed himself in their midst. Nevertheless, in the first few hours and days, children and parents develop habits of living, caring for the baby and relationships that will play a decisive role in shaping their next phase of life. Parents learn here primarily through the example of the midwife, nurses and other mothers. The greatest success comes from repeatedly showing each other and discussing what we do, rather than one-time demonstrations.

After the puerperium
After the puerperium, counseling is transferred to the parental social environment. Nurseries, parent-child, and breastfeeding groups now form the frame of reference, in addition to personal and family contacts. Here it is particularly important to stimulate the parents' perceptive faculties by observing children with different personalities and levels of developmental maturity. Characteristic of the way that parents anxiously compare their child with others is the question "Can my child do that yet?" The person responsible for the group will ensure that such comparative assessments do not lead to early childhood competitive sport or to unfounded fears of developmental disorders. Instead, parents can learn to be amazed about the laws of personality development and can anchor this as a soul quality going far beyond the area of childcare. Advisors to pregnant women and parents are involved in a significant process of social transformation. After the disappearance of extended families and the increasing

isolated suffering of small families, advisors now help parents to develop freely chosen social relationships. Adult education is based on freedom and responsibility, the modern educational maxims of child education.

Essentially, there are six areas in which parents become active in providing care or for which they need support and advice from professional nurses:

- The newborn baby's physical environment
- Clothing
- Body care
- Breastfeeding—nourishment
- The relationship between parents and child
- Education

2.1 The newborn's physical environment

When the baby comes out of the womb, she leaves behind a world of warmth, quiet and weightlessness. Courageous and full of the will to live, she dives into a cosmos of light, sounds, pain and inadequacy. Ideally, parents and nurses should design the transition between these two worlds in such a way that all sensory impressions are adjusted to the child's level. This point of view also guides us in matters of clothing and body care. First, however, we focus on the immediate living space of the newborn.

During the first few hours after birth, the newborn will be very close, ideally in direct skin contact with his mother. Resting on her body or at her side, he breathes her smell, feels her warmth, hears her heartbeat and her voice. The room is darkened to avoid bright light impressions. After some time, he is placed in his own bed or cradle. His bed is equipped with a firm mattress (e.g., coconut) which is covered with a virgin wool blanket.

Virgin sheep's wool offers an ideal microclimate. Wool warms, binds odors and absorbs moisture. In doing so, it doesn't feel wet. The interior of the bed should provide just enough space for the baby to stretch his arms to the side. His head and feet are a hand's width away from the edge of the bed. In larger beds, a small nest can be built with spelt and millet cushions or wool blankets. Especially spelt cushions can easily be adapted to the baby's shape. They surround the small body and convey gentle, snug pressure already familiar from the womb. A peach-blossom-colored silk veil envelops the bed from above. A particularly beautiful color mood can be achieved by hanging plant-dyed blue and pink silk cloths on top of each other. Through this veil light reaches the child in tones similar to in the uterus. A small cotton or linen towel carried by the mother can be the first toy through which the baby feels the smell and closeness of his mother. On the other hand, hanging mobiles should be avoided in the first part of life. They disturb the baby with their incomprehensible movements or fix his attention.

Cuddly toys or other toys do not belong in the bed of newborns either. Becoming aware of his mother and father, experiencing his own body through the play of his fingers, the sounds of everyday life, voices, colors, joy and suffering, hunger and thirst are initially enough stimulation and activity for the infant. The concern of some adults that the baby might get bored is completely unfounded. On the contrary, early habituation to an excessively large range of stimuli will trigger a future desire for distraction and diversion.

The baby's first playing with his hands and eyes can only happen lying on his back or side. In contrast to lying on his stomach, lying on his back supports the free and independent development of movement. A lateral position is recommended during the first days of life for infants who frequently vomit after birth.

In the first year of life, the baby sleeps in her parents' bedroom. Her clothing and blankets are adjusted to the room temperature so that she neither sweats nor freezes. Draftts should be avoided. When the cradle is in the parent's bedroom or living room, the TV and radio remain switched off. Even when the newborn is asleep, such stimuli have a deep effect on the baby's consciousness.

A place to change diapers, near the bed or in the bathroom, offers a protected atmosphere. Toys must not distract from care of the baby. Baby changing equipment that allows parents to work in an upright, back-friendly position are well suited. With appropriate changing equipment, the child can move freely without the risk of falling down. As he gets older, he begins to pull himself up and can be playfully involved in dressing, undressing or washing in a safe environment. The necessary utensils, diapers and clothing are within easy reach.

When the infant sleeps through the night, approximately after one year, it is advisable to move him out of his parents' bedroom.

The process of "cutting the cord" that started with the switch over from breast milk to other foods is now expressed spatially. Difficulties in sleeping through the night can be caused by excessive proximity between mother and child. In that case, an earlier separation is helpful. On the other hand, children in developmental phases or crises (e.g., when they are ill) need greater closeness and can temporarily move back into their parents' bedroom, or one parent sets up a sleeping place in the child's room. (Sometimes it helps parents to assure them that their little ones will move out of their parents' bed on their own volition at the beginning of puberty at the latest.)

The baby's room is designed in mild colors, the bed remains protected by a "sky." When choosing furniture and toys, we should make sure that the baby is not overwhelmed by overcrowding. In general, a child's room is furnished in a child-friendly manner if you do not have to forbid the child to do anything. Gradually, the newborn's range of motion expands. From the timeless perfection of the uterus he enters into the dimensions of our world. Through his senses he seeks his way into the world and learns to understand it. We will pave the way and show him: "The world is kind to you—it is good!"

Tips for room design in hospitals

Special efforts are required to create the conditions described above in a maternity clinic. Parents should be allowed to spend the first hours after delivery in a comfortable room in the care of the midwife. After sucking on his mother's breast for the first time, the baby can fall asleep on his mother's or father's body. His little bed is hung with a "sky."

Parents can bring baby clothes, as well as their own nursing pillows and blankets. If the baby is accustomed to his own clothes, this will make the transition from the maternity ward to home easier for him.

Many maternity hospitals now practice 24-hour rooming-in. The room is equipped with a radiant heater that allows the baby's diaper to be changed in the room. A breastfeeding room allows for the option to retreat when visitors or other distractions interfere with breastfeeding. A family room supports the building of relationships and bonds.

2.2   Clothing—Wrapping

The newborn baby emerges from the uterus and the amniotic membranes unprotected into the light of the world. Only the vernix and some sparse hair protect her a little from cold and dehydration. Seeing the small, naked being we perform a typical nursing gesture almost without thinking about it. We wrap her up, enclose her, give her warmth and protection, because her not-yet mature warmth organism needs care. If she were not enveloped in warmth, the newborn baby would cool down completely within a short time and enter a life-threatening state. She cannot yet protect herself against excessively high outside temperatures either. Her ability to regulate warmth is not sufficient to maintain the core temperature of 37 degrees Celsius (98.6°F) that is normal for human beings. This temperature is required for optimal growth and maturation of the body's organs. Warm feet indicate healthy warmth. We can see that the outside temperature is too high when sweat forms on the baby's neck.

The infant's clothing takes this fact into account. Natural textiles made of virgin wool, silk and cotton are particularly suitable. Fibers extracted from the animal kingdom are closer to humans than plant-based ones. Among them, sheep's wool takes a special position. Its microscopic structure is most like that of human hair. Virgin wool, with natural fat content (greasy wool), can form a uniform thermal envelope, absorb moisture and release it into the outside air in the form of water vapor. Wool acts as a barrier that conducts moisture to the outside while enabling additional warmth. It also repels heat and moisture that comes from the outside. Depending on its quality, virgin wool absorbs 30 to 40% of its own weight in water without feeling wet. It neutralizes ammonia (the product of urine degradation), sweat and odors of all kinds. Skin intolerances to sheep's wool are often caused by chemical treatment (superwash) and moth proofing. Therefore, preference should be given to virgin wool from controlled organic animal husbandry.

Cotton, as a plant fiber, cannot fulfill the physiological functions of virgin sheep's wool, which are similar to those of human hair, but it is characterized by its durability, softness and absorbency. As a hand-picked, certified organic product, it is particularly recommended for allergy sufferers or children with sensitive skin.

Synthetic materials are unsuitable for the clothing of newborns, as they either do not provide sufficient warmth or they accumulate heat and moisture.

We especially want to draw attention to the need for a cap to protect the baby's head from excessive heat loss. A baby's head is very large in relation to the rest of his body.

When the newborn is not asleep, he is completely devoted to his surroundings via his senses. Each sensory stimulus impresses a baby much more directly than it does an adult, who can distance himself. Clothing thus not only serves as a warming covering, it is there to protect the newborn from the environment. This is another reason why it is appropriate to wrap his little head in a virgin wool, silk, or cotton cap. Delicately dyed or natural clothing protects better against an oversupply of sensations than colorfully printed garments.

We also encounter the baby's lack of ability to ward off the outer world in his movements, which are initially uncoordinated. The picture is characterized by the kicking and twitching, jerking and pushing of his arms and legs. Here, too, we can help the newborn to stay with himself more and not lose himself to the environment. Closely wrapping the baby with diapers and cloths (swaddling) limits his involuntary movements and helps him to calm down.

A special feature of newborn clothing is the diaper. Due to the use of disposable diapers, diapers are no longer an issue for many parents. However, anyone who is critical of the use of plastic as a garment will think about "alternatives to airtight packaging."

The following speaks for the use of cloth diapers:

- Cloth diapers are environmentally friendly
- They create a healthy microclimate in the diaper area
- They have a low risk of allergy (if the baby cannot tolerate wool, you can use breathable synthetic fiber pants over the diaper).
- Children learn to use the toilet earlier

In most regions of Germany, diaper services offer the collection, cleaning and delivery of various diaper systems. Diapers can usually also be purchased, borrowed or leased via these services.

Tips for using cloth diapers in maternity wards

Nothing stands in the way of the use of cloth diapers in maternity clinics. Not least from the point of view of waste management, as they can potentially save money. A prerequisite for the introduction of cloth diapers is to train the nurses, who in turn will instruct mothers and fathers. In contrast to cotton diapers, which can be washed at 95°Celsius (203°F), virgin wool diaper pants can only be used in the ward if they are brought by the parents, for hygienic reasons. When fastening cloth diapers in place, care must be taken to ensure that the baby is warmly covered.

2.3   Body care

Our first encounters and touches with the newborn are devoted to body care. Just after birth, we clear the infant's airways, place the baby on her mother's stomach, cut the umbilical cord, and remove amniotic fluid and the remaining blood. The baby's skin still wears a protective layer of vernix, which we do not want to remove. That is why we like to do without the bath that used to be customary after birth.
Body care essentially takes three aspects into account:

- Cleansing and prevention of infections
- The skin as the body's boundary
- Touch and relationships during body care

2.3.1 Cleansing and prevention of infections

For the daily cleansing of a newborn baby it is enough to wash his face, hands and diaper area with clear, warm water and gently dab off. Skin wrinkles on his neck and armpits, including the area behind the ears, are cleaned with a mild oil every day by carefully wiping them out.

We can avoid moisture accumulation as a source of macerations and infections in this way. To remove meconium or other tenacious impurities in the diaper area, we apply a few drops of oil to a damp washcloth or a clean diaper tip. No soap is usually needed for the washing of newborn babies. We also wipe out the nose with a cotton swab soaked in water. If there is a lot of mucus or encrustation, we can use a physiological saline solution. After this, a drop of breast milk can be used to care for dry mucous membranes. If the baby's eyes tend to stick together, wipe them from the outside to the inside with clear boiled water.

A drop of breast milk or

- *Calendula D4* (Weleda) eye drops

will cause inflammation of the conjunctiva to subside. Scabby, sebaceous deposits on the scalp can be gently removed with water. In case of stubborn deposits, we generously oil the scalp overnight with

- *Comforting Baby Oil* (Weleda)

The next day, the deposits are usually easy to remove. Persistent remainders may be left where they are.

2.3.2 The skin as the body's boundary

The skin of newborns has little resistance. The initial protection provided by the vernix is used up after a few days. The skin is now susceptible to dehydration, irritation, infection and allergy. Caring for it is therefore particularly important to us now.

Usually, skin care is done in connection with washing. The cleansings described above protect the skin as well as possible. Nevertheless, the skin often requires additional protection: we protect the face from wind, cold and sun with fatty creams or water in oil emulsions.

- *Calendula Wind & Weather Balm* (Weleda)

- *Rose Day Cream* (Dr. Hauschka)

Problems occur most frequently in the diaper area. Usually it is digestive disorders that lead to irritating diarrhea and then to inflammation. Stress, feverish illnesses and teething also favor a sore bottom, often associated with monilial infections. The most important principle for treatment is to change the diaper frequently. Virgin sheep's wool inserted into the diaper (with a high wool wax content) or cooling farmer's cheese packs will heal the baby's bright red, touch-sensitive bottom. Good healing results are also achieved by coating the baby's bottom with breast milk. It greases the skin and has an antibacterial effect. This is the remedy of choice, especially for hypersensitivities to other substances or for allergy sufferers. The external application of breast milk has also proven successful in newborn exanthem.

The creams mentioned above are naturally based on oils and fats and include the addition of essential oils. Oils and fats have a close relationship to warmth. Plants and animals form them by seemingly compressing sunlight. Another important warmth carrier from the animal kingdom is beeswax. This is another component that is used in body care products (e.g., *Calendula Diaper Rash Cream* (Weleda)). The high capacity of oils, fats and waxes to store warmth stimulates the child's warmth organism. Extracts of chamomile or calendula (marigold) are used in many natural care products. These two plants are characterized by their slightly antibacterial and anti-inflammatory properties. *Chamomile* has a stronger effect on the nerves and senses, soothing and relaxing, while *calendula* tends more to a harmonizing and balancing effect in the metabolism. By using appropriate products, we affect the child's whole organism, as well as the skin.

2.3.3 Touch and relationships during body care
In the first period of a newborn's life, each day consists of sleeping, drinking and being cared for. The baby is gathering his first experiences in having relationships with

other people, particularly through the hands that touch him. The newborn baby feels whether the body care is only being done to get the job done or whether there is a real encounter between him and his mother or father. For example, the use of disposable diapers is justified time and again by the idea that the time saved during diaper changing would allow more time for play and "real" attention. This already predisposes a separation between unpleasant duties, as necessary evils, and pleasant rewards reserved for play and leisure time. Yet body care could become a happy encounter between parent and child. This can be achieved if the adult's attention remains completely focused on the baby and the individual steps of care. The parents will then touch the baby in accordance with her age and include her in their actions according to her abilities. They will announce every step in undressing, washing, drying, applying cream, putting on the diaper and dressing. They will guide the baby with gestures and with their eyes. The baby's bath is a special event. For reasons of cleanliness a bath is not absolutely necessary for the infant, rather it gives the baby intensive sensory experiences: the warmth of the water (37°C or 98.6°F) flowing around the baby's body on all sides, the baby's weightlessness in the buoyancy, the being held by the arms and hands of the mother or father, the letting go and relaxing. The first bath should only be given after about forty days of life. Now the infant is already more deeply connected with the elements of the Earth. The bath must not be given more often than once a week. If it is performed regularly on the same day of the week, at the same time and according to the same sequence, it promotes a feeling for rhythms and gives a sense of security. To avoid removing oil from the skin in the water, add five tablespoons of breast milk or another non-foaming bath additive (e.g., *Comforting Cream Bath – Calendula* (Weleda)) to ten liters of water. After the bath, vegetable oil can be applied to the baby's moist skin.

> *"Our love and care must surround the child like a pleasant, evenly-tempered, warm bath."*
>
> Emmy Pikler (1902–1984)

2.4 Breastfeeding—Nourishment

Newborn babies connect with the world in three ways immediately after birth:
- Through sense impressions
- Through breathing
- Through taking in nourishment

Guided by heat and smell, the healthy newborn baby, when placed on his mother's stomach, usually finds his way to her breast within the first thirty minutes after birth. The first sucking movements stimulate milk production and influence the baby's sucking behavior. Despite this instinctive finding of each other in mother and child, many mothers doubt their ability to breastfeed their baby, or do not want to for social reasons (work, partner). It is therefore decisive for the motivation and success of breastfeeding to counsel the mother already during pregnancy, as well as in the first hours and days after the birth, and to provide rapid counseling and assistance during the breastfeeding period. This gives confidence in the natural ability of every mother to breastfeed her baby. After the birth, the focus is on practical assistance in putting the baby on the breast, regulating milk production, developing observation criteria for adequate nutrition, and prophylaxis against mastitis. Advice for the transition from breast nutrition to healthy baby food concludes the breastfeeding period. The official recommendation of the World Health Organization and UNICEF is to exclusively breastfeed for six months and to continue breastfeeding until the age of two and beyond, parallel to the introduction of complementary nourishment, if both mother and child agree. Rather than the traditional introduction of puréed and mashed food, some parents today choose the path of Baby Led Weaning, which means that the child is offered a selection of cooked food and decides for himself what and how much he wants to eat. Either way it is important that breastfeeding be continued while the baby is learning to eat, so that each type of new food is better tolerated.

2.4.1 Assistance with getting the baby latched onto the breast

The main principle in helping to latch is to disturb mother and child as little as possible in finding each other. First, the mother must settle into a comfortable breastfeeding position. This can be facilitated and stabilized by a nursing cushion. The baby finds the breast or is supported in doing so, under no circumstances do we press the baby's neck or head against the breast. Rather, the breast-feeding counselor, midwife or nurse observes the mother and child from a suitable distance in order to give targeted tips from the calm of their perception if the mother's position or anxiety blocks the child's path to the breast. This perceptive role of the nurse is particularly important when the infant is impetuous, perhaps crying with hunger, and is getting in his own way to the source.

It is important to ensure that the infant grasp the nipple well and enclose the entire mammary gland firmly, his lower lip arched outwards, sucking in. The breastfeeding position must be changed again and again so that the nipple is evenly exposed, to protect it from rhagades. Normally, when one breast is empty, the other is offered to the baby. This stimulates milk production optimally. If milk production is still not sufficient, we can help by putting the baby back on the first breast or by breastfeeding more frequently. If milk production is too strong, the baby is only placed on one breast and the other one is gently emptied. The infant drinks the largest amount of breast milk in the first four to five minutes, but a breastfeeding meal may last longer than thirty minutes. Non-nutritive sucking ensures bonding, a sufficient quantity of milk and a feeling of well-being for mother and child.

2.4.2 Nipple confusion

If the infant does not suck sufficiently on the breast, it may be necessary to give added breast milk or another substitute (glucose or maltose supplements only with a doctor's prescription). If drinking bottles with ordinary nipples are used, the infant will develop sucking behavior that differs considerably from drinking at the breast. This can result in a diminishing of the baby's instinctively correct sucking behavior at the breast. Because of the now ineffective sucking, the frustrated baby may turn away from the breast and favor the "more generous" bottle.

This can be prevented by using a small spoon, a cup or a glass with a rounded edge. The infant absorbs the liquid without choking on it. His natural sucking behavior is not affected. If drinking at the breast is not possible for a longer period of time, special nipples can prevent confusion. These nipples require the infant to use a technique similar to breast drinking.

2.4.3 Breastmilk and milk substitutes

The fact that breast milk is the optimal nutrition for infants has become common knowledge again today. The following overview of the most important arguments in favor of breastfeeding is for those who must nevertheless counsel and convince pregnant women and new mothers about this:

- Bonding between mother and child.
- Immune protection for the child.
- Protection against diabetes and other diseases of civilization.
- The composition and quantity of breast milk adapts optimally to the baby's needs during the entire breastfeeding period.
- Breast-feeding is a source of trust and security for the infant.
- For the mother, breastfeeding provides important training in the relationship.
- Fresh breast milk is germ-free and has an antibacterial effect.
- Breastmilk is safe from industrial contamination.
- Breastmilk is convenient in all situations and is available at the right temperature.
- Breastmilk is the most cost-effective form of nutrition.
- Breastmilk avoids packaging and transport and is thus a contribution to active environmental protection.
- Breastmilk acts as an excellent skin-care substance.

In a few cases, breastfeeding is only partially possible or not possible at all for medical or social reasons.

2.4.4 Introducing other forms of nutrition—Weaning

Breastfeeding keeps the infant physically connected to his mother. Both share close-ness, warmth and moods with great immediacy. Slowly but steadily the baby's attention turns outwards. His sensory activity and movements begin to focus on goals. The intake of food from plants and animals naturally continues this process of opening up. At about six months of age, the baby's physical and mental development has progressed so far that breast milk can be gradually supplemented by other foods.

The right time for weaning is approaching when the mother feels the need to become more independent of the child and/or the child is clearly interested in the food that is being served at the family table. The overall breastfeeding time varies greatly. Often the impulse for weaning comes from the infant himself, when he has found a taste for new food or develops an interest in what parents or siblings are eating. Weaning creates a new relationship between mother and child. The transition from breastfeeding to other food can happen without a bottle, which often prolongs infantile behavior into the first years of life. Babies and toddlers quickly learn to eat with their hands, a spoon and a fork, and to drink from a glass.

Nursing problem	Possible cause	Advice	Helpful measures
The mother does not (yet) have enough milk	Insufficient stimulation of milk production, stress	More frequent breast feeding, the mother should drink a lot (but not more than 2.5 liters), eat carbohy-drate-rich food, breastfeed undisturbed	Breast massage, mustard compress between the shoulder blades, *Nursing Tea* (Weleda), *Phyto-lacca D30* (DHU) dil., 3 x 10 drops
Painful nipples, fissures,	Excessive irritation due to incorrect sucking behavior, sensitive skin type	Relieve nipples, change position-ing, possibly offer only one breast, ensure correct sucking behavior	Nipple protection (Medela) and care (with mother's milk or lanolin), virgin wool, nursing pads made of wool-silk, possibly pump out temporarily

Nursing problem	Possible cause	Advice	Helpful measures
The baby quickly falls asleep at the breast	Tiredness, neonatal jaundice	Stimulate by changing the diaper, massage the feet and hands, place on the breast very often, caution: dehydration!	Possibly combine with breastfeeding kit (Medela), administer breast milk with a spoon or cup
Milk congestion, incipient mastitis	Insufficient emptying of the breast, stress, constipation of the mother	Ensure good emptying of the breast, adjust breastfeeding position (lower jaw of the child points in the direction of milk congestion), warm up the breast before breastfeeding, breast massage, ensure digestion.	White cabbage application, a wrapped farmer's cheese compress on the breast (body warm) *Phytolacca D12* (DHU) dil., 3 x 10 drops, *Silicea D10* (Weleda) trit., 3 x 1 saltspoon (~¼ tsp.)
The baby begins to suck greedily and then tears herself off the breast crying.	Abdominal cramps or flatulence can be caused by ingestion of food	Ensure quiet, put the baby on the breast before she cries with hunger	Rub her belly with *Cuprum metallicum praeparatum 0.1%* ointment (Weleda) or *Oxalis, Folium 10%* ointment (Weleda)
The baby does not latch onto the nipple, drinks little or gives up trying to drink, while crying	Incorrect positioning technique, flat or inverted nipples, possible suction confusion	Patience and calm, patiently put the baby on repeatedly, preform the nipple, avoid bottle nipples, use a spoon or cup	Pumping out, breastfeeding kit (Medela), nipple former (Medela) for flat or inverted nipples

Nursing problem	Possible cause	Advice	Helpful measures
The baby is hungry and yet does not go to the breast	Over-irritation, restlessness in the room, the mother is distracted or tense	Ensure quiet, rub the baby with *lavender 0.1% oil* (pharmacy formula) before breastfeeding; naked bonding, swaddling, calm the mother	Empty the breast by hand, or with a pump, offer milk in spoons, cups
Too much milk	Initial milk formation, excessive stimulation of milk formation	Only nurse on one side, empty the other breast by hand to relieve pressure, do not pump, drink less	Wear milk collection shells, use sage tea, peppermint tea, *Phytolacca D1* (DHU), 10 drops just once is often enough

Chart: Overview of the most important breastfeeding problems and possible self-help measures

2.5 Relationships—Education—Development

A relationship between two parents and their newborn baby is, like any encounter, completely individual. Many parents become aware of this relationship even before their baby is conceived. The new being announces itself in dreams or in deep thoughts that rise up from within. When the baby begins to develop in the mother's womb during pregnancy, the parents and child seek to tune in to their life together. Complaints during pregnancy are often physical and mental expressions of this process. With birth, an individuality enters the world—not a blank page or an entity determined by genetics, as people would often like us to believe. Of course, this individuality needs our care so that it can develop its specifically human capacities: an upright gait, the ability to speak and to think. These lay the foundation for the child to master the "adventure of being human" responsibly and in freedom. Helping the child to develop this foundation is probably our most important educational goal in the first stage of life.

2.5.1 Supporting movement development through everyday care

During the first few days, the infant lives in congenital behavior patterns and reflexes (sucking, grasping, crying). These reflexes must be gradually overcome. This is done by learning to replace involuntary movements with voluntary ones, by imitating human behavior. The child follows her mother's gaze, gestures and facial expressions. Soon she begins to bring her fingers to her mouth and grasp things, or she lets her gaze linger, and listens, smiles.

The baby should be granted time to do this. He may discover new movements, noises, sounds all on his own. Already in the first days of life, some babies succeed in turning their head towards lights or sounds. This is followed by lifting their shoulders and hips. That is how they get onto their side. After about five months they feel the urge to turn from their back over the side onto their stomach. This sometimes looks quite exhausting, and perhaps such efforts seem to sometimes fail. With every effort the baby develops strength and skill for the next step in movement development. As caregivers or parents there is no need to want to help. A healthy baby, after some effort, will certainly manage it. By helping the baby, we take away the experience of being able to achieve something on his own. Verbal "cheering on" also counteracts self-confident development in such situations. For one thing, it distracts the child from his actual intention; for another, it is no longer the achievement of the self-chosen goal that becomes the determining motive for action, but rather the praise and joy of his parents. Thus, apparently insignificant, well-intentioned everyday habits can be used to shape the child's character traits.

Only when the child walks upright has he attained a specifically human manner of movement. This development takes place over many intermediate steps from the supine position into the prone position, via rolling, belly-crawling, crawling on his hands and knees to kneeling and sitting, then standing, walking along railings and finally walking freely. Experiences of touch and movement with one's own arms, legs, head and torso lay the foundation for later intellectual development. The child completes a path from grasping with his hands to grasping intellectually, from standing to understanding! Our attentive, silent accompaniment of the baby's initiative in carrying out movements, our verbal announcement of our care-giving actions, our naming of objects, our waiting for the baby's cooperation, our regaining his attention when distracted—all this describes a caring attitude which strengthens the child's independence and initiative during all phases of his developing movement. In the first weeks of life almost all encounters with the newborn are of a caregiving nature. Therefore, it is important to develop a joyful relationship with the baby during this time. Everyday care for the baby becomes the beginning of his education to freedom.

2.5.2 Cultivating a rhythmic lifestyle

Two views on the rhythms of infants seem to be irreconcilable. One position assumes that a healthy child will always find his own rhythm for drinking and sleeping, if you let him. In practice, babies who are cared for according to this view are nursed when they show desire (on-demand feeding), and are placed in their bed when they are about to fall asleep. The other view is that children do not have their own rhythm, so parents must establish one. These babies usually receive their food every four hours and they are woken up and taken to bed at set times. According to our experience, babies find a rhythm independently when their parents themselves live rhythmically. That is the big exception today. Our independence from the rhythm of night and day, from the seasons and from seasonal food is considered to be a cultural achievement; probably no one wants to forego it anymore. We therefore recommend that people look for a rhythm that meets the needs of the child and the parents, and maintain that rhythm. This means that a rhythm is consistently maintained until there is a developmental change (e.g., when the infant sleeps through the night, in case of illness or when the baby's diet changes). The newly found rhythm must be maintained over and over again. Being responsible for the life-giving power of rhythm becomes a serious task, to ensure that the necessary freedom in the "choice" of rhythm does not degenerate into opportunistic arbitrariness.

A major problem for many parents is to figure out why their baby is crying at any given moment. Is he hungry, did he perhaps not get enough at the last meal, does he have flatulence, does he want attention, is he sick? Breastfeeding or giving a bottle usually has a temporarily assuaging effect. However, if ingestion of food is used to eliminate every discomfort, then no rhythm will be established.

The same applies to children who cry when they are put to bed. Often people pick them up again, carry them around, push them in a stroller or (a common modern method) drive them around in their car seat until they fall asleep. Sometimes the cause of these sleep disorders is air in the gastrointestinal tract or a wet diaper. These problems can be easily solved. The child will soon calm down after a little burp and a fresh diaper, or perhaps a tummy compress with *Baby Tummy Oil* (Weleda). In most cases, however, the cause of sleep disorders is irritation and being overly awake. Who doesn't know this situation: the whole afternoon there were visitors, the baby wandered happily from arm to arm, the parents think that he is now truly tired and will fall asleep easily. The opposite is true. The baby does not calm down, he drinks in restless short gulps and gets flatulence. Mental "digestive disorders" are the cause of the problem of falling asleep in this case. Avoiding such overload is of the utmost importance. Acute cases can be relieved by giving clockwise embrocations around the navel with:

- *Cuprum metallicum praeparatum 0.1% ointment* (Weleda)

- A tummy compress with *Melissa oil* (WALA) or *Oleum aethereum Melissae indicum 10%* (Weleda)

There are not always external causes for crying. Sometimes babies are looking for an intensive experience of self in crying just before falling asleep. Now the baby can be on his own. Intervention by his parents usually prolongs this crying phase. The rule of thumb is: we should not deprive the baby of crying or screaming as an expression of discomfort. We can take care of the cause, knowing that we cannot relieve the baby of all pain or keep away all troubles. With some experience and empathy one can learn to recognize the different expressions in crying. Crying with hunger sounds different from crying with a stomachache, over-excited crying differs from crying as a sleep ritual.

2.5.3 Imitation as a basic principle of education

Children learn until about the age of seven exclusively by imitating their environment. Only then will intellectual learning become possible without having to use organ-building forces for intellectual activity. Movements, gestures, facial expressions, language, tone of voice, daily rhythms, habits, social skills and much more are adopted directly through imitation based on the child's temperament and individual personality. "Fools and children tell the truth," as the saying goes, which means that children reflect their surroundings in the most exact way. They are the educators of adults. Every weakness, every wrong word, but also our strengths (unfortunately parents rarely notice them) appear in the imitating behavior of children. Even newborns seismographically perceive moods such as sadness, joy, restlessness, or calmness. In this sense, education is self-education above all. Our care leads the new earth inhabitant on his way to training and perfecting his abilities. Caring for him is an occasion for caregivers and parents to remember the dignity and task of their own humanity.

Category	Example learning objectives	Recommended learning path
Skills	You are expanding your repertoire of caregiving methods by using natural substances.	A
Your own learning objective		
Relationships	You encourage and advise mothers and fathers in the care of their children.	B
Your own learning objective		
Knowledge	You know how important caring for newborns is for their further development.	C
Your own learning objective		

Further reading

- Bauer D., Hoffmeister M., Goerg, H. *Children who communicate before they are born. Conversations with unborn souls.* Temple Lodge Press, Forest Row 2005.
- Bopp, A., Krohmer B. *Der Baby-Guide fürs erste Jahr.* Kösel-Verlag, Munich 2010.
- Endlich, J. *Das kleine Kind und seine Bekleidung.* Verlag Freies Geistesleben, Stuttgart 1995.
- Fels N., Knabe A., Maris B. *Ins Leben begleiten.* Verlag Freies Geistesleben, Stuttgart 2003.
- Glöckler M., Goebel W., Michael K. *A Waldorf guide to children's health. Illnesses, symptoms, treatments and therapies.* Floris Books, Edinburgh 2018.
- Hassauer, W. *Die Geburt der Individualität.* Verlag Urachhaus, Stuttgart 1995.
- Kühne P. *Säuglingsernährung.* Arbeitskreis für Ernährungsforschung, Bad Vilbel 2012.
- Pikler, E. *Lasst mir Zeit.* Pflaum Verlag, Munich 2001.
- Pikler, E. *Miteinander vertraut werden.* Arbor Verlag, Freiamt 2014.
- Pikler, E. *Friedliche Babys, zufriedene Mütter.* Herder Verlag, Freiburg im Breisgau 2009.
- Soldner, G.; Stellmann, H.M. *Individual paediatrics. Physical, emotional and spiritual aspects of diagnosis and counseling.* Wissenschaftliche Verlagsgesellschaft, Stuttgart 2014.
- Stave, U. *Die Umwelt des kleinen Kindes.* Verlag Urachhaus, Stuttgart 1992.
- Steiner, R. *Educating children today.* Rudolf Steiner Press, London 2008.
- Steiner, R. *Prayers for parents and children.* 4th ed. Rudolf Steiner Press, Forest Row 2012.
- Stadelmann, I. *Hebammensprechstunde.* Selbstverlag, Kempten 1994.
- Vagedes J., Soldner G. *Das Kinder Gesundheitsbuch.* Gräfe und Unzer Verlag, Munich 2013.
- van Houten, C. *Awakening the will. Principles and processes in adult learning.* 2nd ed. Temple Lodge, Forest Row 2000.

Further information on the internet

- Verband der Windeldienste in Europa e.V., www.windeldienste.de
- www.safe-programm.de
- www.stillen-huellen-pflegen.de
- www.stillen.de
- www.naturwindeln.de

CHAPTER XVII

The Concept of Development as the Basis for Anthroposophically Extended Pediatric Nursing

CAROLA EDELMANN

Child development happens in rhythms. Knowledge of these rhythms, which can be subdivided into seven-year cycles, is essential for the treatment and nursing care of typical diseases. It is equally important to perceive and support the relationships that parents have with their child. When we succeed in integrating these aspects into pediatric nursing, we come closer to the nature of children.

→   Learning objectives, see end of chapter

1.   The nature of children

Knowledge of Rudolf Steiner's understanding of the human being deepens pediatric nursing. When we combine scientific training with the understanding of the human being developed by Steiner—which sees the human being as a unity of body, soul and spirit and includes the idea of ongoing development—we can develop a healing understanding of the nature of children. It is necessary to get to know children as beings that are in development:

- How has this child changed from birth onwards through various stages of individual development?
- Are there hidden laws in these changes?
- Is there a connection between the development of this child and his illness?

In his work *Educating Children Today,* Rudolf Steiner described developmental phases that occur in seven-year cycles. These can be summarized as follows:

If we want to recognize the nature of children, we must start by contemplating the hidden nature of human beings. Before being born the growing human being is surrounded by the physical body of his mother and by self-formed amniotic membranes. At birth, the newborn leaves his mother's physical protection and begins to be directly affected by his environment. The strength with which the child emerges from these protective layers already gives a hint of his individuality.

The human physical body is subject to the same laws as the mineral world. This human body is also permeated by an etheric body, which Rudolf Steiner described as follows: "Man has nutrition, growth and reproduction in common with all plants. If he only had a physical body, like a stone, he could not grow, eat or reproduce. So, he must have something in him that makes him able to use physical forces and substances in such a way that they become a means for him to grow and so on. That is the etheric body."

The newborn now begins developing his body's organs and transforming his inherited body into one that is appropriate to his own individuality. He activates his inherited body individually ("epigenetically").

The first seven years
In the first seven years children live entirely in imitation. This imitation of meaningful activity enables them to develop a strong will. This will is activated and developed through the child's own activity. After voluntarily taking control of his body (learning to walk) and then his soul (learning to speak, imaginative play), the child then expands his will activity into the realm of thinking (methodical play).

The second seven-year cycle
In the second seven-year cycle the etheric forces now becoming free can be used to form thoughts. The child is now ready to start school. His focus turns to forming a healthy emotional life, accompanied by the loving authority of the people closest to him.

The beginning of the third seven-year cycle
When the child reaches sexual maturity, his soul body develops. As the carrier of drives, desires and passions, the soul body is something that human beings have in common with animals.

Now the youth's individuality emerges even more. Further training of the ability to think follows the development of will and emotions.

Rudolf Steiner described the following: "The human being has a fourth member of his being, which he does not share with other earth beings. This is the carrier of the human 'I'. When we call ourselves 'I', we refer to ourselves from within our own being. A being that can say 'I' to itself is a world of its own. Religions that are built on spiritual philosophies have always felt this. Thus, they have said: God, who normally only reveals himself to lowly beings from outside—in outer appearances—begins to speak from within with the word 'I'. The 'I'-body is the bearer of the abilities described. This 'I'-body is the bearer of the higher human soul. Through it the human being is the crown of earth creation."

Rudolf Steiner's idea of development encompasses a total of nine seven-year phases, throughout which human physical, mental and spiritual development extends. These phases are not bound to operate according to rigid laws, they are living segments of each person's individual biography.

The following text will describe the developmental phases of childhood along with the relevant laws and problems, in order to determine the nursing care that is appropriate to the child at each stage.

2. The stages of child development, with a view to the associated illnesses and nursing care requirements

2.1 Infants and small children

Regardless of all the medical knowledge now available, childbirth is still always surrounded by a sense of wonder and a feeling of reverence. Even if one initially has the impression that newborns all look alike, on closer inspection and through contact with the baby one soon feels that an individual has been born. Our desire to do justice to this individuality challenges us to recognize this unique 'I' with all our senses.

With the first breath, the baby's soul and spirit are drawn into the body. This arrival requires loving accompaniment and care. The most important prerequisites for the baby to find his way into his own rhythm of life are the presence of his mother, along with peace and warmth. The relationship between mother and child is very close, which is particularly evident in breastfeeding.

The infant, who is completely dependent on care, develops into a purposefully looking and finally upright walking child through persevering practice of romping, turning, sitting, crawling and grasping. His joy at every achievement on the way there is overwhelming.

Parallel to the development of movement we observe the training of speech. In the beginning, parents find it very difficult to interpret their baby's crying. But soon they learn to distinguish the subtle nuances, whether it is hunger, wet diapers or pain that the baby wants to communicate. It is exciting to watch how the baby progresses from making sounds to babbling and then acquires language via delightful word paintings. The word 'no' often appears as a favorite, and the baby's needs are expressed loudly and stubbornly. This stubborn opposition establishes distance from the environment and creates space for the child to experience himself, which is clearly seen in the moment of first saying 'I'.

Almost everything that the child learns from birth is acquired through imitation; he is entirely a sensory organ. Through this openness, all impressions influence the child's development, right down to the physical. This has consequences for our behavior towards the child and for the design of his environment in the broadest sense. It is crucial that the child experience meaningful action and clarity of language and gesture. He learns much more from non-verbal communication than from any instruction, however clever.

The daily routine is based on the baby's rhythm of eating and sleeping. To stimulate the baby's imagination, we shape his environment with materials that are as close to nature as possible in terms of form, color and choice of object. Imitation also has a significant influence on the forming of the baby's organs. This can be supported, for example, by making a doll out of silk cloth: we form the head with a small ball of wool, which we tie into the middle of the cloth. We make the legs by knotting together the respective ends. In contrast to perfectly completed dolls, this simple silk doll stimulates the child's formative forces.

The importance of the environment is illustrated by the following practical example from home childcare.

Example

Mehmet, a six-month-old infant, a former premature baby with bronchopulmonary dysplasia, comes home for the first time. Soon he will be admitted again because he does not drink enough at home. In the clinic he quickly regains his rhythm of eating, puts on weight, and can soon be released. This time the ward doctor asks me to continue accompanying the baby and his family.

During home visits it becomes clear that his mother, who can hardly speak German, suffers from strong homesickness. The family lives with her husband's brother. This housing situation is a makeshift solution; the mother feels that she is merely tolerated and she longs to have a home of her own. Due to the family situation, the mother rarely brought Mehmet to the hospital and is therefore still very insecure in the care of her son.

The bronchopulmonary dysplasia makes Mehmet a child "at risk." This represents a further hurdle for the mother trying to establish an uncomplicated relationship with Mehmet. He is already her second child, but through conversations I learn that her three-year-old daughter was born in Turkey and was mainly looked after by her grandmother there. I try to familiarize Mehmet's mother with the care of her child.

On my first visit to the house, the mother receives me, helplessly pointing at her screaming baby lying on the matrimonial bed kicking—beside himself from so much crying. Turkish women sit all around knitting, while Mehmet's little sister also wants to be heard.

I introduce myself and first take Mehmet firmly in my arms so that he feels support. He calms down more and more, and after a short time it is even possible to make eye contact. I ask his mother for fresh diapers and a bottle of milk, because the baby has not drunk for a long time.

As I change Mehmet's diaper, I tell him what I am doing and try to keep eye contact with him so that he doesn't immediately start crying again. I care for him slowly and pay attention to where he can already respond and help me with what I am doing. To give him the bottle, I sit down relaxed in a quiet place and hold Mehmet snugly in my arms again. I am lucky, he is very hungry and drinks slowly, but perseveringly.

At first the women marvel in silent amazement, but then they try to tell me all kinds of things; I ask them not to disturb Mehmet now. In this way I try, step by step during the following home visits, to give Mehmet's mother certainty in the care of her child. We arrange the surroundings according to Mehmet's needs, starting with a healthy rhythm for eating and sleeping, and setting up a suitable little bed with a canopy. Gradually the mother gains confidence. It is interesting to observe how Mehmet is increasingly becoming a natural part of her life; how she develops a sense for what her infant needs. This can be seen in the way that she moves him without making him "ride a roller coaster," and how she makes sure that Mehmet is always warm enough.

A social worker is trying hard to find an apartment. Ultimately, the long-awaited move confirms my suspicion that the main cause of the problems was the housing situation: having her own apartment gives the mother a new attitude towards life, the situation relaxes and the nutritional problems disappear almost from one day to the next. The baby also makes significant progress in developing his motor skills.

An indirect cause of Mehmet's nutritional problems was that his mother did not feel at home. Mehmet clearly sensed this; he did not find his way into his "new home" either. Because of the long separation of mother and child, the two first had to grow closer together. The surroundings had to be designed in such a way that there was a place for Mehmet too.

Let us look again at the important aspects:

- A newborn baby is an individuality, not a blank page, and he arrives in the world with a deeply hidden intention.
- Mother and child form a unity.
- Imitation determines the child's development up until the time when he is ready to start school.

Mehmet is a child who fought massively against the unfamiliar home environment; in the hospital he felt immediately safe again. With the help of home nursing care, Mehmet's mother gradually built a relationship with her son in her not necessarily happy but familiar environment and got to know him better and better just as he was. She became more confident and relaxed in dealing with Mehmet and brought in more and more of her own ideas.

As the nurse, I set an example and make sure that the baby is not merely cared for routinely, but in a way so rich in relationships that Mehmet feels satisfied afterwards. For example, draping a "sky" over his little bed helps him to "be on his own." With this protection, the baby is not constantly disturbed and distracted by external impressions.

2.1.1 Disease dispositions

The phenomenon of imitation is also reflected in a pronounced openness to infection in the first seven years. At no other age are children as susceptible to infections as at this time. Overcoming childhood illnesses strengthens the immune system and the acquired immunity protects against later infections. Especially skin changes are symptomatic of many childhood diseases. A veritable scaling can take place up to the time of school readiness, revealing the child's own individual shape more clearly. This can be impressively observed with the much-dreaded measles:

At first the child's eyes and nose start to drip, his face is bleary and he is cranky. Then he gets a high fever, is sensitive to light and cold, and longs for rest. Suddenly a fine spotted exanthem begins to spread from his ears downwards. The child now needs bed rest according to his sensitivities, preferably in a darkened room, and sufficient warmth. The high fever should not be reduced unnecessarily. If the exanthem does not erupt fully, a rinse with lukewarm saltwater will help to prevent the disease from "turning inwards"; the rinse prevents complications in the form of pneumonia or encephalitis.

This is a particularly exhausting time for the mother. The child now needs her at the bedside 24/7. But after a few days it becomes apparent that the exertions were worth it. The child emerges from the high fever and his overcoming of the illness as if newborn. If the child looked very much like his parents before, now his own features come forth more clearly. This development can also be seen from the difference in the pictures that the child draws before and after the illness.

In addition to acute illnesses, initial symptoms of possible familial ailments often occur at this age, for example diabetes mellitus, epilepsy and developmental disorders resulting from premature birth. The diagnosis usually initially puts the family into a state of shock. It can be a long, arduous journey from initial resistance to acceptance of the disease, and the family urgently needs support.

2.2 The school child

While small children still have a very pronounced resemblance to their parents, their own personalities come more and more to the fore when they reach school age. Now some of their forces are free for learning reading, writing and arithmetic. The kindergarten child becomes a school child. In addition to the authority of the parents, there is now the authority of the teacher, and it is not uncommon to hear the justification: "But my teacher said...."

School-aged children are marked by contrasting inner states, which often cause them unspoken suffering. Feelings appear right down to the physical level, e.g., in the pallor of shock, and the flush of anger or shame. The child oscillates between joy and suffering, courage and fear. Like the moment when the child first used the word 'I' around the third year of life, the ninth year represents another distinctive moment in the development of the 'I'. The child now feels separation: "Me, and the world." The child experiences this partly as intense loneliness. He doubts many things in the adult world, and it is not uncommon for the question to arise: "Am I really your child?" The child now expects his parents and educators to be people that he can trust.

He requires adults as mediators between himself and his environment. By hearing fables and legends, the child receives soul nourishment through which the laws and secrets of nature shine through before he learns about them in intellectual terms in the classroom. In dealing with schoolmates, the child learns social rules. Unconsciously, children of this age still need an orderly daily routine, even if they are constantly tempted to practice the opposite. The imaginative and loving authority of the people close to them effortlessly fascinates them.

On the one hand this means giving the child generous space to try out his powers while at the same time accompanying him with inner vigilance, on the other hand it is necessary to set limits in certain situations. In this way the child learns to develop an inner balance in accordance with his temperament.

2.2.1 Disease dispositions

Physically the child is quite healthy in the second seven-year cycle. Nevertheless, frequent visits to the doctor or even to a clinic may be necessary. It is not unusual for a failed test of courage to end in the hospital with a broken bone or concussion. The outward appearance of the schoolchild, with gaps in his teeth, suggests what is happening in his soul: old things are disappearing and the new are not yet in sight. This unsettles the child. It is the time of "school ailments." The child's inner instability usually manifests in abdominal pain, loss of appetite, headaches, etc., although it should not be overlooked that there may also be organic causes.

The example of eight-year-old Daniel will give us insight into the mental state of a child in the second seven-year cycle.

Example

Daniel is admitted to the clinic during the holidays because of his overweight condition. He is the only child of concerned parents. The boy seems very unhappy about having to spend part of his holiday at the clinic, and only barely holds back his tears when he learns that he is old enough to stay there without his mother. He gets a bed in a big room where his peers are curiously waiting for him. The nurse introduces Daniel to the children and lets him choose one of the free beds. He indifferently heads for the bed in the back corner.

After the admission interview, the responsible nurse explains the daily routine and the visiting hours to Daniel and his mother. His mother helps Daniel put his things in the wardrobe. After dinner, she says goodbye to him for a week.

First, we give Daniel time to settle in. That is how he gets to know us, and we get to know him, with his needs. Every day he grows more curious about what's going on around him. He does not appreciate his morning bath, which is supposed to stimulate his metabolism and formative forces, at all, especially as he can't dawdle, because afterwards it is time for the morning circle. There they sing in a group to start the day and the ward doctor or educator for special needs tells a story. It is exciting to see Daniel gradually "catch fire," and after a few days he is among the first to arrive at the morning circle.

After breakfast, the educator takes Daniel to the crafts and play group. He used to sit shyly on his bed during rounds, now he proudly presents his handicraft work. At mealtimes, he is still the first to stand by the cart and he can hardly wait to see what is hidden under the cover on his plate. But he must be patient; everyone starts eating together. His appetite varies strongly depending on the dish: he devours his beloved noodles in a flash, while he needs a long time to chew his way through vegetables and grains. Some of his table companions develop compassion for him and secretly give him things.

One of the boys is lying in bed with his foot in a cast. Daniel and he soon become friends, and Daniel always clears away the boy's tray after dinner.

During the midday rest the ability of the nurses to remain consistent and composed is tested and they do not always pass the test. Daniel, too, is increasingly developing a spirit of enterprise when it is time to be quiet.

If artistic therapy such as painting or sculpting is not on the timetable, Daniel can play in the woods with the educator or have a game of ping pong. After dinner everyone tidies up and brushes their teeth.

In the evening Daniel gets a Rhythmical Einreibung treatment with an essential oil, alternating between his belly and his arms and legs. The final activity of the evening is arranged by the educator. The children are usually excited to find out how the story from the previous evening will continue. After a goodnight song, the quiet of night gradually settles in and sometimes homesickness as well.

Daniel has a lot to tell when his parents come to visit him on the weekend. His mother is now permitted to visit him once during the week as well, and then she has an opportunity to talk with the ward team and pick up ideas for home. She gets to know the connections between Daniel's eating habits and his mental condition.

The following problems emerge:
Since Daniel is an only child and his school friends do not live in the neighborhood, he often gets bored at home. This awakens in him the need to nibble and pursue his fondness for sweet drinks.

Although his mother cares for Daniel lovingly, her son no longer accepts her unreservedly. He misses his friends and instead of romping about, he stuffs everything into himself.

Let us recall the core principle of the second seven-year cycle: during this time, the presence of a loving authority figure becomes more important, someone who assists and guides the child in phases of uncertainty.

The clinic therefore focuses on the following areas of care:

- The family has to accept that Daniel is now old enough to be admitted without his mother. How is a child supposed to become self-confident if we do not let him go?
- The topic "food" is only one part of the varied daily routine.

- Daniel makes friends with the three or four patients of the same age. He assumes responsibility by clearing away the tray for his bed neighbor.
- Through the baths and Rhythmical Einreibung Daniel becomes more aware of his body. This stimulates his metabolism and his inner activity.
- He also receives stimulation for his soul through painting and sculpting.
- During team meetings, everyone describes their observations, creating a clear picture of Daniel and developing ideas for appropriate therapy.
- In a conversation with the educator for special needs the mother is shown the connection between Daniel's obesity and his problems and is given recommendations for home.

In Daniel's case they are:

Daniel's eating and getting too fat should preferably not be an issue that is talked about in the family. Rather, value should be placed on lovingly preparing meals that are eaten together. Sweet drinks should be avoided. Rules for candy consumption will prevent Daniel from constantly nibbling. Such agreements can also be made between the boy and "his" pediatrician.

A varied daily routine will distract him from his need for food. If Daniel soon learns to ride a bicycle, he will be able to visit his friends more often.

Ultimately, it is also important that his parents accept that their boy does not need to become an "Ichabod Crane."

2.3   The adolescent

For the sake of completeness, we shall also describe adolescence, even though we do not encounter the third seven-year cycle as frequently in pediatrics.

Puberty is like crossing a threshold. It is a time of differentiation in body, soul and spirit. Physically, in addition to reaching sexual maturity, there is a new spurt in growth. The extremities are not in proportion to the rest of the body. The adolescent looks either lanky—"skinny as a beanpole"—or heavy. He doesn't really know where to put his hands and feet.

His outward appearance does not correspond at all to how the young person feels inside. A soul still easily wounded is concealed behind some of the foolishness and cockiness. Unknown feelings make the teenager quickly fly into a rage. He often doesn't like himself—especially when pimples appear. Everything that awakens an interest in the world is now of great importance for him. In addition to becoming aware of history and experiencing nature and art, it is important that he now become practically active himself, so that he can train and test his abilities. Such experiences help him to find healthy judgement and to form his own opinions. Listlessness and boredom are "deadly," they put the young person in danger of becoming too preoccupied with himself, his wishes and moods. The authority of adults is now completely questioned, his parents' attitudes are put to the acid test and compared with his own.

The young person wants to meet people whom he himself chooses as role models, who live according to "true" values. He wants to know: "What is the world like? Where do I stand in this world?" It is precisely this phase of development that poses a major challenge for adults. How he stands in the world is now particularly important, how well-founded and consistent he can be in shaping his life and whether he can be tolerant in meeting fellow human beings who think differently. In girls—but also in boys—the more or less conscious fear of adulthood increasingly manifests itself in anorexia and/or eating addictions. Young people are characterized by the search for themselves and the meaning of life. Nutritional disorders that manifest in the third seven-year cycle are mostly symptoms of a deep inner crisis. The adolescent is afraid of taking the step to adulthood and urgently needs people or a therapy that awakens self-confidence and courage in him to overcome his fear of this threshold.

It is extremely important to recognize the symptoms in time and to add suitable people as "development workers."

Since we cannot give more detailed consideration of the typical illnesses here, we refer to the detailed work of the educator Henning Köhler on "the silent longing for home" ("Die stille Sehnsucht nach Heimkehr").[2]

Caring for and nursing young people confronts us strongly with ourselves. It depends on how worldly we are. Pubescent behavior must not prevent nurses from taking the young person seriously. The time in which certain rules were accepted solely on the basis of authority is over. The adolescent has a right to be informed about his illness. His active and responsible involvement has a health-promoting effect. Parental work also plays a major role at this age. The gap between parents and adolescents is widening and parents need to understand what is happening inside their child and why. We assume that young people are not only shaped by their environment and upbringing, but that they already began their individual path of life at birth. Since these personal intentions have a decisive influence on the person's biography, we treat the young person with interest and understanding, trusting in his core nature.

3. The professional profile of extended pediatric nursing

The work of nursing children is deepened by the recognition that we require knowledge of childhood development, that education and nursing can have healing effects if they are learned as arts of education and nursing. The individual stages of childhood development require nurses to prove themselves anew at each stage.

Let us always encounter the child with inner questions:

- Where have you come from?
- What are you dealing with through your illness?
- What developmental opportunities do you and your family have through your illness?

If we succeed in developing nursing care that is aligned with the developmental laws of childhood, then our approach will mature from purely symptom-oriented to holistic care.

We will learn to grasp the connection between the child and his or her illness, and perhaps we will also acquire an inkling of the meaning behind it. These insights and experiences will give us additional competence to advise parents regarding their questions and be understanding as we accompany them. Mutual caregiving concepts facilitate our work with parents, enabling trustful cooperation to develop.

We will bring a new self-conception to our profession.

When we work with Rudolf Steiner's idea of development, nursing care proves to be an infinitely exciting field of research.

4.   New areas of activity for pediatric nursing

The much shorter hospital stays of today present new challenges for the nursing of children. Not infrequently, children also need intensive medical care at home if, for example, they are dependent on respiration-supporting measures. This requires good cooperation between the clinic and a nursing service in order to provide all the necessary aids and equipment in the home environment in good time. The transition from hospital to home is a very sensitive process in which experienced pediatric nurses support and accompany the parents learning to care for their child. A good parent-child relationship has fundamental importance for the child's future mental and physical health.

In addition to all medical measures, it is therefore important to create space for "nesting and protecting." The focus of this cultivation of relationships is on gentle initiation of breastfeeding, intensive physical contact (e.g., "kangaroo care") and the quality of the sensory impressions to which the child is exposed.

The child finds support and security during nursing care when eye contact, speaking and action form a unity of undivided attention. This creates space for questions to the child: "Who are you? Which tasks do you bring along for yourself and your environment? What kind of support do you need?"

One concern of home nursing for children is to support parents in all their tasks, to enable them to perceive the individuality of their sick child better and better. Parents need time and patience to become "experts" in the care of their own child.

In addition, it is important to strengthen the family's psychological and social resources and provide any necessary support. This is best achieved when the professional groups involved—such as doctors, pediatric nurses, educators, therapists and social workers—work together and place the needs of the family at the center of their care.

A further area of responsibility in pediatric nursing has opened up as a result of the continuing trend towards inclusion. More children needing intensive medical care, such as tracheostoma or oxygen administration, can now attend regular kindergartens and schools, accompanied by a pediatric nurse. In addition to medical and nursing responsibilities, pediatric nurses now have pedagogical tasks in the large field of social interaction.

A genuine art of nursing can mature when we successfully extend nursing care with our knowledge of children and healthy development.

Category	Example learning objectives	Recommended learning path
Relationships	You can advise parents on how to care for their sick children.	B
Your own learning objective		
Knowledge	You evaluate a child's illnesses against the background of his development.	C
Your own learning objective		

References

1 Steiner, R. *Educating children today.* Rudolf Steiner Press, London 2008.
2 Köhler, H. Die stille Sehnsucht nach Heimkehr. *Zum Verständnis der Pubertätsmagersucht.* Verlag Freies Geistesleben, Stuttgart 2008.

Further reading

- Glöckler, M.; Goebel, W.; Michael K. *A Waldorf guide to children's health. Illnesses, symptoms, treatments and therapies.* Floris Books, Edinburgh 2018.
- Glöckler, M. *Elternsprechstunde.* Verlag Urachhaus, Stuttgart 2014.
- Holtzapfel, W. *Krankheitsepochen der Kindheit.* Fischer Taschenbuch Verlag, Frankfurt am Main 1988.
- Pikler, E. *Friedliche Babys–zufriedene Mütter. Pädagogische Ratschläge einer Kinderärztin.* Verlag Herder, Freiburg im Breisgau 2009.
- Pikler, E. *Lasst mir Zeit–Die selbstständige Bewegungsentwicklung des Kindes bis zum freien Gehen.* Pflaum Verlag, Munich 2001.
- Pikler, E. *Miteinander vertraut sein–Erfahrungen und Gedanken zur Pflege von Säuglingen und Kleinkindern.* Arbor Verlag, Freiamt 2014.
- Soldner, G.; Stellmann H.M. *Individual paediatrics. Physical, emotional and spiritual aspects of diagnosis and counseling.* Wissenschaftliche Verlagsgesellschaft, Stuttgart 2014.

CHAPTER XVIII
Psychiatric Nursing

KLAUS ADAMS

→   Learning objectives, see end of chapter

1. General psychiatric nursing and elements of anthroposophically extended psychiatric nursing

Nearly everyone
confuses you a little –
because he has an I
for every future

Theowill Übelacker[1]

"Psychiatric nursing takes its starting point from the person's everyday life, the people around him, his life story and illness history, and his abilities and limits. Nurses use body-oriented practical access routes, joint activities, conversations and medical and nursing measures. The primary objectives of psychiatric care are to:
- restore and expand the patient's relationship to himself and his environment,
- expand social skills, especially everyday skills,
- foster self-determination, personal responsibility and autonomy,
- help him to learn coping strategies."[2]

1.1   Nursing as relationship work

Psychiatric nursing is primarily relationship work. People affected by psychiatric illness must be accepted as mature partners. We perceive them, show interest and are open for encounters. This facilitates the development of trusting relationships.

It is important to give the patient time to build a relationship—not to pressure him—to let him arrive, to be noticeably there. The quality of active listening plays an important role. Nursing gestures (such as helping the person's being to appear) characterize the attitudes needed [→ Chapter "The Concept of Nursing Gestures as a Model for Nursing Care"].

The nurse is asked to actively deal with how psychiatry is seen in society in addition to developing her understanding of the professional role of the nurse. What is normal? What does it mean to be mentally ill? Why are mentally ill people still stigmatized today (public stigmatization, self-stigmatization, structural stigmatization, e.g., discrimination regarding eligibility for health insurance)?[3]

How do I stand on ethics? Do I use coercive measures to protect patients at risk of suicide? How are we to evaluate such things?

Nursing in inpatient settings includes both working with groups and accompanying individual people in targeted ways. Primary nursing provides the framework for empathic individual support for each patient. A confused person needs orientation (nursing gesture: creating order), a patient who feels inferior seeks to be valued (nursing gesture: nourishing), an anxious, insecure person wants to be accepted (nursing gestures: affirming, enveloping), a suicidal patient needs a safe place (nursing gesture: protecting). It is important to build a sustainable relationship beyond the initial encounter. Our accompaniment throughout the day is shaped between closeness and distance, relieving and challenging, individuality and adaptation, as well as protection and confrontation.

1.2   Milieu therapy and psychoeducation

The external framework for this work is provided by milieu therapy[4], e.g., participating in groups with common meals, morning and evening circles and activity groups. There are a variety of opportunities for encounters in which people can practice respectful, healing cooperation. In addition, nurses conduct therapy groups, e.g., for psychoeducation[5] or social competence training, to support those affected in dealing with their illness.

Example

The psychoeducation group "Depression" at the Friedrich Husemann Clinic (an anthroposophic clinic for psychiatry and psychotherapy in Buchenbach, near Freiburg im Breisgau, Germany).

Sessions begin with a presentation of the clinical picture of a particular illness, the ways it can develop, and the medications that can be used. In the discussion that follows, participants are asked to report on such things as their symptoms, possible causes of their illness and their experiences with treatment. This is followed by an open exchange about typical depressive thought patterns and experiences with different treatments. We encourage patients to know their medications, gather experiences through the clinic's regular daily structure, inner exercises and walks, and draw up personal prevention plans (crisis plans). In addition to appreciating the information provided, participants particularly value the opportunity to talk with other affected people.

Nursing staff are responsible for these groups at the Friedrich Husemann Clinic (exception: doctors explain the medications). This places high demands on the nurses. In addition to having general knowledge of the clinical picture, it requires an ability to moderate and lead a group. It is absolutely desirable to do the presentations in pairs. You can give each other feedback, and inexperienced colleagues can learn from more experienced ones.

In addition to presenting information and perceiving group dynamics, it is important to maintain a conducive overall atmosphere, because with the topic of depression there is always the danger that the mood will become too "heavy"— not only when talking about suicidal tendencies.

For patients, the psychoeducation group is an important part of their therapy— they learn a new way of dealing with their illness, especially if they can classify their suffering as a symptom of depression, including physical problems (especially pain).

Interdisciplinary cooperation between the various professions (doctors, nurses, social workers and therapists) helps with the complex life situations of those affected. The daily work is founded on a comprehensive knowledge of disorder-specific nursing care concepts.[6, 7, 8] Salutogenesis, resilience, empowerment and recovery are health science models and concepts that are intended to bring about the ability to positively influence one's own health.[9]

1.3   Cultivating rhythm, a daily structure, seasonal activities and annual festivals

Biographies are rhythmic. Phases of incarnating into the body are followed by phases of maturity and then degeneration. Seven-year rhythms mark physical, mental and spiritual stages of development through which the 'I' gradually integrates itself into body and soul (incarnation) and detaches itself again (excarnation). A rhythmic lifestyle not only strengthens physical health, it offers a model of incarnation and excarnation. Each day is integrated into the time structure of the week, the month and the year. It is divided into two halves: day and night, with the transitions of morning and evening (sun and moon).

People live between the polarities of waking and sleeping, getting up and going to bed. It is good to have three meals. There are phases of movement and rest, work and leisure. Times of being alone and times with others. In addition, there is everyday life and there are festivals that relate to both the world of the senses and the world of spirit.

In psychiatric patients, the day/night rhythm is often massively disturbed (day/ night reversal). Many suffer from difficulties in falling asleep and sleeping through the night. This is precisely why it is so important to give a rhythmic structure to the course of the day. Rhythmic structuring of the day and year strengthens psychiatric patients.

Example

In the free discussion group of a closed ward, the patients were very upset about the daily routine and the rules they were supposed to observe. They felt patronized and this increasingly escalated into emotional attacks. I listened to what they had to say and looked for ways to bring the discussion circle to a constructive conclusion. I asked the patients for a final round on the subject: what is my daily routine at home? The mood changed immediately and some of them, crying, said that they lacked a daily structure and suffered a lot because of it. This insight led to gratitude for the daily routine on the ward, which gives inner support. The exercise ended with the conclusion that the ability to structure the day is at the core of the personality.

In addition, occupying oneself with the course of the year opens up a greater healthful perspective. Rudolf Steiner described the course of the year as the earth's respiratory process.[10] Annual festivals, which contain forward-looking references to the spiritual development of the world and the human being, are embedded in the earth's breathing process.

Celebrating the annual festivals (Easter–St. Johns Day–Michaelmas–Christmas) offers nice opportunities to become active in many ways. In the inpatient setting of the Friedrich Husemann Clinic there are groups of nurses and patients who meet regularly to prepare the festivals.

Based on the seasons (spring–summer–autumn–winter) we talk about our current "encounters with nature": "What catches my attention in nature today? What can I marvel at?" (Weather: warm/cold, wet/dry, fog, rain, snow, clouds, light, air, smell, stars, plants, animals, etc.)

A second set of questions is directed at our own experience. "How do I feel at this time of year? What do I like? What do I not appreciate? What is characteristic about this season?"

The third level refers to the annual festivals and requires a certain degree of tact. People often lack their own independent connection to the festivals, or it has been overshadowed by negative experiences. The patient group is usually "multicolored" culturally. It takes situational empathy to combine the characteristics of nature and personal experience with the motifs of the annual festivals.

Festival	Motif
Easter	External sprouting and burgeoning— inwardly death and birth
St. John's Day (June 24)	Outwardly going along with the sun, the highest position of the sun— inwardly changing direction ("He must increase, but I must decrease.")[11]
Michaelmas (September 29)	Nature withers externally, seems to be dying— inwardly not dying, but there is a growing power of self-awareness, grappling with the "dragon" within.
Christmas (December 25)	Externally cold, snow, dark— inwardly, the "birth of the World Redeemer"

Chart: The annual festivals and their motifs

It takes courage and a personal connection with the annual festivals to bring this topic into open groups. Songs, stories, fairy tales, poems, pictures and plays offer many possibilities for approaching the respective themes together. A festive table[12] with flowers, a picture and collected materials, as well as handicrafts and baked goods can provide links to the season. A celebration arranged together can strengthen the festive character very much, e.g., through making music, singing, contemplating a picture, a poem and free discussion.

1.4   External applications

External applications offer various possibilities for supporting people who are grappling with psychiatric illness. Often the well-being of the affected people is clearly improved by the treatment, enabling them to come to themselves and feel themselves. Where there is tension, external applications help to relax, where there is physical heaviness, they convey lightness, and where there are dissociative states they strengthen the experience of one's own body boundaries.

Warming through plays an important role, but there can also be cool applications. Compresses, baths and Rhythmical Einreibung according to Wegman/Hauschka are used both for ongoing treatment and to meet acute needs.

The type of application (e.g., liver or kidney compress) and the substance to be applied (e.g., yarrow or ginger) depend on the constitution of the patient and/or her mental condition. If changeable emotions or emotional states of tension predominate, we are more likely to choose a ginger kidney treatment. If compulsive abstract thoughts predominate, we aim to treat the lungs. If the person is rather inhibited and exhausted,

SPECIALIZATIONS IN NURSING

we administer a yarrow liver compress [Instructions → Chapter "From the Question of Meaning in Cancer to the Cultivation of the Senses"].

Many patients suffer from sleep disorders and experience worried, anxious moods before falling asleep, which can be alleviated with *Aurum/Lavandula comp.* cream (Weleda) heart compresses. The person can sleep better. Other sleep-promoting applications are:

Footbaths, with	
Mustard powder (pharmacy)	To support the patient in letting go and coming to himself
Lavender Relaxing Bath Milk (Weleda) or *Moor Lavender Calming Bath Essence* (Dr. Hauschka)	To promote relaxation in case of nervous tension

Rhythmical Einreibung of the feet, with	
Red Copper Ointment (WALA) or *Cuprum metallicum praeparatum 0.4% ointment* (Weleda)	Has a strong warming effect and relaxes deep into the body
Lavender 10% oil (Weleda), *Lavandula, Oleum aethereum 10%* (WALA) or *Solum oil* (WALA)	To relax and envelop in case of nervous tension

1.5 Soul exercises (attention and mindfulness)

[→ Section "3. Soul exercises"]

Soul Exercises are therapeutic measures in nursing care that invite the patient to engage in targeted, regular practice. The person seeking help can find invigoration and security in contemplating an object, a plant, an image, the weather, the day, in listening to sounds, in hearing birdsong, in smelling, touching, balancing. These can be individual and group exercises. The patients are guided to practice on their own or we do the exercises together with them.[13]

1.6 Dealing with medications

Medications have a high priority in psychiatry. Treatment with psychotropic drugs (neuroleptics, antidepressants, tranquilizers, hypnotics, etc.) requires the nurse to acquire a general overview of their effects (desired and undesired) in order to be able to accompany the patient in a targeted manner and administer them exactly as needed.

With anthroposophic medications—whether oral, injected or applied externally—the nurse's task is to establish an inner relationship with the mineral, herbal or animal substances used, that is, to consciously support the healing process.

1.7 Work with the twelve nursing gestures

Part of the work of psychiatric nursing is to cultivate intensive relationships with patients. We can support patients with the help of nursing gestures. If the person's 'I' is responsive, e.g., in people with anxiety or personality disorders, we are more likely to consider using activating gestures (from stimulation to uprightness). If the 'I' is barely responsive, e.g., in people with severe depression or severe psychosis, we use substituting gestures (helping the being to appear until balance is restored) [→ Chapter "The Concept of Nursing Gestures as a Model for Nursing Care"].

Example

A 47-year-old woman with recurrent depressive and post-traumatic stress disorder, with flashbacks, suffered from chronic sleep disorders and was suicidal. Her thinking went around in circles, her feelings were easily vulnerable, she closed herself off and she wanted to be asked. Her will was constrained, and she withdrew. The patient was treated on the closed ward (nursing gesture: protecting). Heart compresses with *Aurum/Lavandula comp. cream* (Weleda) and Rhythmical Einreibung treatments of her back were used to relax her and promote sleep (nursing gesture: enveloping). The aim of the treatment was to stabilize the patient so that she could subsequently undergo trauma treatment (nursing gesture: uprightness).

1.8 The therapeutic attitude

"Nursing care is apparently an activity that is essentially aimed at ensuring the basal therapeutic milieu. Although nurses also use specific therapeutic instruments, they do not do so primarily to treat patients, but to facilitate the basic therapy (of all therapists, doctors and nurses) or to enable patients to make constructive use of their inpatient stay in psychiatry. This creation of a therapeutic milieu is an "activity mediating between the patient and therapy."[14]

The psychiatrist Friedrich Husemann[15] (1887–1959), founder of the Friedrich Husemann Clinic now named after him, wrote in 1929 in a letter to friends:

"Based on our experience we can say: [...] anthroposophy creates the atmosphere of peace and trust in the spiritual world which in a sense must be the atmosphere of a healing institution, right into the shaping of practical life, right into apparent outward appearances. Such an atmosphere makes it possible to build a bridge

of trust, understanding and helpfulness from person to person, the absence of which is noticeable in all areas today. [...] Whoever feels the positive aspect of the healing milieu will also maintain it vis-à-vis other ill people, for example, when experiencing a bad mood or a nagging wish to disturb the process of building people up. Very often guests have provided us with valuable services of this kind. I've often thought: if there were no diseases, how many positive relationships between people would never have come about! Illness always has a social task. It requires the doctor and the helper to deepen their knowledge, to increase their ability to love, and the patient to overcome their preoccupation with their own personality. So, more and more in a sanatorium the attitude can develop: illnesses are shared tasks. Of course, the ill person initially wants to become healthy for very personal reasons; but he will never be able to become whole if the desire for health remains a purely selfish one. The ill person and the healer should feel that they are participating in an objective event, in fact in the whole world process, when they transform a symptom into health."[16]

Recently, a patient in his early 30s, with paranoid hallucinatory schizophrenia and autism, was asked what he thought nurses in training should learn to prepare for ward duty. He responded: "I would teach them to respond to people, communicate, listen properly and understand, but also to explain the rules, clearly define tasks and show cohesion (between patients and nurses)."[17]

2. Anthroposophic aspects of the treatment and nursing care of common psychiatric diseases

According to Rudolf Steiner, the following fundamental aspects result from our understanding of psychiatric diseases and their treatment:[18, 19]

... it is ridiculous to use this term ('Geisteskrankheit' or 'illness of the spirit' in German) because the spirit is always healthy and incapable of falling ill. [...] What happens is that the spirit's ability to express itself is disturbed by the physical organism. There is never any real illness in the life of the spirit or soul. Symptoms appear, but that is all."[20]
"Especially in so-called psychiatric disorders, it should occur to us to implement physical methods of treatment. It may seem contradictory that spiritual science would lead, on the one hand, to physical treatment in so-called psychiatric disorders, while on the other, pointing to the soul's role in recovery from physical ailments."[21]

An expanded view of the human being arises from seeing people as beings who go through repeated lives on earth and experience destiny. Their higher selves shine over their life on earth without immersing themselves in it. The 'I' in life on earth (the everyday 'I')[22]—appears as an expression of the current individuality and may be masked or obscured by illness—but the higher 'I' cannot fall ill.

This view gives us inner strength, e.g., when dealing with a person who has severe schizophrenia, to address his healthy higher self.[23]

The patient's biography can awaken an understanding of the life context of his illness.[24, 25] Our view of the disturbances, crises and illnesses expands to a meaningful integration of them into the laws of biography[26, 27] [→ Chapter "Illness and Destiny"].

2.1 Depression

Depression is one of the affective disorders, i.e., a pathologically altered mood is at the forefront of the symptoms: too elevated in mania, too depressed in depression. The illness can be classified according to its severity (mild—moderate—severe) and the course of the illness. Sometimes psychotic or somatic symptoms occur.

The incidence of depression requiring treatment in Germany is 5 to 10% (about four to eight million people). Between 10 and 20% (8 to 12% of men, 10 to 25% of women) develop depression at some time in their lives.[28]

Besides a depressed mood, the main symptoms are inhibited thinking and drive, as well as physical-vegetative disorders (especially sleep disorders).

Depressed people are often afraid, hopeless. Their inner unease can increase to an agonizing mood of "numbness" and hopelessness. Their thinking is mostly past-oriented, unfocused, fixed on problems and brooding ("like on a hamster wheel"); sometimes delusional experiences occur (especially delusions of guilt, sin or impoverishment). Forgetfulness can develop into pseudodementia. The will seems paralyzed, the person withdraws, cannot decide, is without interest, joy and initiative; but the person can also be agitated and feel driven.

The dynamics of severe depression resemble a downward spiral in whose depths suicidality emerges. 15% of people with severe depression commit suicide, 20 to 60% have suicide attempts in their medical history and 40 to 80% suffer from thoughts of suicide during depression.[29]

To date, the causes of depression have not been fully clarified. It is believed that many different factors are involved in the development of the illness.

There is much to suggest that the epidemic prevalence of depression makes it an illness of modern times. The demands of our modern society are increasing—with fear of unemployment, stress at work, changing family life and even stress during leisure time, which can cause depression. Increasing consumption of alcohol, nicotine, psychotropic drugs or other addictive substances weakens the life of the soul.

Another point that is often overlooked is the disregard of inner rhythm. Modern technology, especially the invention of electric light, has made it possible to shift the rhythm of life. In the old days you would get up when the cock crowed and go to bed when the sun went down. Nowadays you get up in the middle of the night and go to sleep in the middle of the night. This causes a misalignment of your internal clock, which is also a trigger for depression.

The appearance of a depressed patient can be described as follows:
He is falling into heaviness, which is physically visible in his lack of uprightness. The person prefers to huddle alone and in seclusion; he often neglects body care; a cold feeling prevails. His life processes slow down.
There are many functional and physical symptoms:

- General exhaustion, fatigue
- Sleep disorders (difficulty in falling asleep and sleeping through, early awakening)
- Loss of appetite, stomach pressure, weight loss, constipation
- Headache (diffuse, oppressive, dull)
- Feeling of tightness or pressure in the throat (globus sensation) or chest
- Dizziness, flickering in front of the eyes, impaired vision
- Muscle tension
- Diffuse neuralgic pain
- Irritated bladder
- Loss of libido, impotence, frigidity
- Suspended menses
- Strong daily fluctuations of well-being (mostly a morning low)

Perception is experienced as being dull and colorless. The soul falls into darkness. The 'I' shines like a sun shrouded behind many clouds.[30]

Example 1

A 29-year-old man with thalidomide damage (dysmelia of both arms) came to an open ward for inpatient treatment with severe post-psychotic depression (condition following paranoid-hallucinatory psychosis). Previously, he had been discharged from a university hospital as "untreatable." The patient was well oriented, complained of concentration problems, heavy brooding, inhibition of drive and self-esteem problems. Socially, he withdrew very much.

He refused almost all therapies, had a pronounced morning low, which made any attempt to get him to stand up before ten o'clock impossible. The only thing that ever drove him out of bed was his nicotine addiction.

He was prescribed oil dispersion baths with *equisetum oil* (*Equisetum ex herba W 5%, Oleum* (WALA)) for stimulation and structuring, and experienced a positive effect, so that he accepted this treatment.[31] The patient received one to two baths a week over the next three months, a total of 22 baths.

The time of the baths was the only time he felt comfortable. He could not give any exact information about the effect, but he relaxed in the bathtub and his mood improved every time. After eight to ten baths there was a slight but clearly visible improvement. The patient didn't seem to be so pent-up (tense) anymore, he seemed freer and more accessible in conversation, and he developed a little more drive for artistic therapies, walking, etc. There were repeated relapses. Sleep was usually subjectively better after the baths.

Example 2

A medium-sized, stocky woman, in her early 50s, came to the open ward for treatment from another clinic with severe chronic depression. She had a heaviness in her posture, her gaze was lowered, her facial expressions were rigid, her handshake without strength, her gait dragging. She had a strong tendency to retreat into bed. Her will to live was extinguished, her husband at a loss. Various psychopharmacological treatments remained without visible success, as did a longer series of electroconvulsive treatments; she was regarded as "untreatable." Neuroleptic treatment was initiated in addition to an existing antidepressant. After clarification of her circulatory stability, the patient was prescribed a sweat bath with a subsequent series of overheating baths.[32] During the third of six baths, the patient recalled an event of abuse in her childhood. Through trusting conversations, she gradually opened herself up. She increasingly participated in the structured daily routine (common meals, therapies). Above all, the warmth therapy (baths, yarrow liver compresses) [Instructions → Chapter "From the Question of Meaning in Cancer to the Cultivation of the Senses"] and Rhythmical Einreibung of her feet with *Red Copper Ointment* (WALA), as well as human warmth in conversations and in interacting with the people on the ward, enabled her to develop a certain joie de vivre.

Example 3

A 43-year-old woman, married with two children, was about to become self-employed. She suffered from severe relapsing depressive episodes with feelings of failure and guilt, as well as strong anxiety. Disturbances in sleeping and falling asleep were a nuisance. There was no suicidal tendency. The patient came to a small closed ward after she "cracked" mentally at home—she had been discharged from an open ward one week before. Her gaze was rigid, desperate, her handshake limp, her gait slow and heavy, her posture weighted down, her self-esteem diminished. She showed a lack of self-perception and was "very much in her head." She felt "devastated," was ambivalent (e.g., about taking medication), restless, anxious and could not take any time for treatment. The patient lacked drive, had warm extremities and felt a lot of strength—but seemed to be "blocked." For the treatment she saw no goal.

She couldn't accept herself in her depression and complained a lot when talking with her husband on the telephone. The telephone contact was then limited to five minutes a day and at the same time a visit was planned for the weekend. However, this did not go well, as the patient experienced herself as if "wrapped in padding" and could not be happy about her family. Among other things she received weekly oil dispersion baths with *Melissa ex herba W 5%, Oleum* (WALA). The baths touched her very much, as she was not used to someone taking care of her. She took regular walks. Her gaze became increasingly one of seeking help. Because of sleepless nights due to strong anxiety, she received diazepam for a time. Gradually she was able to get more involved with the whole treatment. She found it difficult to purposefully carry out what she had decided to do. A written daily preview supported her with structure.

In arts and crafts therapy, she carved with increasing feeling for what she was doing. In music therapy she sang properly without being able to hear it herself.

In addition, she regularly practiced various soul exercises. During a writing exercise—*mindful handwriting*—she was able to collect herself well and saw clearly from the changes in her writing when she digressed. Her concentration was challenged more when she wrote single letters in an intentionally altered way. *Balancing* on a roof batten laid out on the ground (see soul exercises) provided her with clarity and she applied it as needed when she could not grasp herself inwardly. She practiced going forwards and backwards, even with her eyes closed. She later did the exercise regularly at home. During the *"sun book"* exercise she had a hard time finding any positive experiences ("If you don't want to discover anything, you won't find anything"). She copied a poem as an alternative. In the last two weeks of her stay she easily managed to find something positive to write down every day.

The patient experienced the rhythmic order of the day as a great support for her nightly sleep. Strengthening the lower senses [→ Chapter "From the Question of Meaning in Cancer to the Cultivation of the Senses"] gave her something to hold onto in herself. After a successful weekend stress test at home, she ended her stay after two months with great gratitude. A few months later she reported that the positive effect of the treatment continued and that she had become self-employed.

2.1.1 Nursing aspects for the treatment of depression

In the nursing care of depressed people, the first thing to do is to establish a sound relationship. The person may not feel worth paying attention to—our task is to draw him into everyday life (daily structure). It is important to approach the patient with understanding, to motivate him to get up and have breakfast despite a bad night's sleep. He must not remain in a brooding retreat in bed, we must work towards a clear rhythm of day and night. If exhaustion is in the foreground, though, we grant sufficient rest periods and time for lying down.

If the affected person needs support in the activities of daily life, such as drinking, eating, excretions, body care and clothing, then our loving, patient, continuous support is necessary.

Warmth and movement are key qualities. They are reflected in the nursing gestures of substituting and stimulating [→Chapter "The Concept of Nursing Gestures as a Model for Nursing Care"].

Plant observation is very helpful as an inner exercise, to experience invigoration through engaging with growth processes.

Example

A woman in her mid-50s with delusional depression retired very much to her bed. She increasingly refused to participate and only irregularly took part in artistic therapies; she seemed indifferent. For her first prescribed plant observation, I had to get her out of bed and instruct her to get a flower from the adjoining garden. Discontented, she came back with a petiolate leaf, sat down and said, "Stem, leaf," and stood up to walk away. I thanked her for her plant observation. She went to bed. Her resistance against observing plants became less with time. Her depression subsided increasingly and, at the end of her four-month treatment, plant observation had become a daily climax. She sensitively described individual plants and it turned out that she cultivated a large flower garden at her holiday home. This regular observation of plants helped her to connect more strongly with the world and to get herself moving inwardly, for which she thanked us very much when discharged.

Organ treatment focusses on the liver and gall bladder system, to overcome the stagnation and paralysis of the will.[33]

External applications aim at warming, relaxing, and releasing effects, to bring processes back into flow and to promote inner lightness. Many people find yarrow liver compresses beneficial [→ Chapter "From the Question of Meaning in Cancer to the Cultivation of the Senses"].

Example

A 56-year-old woman with severe depression, anxiety and post-traumatic stress disorder responded to the question of whether she was looking forward to the yarrow liver compress: "When I get that compress, that's the best thing—better than any conversation—I feel like a comfortably warm, contented child; I'm looking forward to the compress." She said this with a happy look.

Summary of accompanying nursing treatments

- Footbaths with *Lavender Relaxing Bath Milk* (Weleda) or *Moor Lavender Calming Bath Essence* (Dr. Hauschka) in the evenings encourage sleep. Footbaths with *Rosemary Invigorating Bath Milk* (Weleda) help patients start the day.
- Rhythmical Einreibung helps the person to feel comfortable in his body and to come to himself, e.g., through treatments of his back, feet or whole body.
- Regulation of rhythm, diet and exercise.
- On a soul level: milieu therapy, soul exercises.
- Oil dispersion baths, e.g., with *Hypericum ex herba 5%, Oleum* (WALA) encourage gentle warming.

In addition, we stimulate the patient's warmth organism by administering sweat and overheating baths, up to the point of eliciting short-term fevers.

SWEAT BATH: The patient drinks a sudorific tea (elderflower or lime blossom tea) before and during the bath. The bath lasts up to 20 minutes, the temperature is increased from 37°C (98.6°F) to a maximum of 40°C (104°F) by continuous water supply (not with the first bath). The aim is to make the patient sweat profusely. The patient is then wrapped for half an hour to a full hour in preheated cotton and flannel cloths for a post-treatment rest. After that there will be about an hour of quiet in the patient's room.

OVERWARMING BATH: The patient bathes with warm feet (possibly a footbath beforehand) at a water temperature of initially 37°C (98.6°F). After a full body brushing for hyperemia (e.g., with sisal gloves), we measure the patient's pulse and body temperature (the bath must be stopped at a pulse frequency of >150/min.). Then the water temperature is increased by one degree (1.8°F), another full body brushing is carried out and we measure pulse and temperature. This process is repeated three to four times and lasts 10 to 15 minutes. The first bath ends at a water temperature of 39°C (102.2°F). During the course of the bath series, the temperature is increased up to a maximum of 41°C (105.8°F), depending on the patient's disease process and condition. The total duration of the bath should not exceed 50 minutes. The patient lies in water all the time (including the back of the head) and experiences a fever. The patient's circulation must be checked, and the patient must be closely accompanied, as the treatment often releases mental processes in the soul. After the bath, the patient is wrapped in preheated cotton and flannel cloth and rests for 45 to 60 minutes, while continuing to be cared for by the nurse. The pack is then ended, and the patient should rest in bed for about 3 to 4 hours until his elevated body temperature has dropped to normal.[34]

Overheating baths are contraindicated in the presence of cardiovascular disease such as hypertension, heart failure, coronary heart disease, cardiac arrhythmia. If in doubt, consult a doctor.

Summary of the concept for treating depression

- Therapy often includes the use of psychotropic drugs
- Treatment of the patient's constitution[35, 36] and organ building processes[37]
- Psychotherapeutic basic treatment, with individual and group therapy, psychoeducation, work with relatives, social psychiatric help, milieu therapy, work therapy, arts and crafts therapy, as well as soul exercises
- Biographical work to stimulate 'I' activity, addressing spiritual borderline experiences and making cultural offerings available[38]

The deeper meaning of depression is reflected in the following quote:

> "It is one of the most widespread misconceptions today to think that happiness, joy and health are to be understood as rewards, while misfortune, suffering and pain are a punishment of some kind. This cultural repression and negation of the supposedly negative creates an enormous psychological and social potential for

misery. The fact that suffering and grief can also become tests, challenges, insight into destiny, etc., is hardly understood or sought today. Symptomatically, the advertising of a large pharmaceutical company reads: 'Just suck the pain away.' But if one wants to experience the deeper connections between happiness and misfortune, joy and sorrow, laughter and crying, etc., then it is necessary to consider the religious and spiritual development of mankind. All these basic categories of human existence refer to the meaning of our existence and to deeper contexts of destiny, which have always been understood religiously or spiritually. Having strong faith was for the most part identical to the ability to endure suffering, sorrow and misfortune and to transform them into wisdom."[39]

2.2 Psychosis

People who suffer from psychosis show qualitative changes in consciousness. Contents alien to reality, some of which are very determining and fearful, are superimposed on everyday life. The people affected live very much in the present and are looking for support and orientation.

Their perception can be marked by hallucinations. Hearing voices and seeing things that are not there are the most common. Various delusions determine the content of the person's thoughts, e.g., delusions of persecution or impairment, relationship delusions, religious delusions, megalomania and love delusions. Delusions are characterized by the fact that the person's judgement about the world is pathologically disturbed; they occur with subjective certainty and regardless of experience. In addition, the experience of the self can be disturbed, e.g., thought insertion, thought withdrawal, thought diffusion, depersonalization, derealization and autism. Disturbances of the 'I' are ones in which the 'I'-like nature of experience is changed or in which the boundary between self and the environment appears permeable.[40]

The person's thinking can be disjointed, it can come to the point where thinking breaks down or is blocked. In the area of feeling, the affected person is sometimes not very present and seems to be withdrawn. The following can also occur: internal and external agitation, emotional impoverishment, inappropriate affects, distrust, dysphoria, irritability, aggressive tension, anxiety, panic, lame behavior, euphoric and depressive moods. Drive and action are often strongly disturbed: interest reduction, apathy, stereotypes, agitation, mannerisms, stupor, mutism, and catalepsy. The person's actions may be dominated by imperative voices that pose a great threat regarding suicidal tendencies. Very unpleasant symptoms include coenesthesias (body hallucinations). In addition, there are often vegetative symptoms: sleep disturbances are frequent, as well as lack of appetite (e.g., in case of poisoning delusions), etc.

In addition to organic and affective psychoses, the term psychosis also includes individual psychotic episodes that do not become chronic. The word schizophrenia stands for a chronic form of psychotic disorder. The three main types of schizophrenic psychosis are paranoid-hallucinatory schizophrenia (where delusions and hallucinations are in the foreground), elevated schizophrenia (affective changes) and catatonic schizophrenia (psychomotor disorders such as agitation or numbness). The symptoms are very different and varied.

About one percent of people suffer from schizophrenia in the course of their lives.

Example

A 20-year-old slim, tall man, of leptosomic body type, came to the closed ward with paranoid-hallucinatory schizophrenia. He neglected his everyday life, no longer took part in his studies and was highly sensitive to any outside influence. He often threw himself on the ground and demanded freedom. He was living in delusional misjudgment. He crowded us nurses at the exit door. He refused all medication. He was willing to allow Rhythmical Einreibung and received a full-body treatment with *Lavender 10% oil* (Weleda) three times a week before lunch. This brought him back to himself, he became calm and relaxed for about two hours. Then his restlessness and feelings of compulsion came back. After about three weeks, he asked the doctors to free him from his horrible states. Now he accepted neuroleptics and was able to participate in artistic therapies. He was grateful for the medication. One Sunday morning, instead of going to a scheduled cultural event, he took advantage of an opportunity to escape and took the train home. He continued to adhere to his objective of undergoing rehabilitation measures.

2.2.1 Nursing aspects in the treatment of psychoses

The focus of nursing activities for people suffering from psychosis is on everyday support. These patients often lack insight into their illness. In experiencing the symptoms, they usually circle in fixed ideas, partly out of delusion. Others are diverted by their experience of hallucinations. Some people talk about the content of their hallucinations; others are very guarded and don't like to be pressed with questions. Perhaps a voice forbids them to communicate what they are experiencing. The key often lies in building relationships based on trust, especially through repeated brief encounters. Having a fixed reference person creates security. People are often very truthful, and they feel whether the other person is too. They appreciate reliability. If, for example, you forget an appointment, they often hold back, but are grateful if you speak to them later and apologize. Your apology is an expression of a respectful attitude that schizophrenic people often miss. In conversation, it is important to express oneself clearly, which helps patients to orient themselves in their efforts to be realistic, despite their concentration difficulties. During the conversation one should pay attention to the ability of the other person to concentrate. Shorter but regular conversations have proven helpful. It is important to integrate the other person lovingly into everyday life, to meet him openly and to perceive him consciously. Concrete questions should be addressed, such as by talking about action-oriented plans for the day (e.g., tasks in the ward, walks, handicrafts, games).

If the patient neglects his or her personal hygiene, it helps to address the problem during individual contact and to define meaningful action in concrete terms (e.g., showering every two days).

In the acute phase of psychosis, we use substituting nursing gestures: relieving, protecting, enveloping, creating order and nurturing. The affected person often seeks the 'I' of the person accompanying him as support!

In psychotherapy, it is fundamental to have a sustainable patient-doctor relationship and the involvement of relatives. The treatment is supportive and structuring. It attempts to develop an understanding of the illness that leads to a realistic self-image and shows patients their own possibilities for action. Psychoeducation in groups has increasingly proven itself in recent years.[41]

However, if the psychotically ill person experiences his delusions (e.g., delusions of love) or hallucinations as pleasant, he may block treatment for years.

The soul exercise of *observing objects* challenges the person to describe outer forms in a structured way. This exercise helps psychotically ill people to find clarity within themselves. The soul exercise of the *daily review* gives the opportunity to connect with the experience of the day, by the patient telling the nurse what happened that day—possibly only in key words.

External applications allow the psychotically ill person to feel noticeably present in his body. *Mustard powder calf compresses* "anchor" the upwardly flighty person into his corporeality.[42]

Example

A young man with paranoid hallucinatory schizophrenia became acutely delusional one Sunday morning. He was very agitated and occupied with his delusions. Instead of applying an additional neuroleptic dose, the doctor ordered a mustard powder calf compress. Already after two minutes the patient's gaze cleared up, he looked at me in a relaxed way and talked realistically. Afterwards he went to the cultural event and remained in a state of conscious clarity.

Mustard powder foot baths also cause the person to come into his corporeality, they calm him and are thereby sleep-promoting. A footbath with

- *Lavender Relaxing Bath Milk* (Weleda)

- *Moor Lavender Calming Bath Essence* (Dr. Hauschka)

has a relaxing effect on nervous restlessness and helps the person to fall asleep. A compress with

- *Plumbum metallicum praeparatum 0.4% ointment* (Weleda)

as a "plumbum cap" (plumbum ointment cloth on the head (parietal region))[43] helps patients with a strong opening "upwards" to shield themselves from psychotic influences. In cases of severe inner restlessness, excitement and tension, a

- Mustard *powder kidney compress*

helps the patient to relax. A compress with

- *Aurum/Lavandula comp. cream* (Weleda)

helps the patient to fall asleep. Patients have very positive experiences with Rhythmical Einreibung treatments, if they can accept them. An evening Rhythmical Einreibung of the feet, with

- *Red Copper Ointment* (WALA)

- *Lavender 10% oil* (Weleda)

- *Lavandula, Oleum aethereum 10%* (WALA)

or a rhythmical Einreibung treatment of the back, with

- *Solum oil* (WALA)

- *Blackthorn Toning Body Oil* (Dr. Hauschka)

helps people to come back to themselves. Whole-body Rhythmical Einreibung, e.g., with

- *Lavender 10% oil* (Weleda)

- *Lavandula, Oleum aethereum 10%* (WALA)

- *Solum oil* (WALA)

- *Blackthorn Toning Body Oil* (Dr. Hauschka)

causes an even stronger experience of being fully present in oneself. Overall, the aim is to achieve warming enveloping, deeper breathing and a feeling of well-being.

2.2.2 Therapeutic aspects

Targeted neuroleptic treatment reduces the symptoms in individual cases to a symptom-free status. The more recent neuroleptics (e.g., Quetiapine (*Seroquel*), Olanzapine (*Zyprexa*), Aripiprazole (*Abilify*)) have significantly fewer extrapyramidal motor side effects than first-generation neuroleptics (e.g., Butyrophenone (Haloperidol), Phenothiazine (Promethazin)). In addition to vegetative side effects, metabolic disorders such as obesity can also occur.

Anthroposophic medications have a supporting effect, eurythmy therapy is healing right into the body, e.g., via the holding quality of the sound 'B'.

In arts and crafts therapy, the structuring aspect is in the foreground, which is directly given in the activities of weaving and braiding. In drawing therapy, the drawing of forms helps to structure, in sculpting it is the work on platonic solids (tetrahedron, hexahedron, octahedron, dodecahedron, icosahedron).

Work therapy that neither demands too much nor too little provides meaningful integration into the world for psychotically ill people. Especially gardening and agricultural activities offer various possibilities.

Social workers deal with questions that concern work, housing and finances. Clarifying matters in these areas is a great help. It is important to focus on continued care at an early stage in order to initiate targeted measures as far as possible. Rehabilitation, assisted living or day-structuring activities (e.g., in day-care centers) must be clarified—unfortunately the waiting periods for people seeking help are often months long.

Treatment usually leads to an easing of the illness rather than complete healing. It is a great challenge for those affected to accept the illness as part of their lives. Sometimes this causes deep humility and modesty towards life.

Anthroposophic points of view on schizophrenic psychoses are very complex and will be given here to a certain extent, using excerpts from an essay by the psychiatrist Wolfgang Rissmann:[44]

> *In delusional life, the human power of judgement appears altered and subdued, meaningful human action is made more difficult, and in extreme cases can lead to neglect, suicide or acts of aggression against others. The power of judgement is one of the central abilities through which human beings establish their humanity. It is an immediate expression of 'I'-activity. In the process of judging, the 'I' realizes itself and creates a bridge to reality. [...] Disturbed formations of judgement therefore always have bodily reasons in pathological changes of the etheric body—or, more precisely expressed—in incorrectly performed reflections of the 'I' in the etheric body. [...] The immediate impression indicates that the 'I' has lost control over the processes of the soul and over the body. Thinking, feeling and willing become independent and lose their connection. Physically, there are vegetative changes, such*

as appetite disorders and sleep disorders. The upright gait is discreetly altered in such a way that it appears too light or the movements are not guided by the 'I' [...] According to Steiner's explanations in the 13th lecture of his first medical course (1920), the brain is actually affected. [...] However, Steiner emphasizes that the brain disorder is not primary but secondary in nature. He sees the primary causes in the metabolic processes of the organs of the lower human being, above all in the processes of the lungs, liver, kidneys and heart. Steiner speaks of 'organ formation processes' that are disturbed. This does not refer to the biochemical metabolism of the organs or even anatomical-histological organ structures, but to the processes that continuously maintain organ structures and organ physiology. These are the etheric formative processes in interaction with the physical force structure of the organs. Biochemical metabolic processes are the result of these image processes.[45]

These organ-building processes—according to Steiner—become defective, the etheric formative power of the organs does not remain active in the organ, it is squeezed out like a sponge and floods the life of soul. So, when we have psychopathological processes of hallucinations, delusions, states of excitement, etc., we are dealing with dislocated image forces of the organs. This is where the primary processes of the disease process lie. The etheric spiritual aspect of the organs has entered the soul space and thus comes to consciousness in a pathological way. [...] What does such illness mean for the destiny of the person affected, who struggles throughout his life for the maintenance of his 'I'-consciousness, who lives continuously between delusion and reality and who is constantly hindered in his ability to make judgements? What are the underlying causes? What inner abilities are being developed in this way for the future? Such questions arise directly in dealing with those affected. [...] Psychotic delusional experiences and also spiritual experiences are an existential challenge of one's own power of judgement. A comparison between psychosis and spiritual experiences sharpens our view for both fields of human experience, which deviate from usual everyday consciousness and represent borderline experiences. Throughout his oral and written work, Steiner never tires of presenting the cultivation of healthy judgement as the central task of contemporary human beings. Anthroposophy can help with this."

When examining the clinical picture of psychosis, the question of normality arises. Where does illness begin? What connection do I have to spirituality? Consider the following patient description:

"After a lecture about Saint Brigid from Ireland, a group of patients fell silent when I joined them. I address the silence and a man suffering from paranoid-hallucinatory schizophrenia responds: "There's talk of visions, but when I report my experiences in the rounds, my neuroleptics are increased."

"There is no life without fear of the other; because without this fear, which is our depth, there is no life; only from the nothingness that we suspect do we understand for moments that we are alive. You enjoy your muscles, you enjoy walking, you enjoy the light that reflects in your dark eye, you enjoy your skin and the nerves that make you feel so much, you enjoy yourself and with every breath you breathe you know that everything that is, is grace. Without this mirroring wakefulness, which is only possible out of fear, we would be lost; we would never have been..."

Max Frisch (1911–1991)[46]

Fear is a feeling and it belongs to human development to a high degree. It calls on us to be more vigilant when we find ourselves in dangerous situations. Fear can intensify to such an extent that it reaches the level of an illness, and the person suffers from it and is only able to cope with everyday life to a limited extent. Fear focuses on the future by expecting the bad, the danger, the punishment, etc., and prevents the patient from being present in the present. In addition to mental symptoms, a variety of physical symptoms occur.

Basically, there are five types of anxiety disorders:

- People who suffer from *agoraphobia* are afraid of large open spaces, crowds, or situations in which they leave their familiar surroundings (traveling, driving, etc.). Their avoidance behavior can lead to being isolated in their home. Agoraphobia is often combined with a panic disorder.
- People who suffer from a *social phobia* are afraid of situations in which they may be the focus of attention. They blush easily, usually avoid eye contact, tremble and sweat, have an urge to urinate and suffer from nausea. They know that their fear is exaggerated and unfounded. They often tend to exhibit pronounced avoidance behavior.
- People suffering from *specific phobias* are afraid of certain objects and situations: certain animals, e.g., spiders or dogs, fear of heights, claustrophobia (fear of staying in closed rooms, such as elevators), fear of thunderstorms, etc. Their fear of the phobic object increases with approach and those affected tend to avoid it. A diagnosis is only made in cases of considerable suffering.
- People with a *panic disorder* suffer from recurring panic attacks that occur suddenly and not in specific situations. They experience strong fear, with sweating, tachycardia, palpitations, chest pain, choking, dizziness, feelings of alienation, fear of death, etc. The symptoms can resemble a heart attack, which is why those affected are repeatedly taken to the emergency room. Panic attacks usually last from ten to thirty minutes, but they can also last for two minutes or for hours. They often lead to fear of fear.

- People suffering from a *generalized anxiety disorder* have a general and long-lasting anxiety that is not limited to specific situations; it is free floating. The person is marked by unrealistic fears, he worries, is tense, and is vegetatively overstimulated.

Fifteen percent of people fall ill with an anxiety disorder in the course of their lives. Women are affected twice as often as men. Anxiety disorders often occur in combination with other illnesses, such as depression and addiction. Anxiety disorders are often only diagnosed after many years (five to fifteen).

> *"All alone, I climbed up to the highest part of the cathedral tower and sat in its so-called 'neck,' under the knop or 'crown,' as it is named, for a good quarter of an hour, until I dared to go back out in the open air and stand on a platform that is hardly a yard square and has hardly any handhold. [...] I exposed myself to similar fears and torments often enough so that I became quite indifferent to the impression they made, and later during geological studies on mountain journeys, and on tall buildings, I raced over exposed beams and cornices with carpenters [...] having gained great advantage from those exercises."*
> J. W. von Goethe (1749–1832): Poetry and Truth[47]

Anxious people often look younger than they are and seem graceful. They take great care of their appearance. When encountering other people, they initially remain noncommittal. It is difficult for them to get involved in new situations, e.g., in a hospital ward. Thus, in addition to building a relationship, the nurse's work initially consists in supporting then in arriving and in adapting to their new daily structure. This includes mandatory participation in ward activities (e.g., common meals, morning circles) and agreed therapies.

Anxiety manifests in many physical and mental symptoms. The following vegetative disorders frequently occur:

- Breath: pressed, held—accelerated, flat
- Blood pressure: hypertension—hypotension
- Pain: palpitations, racing heart, heart pains
- Redness, paleness, warmth, cold
- Muscle tension: trembling, eye spasms, rigidification
- Sweating (possibly cold sweating)
- Salivation—dry mouth
- Urinary retention—increased urination
- Bowel movements: constipation—diarrhea
- Diet: no appetite or eating much too fast, with subsequent stomach pain
- Sleep: disturbances in falling asleep and sleeping through
- Nausea, vomiting, abdominal discomfort
- Dizziness, weakness

Possible mental disturbances:

- Perception: objects are more and more lost sight of or else overvalued.
- Thinking: empty, confused–fixed
- Feeling: constricted–unwound
- Willing: rigor–flight

Overall, tendencies towards powerlessness, fear and flight are discernible.

2.3.1 Nursing aspects in the treatment of anxiety disorders

The symptoms of anxiety disorders result in a broad spectrum of external applications: Rhythmical Einreibung as partial or full-body treatments with various oils and ointments, footbaths with mustard powder or bath additives, full baths as oil dispersion baths (e.g., with *Melissa ex herba W 5 %, Oleum* (WALA)).

BATH ADDITIVES:

- *Rosemary Invigorating Bath Milk* (Weleda)

- *Lavender Relaxing Bath Milk* (Weleda)

- *Moor Lavender Calming Bath Essence* (Dr. Hauschka)

- *Citrus Refreshing Bath Milk* (Weleda)

- *Lemon Lemongrass Vitalising Bath Essence* (Dr. Hauschka)

Ginger kidney compresses [→ Chapter "From the Question of Meaning in Cancer to the Cultivation of the Senses"] and *Aurum/Lavandula comp. cream* (Weleda) heart compresses are often used. Cool citrus wrist wraps help with acute anxiety.

INSTRUCTIONS: Add 5 ml *Citrus Refreshing Bath Milk* (Weleda) or fresh lemon juice to 200 ml water (body temperature, or cooler when the patient's hands are warm). Then soak two cotton cloths (about 8 cm wide) in the lemon water, wring them out moderately and wrap them around the patient's wrists. Cover the damp inner cloths with approx. 12 cm wide flannel cloth and attach in place with sticking plaster. Now the patient can go about his activities and, when necessary, replace the inner cloth when it has dried out.

Pentagram Rhythmical Einreibung, with

■ *Aurum/Lavandula comp. cream* (Weleda)

brings the patient to himself in a beautiful way [→ Chapter "Rhythmical Einreibung According to Wegman/Hauschka"].

Soul exercises specifically support people with anxiety disorders. Fear phenomena occur because the 'I' is not properly anchored in the body. Thus, the patient first needs to practice using the lower senses[48], to give the 'I' steadiness and security in the body. Exercises such as *tactile perception, balancing, juggling* and *rod exercises* are particularly suitable for this.

> ### Example
>
> A 60-year-old, depressed, anxious woman comes to her first *tactile perception exercise*. She avoids eye contact. I show her how to do the exercise. She remains tense and thinks that she can't do it well. She closes her eyes and I give her an object. She describes a few tactile impressions and then falters. With the help of calm, targeted questioning, she becomes increasingly involved in the exercise and can describe her tactile perceptions in more detail. At the end of the exercise she looks at me and is amazed that she has become quite calm.

In addition, we need to support the patient's rhythmic processes, whereby any rhythmic activity is helpful. A good exercise is conscious, rhythmically swinging walking, which also leads to deeper breathing.

Writing exercises, plant observation, picture contemplation and other soul exercises promote the presence of the 'I' through the effort of attention and concentration, thus strengthening inner clarity.

Among the nursing gestures, the gesture of *awakening* is primary. The person affected by the anxiety disorder must recognize himself in his fear, see through his avoidance strategies and be prepared to actively overcome his fears. In this way he can come back to himself and feel strengthened. In addition to awakening, we use the nursing gestures of *challenging* and *stimulating* to persuade the patient to practice concretely. A trusting relationship must be established and is the basis for making demands on an ill person.

2.3.2 Therapeutic aspects

SSRI antidepressants (selective serotonin reuptake inhibitors) are used. *Bryophyllum 50% powder* (Weleda) is a proven support in cases of anxiety.

Psychotherapy is an important pillar of treatment, especially behavioral therapy with exposure training.

Our lives are constantly changing from childhood to old age, from birth to death. It is challenging to deal with change. Fear shows us that in our 'I' we do not yet have the strength to cope with the demands. Questions arise that are greater than our answers.

Grappling with them is one of our elementary life tasks. As human beings we can actively support each other in this process of searching.

The times are all so wretched!
The heart, so full of cares!
The future, far outstretched,
A spectral horror wears.

Wild terrors creep and hover
With foot so ghastly soft!
Our souls black midnights cover
With mountains piled aloft.

Firm props like reeds are waving,
For trust is left no stay;
Our thoughts, like whirlpool raving,
No more the will obey!

Frenzy, with eye resistless,
Decoys from Truth's defense;
Life's pulse is flagging listless,
And dull is every sense.

Who hath the cross upheaved
To shelter every soul?
Who lives, on high received,
To make the wounded whole?

Go to the tree of wonder;
Give silent longing room:
Issuing flames asunder
Thy bad dream will consume.

Draws thee an angel tender
In safety to the strand:
Lo, at thy feet in splendour
Lies spread the Promised Land!

Novalis (1772–1801): Translated by George MacDonald, in: MacDonald G. Rampolli. *Growths from a long planted root.* Nabu Press 2010.

2.4 Personality disorders

Personality disorders often occur in connection with other illnesses and are not easily distinguished from conspicuous personality traits.

The most common diagnosis is borderline personality disorder, which has played an increasingly important role since the middle of the last century. It can be classified as an illness between neurosis and psychosis. The people affected are "border crossers" in today's modern world. They lack inner security and orientation. Among other things, they suffer from inner conflict and massive fears of being alone. This dynamic is also reflected in their environment, e.g., when teams of colleagues providing treatment split into those who are for and those who are against the patient.

In psychological-psychiatric linguistic usage, "personality" is defined as the totality of (psychological) qualities and behavior patterns that give the individual a characteristic, unmistakable individuality of his or her own. It is a largely stable and long-lasting structure of individual characteristics in terms of character, temperament, intelligence and basic physical conditions. "Temperament" describes the kind of drive and activity that manifests in the form of feelings, will formation and drives.

"Character" refers to largely constant attitudes, ways of acting and above all values of a person throughout his or her life.

Personality disorders are deeply rooted and long-lasting behavioral patterns that manifest as rigid and non-adapting reactions in personal and social situations. Reference is made to an average norm that applies to most of the population or cultural group concerned. The deviations are particularly evident in perception, thinking, feeling and in relationships with others. This deviation from the norm is not so much a single aspect of behavior and experience, it is the way in which the behavior dominates, which can be expressed in both a lack of social adaptation and in subjective complaints.

General diagnostic guidelines for personality disorders (ICD-10 F 60):[49]

- Clear imbalance in attitudes and behavior in multiple functional areas, such as affectivity, drive, impulse control, perception and thinking, relationships with others
- Uniform, persistent patterns of behavior not limited to episodes of mental illness
- Deeply disturbed, in many personal and social situations clearly inappropriate behavior patterns
- Beginning of the disorder in childhood and adolescence, permanent manifestation in adulthood
- Significant subjective suffering and/or significant impairment of occupational and social performance
- The disorder is not due to severe brain damage, brain diseases or other mental disorders

Specific personality disorders and their essential characteristics:

- Paranoid personality disorder (suspicious, quarrelsome, resentful)

- Schizoid personality disorder (emotionally cool, distant, solitary)
- Dissocial personality disorder (irresponsible, aggressive, disregarding norms)
- Emotionally unstable personality disorder (unstable mood, impulsive action regardless of the consequences)
- Histrionic personality disorder (dramatizing, theatrical, manipulative)
- Obsessive-compulsive personality disorder (conscientious, rigid, pedantic, perfectionistic)
- Anxious (avoiding) personality disorder (constantly tense, worried, insecure)
- Dependent personality disorder (weak decision-making, dependent, helpless, yielding)
- Narcissistic personality disorder (arrogance, excessive sense of greatness, need for excessive admiration)

People with an emotionally unstable personality disorder (F 60.3) have the following symptoms: unstable mood, impulsive action regardless of the consequences, lack of planning in advance, outbursts of intense anger and violent explosive behavior, triggering easily when criticized or hindered by others.

This disorder is further differentiated into two subtypes:

- *Impulsive type* (F 60.30): emotional instability and lack of impulse control are in the foreground, often violent and threatening behavior, especially when criticized by others.
- *Emotionally unstable personality disorder, borderline type* (F 60.31): The characteristics of F 60.3 and additionally: self-image, goals and preferences, even sexual ones, are unclear and disturbed, suffers from a chronic feeling of inner emptiness, relationships are often intense but unstable, frequent emotional crises, suicidal, parasuicidal and other self-damaging actions, free-floating fears, dissociative reactions, depersonalization, addictive behavior and short-term psychotic decompensations.[50]

Example

A 20-year-old woman came to the closed ward for admission. She had attempted suicide with tablets and called the emergency doctor herself. In the weeks before, she repeatedly cut her arms. She hadn't talked to anyone about her suicidal tendencies. She also suffered from the persistent idea of having to kill someone. She had begun her studies and moved into her own apartment but was busy with her suicide plan. A few years previously, she had undergone twelve months of psychiatric treatment.

She was very "in her head" and seemed cut off from her feelings. She was used to withdrawing and "bottling up" her problems in herself. Verbally, she sometimes acted quite aggressively as a way of massively refusing to make contact.

The patient slept poorly due to inner agitation (problems falling asleep and sleeping through) and she mostly had cold hands and feet. She drank too little and had a lack of appetite. She hadn't pursued her own interests lately.

She was initially very hostile towards taking medication, but then increasingly accepted it.

We agreed on hourly contact with her, if she didn't come, we went to her. She experienced this as giving her stability. After her acute suicidal tendency had subsided, we agreed on one contact per shift. We accompanied her during her daily routine, at meals, kept track of her drinking and went for a walk with her once a day.

She experienced the ginger lung compresses as warming and soothing. In the evening she received a Rhythmical Einreibung treatment of her feet with *Red Copper Ointment* (WALA); her perception of her feet became increasingly differentiated.

The patient could not relate to the soul exercises *review of the day* and *sun book* and only reluctantly performed them. Towards the end of her seven-week stay she took up a suggestion and memorized two poems via their pictorial content and recited them in the morning circle.

She increasingly trusted us and actively spoke to us to discuss problematic thoughts. She became more independent in the daily rhythm and her sleep improved considerably. Suicidal thoughts continued to emerge, but she was able to distance herself from them. She let her studies rest and started rehabilitation measures near the residence of one of her parents.

A person suffering from a borderline disorder is constantly searching for his center. He is suffering from a lack or absence of identity on a physical, psychological and spiritual level. The ill person is looking for orientation regarding the "thread running through his life," his choice of partner, his profession and his lifestyle. He tends to wishful thinking and lives in "friend-foe" imagery—idealizing himself and devaluing his fellow human being in alternation with idealizing his fellow human being and denigrating himself. He seeks the fault for his sense of being overwhelmed outside of himself and perceives the weaknesses of others more than clearly. A person suffering from a borderline disorder sees things in black and white—his thinking is shaped by this. He often has a low tolerance for frustration, anxiety and stress. He is very irritable; his mood is subject to an endless "roller-coaster ride." The patient suffers from various physical complaints due to increased tension. He has a poor connection with his body and his needs. Self-harm can break through his lost ability to feel himself. Some extreme consequences of this are cutting his skin with razor blades or other sharp objects, taking drugs, and high-risk activities. For the majority of those affected, serious abuse or emotional neglect are among the causes of the illness.

"In the soul there is an insurmountable abyss between the 'ideal heavenly, cosmic I' and the 'earthly, daily responsible I'. The borderline patient can connect and identify with the cosmic 'I', but not with the polar opposite earthly-active self,

who is responsible for his actions. The biographical earthly aspect is 'done to him as suffering,' it is 'not self-chosen,' it is even perceived as false, as a deception or a lie. Such non-identification leads from anger and rage against earthly-biographical aspects, through rejection of the body (in various forms of self-neglect and self-mutilation) to destructive gestures and suicide attempts, [...] with a deep longing to spiritualize earthly existence and at the same time—caused by disappointment—an inability to endure the earthly. [...] Let us turn to the second division, the one between 'inside' and 'outside': Not a few borderline personalities complain about inner emptiness. Physically, this manifests in constricted breathing or constant pain in the heart-lung area, often accompanied by cold sensations and the feeling of a gaping inner hole; a mood of death fills the person, or he feels a space full of splitting forces and in it a struggle between life and death. The 'internal/external' problem includes, as a serious phenomenon, the reversal of the relationship between the 'I' and the environment (point and circle), in such a way that the environment becomes the 'I'—the 'I' becomes the environment. The resulting social chaos affects not only the borderline personality himself, but also—and to no small degree—all of the people involved with him."[51]

2.4.1 Factors in the nursing care of people suffering from borderline illnesses

When accompanying borderline patients, nurses need a willingness to meet the other person in an open and honest manner. In developing a trusting relationship, it can be helpful to inwardly cultivate the nursing gesture of *helping the person's inner being to appear*. Otherwise, it is always about the nursing gestures of *relieving* and *uprightness*. A rhythmic daily schedule gives the patient great support. Dealing with closeness and distance must be continuously explored anew.

Example

A 32-year-old borderline patient retired to her room in a crisis. Our contact was rather difficult due to some arguments. At our last meeting before what would be my free weekend, she asked me urgently what I had planned for the weekend. I was perplexed and at first, I distanced myself, because I found the question too personal. Then I felt the need of the patient—she was so disoriented, desperate. I briefly inquired as to the reason for her question. She said that she wanted to know what a healthy person does on a weekend. I then told her my plans, she thanked me. After that, our relationship improved significantly and was sustainable even in severe crises.

Rhythmical Einreibung according to Wegman/Hauschka has great importance as an external application for this illness. Initially, it is a question of whether the patient will allow touch at all—Rhythmical Einreibung treatments of the feet or back are gradually increased up to whole-body treatments. Patients then relax better; they gain a positive connection to their body.

often provide good relaxation in the warmth that develops.

In terms of soul exercises, the lower senses come first: *balancing* and *tactile exercises*. The *writing exercise* helps many to come back to themselves. Those affected like to do it several times a day. The *review of the day* makes it possible to reflect on the day's events from a certain distance. The *sun book* can develop into a joyful companion throughout the day, it can be updated continuously.

Example

A woman in her late 30s, dressed in black leather and tattooed in several places, had experienced little care and appreciation in her childhood. Early in her life, at the age of 17, she lived alone; alcohol and changing partnerships with women shaped her everyday life. When she came under pressure, she cut herself. After years she gained more endurance, she found support through intensive fitness sports. Partnership disruptions caused some relapses. She had a lot of friends. She came without hope to an open ward for treatment during a suicidal crisis. She needed time to develop trust in her doctor and primary nurse, she felt valued and taken seriously. She often thought about her ex-partner, texted her and thereby intensified her inner turmoil. The *balancing* exercise and the whole daily structure gave her stability. She reflected on her behavior in regular conversations with her key caregiver. The *sun book* as a soul exercise struck her like lightning. It helped her get out of her narrow, negative thinking. She meticulously wrote down her "sun experiences" every day and recommended the *sun book* to people in her circle of friends. After six weeks she felt stabilized and was released with more confidence.

2.4.2 Therapeutic aspects

Medication is used for stabilization, which is usually possible with a relatively low dosage of an antidepressant or neuroleptic (side effects are often very noticeable).

The most proven method in the treatment of people with borderline personality disorders today is Dialectic Behavioral Therapy (DBT) as developed by Marsha Linehan. Abnormal behavior, e.g., self-injury, is regarded as an attempt to overcome a problem. In a very structured framework, patients are trained to deal well with their emotions and states of tension. Great importance is attached to the practice of mindfulness and targeted skills.

The aim of treatment is:
"When we look at the relationship between the 'I' and the three soul forces, the overall characteristic is that the ability of the 'I' to harmonize thinking, feeling and willing is severely impaired. The soul forces seem to be isolated; they often work against each other and block each other's effectiveness. The aim of treatment must therefore be to

strengthen the 'I' forces so that they intervene in the soul forces in an orderly and harmonizing manner."[52]

'I'-like activity is specifically promoted in arts and crafts therapy; in eurythmy therapy it affects the formation of the physical body.[53]

In our accompaniment of people with borderline disorders who have gone through severe suicidal crises, the question may arise—what gives these people the strength to still be alive? Great respect for their achievements in struggling with their biographies is expressed in the following poem:

> *Development*
> *I look back,*
> *what was there is good:*
> *the firm ground,*
> *on which everything rests.*
>
> *I look at my fate,*
> *see deep within,*
> *and I understand:*
> *What is, must be.*
>
> *I turn my gaze*
> *to what is becoming:*
> *and know I'm awakening*
> *to 'I am'.*   Ursula Burkhard[54]

3.   Soul exercises

Soul exercises are therapeutic nursing care measures through which people can inwardly strengthen themselves. They are mainly exercises in perception. Attention is focused on an object and this process is accompanied by concentration. In doing so, the person strives for mindful engagement. The term 'soul exercises' incorporates the idea of daily hygiene for the soul.

Already Rudolf Steiner gave suggestions for soul exercises, e.g., in *Overcoming Nervousness, Practical Training in Thought, How Know Higher Worlds*, and *An Outline of Esoteric Science*.[55, 56, 57, 58]

Soul exercises are used in psychiatric or psychosomatic treatment. For about fifteen years, nurses have been increasingly leading the work with soul exercises.[59]

The practice of mindfulness is widespread worldwide, with similar indications. Harald Haas and Theodor Hundhammer developed a mindfulness program within the anthroposophic framework.[60]

At the Friedrich Husemann Clinic the following soul exercises are the main ones practiced.[61] The exercises marked with an asterisk will be described in more detail below:

- Object description*
- Plant observation*
- Writing exercise*
- Tactile exercise*
- Smelling exercises (perceiving and naming different scents)
- Listening exercises (noises, music, bird calls, rhythms)
- Picture contemplation (describing a picture in three stages: What do I see? How does the picture affect me? What is the meaning/title of the picture?)
- Weather observation (describing the current weather, with temperature, humidity, brightness, colors, clouds, etc.)
- Balancing*
- Juggling (increasingly difficult exercises with one, two or three balls)
- Rod exercise (partner exercise with two rods—engaging in a non-verbal exchange)
- Review of the day (chronological, non-judgmental remembering of all the day's events)
- Sun book*
- Pros and cons (note pros and cons side by side when making decisions)
- Conscious placement of objects (objects such as glasses or keys are intentionally and deliberately placed in absurd places)

Tactile exercise

The patient closes his eyes and receives an object. Alternatively, the object can be hidden under a cloth. After quietly feeling it for a few moments, he describes the object to the other person according to its size, weight, shape, surface and temperature. Terms that refer to the material, such as "wood," "plastic," "metal," etc., should not be used. The methods of the exercise are to get involved with the object, touch it, and describe it. The goal is to experience trust in oneself, to center oneself, to let go of illness-related one-sidedness, e.g., to gain distance from oppressive feelings and thoughts, to take control of one's inner space.

Example

A 58-year-old woman, in treatment on a closed ward, came to her first tactile exercise. She suffered from severe depression with great inner agitation. This had been preceded by an attempt at suicide. She didn't see any future prospects at all. We sat down in a room and she was almost in meltdown and didn't know what to expect. I quietly explained the exercise to her and showed her how to do it. She said immediately that she could not describe so much herself. She was going to try. She uneasily described a few aspects and after two minutes knew nothing more to say. Quiet questions helped her to immerse herself more deeply. It ended after seven minutes. I was just about to ask what the exercise had done for her when she suddenly exclaimed in surprise: "I'm completely calm!" She performed the tactile exercise with great pleasure during the further course of treatment and experienced a strengthening of her self-esteem.

Object observation
The patient receives an object and takes a close look at it. Then he describes it to the other person exactly, according to shape, color, size (in centimeters), weight (in grams) and surface. The description should be as elementary as possible (without using the terms "wood," "plastic," "metal," etc.). The other person ensures that the one describing does not digress. In addition, she supports the patient by asking concrete questions. The aim of the exercise is to focus attention on the object, to distance oneself from oneself, to become awake and clear (structured).

Plant observation
The patient brings a plant (or part of a plant, e.g., a leaf) to the exercise. He quietly looks at it and describes it according to the following aspects: shape and color, smell and possibly taste, size, transitional changes (e.g., from the leaf area to the flower), and at the end possibly the name of the plant. The aim is to arrive at a comprehensive perception, to connect with something living, to vivify oneself.

Writing exercise
The patient writes a text on an unlined piece of paper with full attention and concentration, using a fountain pen or soft pencil. She forms every letter very consciously and beautifully and tries to get into a flow while writing. She makes sure that she doesn't cramp her fingers. She makes sure to take enough breaks. At the end she looks benevolently at what she has written, without judging it.

To increase concentration, the patient can write a short text repeatedly in the above way, deliberately changing the way she writes one letter. She writes fluently and varies the selected letter within the flow. She does not correct anything afterwards. This procedure can be very much intensified with two, three or four changed letters. At the end, she looks lovingly at what she has written. Other variants are to write with the other hand, write with a foot or write with one's mouth.

The aim is to practice patience, overcome nervousness, find peace in oneself, change one's habits, strengthen one's life forces, center oneself and hold one's attention.

Balancing
The patient walks along a roofing batten lying on the floor. He looks straight ahead and feels himself in his feet. His arms hang loosely down and his breath flows. Initially he walks quietly next to the batten, then next to the batten while crossing one foot in front of the other; then he walks on top of it. In case of uncertainty and wobbling he can take a step next to the batten, collect himself and then continue on top of the batten. Then he does the exercise backwards. When walking on the batten, it is often helpful to get someone to steady you. In longer periods of practice, the exercise is also

performed with the eyes closed. The aim is to consciously grasp the lower senses, to let go of oppressive feelings and thoughts and to find trust in oneself.

Example

A young woman, in her mid-20s, attempted suicide after a sudden infant death. A short time later she came to the closed ward for treatment. She balanced daily. She found her way out of her life crisis and described how balancing was a great help to her. First, she regained the "ground under her feet" and then her self-confidence gradually grew.

Sun book

In the evening, the patient reflects on the events of the day and looks for experiences that appealed to his heart. These can be impressions of nature, a bird, a plant, a cloud, a certain light, an encounter, a smell, a food, a poem, a picture, a touch, etc. He selects an event and enters it into a booklet or book. He freely designs the way he does it, expresses himself descriptively or in a poem, he can draw it or glue it onto the page as a collage. The aim of the exercise is to arouse interest in the individual day, to open his senses, to stimulate sensations and feelings and to connect with something.

> *For Many*
> *How much beauty is scattered*
> *inconspicuously on earth;*
> *I want to notice it more and more.*
> *How much beauty, shy of the day's clamor,*
> *in humble hearts, old and young!*
> *Even if only the scent of a flower,*
> *it makes the earth's fields lovelier,*
> *like a smile through many pains.*   Christian Morgenstern (1871–1914)[62]

Example

A 64-year-old woman came with depression and anxiety to the closed ward for treatment. She had suicidal thoughts; her self-esteem seemed very low. She was retired, had until recently enjoyed working as a teacher and no longer understood the world. At first, she could not do the sun book exercise because she did not find any positive heart experiences. Negative feelings prevailed. She wrote a saying or a poem every day to bridge the gap, because she normally loved these texts. As her condition improved, she was able to find positive day experiences and entered them into the sun book in various creative ways. The sun book became her joyful support.

Work with soul exercises is possible with patients who are able to act purposefully (possibly with concrete accompaniment). When working with severely ill people, we begin with preliminary low-threshold offers in the sense of "doing things together" (playing, walking and observing, etc.). Soul exercises of this kind are to be distinguished from engaging in a personal path of development (meditation), which each person can only pursue out of their own free decision.

The soul exercises can be expanded in many ways once the inner direction of the exercises has become clear. It is helpful to have an understanding of what it means to be a human being in our time.

Human beings live in an environment in which they actively participate. Their experiences give them ideas for personal development.

From a historical perspective, people have freed themselves more and more from the guidance that used to bind them into communities. People have become more individual. They are increasingly breaking away from traditional ties such as family or religious beliefs, so people are more and more on their own, it is up to each one to shape his or her own life. Each one struggles independently with this, finding his own inner orientation, in order to master his tasks by virtue of his personality. Each adult must act independently and be his own leader in life.[63]

People are always faced with finding their inner balance anew. To this end, it is necessary to "actively take control of one's own soul life and thus take responsibility for one's own health."[64]Soul exercises can be a support in this endeavor. They challenge the person on the one hand to consciously open themselves to the outside world and on the other hand to perform specific mental processes within.

People find access to the world—including their own corporeality—through the portals of the senses. Rudolf Steiner described twelve senses.[65] The process can be intensified by directing one's attention to the object of perception and remaining concentrated on it. In this way one can distance oneself from dissipating thoughts, nervous restlessness and stress-related fears.

When we let go of the sensory impressions of direct perception and surrender to our imagination or feelings, we withdraw from the world and turn to our inner being, to our own soul. Visualization, thinking, feeling and willing form the content of our inner life of soul. By means of perceptions, we develop enriching experiences. We can increasingly penetrate this wealth of experience with our own reflective thoughts—intellectually and through feeling it more deeply. This brings us to a clear realization. We connect ourselves with the world through our purposeful activity within it. These inner soul processes are guided by our 'I'. Thus, we stand in life in three ways: through our body (senses), through our soul (thinking, feeling and willing) and through our spirit ('I').

When we consider the soul exercises, we can differentiate between four qualities. Some of the exercises refer to:
- sensory objects (object description, plant observation, tactile, olfactory and auditory exercises, picture observation, weather observation)
- concrete actions (balancing, juggling, writing and rod exercises, deliberate placement of objects)
- a limited period of time (review of the day, sun book)
- a targeted project (pros and cons)

The exercises should be understandable, feasible (manageable) and meaningful. They have an effect on the person's feeling of coherence and thus strengthen the person's core in the sense of salutogenesis. The therapeutic effectiveness of the soul exercises can be summarized as follows:

They challenge the patient to focus his attention on the content of the exercise and stay focused. At the same time, he is freeing himself from illness-related one-sidedness. Through regular practice he strengthens his willpower. This stimulates the patient's interest in what he is doing. The exercise should be as successful for him as possible and strengthen his self-esteem. In this way, the patient develops more confidence in himself. The power of the 'I' connects more intensively with the person's actions. His life of soul unfolds more harmoniously. His life forces are strengthened and thus also provide for recovery in the body. According to Rudolf Steiner, these exercises are "a remedy."[66] Furthermore, they are an everyday support for all people to master the challenges of today's world.

Category	Example learning objectives	Recommended learning path
Skills	You have practiced some of the soul exercises yourself.	A
Your own learning objective		
Relationships	You can lead a discussion group or a morning circle.	B
Your own learning objective		
Knowledge	You know the typical manifestations of depression, psychosis, anxiety disorder, personality disorder.	C
Your own learning objective		

References

1   Barz, B., Dellbrügger, G. *Pfingsten.* Verlag Urachhaus, Stuttgart 1991, p. 16.

2   Schädle-Deiniger, H. *Basiswissen. Psychiatrische Pflege.* Psychiatrie-Verlag, Bonn 2008, p 12.

3   http://berger-psychische-erkrankungen-klinik-und-therapie.de/ergaenzung_ruesch.pdf (checked June 2020).

4   Sauter, D.; Abderhalden, C.; Needham, I.; Wolff, S. (ed.). *Lehrbuch Psychiatrische Pflege.* Verlag Hans Huber, Bern 2004, pp. 419–435.

5   Adams, K. *Verband für Anthroposophische Pflege. Erfahrungen aus der Psychoedukationsgruppe Depression in der Friedrich-Husemann-Klinik.* Pflege-Perspektiven, Herbst 2012, pp. 26–28.

6   Sauter, D.; Abderhalden, C.; Needham, I.; Wolff, S. (ed.). *Lehrbuch Psychiatrische Pflege.* Verlag Hans Huber, Bern 2004, pp. 633–992.

7   Schädle-Deininger, H.; Villinger, U. *Praktische Psychiatrische Pflege.* Psychiatrie-Verlag, Bonn 1996, pp. 183–411.

8   Schädle-Deininger, H. *Fachpflege Psychiatrie.* Urban und Fischer Verlag, Munich 2006, pp. 241–409.

9   Huck, G.; Schmidt, S. Förderung von Gesundheitskompetenz. *Praxiswissen Psychosozial* 2014, (18), p. 50.

10   Steiner, R. *Der Jahreskreislauf als Atmungsvorgang der Erde und die vier großen Festeszeiten* (GA 223). Lecture of March 31, 1923. Rudolf Steiner Verlag, Dornach 1985, p. 11.

11   John 3:30

12   Barz, B. *Feiern der Jahresfeste mit Kindern.* Verlag Urachhaus, Stuttgart 2004.

13   Adams, G.; Roknic, M. Die Arbeit mit den "Seelenübungen" in der Friedrich-Husemann-Klinik. *Weihnachtsbrief der Friedrich-Husemann-Klinik* 2007, pp. 20–25.

14   Roknic, M.; Bertram, M. Pflegeforschung in der Friedrich-Husemann-Klinik. Verband für Anthroposophische Pflege (ed.). Rundbrief Frühjahr 2005, pp. 22–26.

15   Husemann, F., Priewer, W. *Friedrich Husemann—Eine Biographie.* Verlag am Goetheanum, Dornach 2008, p. 184 f.

16   Husemann, F., in: *Verband für Anthroposophische Pflege*: Rundbrief Ostern 1992.

17   Adams, K. Krankenpflegeschülerinnen in der Friedrich-Husemann-Klinik. Verband für Anthroposophische Pflege (ed.). *Rundbrief Frühjahr* 2005, pp. 27–29.

18   Heusser, P. Der wissenschaftliche Ansatz der Anthroposophischen Medizin und Psychiatrie und das Leib-Seele-Problem. In: Rißmann W. (ed.). *Was heißt seelische Gesundheit?* Verlag Königshausen & Neumann, Würzburg 2011, p. 58.

19   Menne, M. Heute auf dem Sofa: Marina Menne. *Psych. Pflege Heute* 2014, 20 (4), p. 187.

20   Steiner, R. *Introducing anthroposophical medicine.* SteinerBooks, Great Barrington 2011.

21   ibid., p. 378.

22   Wais M. Ich bin, was ich werden könnte. Entwicklungschancen des Lebenslaufs. *info 3 Verlag,* Frankfurt am Main 2011, p. 21–32.

23   Steiner, R. *Introducing anthroposophical medicine.* SteinerBooks, Great Barrington 2011.

24   Hofmeister, S. *Wo stehe ich und wo geht's jetzt hin. Wie Sie den roten Faden im Leben finden.* Graefe und Unzer Verlag, Munich 2014, p. 12.

25   Burkhard, G. *Das Leben in die Hand nehmen. Arbeit an der eigenen Biographie.* Verlag Freies Geistesleben, Stuttgart 1993, p. 7.

26   Lievegoed, B. *Lebenskrisen—Lebenschancen. Die Entwicklung des Menschen zwischen Kindheit und Alter.* Kösel Verlag, Munich 1981, p. 9.

27   Treichler, R. *Die Entwicklung der Seele im Lebenslauf. Stufen, Störungen und Erkrankungen des Seelenlebens.* Verlag Freies Geistesleben, Stuttgart 2012, p. 9.

28   Möller, H.; Laux, G.; Deister A. *Psychiatrie und Psychotherapie.* Thieme Verlag, Stuttgart 2005, p. 77.

29   ibid., p. 83.

30 Kuiper, P.C. *Seelenfinsternis—Die Depression eines Psychiaters.* Fischer Verlag, Frankfurt am Main 1991.

31 Roknic ,M. *Das Öldispersionsbad bei psychiatrischen Erkrankungen. Studie aus der Friedrich-Husemann-Klinik. Äußere Anwendungen—Werkstattberichte und Studien.* Heft 1. Verband für Anthroposophische Pflege (ed.) 2000, pp. 12–19.

32 Riches, D.; Conens, M. *Das Überwärmungsbad bei psychiatrischen Erkrankungen. Studie aus der Friedrich-Husemann-Klinik. Äußere Anwendungen—Werkstattberichte und Studien.* Heft 1. Verband für Anthroposophische Pflege (ed.) 2000, p. 11–19.

33 Rißmann, W. *Depression und seelische Verstimmungen—Wege zur Selbstfindung?* Gesundheit aktiv, Berlin 2012, p. 30.

34 Riches, D.; Conens, M. *Das Überwärmungsbad bei psychiatrischen Erkrankungen. Studie aus der Friedrich-Husemann-Klinik. Äußere Anwendungen—Werkstattberichte und Studien.* Heft 1. Verband für Anthroposophische Pflege (ed.) 2000, p. 11–19.

35 Steiner, R. *Introducing anthroposophical medicine.* SteinerBooks, Great Barrington 2011.

36 Rißmann ,W. *Was heißt seelische Gesundheit? Anthroposophische Psychiatrie als integrativer Ansatz—mit Hinweisen auf die Behandlung depressiv Erkrankter.* Verlag Könighausen & Neumann, Würzburg 2011, p. 78.

37 ibid., p. 79.

38 ibid., p. 75.

39 Koob, O. *Die dunkle Nacht der Seele. Wege aus der Depression.* Verlag Freies Geistesleben, Stuttgart 2007, p. 111 f.

40 Möller, H.; Laux, G.; Deister A. *Psychiatrie und Psychotherapie.* Thieme Verlag, Stuttgart 2005, p. 143.

41 Rißmann, W. Wahnerleben und geistige Erfahrung als Herausforderung der eigenen Urteilskraft—Die verstärkte Suche nach wahrer Wirklichkeit. *Der Merkurstab* 2013; 66 (4), p. 305.

42 Fingado, M. *Compresses and other therapeutic applications. A handbook from the Ita Wegman Clinic.* Floris Books, Edinburgh 2012.

43 ibid., p. 117.

44 Rißmann, W. Wahnerleben und geistige Erfahrung als Herausforderung der eigenen Urteilskraft—Die verstärkte Suche nach wahrer Wirklichkeit. *Der Merkurstab* 2013; 66 (4), pp. 296–309.

45 Steiner, R. *Introducing anthroposophical medicine.* SteinerBooks, Great Barrington 2011.

46 Frisch, M. Tagebuch 1946–1949. Suhrkamp Verlag, Frankfurt am Main 2007, p. 157.

47 Möller, H.; Laux, G.; Deister A. *Psychiatrie und Psychotherapie.* Thieme Verlag, Stuttgart 2005, p. 115.

48 Steiner, R.; Lindenberg, C. (ed.). *Zur Sinneslehre.* Verlag Freies Geistesleben, Stuttgart 1994, p. 83–85.

49 International Statistical Classification of Diseases and Related Health Problems 2012.

50 Freyberger, H.J.; Stieglitz, R. *Kompendium der Psychiatrie und Psychotherapie.* Karger Verlag, Basel 1996, pp. 218–222.

51 Dekkers, H., in: Beck, D.; Dekkers, H.; Langerhorst, U.S. (ed.). *Borderline Erkrankungen.* Verlag Freies Geistesleben, Stuttgart 2001, p. 61–64.

52 Junker, B., in: Reiner, J. (ed.). *In der Nacht sind wir zwei Menschen. Arbeitseinblicke in die anthroposophische Psychotherapie.* Verlag Freies Geistesleben, Stuttgart 2012, p. 199.

53 Treichler, R. *Die Entwicklung der Seele im Lebenslauf.* Verlag Freies Geistesleben, Stuttgart 2012, pp. 271–273.

54 http://www.christengemeinschaft.de/fix/1817/doc/20131106_Weihnachten_Bote.pdf (checked December 2014).

55 Steiner, R. *Nervosität und Ichheit. Stressbewältigung von innen.* Rudolf Steiner Verlag, Dornach 2010.

56 Steiner R. *Practical training in thought.* Rudolf Steiner Press, London 1968.

57 Steiner R. *How to know higher worlds—a modern path of initiation.* Anthroposophic Press, Great Barrington 2002.

58 Steiner R. *Occult science. An outline.* Rudolf Steiner Press, London 2013.

59 Adams, K.; Roknic, M. *Die Arbeit mit den "Seelenübungen" in der Friedrich-Husemann-Klinik.* Weihnachtsbrief Friedrich-Husemann-Klinik, Buchenbach 2007, pp. 20–25.

60 https://www.bewegteworte.ch/ (checked May 2020).

61 *Soul exercises: nursing standards in the management handbook of the Friedrich Husemann Clinic,* Buchenbach 2011.

62 Translated from: Morgenstern, C. *Melancholia.* Zbinden Verlag, Basel 1972, p. 62.

63 Vandercruysse, R. *Ich und mehr als ich–Grundübungen einer Kultur der Selbstführung.* Menon Verlag im Friedrich von Hardenberg Institut, Heidelberg 2011, p. 41 f.

64 Vandercruysse, R. Ich-Mangel. Störungen der Aufmerksamkeits-und Impulskontrolle. *Das Goetheanum* 2007; (44), p. 1.

65 Steiner, R. *Riddles of the Soul.* Mercury Press, Spring Valley 1996.

66 Steiner, R. *How to cure nervousness.* Rudolf Steiner Press, London 2008.

CHAPTER XIX

From the Question of Meaning in Cancer to the Cultivation of the Senses

BERNHARD DECKERS

Despite an immense amount of research, it has not yet been possible to conquer cancer. Hardly any other disease confronts patients with the topic of death in a comparable way. Cancer confronts patients themselves, and also their relatives and companions, with the question of the meaning of life. This illness involves a withdrawal of the person's 'I' from the body, which often begins long before the outbreak of the disease and can also be found on a cellular level. Starting from the pathology of cancer (from the point of view of Anthroposophic Medicine), this chapter will look at how nursing care can help in the accompaniment of cancer patients. It will be shown how care of the senses brings about concrete improvements in the quality of life and supports the patient's will to change and heal.

→   Learning objectives, see end of chapter

1.   About our encounters with cancer patients in nursing care

> *"What I first became aware of was the actual significance, the inescapable nature of this disease. Before having cancer, I had several life-threatening cardiovascular diseases. Now I noticed an interesting change in my reaction to this new illness. While I had never hesitated to say that I had rheumatic fever or a heart attack or anything else when asked about it, for some reason I had inhibitions to say: I have cancer."*[1]

The enigma of cancer, the wall of silence that builds up around it, seems at the same time to express something essential about it.

Three characteristics in particular stand out when encountering cancer patients:

- The course of the disease is usually very idiosyncratic, not predictable, plannable or standardizable.
- The questions that cancer patients ask—spoken or unspoken—are radical: they concern dying and euthanasia and the meaning of life, disease and death.
- Nurses' memories of cancer patients are often more vivid and "colorful," than what they remember of many other patients.

The localization and progression of tumors causes a wide variety of symptoms and complaints, so that therapists and nurses run the risk of getting bogged down and losing themselves in it all. On the one hand, cancer has a very varied appearance, because it can occur almost anywhere in the organism, on the other hand it raises questions of a radical, fundamental nature. Nursing care that is completely oriented towards symptoms, findings, effects and side effects of treatment remains superficial and stands in barely tolerable contrast to the life questions that present themselves. This chapter will draw attention to the finer processes in the organism and place them in relation to the human body, soul and spirit. Such an understanding of cancer can give rise to a presence of mind that make us capable of action in many moments of everyday nursing life. The aim is not to add even more techniques to the universal responsibility of nursing care ("One treats cancer cases by..."), rather, our aim is to deepen our understanding of the disease and provide help and encouragement for patients and nurses.

2. The process by which cancer develops

Two life principles can be observed in the human organism, which interact with each other in a healthy way, complementing each other to form a unified whole: the principle of growth and the principle of shaping or forming. In the case of a wound, these two principles can be observed in the course of wound healing. On the one hand, tissue quickly reproduces, on the other hand this growth is slowed: so that the new tissue is not arbitrary but is an imitation of what was before. Growth stops at certain boundary lines, enabling the original form to be restored. At most, there is a final or temporary keratinization or scarring, but this does not exceed certain limits.

The cell principle of dividing and multiplying leads, if left to its own devices, to proliferation and chaos. This pure growth principle is opposed by a force of a higher order: the formative principle which gives the growth process a direction, a profile, a face. It follows from this that cells are differentiated in their structure and function. "A cell is something that stubbornly asserts itself in its own growth and its own life, in opposition to what the human being really is."[2]

The principle of differentiation and the creative power that works within it give a new, higher "meaning" to the "obstinance" of cells. Interesting in this context is the fact that the malignancy of a cancer cell is also measured by the degree of its "dedifferentiation." This means that the less a cell subordinates itself and assumes a certain task within the whole, the more it directs its activity against the organism. It is remarkable that cancer, more precisely carcinomas, develop in epithelial or covering tissues. This type of tissue forms on the borders between the inside and the outside of organs and represents the shell or skin, which protects what is inside and determines what belongs there and what does not. This "skin" also reveals the characteristic shape of an organ. It is a border crossing through which substances, on the one hand, and stimuli or signals, on the other, pass back and forth. To make the latter possible, special perceptual organs (receptors) are integrated into this boundary. In the case of the outer skin, it is the sensory organs that present themselves to light, warmth, sound, touch, etc.

If degenerate cells from epithelial tissue form a proliferation or protrusion, this happens because the organism has reduced its powers of integration and formation at that location. The growth is not perceived, the organism is quasi "blind" to it. Everyone is confronted with such growth tendencies in the course of their life. The healthy organism recognizes these formations as foreign, it distinguishes between what belongs to it and what remains foreign. This healthy power of the organism can be impressively experienced in inflammation as a parenteral digestive process, where recognition and differentiation are followed by digestion (phagocytosis) and excretion. Inflammation is similar on a physical level to how the human 'I' can get enthusiastic about an idea and adopt it as its own.

In addition, "it is not the tumor that primarily grows through the basal membrane, as an accumulation of atypical cells, but rather the capillaries of the connective tissue under the basal membrane that dissolve the membrane and grow into the tiny cluster of atypical cells. Only after it has been supplied with blood by the organism does the initially small malignant heap of cells acquire the potency for powerful, border-bursting growth. The group of cells also remains dependent on the capillary system of the organ, which it destroys. Where the organ's capillaries do not grow towards it, penetrate it and feed it, the tumor cannot continue to grow."[3]

Without perception, the organism meets the tumor process "blindly," as it were, it is attracted to it and finally succumbs to the process. Cancer thus ultimately destroys its own basis for life. The "host" suffocates in the chaos that it fed but did not shape. To say it in a picture: an uncontained well allows water to flow unused until it dries up.

The human 'I', which constitutes the individuality of human life, gives the body its characteristic shape down to its (genetic) fingerprint. The 'I' has the possibility to connect with an idea as a task and to inspire the soul to unfold the power to turn the idea into action. In cancer, this 'I' appears weakened compared to the autonomous growth forces in the body. The 'I' loses itself in life processes that only live by constantly multiplying their own substance, reproducing themselves: "Whoever loves his life loses it, and whoever hates his life in this world will keep it for eternal life."[4] This life, which only wants to preserve itself, occurs unnoticed, because it does not communicate with the environment and only comes to consciousness when it destroys the organism.

In cancer, the shape-forming force in the organism, ultimately the human 'I', thus appears diminished compared to the forces of pure growth. The carcinoma develops on the boundary layers of the body, where the formation of form becomes particularly apparent, and where the separation and perception of the inner and outer world take place. The power to distinguish and repel, as well as to integrate, is seemingly absorbed by the cancer process and is in danger of foundering in it. In our approach to nursing and therapy, the task arises to support the patient in the formation and shaping of boundaries. On the one hand, the patient's inner world needs protection and shelter from the outside world. On the other hand, the digestive activity of the organism must be strengthened so that "nourishment," e.g., including sensory impressions, can be utilized in its favor.

3. The experience of cancer patients

"I feel like I've been trying to climb a very steep mountain all my life. There are sometimes rocky outcrops where I can rest, experience some joy. But I have to keep climbing, and my mountain simply has no summit I would ever reach." "I couldn't stand my work at the union. But I was too old to return to music, even though I tried. I knew I had to stay where I was. There was no way out, no matter how I looked at it."

"The more I tried to tear it down, the higher and denser the wall of thorns that I had built around me became. I couldn't get through, I couldn't reach anybody. I feel like Sleeping Beauty, but the forest has become so impenetrable that nobody will find me. The path is completely overgrown by a thicket, it can never be used again."

"Whatever I started, nothing worked. I couldn't (write) any more, and neither could Tom. And the more desperately we tried, the worse it got. I gave up everything for him, and today I know that this destroyed us. We suffocated each other. There just didn't seem to be any way out... I've often thought: 'I won't get out of here until I'm dead.'"[5]

According to Lawrence LeShan, an American psychotherapist with over 40 years of experience in caring for cancer patients, these statements by cancer patients are characteristic of people who tend to hold back internally in situations of conflict, who are afraid to engage in disputes when things become difficult, and who prefer harmonious conditions. This attitude of retreat, this inability to participate in the world, this "I already know this," "I'd rather not" or "It is no use anyway" has the consequence that the person takes everything from outside into himself without actively accompanying it, without "digesting" it. So, he cannot profit from his experiences and mature through them. The human 'I', which develops and strengthens itself precisely when it has to differentiate, defend and integrate, weakens itself by withdrawing from conflict. LeShan speaks of prevented "inner growth"; he means spiritual-emotional, non-bodily growth.

Impressions that were not accepted and processed by the soul, but were possibly pushed back for decades, seek their way out in the physical and make the person ill. Life seeks in the physical that which in the soul has striven in vain for further development. A revealing account of these connections can be found in a book published by Andreas Goyert (internist). Particular reference is made here to the contributions of Goyert and Treichler.[6]

3.1 The question of the meaning of life in cancer patients

The question of cancer is immediately regarded as a question of life or death. The cancer patient asks herself: "Why me?" "What is the reason for this—isn't it pointless?" "What have I done wrong?" There are cancer patients who are not aware of these questions, who suffer silently. Sometimes such questions will become tangible when, for example, a bewildered relative verbalizes them.

With others the questions appear rather in the form of inner moods. The questions are written all over their faces, but the people affected are internally too flooded with fear and despair to express them. An unbearable situation—also for the people around them!

Some patients address such topics spontaneously and very clearly. Ultimately, they ask the basic life question: Who am I? It becomes clear that the question of the meaning of life and illness is related to the question of human identity. The following sentence is found in the story of the resurrection of Lazarus in the New Testament: "This illness does not lead to death. It is for the glory of God, so that the Son of God may be glorified through it."[7] So we are talking here about revelation through illness. What or who should be revealed through illness?

> *"Man's illness is not what it seemed, a machine defect. It is nothing but himself—*
> *better: it is his opportunity to become himself."*
>
> Viktor von Weizsäcker (1886–1957)

Thus, the question of the human 'I' becomes a fundamental therapeutic question, especially in the case of cancer, and it is important to track down and strengthen this 'I', which is in danger of succumbing. It is about "finding and confirming the individuality of the patient and praising it as something unique."[8]

In the nursing care of cancer patients this means to arrange everyday life in such a way that the patient can find himself again through discovering interest in the world.

4.   Care of the 'I'—care of the senses

In summary, the processes of soul and spirit present the following picture in cancer: the soul and spirit, with the 'I' as their core, are not fully engaging in a confrontation with the world. Perception and action are not happening with full inner participation. The human soul needs precisely this contact, this friction with the outside world (which begins with defiance in childhood), so that it can develop its own individuality and recognize its identity. But the soul is afraid to be individual because it fears it may become unsympathetic. Or else it wants to be completely autonomous and then appears in its social environment as a dominant personality, which in reality is a masking of inner insecurity.

This inability to immerse oneself completely in life and emerge from it enriched leads to isolation and retreat. Out of disinterest arises resignation, despair, fear, while creative forces are inhibited and remain effective only in the physical. The weakened 'I' no longer shapes its life, but leaves it to overflowing, uncontrolled life processes. How can the 'I' of the cancer patient be addressed, strengthened and brought back into life? How does the soul regain interest in the world to warm and nourish itself? How does the person get back into a fruitful relationship with life? The human soul experiences the world through the senses. The soul works with sensory impressions, makes them its own, makes them its treasure trove of experience and can then use them productively. Tasting, smelling, touching, hearing and seeing are activities which, through the active involvement of the person, elicit a wide variety of emotions. Rudolf Steiner described a concept of twelve senses, whose reality is gradually now being confirmed by modern sensory physiology and epistemology.

The following description of the various sensory activities describes approaches for working with patients.[9]

Perceiving the 'I' of the other person	
Perceiving thoughts	The senses are predominantly directed
Experiencing speech	towards the person's spiritual nature.
Hearing	

Perceiving warmth	
Seeing	The senses primarily touch the person's
Smelling	emotional life.
Tasting	

Experiencing balance	
Experiencing movement	The senses are primarily directed towards
Perceiving one's state of health	the person's own body.
Touch	

Chart: The twelve areas of experience conveyed through the senses

4.1 Touch

In the nursing profession we feel at home with touch, as touching is an essential part of our work. It has special significance because people grow up in a rather touch-hostile culture in which many surrogates, such as technology or media, interfere with human relationships and experiences.

If we separate the qualities of warmth, movement, hearing and seeing from tactile experiences, then we arrive at a double aspect of the sense of touch: on the one hand, my body feels an impression, a shift of the skin and the underlying tissue; it is therefore primarily a matter of becoming aware of the surface of my body and my body's boundary: "This is where I start." "This belongs to me." "This is me." When we experience something unbelievable, we sometimes wonder if we are imagining it. We feel the need to touch ourselves, to pinch ourselves, to rub our eyes: "Am I still here?" This is also the case with nervousness and excitement: people unconsciously try to make sure of themselves through nervous shifting, scratching, chewing on hands and lips.

On the other hand, touch gives us a sense of the other, of the foreign, of that which does not belong to us, the hard or the soft, the pointed or the angular, etc. How exciting it can be to feel something with closed eyes, without the sense of sight's "I already know what this is." It is important for cancer patients to arouse their interest, their attention towards their own body through touch. Conscious, guided touch during physical contact during nursing care and during external applications conveys an experience of the body's boundary, as well as a sense of envelopment and protection. We promote a feeling for the border between inside and outside, for what belongs to the person or not. The experience of "This is me," which the touch evokes, alleviates feelings of fear and pain.

4.2   Perceiving one's state of health

Our sense of life conveys to us something about our inner bodily state and only becomes conscious when a feeling of discomfort becomes concrete, e.g., when we feel hunger or thirst. Conversely, a feeling of general well-being can increase into an experience: "I'm fully present and my body is entirely at my disposal."–"My body and I are one."

The sense of life tells me something about whether my life processes–such as breathing, nutrition and excretion–are in harmony with each other and whether I am "master of my house," or whether something is binding my attention and irritating me. My conscious, clear perception of my physical condition is an important process.

The daily exercise of asking about the patient's condition ("How are you?") becomes particularly important if this is accompanied by keen interest on the part of the questioner. Our regular recording of temperature, pulse, bowel movements, etc., promotes the patient's alert awareness of his body. It is particularly important to pay attention to healthy life processes with patients who tend to hypochondria.

The cancer patient's attitude towards life is often marked by a lack of desire, drive, appetite, as well as weakness. As unspecific symptoms they are expressions of the self's inner retreat from the environment. If, for example, an individually and lovingly prepared meal allows the patient to enjoy a small amount of pleasure; if the room can be ventilated or the patient washed for refreshment; or if the patient can create moments of relaxation during an undisturbed midday rest, then he can feel more at home in his own body.

4.3   Sensing movement and experiencing balance

Our sense of movement refers to the position, posture and movement of our body and limbs in relation to each other. We recognize the significance of this, for example, when a movement was wrongly "gauged," and we knock something over or overshoot the target. In movement, people experience freedom in their bodies; they enjoy it when, for example, they master motor skills in sports, dancing or the arts. It proves to be problematic when the same movements, the same repetitive actions are always carried out in the same way, so that the person functions like a machine and no longer actively guides the movement. He then appears to be manipulated like a puppet from the outside.

The sense of balance refers to our orientation in the dimensions of space. For example, it requires ongoing activity of the sense of balance for people to be able to straighten themselves upright. Each of us knows the feeling of panic when sudden dizziness occurs or when we lose orientation under water. Our sense of balance gives us inner security.

For example, patients clearly show how much external immobility corresponds to internal rigidity in depression: their thoughts become heavy and immobile, they keep thinking the same things over and over. In the physical this corresponds to a lack of movement, to a slowing down, to "paralysis" of movement, which can lead to a solidification of the body's life processes, e.g., in constipation. In cancer, very similar phenomena occur when, for example, "thinking loses its elasticity, creativity and productivity" and the person forms "fixed ideas."[10]

Any stimulation of the person's own activity helps to release inner rigidity and heaviness. The liberating experience of movement and uprightness of the body promotes the overcoming of mental paralysis and entrenched thinking.

A cancer patient who was admitted to the hospital said he had to fight. Where and how was he to fight? Most of the time he brooded dully and turned his attention inwards to his physical condition. One morning there was singing in the hall in front of his room. He tore open the door, plunged into the hallway and showed himself joyfully moved. For a brief moment he had become a different person.

4.4   Taste

When human beings become interested, i.e., when they approach something inwardly, this begins with them developing a "taste" for it. In the morning, after getting up, we feel the need to remove the stale taste in our mouth and get "a taste of the world," something fresh, awakening, stimulating, which enlivens our sense of taste. When our bland self-taste is overcome, we develop an appetite for something that corresponds to a concrete inner need: an appetite for sweet, salty or savory food.

One evening a cancer patient, who struggled with nausea and loss of appetite, expressed a "craving" for Toast Hawaii. It was possible to satisfy her "desire" with some effort on the nursing ward. This food agreed with the patient very well, and, in the days that followed, her appetite improved and she gained strength. They had succeeded in reversing a process characterized by growing nausea and loss of appetite. It is certainly desirable that nursing staff should be able to better individualize patients' meals.

There are a few things to consider in this context:

- The timing of the meal should be adjusted to the patient. Many cancer patients do not feel able to eat until later in the morning.
- The food is to be prepared with inner attunement ("food ritual").
- A bittering agent (e.g., *Gentiana comp. pillules* [WALA]) will stimulate the appetite and digestive secretions.
- At first only small or smallest, beautifully arranged quantities should appear on the plate.
- A moist-warm compress, e.g., a yarrow liver compress, will support digestive activity.

INSTRUCTIONS: Pour freshly boiled yarrow tea (pharmacy) over the compress cloth (folded cotton diaper or the like) and wring it out as vigorously as possible (wear insulating gloves because of the hot tea or leave the two ends of the cloth dry when pouring the tea, so that you have something to hold). Now place the compress with its "dry" heat, as hot as the patient can tolerate it, over the liver area, cover with another diaper or terrycloth towel and wrap a wide woolen cloth around the patient's whole body. Then put an additional hot water bottle on the compress from the outside. The treatment lasts for about 30 minutes. Ensure that the patient's feet are warm (use a hot-water bottle if necessary).

4.5 Smell

When using their sense of smell, people extend themselves beyond the activity of tasting, but unpleasant smells cause them to contract into themselves and hold their breath. Bad smells can even make them nauseous to the point that they lose consciousness. It is difficult to distance oneself from an odor. This is all the more reason for people to sometimes express their feelings with this German saying: "I can't stand the smell of you!"

With the sense of smell, we experience how much the human soul expands with sympathy and withdraws with antipathy. But how pleasant it is when our breathing becomes free and we can take a deep breath or even sigh. The olfactory environment, the atmosphere around a cancer patient, can physically, mentally, and spiritually prevent him from exhaling, letting go, giving something of himself. In this respect, our choice of body-care substances and even cleaning and disinfecting agents is important. How uninspiring the smell in hospitals often is, and sometimes also the personal odor of a patient!

Seeing is the sensory activity that dominates human consciousness.

Yet the eye is also an organ of our sense of movement. It follows contours, moving along them in the process, and this movement is perceived. So, it makes quite a difference whether people constantly surround themselves with rectangular, linear architecture, or whether their eyes seek to follow the pointed arches of a Gothic cathedral. And it makes sense, especially for bedridden patients, that the wall opposite the bed not be monotonous and monochrome but animated by various shades of color. The designations 'cold' and 'warm' colors have their justification. Warm, luminous color tones can transform into inner light and warmth.

Thus, it becomes a nursing task to arrange for the lighting conditions in the room and the handling of pictures, because, to cancer patients, the world and their own life often appear colorless, grey in grey, and they lack the ability to allow color to emerge within them, e.g., from their own memory.

A young cancer patient noticed the daily autumn changes in the leaves of a tree in front of his window and documented this development by photographing it. It was his special gift to "enjoy" such things.

4.7   Perceiving warmth

The extent to which the sensation of warmth is disturbed in many people can be seen from the fact that they often hardly notice whether they have cold or warm feet, for example. Also diminished is their feeling for the quality difference in the way heat is generated, whether by electric heating or a wood stove. On the other hand, we feel exactly how important warmth is for our inner mood. This "warming" to something, and perhaps getting "fired" with enthusiasm, forms the immediate preliminary stage to "setting oneself in motion." Warmth is the element in which something can grow and mature. Cold hands and feet, trembling and shivering with excitement, nervousness and fear correspond to an inner retreat of the soul.

When administering external applications and Rhythmical Einreibung in nursing care [→ Chapter "Compresses"] it is of quite crucial importance whether one encounters a resonance or reaction to warmth in the patient. The warmth with which we confront the patient depends on the patient's ability to react. Only when the warmth is taken hold of by human activity does it become animated, does the person become present within it. This is an essential difference to mechanical movement.

Warmth generation and malignant degeneration are two opposing processes: The warmth organism of the cancer patient is disturbed at the place where foreign life is proliferating. In the history of these patients, one often finds a lack of fever reaction in infections, a rather overcooled warmth organism and a lacking daily rhythm in body temperature.

The anthroposophic treatment of cancer therefore finds an essential approach in its stimulation of the warmth organism using mistletoe as a specific cancer medication.[11]

All the more important, next to the cool, rational objectivity of the medical profession, is warmth as the active and activating element of nursing care. We perceive the warmth of the patient together with him and we care for the patient by attending to everything from creating a warming mantle of protection to actively stimulating his warmth organism. On the one hand, we can consider hygienic measures, such as:

- Warm clothing
- Raising the patient's awareness of subjective and objective thermal conditions
- Avoidance of prolonged exposure to cold

On the other hand, we can recognize the need for targeted nursing and therapeutic measures, such as:

- Rhythmical Einreibung treatments with oil, e.g., *Solum oil* (WALA)
- Oil dispersion baths. Using a glass dispersion device (Jungebad),[12] add approximately 3 to 5 ml of an oil (e.g., rosemary oil: *Rosmarinus, Oleum aethereum 10%* (WALA), swirled in the bath water, so that the skin can better absorb the fine oil droplets. This can lead to an activation of the patient's warmth metabolism.
- Ginger kidney compresses

INSTRUCTIONS: Add a heaped tablespoon of dried ginger powder (Pulvis Zingiberis) to about 250 ml of hot water, dip a compress cloth (e.g., folded cotton diaper) into it and wring it out well. Then place it across the kidney area, cover it with an additional terrycloth towel and fix it in place with a wide woolen cloth wrapped all around the body, or similar. The compress should stay on between 20 and 30 minutes, followed by rest for at least 30 minutes. The patient should have warm feet (hot-water bottle) at the beginning of the application and should remain undisturbed throughout.

Warmth as a quality of body, soul and spirit around the patient is a prerequisite for the person to develop their personality.

4.8 Hearing

The four upper senses—perceiving the 'I' of the other, perceiving thoughts, experiencing speech and hearing—require activity on the part of those who are accompanying the cancer patient. For it is precisely here, where sensory perception qualitatively moves outwards the farthest, where we become listeners, freeing our own inner space for the other, that the cancer patient is most likely to be overwhelmed. His perception, his attention, are too much bound to bodily processes, his interest in other people is paralyzed by introspection. It is necessary to release the soul from being excessively occupied with perceiving the body.

We experience in music just how much what we hear fills us inwardly in our soul. Our inner "acoustics," our inner space of resonance, is set into vibration even more intensively through hearing than is the case when we experience light or warmth. You must be free inside to be able to lend your ear to the sounds of the other person. How much attentive listening is already disturbed by background noise! Can we create an interior for listening in the way we provide nursing care, or does the beat of our work shape the music?

A cancer patient who had already received several injections of a painkiller said in a weak voice to the nurse: "I don't want any more shots like that!" Hearing this, a relative said, "Don't listen to him. He needs them." Sometimes it can be necessary to listen carefully and make an effort, especially when the person's voice is quiet and weak. Conversely, something spoken into the room can reach the sick person better when it is not done casually, but when we turn our full attention to the person while saying it.

4.9   Experiencing speech and perceiving thoughts

With the three upper senses—the senses of perceiving speech, thought and the 'I' of other people—it seems most difficult to assign one sense organ to each. One reason for this may be the problem of distinguishing the sensory zones from each other. It is essential to pay attention to the conditions needed to develop the sensory organs concerned. The sense of thought, for instance, develops through encounters with the thought world of other human beings.

The way in which the mother tongue is cultivated is decisive for growing children. When people only "mumble," they can hardly develop a sense for language and its right sound. When the word 'silence' is reduced to a mere carrier of information, for instance, that "silence equals discipline," then the timbre of speaking cannot be having an effect. It is quite different when someone impatiently shouts "Silence!" Poetry unfolds its full effect only when spoken. Think of the poem "Waterfall by Night" by Christian Morgenstern (1871–1914):

> Stillness, stillness, deep stillness.
> Silently slumbering people and animals.
> Only the summit's glacial hush
> pours water down to the valley ...

What creative power is needed to make the sound aspect of this poem resound! It takes courage to overcome oneself, to make language resound, to grasp it in a formative way. Embarrassed shy whispering behind raised hands is part of the wall of silence and repression that surrounds patients. Do we have the courage to make a sonorous (not loud!) "Good morning" sound at the patient's bedside? It is precisely with these everyday words that it is time and again possible to mobilize the strength of the sick person, so that she herself resonates with the objective sound of the word and for a moment overcomes the severity of her illness.

Understanding another person is not only dependent on language, it is also promoted by gestures and facial expressions. It is possible to express thoughts without saying a single word. In order for a person to be able to absorb what the other person wants to say, he must put his own thoughts back and try to understand the other person's train of thought. This is more than just an intellectual ability, because even if what is said is illogical, it can still be true or have meaning. When people have a tendency towards abstraction, when they have a tendency to press everything the interlocutor says into certain definitions and models, this hinders true encounter. Maintaining a cool head, which is justified in certain situations, does not allow the whole person to participate in the exchange. The human heart has spiritual powers of perception; this is indicated in the English and French languages by the words "by heart" and "par coeur." And the Bible says: "She kept his words in her heart." How do words get "into" a heart?

> *"When it is said that thoughts are pale, one should not draw the conclusion that one does not need thoughts in order to live as a human being. Thoughts just shouldn't be so weak that they remain stuck up in the head. They should be so strong that they flow through the heart and the whole person down to their feet; for it is truly better when thoughts pulsate through our blood instead of red and white blood cells only. It is certainly valuable that the human being has a heart and not just thoughts. But the most valuable thing is when thoughts have a heart. Yet we have lost that completely."*[13]

The quote at the beginning of this chapter described the "inhibition" of cancer patients to speak about their disease. Exercising our sense of thought is essential to understanding what the patient actually wants to say. Our sense of thought breaks through the wall of silence. The more I understand the patient, the more he learns to use his sense of thought. And only then does an encounter really take place.

4.10 Perceiving the 'I' of the other person

One of the most primal experiences of human encounter is the shock at discovering that the other person is completely different from me. It is not easy to accept the abyss between Me and You; people prefer to speak of a "we feeling" and they think they must adhere to common habits and external signs of belonging together. Loneliness as the primordial experience of the 'I', and being different from other people, belong substantially to human encounter, for it is precisely in this that we can experience the quite authentic, the unmistakable, the essence of the other person. Cancer patients, after a phase of fear, shyness and modest restraint, occasionally make claims upon us, friction arises, we feel their aggression. They are expressing a kind of "just" anger. Behind this lies an attempt to infuse life with a new character, and we are amazed at the strength of their personality ("I didn't know this side of him!").

We do not overcome the cancer patient's self-centeredness and isolation by distracting him from himself and his problems. But we can encourage him to grow beyond himself through our loving interest. The self that feels perceived receives an incentive to grow, because it is being sought: "The human being becomes an I through meeting a You" (Martin Buber, 1878–1965).

The nurse's inner effort to discover the patient's 'I' consists in asking herself questions: "Who is he? Where is he? What does he want?" Or more concretely: "What is his question? What is on his mind?" Sometimes we must have the courage to ask a question. For example: "Why do you think you got sick?" Then a meeting can take place in which the person being asked experiences: "I feel understood!"

5. Concluding remarks

This chapter has illustrated how the sensory world of the cancer patient is also a task for nursing care. The patient should be helped to establish an active relationship with his environment. He must be supported in overcoming his inner paralysis and isolation in order to take the shaping of his life back into his own hands. For nurses, the task results in paying greater attention to the everyday, seemingly unimportant things of life. In particular, we focus on sources of experience that tend to be closed to the patient. Thus, by joining the patient in actively cultivating her senses, we enable her to exercise a creative power which will benefit her diseased organism.

Category	Example learning objectives	Recommended learning path
Skills	You can improve the quality of life of cancer patients by stimulating their twelve senses.	A
Your own learning objective		
Relationships	You support cancer patients in their search for a task and purpose in life.	B
Your own learning objective		
Knowledge	You understand the significance of the question of meaning for healing and for living with illness.	C
Your own learning objective		

References

1   Juchli, L. *Krankenpflege*. Thieme Verlag, Stuttgart 1991, p. 912.
2   Steiner, R. *Introducing anthroposophical medicine*. Steiner Books, Great Barrington 2011.
3   Schürholz, J. Krebskrankheit—eine Allgemeinkrankheit? *Deutsche Krankenpflegezeitschrift* 1992;
    45 (2), p. 84.
4   John 12:25
5   LeShan, L. *Diagnose Krebs. Wendepunkt und Neubeginn*. Klett-Cotta Verlag, Stuttgart 2013, p. 125.
6   Goyert, A (ed.). *Der krebskranke Mensch in der anthroposophischen Medizin*. Verlag Freies Geistesle-
    ben, Stuttgart 1989.
7   John 11:4
8   LeShan, L. *Diagnose Krebs. Wendepunkt und Neubeginn*. Klett-Cotta Verlag, Stuttgart 2013.
9   Steiner, R. Zur *Sinneslehre*. Verlag Freies Geistesleben, Stuttgart 2014. English book on a similar
    topic: Aeppli W. T*he care and development of the human senses. Rudolf Steiner's work on the signif-
    icance of the senses in education*. Floris Books, Edinburgh 2013.
10 Schürholz, J. Krebskrankheit—eine Allgemeinkrankheit? *Deutsche Krankenpflegezeitschrift* 1992;
    45 (2), p. 84.
11 Simon, L., in: Goyert, A. (ed.) et al. *Der krebskranke Mensch in der anthroposophischen Medizin*.
    Verlag Freies Geistesleben, Stuttgart 1989.
12 Öldispersionsbäder nach Werner Junge. WALA Heilmittel GmbH (ed.), Bad Boll 2008.
13 Steiner, R. *Becoming the Archangel Michael's companions. Rudolf Steiner's challenge to the younger
    generation*. SteinerBooks, Great Barrington 2007.

Further reading

- Fingado, M. *Compresses and other therapeutic applications. A handbook from the Ita Wegman Clinic*. Floris Books, Edinburgh 2012.
- Girke, M. *Internal medicine. Foundations and therapeutic concepts of Anthroposophic Medicine*. 1st
  ed. Salumed, Berlin 2016.

CHAPTER XX
Anthroposophic Oncology Nursing

JANA SCHIER

Thinking, penetrating the dark,
working, weaving in warmth,
lovingly experiencing the light.   Herbert Hahn (1890–1970)

1.   Historical aspects

Cancer is by no means just a phenomenon of today's industrialized world. The probably oldest description of this disease was found on an Egyptian papyrus from the 16th century before Christ.

Hippocrates (460–371 BC) began to distinguish between benign and malignant tumors. At that time, it was assumed that breast cancer, for example, was caused by melancholy. He was probably the first to introduce the word cancer–*karkinos*–in Greek.

The development of cellular pathology in the 19th century marked a turning point in the study and investigation of cancer. With this method it was possible to prove that tumors originate from the body's own tissue, i.e., cells, and are characterized by non-subordination to tissue-specific structures. Scientists are still conducting research in this field today and are trying to understand cancer down to the smallest molecule in every gene.

Rudolf Steiner showed how tumor disease can be considered in a more comprehensive context. He laid the foundation for us as nurses to accompany people affected by the disease in a way that takes their whole being into account, including their physical body, etheric body, soul body and spirit.

2.   The anthropological basis for understanding cancer

Every healthy human cell is differentiated according to its organ or tissue, e.g., as a nerve or liver cell with a particular task. There in the cells presides the ordering principle of the fourfold human being—the physical body, etheric body, soul body and I-organization— and the cells also form the border between inside and outside.

Cancer is characterized by a loss of the principles of formation and order. The spiritual core of the person has withdrawn from the body's life processes, pulling back from its activity as a formative and individualizing element. The etheric and physical bodies have thus lost the power which orders, shapes, structures, and guides them.

433

When we look at malignant tumor diseases, we can identify specific characteristics, such as dynamic, uninhibited, cross-border growth, a falling out of the context of the entire organism, and dedifferentiation, as expressions of autonomous action.

> *"We are faced with the fact that it is simply shown to the eye that the etheric body is working too strongly in an organ. The soul body and 'I'-organization (the soul organization through degenerating activity, the 'I'-organization through revitalizing activity) are not able to control this overriding process of the etheric body in the affected organ. So we are facing a soul organization that has become too weak, and perhaps also an 'I'-organization that is directed too feebly—the etheric body predominates. It brings processes of growth, of nutrition, to whatever organ in such a way that the organism is held together too little by the ruling soul body, by the ruling 'I'-organization."*[1]

3. The four phases of the disease

Let us consider people affected by a diagnosis of cancer. The idea of possibly having malignant tumor disease, even more so to have it confirmed by a diagnosis, places the patient, as well as his relatives, into an exceptional situation, especially psychologically.

In this life situation we often experience people in deep shock, desperate, anxious, sad, sometimes disoriented. They seem to have temporarily lost the thread of their life.

In consultation with their physician, patients are shown the possibilities for intervention in the form of surgery, radiation therapy, chemotherapy and/or complementary therapies.

After the personal decision of the patient, the path through treatment begins, which can last several weeks to months, sometimes even years.

Depending on the stage of the disease, oncology differentiates between four therapeutic approaches, which may overlap. Treatment with curative intent (Lat. *curatio*, meaning "healing") has the goal of healing. Adjuvant therapy (Lat. *adjuvare*, meaning "support") is intended to reduce the risk of relapse, mostly through postoperative, partly combined radiation therapy and chemotherapy. The third form of therapy is neoadjuvant treatment. Any reduction of tumor tissue serves to improve operability. Radiation and/or systemic therapies are used for this. The fourth approach concerns palliative treatment.

Depending on the progress of the illness, the aim is to achieve tumor remission with curative intent, or relief from tumor-related symptoms and an improvement in the individual quality of life.
Here it is an art and a challenge for the cancer patient—but also for her relatives—to integrate the illness into her everyday life, her life situation, her biography, i.e., to take up the thread of life again.

The progression of the disease cannot be stopped in every case. Palliative treatment is more about alleviating the discomfort and suffering caused by tumor growth on a physical level, and giving the patient a high degree of autonomy and quality of life. Patient care in this phase means life support to the end of life under consideration of social, psychological and spiritual aspects.

Phase 1	Support before/after diagnosis, coping with helplessness
Phase 2	Supporting therapy and alleviating its consequences
Phase 3	Living with the disease, integrating it into everyday life
Phase 4	Palliative phase: symptom control and coping with fate

Chart: Tasks in oncology nursing[2]

4. The nurse's case history based on an anthroposophic understanding of the human being

The nurse's patient interview represents a fundamental action in outpatient and inpatient care.

In anthroposophic nursing care, the case history can be expanded by looking at the interaction of the members of the fourfold human being, which helps to make sense of our perceptions of the patient and grasp the person as a whole.

> *"People will get to know each other as an 'I' by really learning to look at each other."*[3]

From the case history we can see what the person opposite us requires in terms of nursing care and action. The conversation is very individual and not always all aspects can be examined during the first meeting. People need time to arrive, to find trust and to open up. The following overview, oriented towards examining the fourfold constitution of patients, gives us nurses an impulse to become active as helping, healing, supporting powers in people's lives and to nurse them creatively. What we require is alert perception, clear thinking, combined with warm, lively feeling from the heart. The perceptions and symptoms that will be mentioned here are meant as suggestions and are by no means to be regarded as complete.

4.1 The physical body

We identify with our physical body and appear through it. Our etheric body, soul body and 'I' express their activity within it, that is, the physical body reveals impressions of life processes, soul activity, and our unique individuality. The physical body is assigned to the element of earth—the mineral kingdom.

Perceptions of the physical body can be recorded in the case history as:

Areas of perception	Examples
Dominant first impression, appearance of stature and physique, posture, gait	Walking insecurity due to neuropathic complaints under cytostatic therapy, mobility aids, danger of bedsores, contracture, falling
Measurable values such as size and weight	Loss of weight, tumor cachexia weight gain, fluid retention in tissue and/or body cavities
Physical peculiarities, e.g., conspicuous skin features	Surgical scars, pronounced acne due to tumor therapy, tumor ulcerations, wounds
Prostheses, implants, drainage, etc.	Port system (central venous catheter), artificial anus, probes and catheters, e.g., PEG (percutaneous endoscopic gastrostomy) tube, pleura catheter, ascites drainage

Chart: Perceptions of the physical body

4.2   The etheric body

Our physical body, which connects us to the earth, is permeated by an etheric body, which is the organizer of our life forces. The etheric body is characterized by rhythm, movement and flow, like the element water. The etheric body forms the basis for all our life processes and finds expression in seven specific life processes: breathing, warming, nourishment, excretion, growth, maintenance und reproduction.

Life process	Observation	Examples
Breathing	Qualities in breathing rhythmic, faltering, deep, shallow	Cough, dyspnea, lung metastases, tracheostoma, pleural effusion
Warming	Temperature regulation: need for warmth, warmth distribution in the body	Agreement between subjective perception and objective temperature measurement, development of the warmth organism under mistletoe therapy, recallable fever, warm/cold experience during chemotherapy
Nourishment	Habits, special diets, intolerances, weight progression	Impairment of food intake due to tumor-related symptoms or drug side effects, such as loss of appetite, changes in taste, nausea, vomiting, mucositis.
Secretion	Discharge, excretion	Constipation with opiate intake, ileus symptoms, fluid congestion, salivation, night sweats
Growth	Wound healing	Postoperative wound healing, healing of fungating tumors
Maintenance	Skin condition Waking/sleeping	Fatigue, disturbed sleep rhythm, e.g., because of pain, circling thoughts
Reproduction	e.g., menstrual cycle	Changes in the cycle, cytopenia under antitumor therapy

Chart: The seven life processes as an extended basis for taking medical histories

4.3 The soul body

The soul interacts with the outside world through the body's sense organs, from which it receives sensory impressions, and responds with sympathy and antipathy.
We experience body-bound soul expressions as pleasure and displeasure or pain.
Air is the element of the soul body.

Areas of perception	Examples
Facial expressions, gestures and posture	Bent gait, hunched shoulders, mask-like face
Consciousness, alertness	Has great importance, e.g., in pain therapy, brain metastases, brain edema
Dealing with one's feelings/moods, relationships with other people, e.g., family members	Grappling with the effect of tumor disease in one's biography
Mood swings	Irritability, impatience, lack of control, possible amplification due to analgesics or chemotherapy
Mental rigidity, fear, anxiety, shock	After the diagnosis and as the disease progresses
Relationship between strain/tension and relaxation	Tendency to tension, moments of inner contemplation and reflection, phases of quiet in everyday life
Pain	Localization, intensity of pain (VAS= visual analogue scale), course of pain, character of pain

Chart: The soul body in medical histories

4.4 The I-organization

The 'I', the inner core of the individuality, is what shapes the human being as a whole.

"The 'I' lives in the soul. Even though the highest expression of the 'I' belongs to what is called the 'consciousness soul,' it must be said that the radiating power of this 'I' fills the whole soul and through the soul expresses itself in the body. And the spirit lives in the 'I'."[4]

Warmth forms the basis for the 'I' to be present in the ensouled, enlivened, physical body.

Areas of perception	Examples
Profession, current situation, perspectives	e.g., work disability, inability to earn a living, possibly supported by clinical social work
Social situation	possibly supported by clinical social work
Biographical events, existing conflicts	Biography work, psycho-oncological accompaniment, pastoral care
Interests, hobbies, creativity	possibly support with implementation

Areas of perception	Examples
Personal attitude towards the illness	e.g., illness as a journey or chance to change, or granting no space to the illness, repressing it: "I don't have time to be sick."
Religious/ideological orientation, spiritual background	If desired, accompaniment by a pastor, priest or pastoral care

Chart: Aspects of the 'I' in medical histories

In the nurse's interview, we discuss any external applications that have been administered so far, enabling us to evaluate them.

The nurse's taking of the patient's history can have an awakening and clarifying effect on the patient. Resources, sources of strength and goals can be formulated together. It is not uncommon for the sick person to raise the question of the meaning of the disease and express his or her desire for healing.

5. Finding meaning and healing

Many people with cancer have questions about the meaning of tumor disease for their own biography, wonder about their identity, ask "Why me?" and also "Why now?"— all of which refer to the aspect of destiny. There are no and cannot be universally valid answers to these questions. However, we should encourage patients to go in search of answers, to overcome passivity, rigidity and powerlessness, to become active. Our nursing care of cancer patients does not lead directly to healing. We endeavor to create the conditions enabling the patient to pursue the path of healing with the aim of recovery. Often, it is helpful for patients to be accompanied by a psycho-oncologist or have pastoral conversations.

Healing in the actual sense means "becoming whole again"; it involves integration on the bodily level and healing in soul and spirit.

People create latitude for healing by activating their resources on the level of soul and spirit, such as through inner reflection and contemplation, thinking about oneself and one's life, cultivating feelings of hope and faith. These enable processes of maturation, development and insight. Abilities and possibilities arise to grasp and transform the destiny impacting them through the disease, to follow an inner path of healing.

Healing always means passing through a creative, individual process of shaping and transforming oneself. Thus, tumor disease can be regarded as an opportunity for self-contemplation and self-perception. In conversations with patients, we repeatedly hear descriptions in which the person expresses gratitude for the onset of the disease. It seems to have the character of a stop sign in the person's life. The person suddenly finds himself thrown back on himself, his established routines get disrupted, he reexamines previously secondary occupations and redefines his life goals.

"Classical" medicine focuses on the treatment and, if necessary, elimination of the tumor, i.e., health and healing are usually limited to the physical level. Yet the goal of healing is attainable in relation to the dimensions of soul and spirit, even when the tumor cannot be removed in this lifetime on earth. With a view to the essential inner nature of the human being, it may be understandable if we speak in integrative medicine of the possibility for the patient to live healthily, even with a tumor. Healthy despite his tumor, he crosses the threshold and lays down the shell of his physical abode.

The question of the meaning of illness therefore does not always mature in this life, but perhaps unfolds only during life after death, entirely in preparation for a subsequent life on earth.

> "It is precisely a matter of organizing healing in such a way that the balancing forces can intervene as favorably as possible; that is to say, that we do as much as we can for real healing, regardless of whether healing occurs or not. [5]

6. Nursing—mediating—accompanying

When we consider the nurse's fields of action, we can identify three important pillars:

We *nurse* the person's *body*,
mediate on *the level of soul* and address the qualities of thinking, feeling and willing,
accompany the person as an *individuality*, as a striving human spirit who is in development, and stand by him.

Nursing—mediating—accompanying means to build bridges and create connections between the physical and the soul and spirit.

Nursing actions and processes that are supported by rhythm, structure, clarity, I-presence and authenticity provide the essential foundation in our accompaniment of cancer patients. They form the antithesis to typical tumor characteristics, such as dynamic growth, chaos, loss of structure, hardening tendencies and dedifferentiation.

These nursing principles have a healing effect and touch the person affected by tumor disease as balancing, stabilizing elements on the level of body, soul and spirit. In this way, the ground can be prepared, the patient can arrive, and with the help of creative and transformative forces can achieve inner uprightness and competence in coping with the disease.

7. Anthroposophic nursing accompaniment of cancer patients

In our accompaniment and care of sick and severely ill people with oncological ailments, it becomes clear how multifaceted cancer is and how multi-layered the need for therapeutic nursing care can be. We encounter patients in different phases of the illness and are called upon to offer ourselves as conscious counterparts with a clear inner attitude.

Nursing care helps the sick person to regain a conscious, positive experience and perception of his physicality and individuality. Nursing applications give the person's soul body and 'I' the possibility to take hold of the physical body as a dwelling place and they impart a healing impulse.

7.1 Shock, bewilderment, speechlessness

> *"I experience anthroposophic nursing care as protective, trusting, warm-hearted, understanding, it catches me. In the repeated situation of progressive tumor disease, I am angry and alien to myself. It takes me a few weeks to get halfway back into balance. Each time this becomes more difficult as I move further and further away from becoming the same as before with my body. When in hospital I receive new, valuable impulses for my path."*

These are the words of a young woman who repeatedly received the news that her tumor was growing.

The confrontation with the diagnosis of tumor disease, as well as the news of the tumor increasing in size or recurring, results in a situation of shock for the affected person, which she experiences as an existential crisis. The experience of shock can last for days or weeks. The sick person needs time to organize the chaos in her thinking and emotions, but in this situation she is often called upon to make important decisions, e.g., with regard to what treatments should be administered. In our encounters we experience the patient with all her worries, needs and fears, and we observe that many people in this situation can only be reached on the level of their emotions. Thus, some patients can only dimly remember medical facts about the disease or the possible further procedure after consulting with their doctor.

From a nursing point of view, it is important to listen to those affected and to see what they need. Perhaps the patient would like to be alone with his perplexity or maybe grief, for the time being, and he will only open himself to talking about it later. He should feel listened to, well-received and protected, in no case lonely or at the mercy of his illness.

External applications are a great help in this situation. They touch the soul and open the door to the person within, they create trust and provide sheltering envelopment. When in shock, people often experience a feeling of inner coldness, a hindrance to the flow of warmth in the body.

By means of external applications, we give the warmth in the organism the possibility to flow again.

Shock causes the etheric body to be loosened from the physical. Oxalis (wood sorrel), leads the soul and spirit back into the physical. It strengthens the upbuilding powers of the etheric body as the opposite pole to the degenerating effect of the soul body and the 'I'-organization.

- Rhythmical Einreibung of the abdomen with *Oxalis, Folium 10%* ointment (Weleda)

- Abdominal ointment compress with *Oxalis, Folium 10%* ointment (Weleda)

- Abdominal ointment compress with *Oxalis Essence* (WALA) or *Oxalis, Folium 20%* tincture (Weleda)

- Abdominal compress with *Oxalis e planta tota W 10%, Oleum* (WALA)

Aurum (gold) combines the qualities of light and heaviness. Rose has a harmonizing effect, lavender warms gently and relaxes the respiratory system. The ingredients of Aurum/Lavandula comp. have a simultaneously strengthening, harmonizing and calming effect.

- A heart ointment compress with *Aurum/Lavandula comp. cream* (Weleda)

Mallow grows up high quickly and combines mobility with firmly rooted stability. It gently envelops, warms, strengthens and counteracts mental rigidity. In the mallow plant we can see an upright power between heaven and earth.

- Rhythmical Einreibung of the feet/back with *Mallow oil* (WALA)

Other components include St. John's wort (light), elderflower and lime blossom (warmth).

In cases of shock and perplexity it has also proven helpful to give:

- A sounding bath [→ Chapter "Variations on Whole-Body Washing"]

- Rhythmical Einreibung of the feet with *Lavender 10% oil* (Weleda), *Lavandula, Oleum aethereum 10%* (WALA), *Moor lavender oil* (Dr. Hauschka), or *Solum oil* (WALA).

If the patient is "beside himself," the following is helpful:

- Mustard powder foot baths [→ Chapter "Compresses"]

- Salt water washes (sea salt)

- Rhythmical Einreibung of the feet/legs with *Rosemarinus 10% ointment* (Weleda)

In case of inner gloom it is recommended to give a Rhythmical Einreibung treatment with:

- *Hypericum, Flos 25% oil* (Weleda)

- *Hypericum ex herba 5%, Oleum* (WALA)

7.2 Fear with agitation

Fear is a basic human feeling that sharpens the senses, increases attention, awakens and urges caution. In fear, people find themselves thrown back on themselves.

Fear appears in various contexts in the accompaniment of cancer patients.

The diagnosis of tumor disease means for many affected people the feeling of facing an existential threat. The person feels fear of the future, fear of being abandoned, fear of losing their identity, fear of being isolated and lonely, or fear of becoming a burden to their family. With regard to their own mortality, patients often express fear of dying.

In addition, there is the fear of bodily symptoms of the disease and the fear of side effects of antitumoral therapy.

Fear has to do with narrowness, constriction, distress. It finds expression in somatic complaints such as chest tightness, increased breathing frequency, tachycardia, tension, abdominal pain and sweating, accompanied by internal and/or external agitation. Nursing support in such a situation should be characterized by circumspection, calmness and attentiveness.

External applications can be given in addition to allopathic and anthroposophic medication to calm the patient, relieve anxiety and induce a sense of being protected.

- A heart ointment compress with *Aurum/Lavandula comp. cream* (Weleda)

- A Rhythmical Einreibung of the legs/feet or back (with back strokes), using *Lavender 10% oil* (Weleda), *or Lavandula, Oleum aethereum 10%* (WALA)

- A Rhythmical Einreibung of the back with *Mallow oil* (WALA)

- A footbath with *Lavender Relaxing Bath Milk* (Weleda) or *Moor Lavender Calming Bath Essence* (Dr. Hauschka)

- A Rhythmical Einreibung of the back with *Solum oil* (WALA)

The active ingredients of Solum oil are moor extract, chestnut, horsetail and lavender oil. This oil creates an enveloping and warming effect, it is calming and relaxing.

Copper mediates between the etheric and soul bodies. It tends to create a balance between the two. Through its relationship to warmth, copper offers the I-organization the possibility to integrate itself into the other members of the person's fourfold constitution.

- Rhythmical Einreibung of the feet with *Red Copper Ointment* (WALA, or *Cuprum metallicum praeparatum 0.4%* (Weleda)

Rose gently envelops, harmonizes, strengthens and conveys light.

- Rhythmical Einreibung of the back with *Rosa e floribus 10%, Oleum* (WALA)

A tea made of lavender blossoms, valerian root or lemon balm leaves, if necessary slightly sweetened with honey, helps stop inner agitation.

Reading a suitable fairy tale or poem, saying a prayer or placing a candle for the patient will address him as a being of soul and spirit and alleviate fear and agitation.

First and foremost, however, is to talk with one another. Here, nurses can work with patients to identify the cause of their worries and take action to alleviate the problem.

7.3 Dysregulation in the warmth organism

Warmth permeates everything. By feeling warmth we put ourselves in relation to the world around us. Warmth in the organism forms the basis for the higher members of the fourfold constitution (the I-organization and soul body) to integrate themselves into the etheric and physical bodies. It is through warmth that the 'I' delves into the lower members (etheric and physical bodies) in a formative way.

When a person with cancer is asked about his warmth organization (his feeling of warmth and cold), he may report, for example, that he feels cold inside, is quick to shiver, and has night sweats with freezing. When nurses draw the patient's attention to the distribution of warmth in the patient's hands and feet, many people notice that their warmth hardly reaches the periphery, i.e., their hands and feet are cool to cold, without the person having consciously noticed this beforehand. Tumor-related symptoms, such as edema of the legs, lymphedema of the arms after surgery and ascites can increase the sensation of cold. In advanced stages of cancer it is possible that patients will feel like they are burning internally and will express the need to cool their body.

Nursing care appeals to the patient's warmth organism on different levels, so that warmth can reappear and flow. On a physical level, nurses may use external applications such as Rhythmical Einreibung, compresses, a balanced, rich diet, exercise and adequate clothing.

When we wish to address the soul and spirit, we can provide warming by arranging the room in an appealing way, creating a warm-hearted atmosphere and cultivating enthusiasm for something. Sincere, authentic encounters from Me to You awaken the 'I' in warmth.

When we do something to warm or cool the body, the whole organism responds.

Ginger has a gentle and long-lasting warming effect. The body's response to a ginger application is warmth from within, which spreads throughout the body[6] [→ Chapter "Compresses"].

- Ginger kidney compress

Mustard causes inflammation of the skin, i.e., it stimulates metabolic activity and increases blood circulation in the treated area. Mustard has a strong warming effect [→ Chapter "Compresses"]

- Mustard powder foot baths

- If a footbath is not possible, apply mustard powder compresses to the calves

In case of internal cold, freezing or chills:

- A kidney compress or Rhythmical Einreibung treatment of the feet with *Cuprum metallicum praeparatum 0.4% ointment* (Weleda), or *Red Copper Ointment* (WALA)

- Abdominal compress, e.g., with *Chamomilla e floribus W 10%, Oleum* (WALA)

Use lemon, which structures and refreshes in cases of hotness, with and without fever; peppermint cools at the same time:

- Washes with *Citrus Refreshing Bath Milk* (Weleda), or *Lemon Lemongrass Vitalising Bath Essence* (Dr. Hauschka) or cooled-down peppermint tea

- A partial Rhythmical Einreibung treatment with *Citrus, Oleum aethereum 10%* (WALA)

- Lemon slices on the soles of the feet

- Calf compresses with lemon water (only if the extremities are warm)

7.4   Pain

"And I feel this pain, quietly in my heart, secretly forming violence."

J.W. von Goethe (1749–1832)

Pain is an experience of disharmony in the soul and at the same time a borderline experience. The confrontation with pain enables development and transformation.

Pain first reveals itself in the physical and makes us aware of our limitation in the physical. In pain, the soul body dives too strongly into the etheric and physical bodies; the feeling of pain is consciousness in the wrong place.

Physical pain in cancer patients is caused by compression and displacement of organs and tissue structures due to tumor and/or metastasis growth, or undesired effects of antitumoral therapy. Pain on the level of soul and spirit can be caused by conflicts between I and You or between I and the world. Anxiety, depression, social isolation, disorientation in the course of the disease are components that lead to an increase in pain. On the other hand, social integration, affirmation, trust and clarity have pain-relieving potential. That is why conversations are anxiolytic, liberating and at the same time "analgesic." How good it can be when you feel someone's hand on your shoulder–protective, understanding and trusting–or your own hand perceiving closeness!

Medications play an important role in pain therapy. Individually adapted pain therapy is the basis to counteract the development of pain, to relieve pain or to repress it. The use of pain medication (e.g., opiates) is not a causal therapy, it has the effect of lowering consciousness in the body. Analgesics lead to an increased detachment of the higher members of the fourfold constitution (soul and spirit) from the etheric and physical bodies. This can be seen in the often-occurring tiredness, nausea and constipation. We repeatedly encounter patients who, despite severe pain, do not want to take any, or only minimally dosed, analgesics in order to consciously face the pain. Complementary treatment and accompanying measures can reduce the need for painkillers or even replace them completely at times. As an example case, there was a young patient with testicular carcinoma, who suffered from back pain (not caused by tumors) for weeks and who received painkillers that had unfavorable effects on his physical sensation of warmth. This was recorded in the nurse's history and the patient received nighttime back compresses with *Aconite Nerve Oil* (WALA). After regular use of the compress, the patient no longer had to resort to his pain medication. He was instructed on how to apply the compress, so that he could use it at home as needed.

Aconite Nerve Oil contains blue monkshood, camphor, lavender and quartz. It is an oil that stimulates the patient's warmth organism, and has a calming and forming effect.

- Rhythmical Einreibung or oil compress with *Aconite Nerve Oil* (WALA)

Solum oil counteracts pain associated with congestion processes. It envelops and structures the body's fluid organism.

- Rhythmical Einreibung of the back with *Solum oil* (WALA)

Flax is characterized by its high content of fatty oils and a particularly pronounced capacity to store warmth. When used for chronic pain or bone metastases, flax has a long-lasting warming effect and is therefore relaxing and pain-relieving.

FLAX POULTICE: Bring five tablespoons of flax to a boil in about twice that amount of cold water and let it simmer over a low heat until a slimy paste forms. Spread the paste about one centimeter thick on a cloth and fold it into a small pack. Apply the pack and cover with additional padding for warmth. The duration of treatment is about one hour, or as long as it feels pleasant to the patient. CAUTION: The freshly prepared poultice can be very hot—there is a risk of burns!

Melissa oil (WALA, with melissa, caraway and marjoram) stimulates the warmth organism, harmonizes and relieves cramps and flatulence, especially in the digestive tract.

- Rhythmical Einreibung of the abdomen, or oil compress with *Melissa oil* (WALA)

Chamomile has an intense warmth quality. This medicinal plant harmonizes the members of the fourfold human being. It warms the organism with an antispasmodic, analgesic and calming influence.

- Rhythmical Einreibung, or oil compress with *Chamomilla e floribus W 10%, Oleum* (WALA)

- Abdominal compress with chamomile tea

In case of liver capsule pain, administer a yarrow compress.

LIVER COMPRESS WITH YARROW TEA: Pour 500 ml boiling water over two tea-spoons of yarrow. Let the tea steep for seven minutes. Fold the inner cloth to the size of the organ to be treated and roll it up, then soak it with tea and firmly wring it out. Apply the compress as hot as possible. It is essential to consult the patient to avoid burning. Now cover the inner cloth with an intermediate cloth. After wrap-ping the patient snuggly in an outer cloth (laid out under him beforehand), we place a hot-water bottle over the compress. After approx. 30 minutes, remove the inner and intermediate cloths, snuggly re-wrap the outer cloth and leave the hot-water bottle in place for a further 30 minutes of rest.

7.5 Fluid congestion processes in the organism

When the ordering, shaping, integrating activity of the higher subtle members disen-gages, this can lead to processes of fluid congestion in the organism. Fluids moving in the animate physical body then succumb to forces of gravity, are sedimented out and become alien to the organism. In patients we experience this particularly in advanced stages of the disease, in the form of edema of the extremities, anasarca, ascites and pleural effusions. Due to the displacing power of the fluid deposits, the affected peo-ple often experience shortness of breath, pain, a feeling of pressure, and dysregula-tion in the excretion processes of the digestive and urinary tracts. For the patient, these complaints often lead to significant restrictions in mobility, combined with a weakening of the strength to be upright, and associated reduced experience of their 'I'.

From a nursing perspective, we support those affected through conscious posi-tioning and mobilization. When we stimulate the warmth organism we strengthen the effectiveness of the members of the fourfold constitution, which enables them to take hold of the bodily processes and integrate deposited, alienated fluids back into the organism.

Here, too, external applications provide essential support.

Farmer's cheese (low-fat) has a relieving and pain-assuaging effect on congestion processes in fluids. Farmer's cheese applications create a gentle suction effect in the treated body region. Depending on the indication, essences can be added to the farm-er's cheese to enhance the specific effect.

- Farmer's cheese compresses

- Farmer's cheese compress with *Borage Essence* (WALA) or *Aesculus/Prunus comp. Essence* (WALA)

Borago officinalis, better known as borage or starflower, has a balancing and cooling effect. This medicinal plant, with its formative and structuring forces, is able to restore the flow of fluid that has come to a standstill.[7]

- Compresses with *Borage Essence* (WALA)

The following applications have proven themselves in the treatment of ascites:

- Abdominal compresses with body-warm farmer's cheese

- Kidney compresses with ginger powder or Equisetum tea

- Abdominal compresses with white cabbage leaves [→ Chapter "Compresses"]

The relieving and decongestant effects of white cabbage are the opposite of the aqueous, dense gravity of ascites.

Recommended for pleural effusions are:

- Chest compresses with body-warm farmer's cheese

- Rhythmical *Einreibung with Plantago Bronchialbalsam* (WALA)

7.6 Identity as a man or a woman

One aspect that is often repressed is the way that we deal with sexuality, the tension between illness and the desire to have children, feelings such as "feeling like a man" or "feeling like a woman." Sexuality and the experience of identity include physical lovemaking, allowing closeness, touching oneself and being attractive to oneself and to others. People affected by cancer, as well as nurses and doctors, often shy away from dealing with this topic openly, out of shame and uncertainty. If the nurse who is accompanying the struggling individuality addresses this matter with respect and empathy, he can often clearly sense relief in the patient.

Due to accompanying symptoms of tumor disease, patients report aversion to their own body, self-doubt, loss of self-esteem; they may suffer from social withdrawal, isolation and depression. One patient described how he felt disgusted with himself and had to vomit when he looked at his urinary drainage in the mirror. Another patient expressed how much her partnership suffered from the fact that she now had an artificial anus, which made it impossible for her to allow physical closeness. Restrictions in the experience of identity as a man or woman arise, among other things, from the undesired effects of drugs, e.g., alopecia due to cytostatics, menopausal symptoms under antihormonal therapy, loss of libido and potency, organic or physical changes due to surgical interventions, e.g., the placement of drains, and mastectomies, which are common.

The people affected can be helped by conversations with the patient's partner, family, nurses and doctors, as well as by allowing space for a couple to be alone together, to grieve together. Where appropriate, contact with specialized therapists may provide important support.

With regard to family planning, there is the possibility of cryopreservation, i.e., the freezing of sperm or ova. Receiving information about this is part of the medical consultation before surgery, radiation or systemic tumor therapy which affects human germ cells.

7.7 Anthroposophic nursing accompaniment of patients undergoing radiation therapy and/or chemotherapy

Besides surgical intervention, radiation and chemotherapy are common, mostly standardized forms of tumor therapy today.

Radiation therapy and chemotherapy can have a corrective effect on tumor growth, but do not transform the actual disease process. The aim of anthroposophic medical and nursing care is to integrate tumor therapy into a holistic concept, i.e., to support and strengthen the patient in a process of healing and recovery.

The ability of tumor cells to divide is the starting point of classical oncological therapy. By inhibiting proliferation, the growth of malignant cells should be suppressed or apoptosis achieved. Newer drugs such as antibodies do not directly influence cell function, but usually regulate the corresponding messenger substances by blocking the receptors. Drug therapies in the treatment of malignancies usually do not only affect the tumor cells, but also the system, i.e., the whole organism, and predominantly tissues with high proliferation rates. These include, for example, the mucous membranes, germ cells, the haematopoietic system and the hair roots, from which the undesirable effects of cytostatic therapy frequently come. The side effects associated with chemotherapy are due to an impairment of the etheric body (life forces), which cannot be effective in the organism in the right way, as well as to changes in soul and spirit.

Effects on soul and spirit	Cancer fatigue syndrome, pain with polyneuropathy, whole body pain, impaired concentration, mood swings, irritability, the feeling of standing beside oneself.
Expressions of impaired life forces (etheric body)	An internal cold feeling, which has often already existed over a longer period of time and appears intensified due to therapy; mucositis, diarrhea and constipation, nausea and vomiting, delayed wound healing, cytopenia, amenorrhea, alopecia.

Chart: Possible side effects of chemotherapy

The force of cytostatic therapy, which has a deep and powerful affect on people, confronts patients with a difficult decision and presents nurses with special challenges.

We must face chemotherapy consciously and alertly. This is by no means easy. It may be possible to create a counterbalance to chemotherapy by offering warming, light-filled forces, empathy and respect that appeal to the person's 'I'. Our efforts in nursing must lie in strengthening the patient's etheric and soul bodies, as well as the patient's I-organization, in such a way that these members can intervene effectively again at the site of tumor formation. Essential pillars of the complementary treatment concept are eurythmy therapy and artistic therapies.

The following section highlights the tasks involved in accompanying patients during chemotherapy and radiation therapy, which can last from several weeks to months.

7.7.1 Prophylactic and therapeutic nursing applications in tumor therapy

We see in front of us the person with cancer who has decided to undergo chemotherapy and/or radiation therapy after a detailed medical consultation. The patient should be given enough freedom to deal with the question of therapy and to make a valid and coherent decision. Only in rare cases is there a medical necessity to urge an immediate start of tumor treatment.

Especially the first dose of medication is perceived by many patients as being very threatening. We then experience the patient's fear and insecurity; tears often flow in such moments, expressing their strong emotional distress.

Our nursing care and accompaniment can help with this, as an upright, enveloping and protecting power. The therapeutic need for nursing care can be seen from the nurse's extended patient history. This will be taken again for each stay. Our communication of clear, honest information about the treatment and making ourselves available to talk about it allow the patient to participate. It gives him the opportunity to help shape this stage of his life out of his own powers. For instance, experiencing a healing compress, a warming footbath or a pain-relieving Rhythmical Einreibung treatment can support the cancer patient in his own activity and strengthen his autonomy. Consider the important role of relatives in the course of illness and therapy in this context. Relatives often feel helpless in the face of this situation and fear that they are not doing the right thing. If, for example, we give them an opportunity to express their concerns or if we show them how to administer external applications, they can experience a new security and it can be easier for them to accompany the sick person on his way.

7.7.2 Nursing support before the start of therapy

Warmth is an essential element in accompanying treatment. In addition to external applications, the patient's warmth organism can be stimulated and healing preparation can be given via metal color light therapy,[8] eurythmy therapy, music therapy, rhythmical massage therapy according to Wegman/Hauschka, and a warmth/light meditation. This stimulation enables the soul to breathe and offers the I-organization the possibility to intervene in the corporeality in a formative and structuring way.

To accompany therapy, a healing prayer or poem (e.g., the Lord's Prayer or Psalm 23) can be spoken for or with the affected person, leading to balance and inner peace.

I bear calm within myself,	*The good and bad lots for my soul*
I bear within myself	*rest quietly*
The forces which strengthen me.	*in the womb of the future.*
I want to fill myself	*What good flows daily to me,*
With the warmth of these forces,	*I will notice;*
I want to pervade myself	*by it I am shown,*
With the power of my will.	*what gods make out of me.*
And I want to feel	*What bad sometimes flows to me,*
How calm spreads	*I want to bear;*
Through all my being	*by it I am shown,*
When I strengthen myself	*what I can still make of myself.*
To find calm as	*I thank my good fate*
The force within me	*for the way I live now.*
Through the power of my striving.	*I thank my strength in challenging situations*
Rudolf Steiner[9]	*for the force that can lead me upward in life.*
	Whoever believes that only good fate advances us,
	and that only bad things bring us down,
	does not see the year, but
	only the day.
	Rudolf Steiner[10]

If the patient seems to have lost his "center" in the way the members of his fourfold constitution interact, we can use the following applications:

- Whole-body Rhythmical Einreibung, e.g., with *Solum oil* (WALA), *Prunus spinosa e floribus W 5%, Oleum* (WALA) on the evening or morning before chemotherapy

- Pentagram Rhythmical Einreibung on the evening or morning before chemotherapy [→ Chapter "Rhythmical Einreibung According to Wegman/Hauschka"]

- A heart ointment compress with *Aurum/Lavandula comp. cream* (Weleda)

To stimulate the warmth organism:

SPECIALIZATIONS IN NURSING

- Rhythmical Einreibung of the feet, kidney compress with *Red Copper Ointment* (WALA) or *Cuprum metallicum praeparatum 0.4% (Weleda)*

- *Rhythmical Einreibung of the back, with Solum oil* (WALA), combined with a "back strengthening" gesture

- Mustard powder footbaths (in outpatient therapy, the patient can be shown how to do the footbaths at home in the mornings)

- Ginger kidney compresses (in outpatient therapy, the patient can be shown how to apply the compress at home in the mornings)

- Abdominal compresses with *Oxalis e planta tota W 10%, Oleum* (WALA)

7.7.3 Nursing support during and after therapy

During the treatment the patient requires attentive, fully present accompaniment. It is just as important to remain close and responsive to the patient in the time after treatment. We can observe impairments in the threefold functioning of the patient's organism when we consider the spectrum of undesirable side effects. In the patient's motor-metabolic system, this may manifest as diarrhea or vomiting. The cardiac and pulmonary toxicity of some cytostatic drugs are related to the patient's rhythmic system. Undesirable drug effects in the patient's neurosensory system are expressed in polyneuropathic complaints or ototoxicity.

Anthroposophic nursing-care applications address the patient as an individual, with a body, a soul and a spirit, and it may be possible to prevent and/or alleviate side effects of antitumoral therapy. People experience prophylactic applications, such as yarrow liver and ginger kidney compresses, as being beneficial and strengthening. Our aim is to support patients on their way through the therapy, to focus their attention on healthy forces and thus activate their resources and self-healing powers.

The following is a selection of applications that are both prophylactic and symptom-oriented. The applications should always be adapted to the specific side effects of the cytostatic drugs.

A) To create a mantle of enveloping warmth

- Rhythmical Einreibung of the feet, kidney compress with *Red Copper Ointment* (WALA) or *Cuprum metallicum praeparatum 0.4% (Weleda)*

- *Rhythmical Einreibung of the back, with Solum oil* (WALA), combined with a "back strengthening" gesture

- Mustard powder footbaths (in outpatient therapy, the patient can be shown how to do the footbaths at home in the mornings)

- Ginger kidney compresses (in outpatient therapy, the patient can be shown how to apply the compress at home in the mornings)

- Upper abdominal compresses with *Oxalis e planta tota W 10%, Oleum* (WALA)

In cases of intravenous drug administration, we can mitigate the patient's perception of the treatment with a warm grain pillow placed under the arm, a warm (not hot!) hot-water bottle and, if necessary, an additional covering with a light cotton cloth.

On the level of soul and spirit, we can strengthen the sense of enveloping warmth through conversations and trusting nursing care.

B) To support liver metabolism, prophylaxis and therapy for nausea, vomiting, loss of appetite and taste changes

- Liver compresses with yarrow tea at midday; consider use in the evening if nightly nausea or evening nausea occur.

- Liver compresses with yarrow oil (*yarrow 5% in olive oil*) (Dr. Heberer bath oils). These are particularly suitable for outpatient therapy

Yarrow has an invigorating and structuring effect on metabolic processes. When used, it can be experienced as warming, antispasmodic, toning and invigorating.

C) Constipation, diarrhea, convulsive abdominal pain

- Abdominal compresses with *Oxalis, Folium 20% tincture* (Weleda)

- Abdominal compresses with *Oxalis e planta tota W 10%, Oleum* (WALA)

- Rhythmical Einreibung of the abdomen, or oil compress with *Melissa oil* (WALA)

- Rhythmical Einreibung or oil compress with *Chamomilla e floribus W 10%, Oleum* (WALA)

D) To support renal activity

The obvious structured, formative powers of common horsetail, as well as its affinity for light and water, make the plant a valuable healing substance.

- Kidney compresses with Equisetum tea or ginger powder

- Kidney compresses with *Equisetum ex herba W 5%, Oleum* (WALA)

- Equisetum tea, taken internally

E) To use in case of anxiety or concomitant to chemotherapeutic agents with cardio-toxic components

- Heart ointment compresses with *Aurum/Lavandula comp. cream* (Weleda)

F) Mucositis prophylaxis and therapy

Rinsing the mouth with natural substances can prevent or treat inflammation of the mucous membranes. Selected medicinal plants in the form of teas are suitable for this purpose, depending on the indication and appropriate preparation. Drinking such teas also has a beneficial effect on the digestive tract.

Type of tea	Preparation	Effect	Application
Chamomile	Pour 150 ml very hot water over 1 teaspoon chamomile blossoms, allow to steep for 2 min.	antibacterial, anti-inflammatory, wound healing, analgesic	Inflammation of the oral cavity and the pharynx
Sage	Pour 150 ml boiling water over 1/2 teaspoon sage leaves, allow to steep for 3 min.	antibacterial, antiviral, astringent, may have a desiccating effect	Inflammation of the oral cavity and the pharynx, evaluate carefully in case of dry mouth
Thyme	Pour 150 ml boiling water over 1/2 teaspoon thyme leaves, allow to steep for 3 min.	antibacterial, antimycotic, deodorizing, stimulates blood circulation	Inflammation of the oral cavity and the pharynx, supportive treatment for oral thrush and halitosis (mouth odor)
Calendula	Pour 150 ml very hot water over 1 teaspoon calendula blossoms, allow to steep for 2 min.	antibacterial, anti-inflammatory, wound healing, mucosa soothing	Inflammation of the oral cavity and the pharynx, xerostomia (dry mouth)
Marsh mallow	Add 2 teaspoons of marsh mallow root to 300 ml of cold water and let swell for about 2 hours, briefly bring to a boil and sieve off.	Anti-inflammatory, wound healing, hemostatic, soothing and protective for the oral mucosa due to high mucilage content	Inflammation of the oral cavity and the pharynx, xerostomia, bleeding tendency
Tormentil	Pour 150 ml boiling water over 1 teaspoon tormentil roots, allow to steep for 5 min.	anti-inflammatory, wound healing, astringent, hemostatic	Inflammation of the oral cavity and the pharynx, bleeding/tendency to bleed, evaluate carefully in case of dry mouth

- Mouth rinse with *Rathania comp.* (Weleda), *Calendula Essence* (WALA, Weleda)

- *Calendula ex herba D3* (WALA) amp. s.c.   1–3 x daily

- Frozen pineapple pieces (CAUTION: Oxaliplatin can cause painful dysesthesia and/or paresthesia when exposed to cold!)

- Local application of honey before and after radiation therapy in the area of the oral cavity, throat, esophagus, to protect against radiogenic mucous membrane damage.

G) Fatigue/weakness

Fatigue can be prevented or alleviated by regular, persevering physical exercise and targeted training (no overexertion!).

The healing effect of blackthorn (Prunus spinosa) can be seen in a strengthening of the patient's upbuilding and regenerative powers.[11] Blackthorn has an invigorating and strengthening effect. "... the patient is thus enveloped in a protective blue mantle, in the warmth of which he can recover."[12]

- Rhythmical Einreibung of the arms with *Prunus spinosa e floribus W 5%, Oleum* (WALA)

- Partial Rhythmical Einreibung treatments with *Mallow oil* (WALA)

- Partial Rhythmical Einreibung treatments with *Rosa e floribus 10%, Oleum* (WALA)

H) Polyneuropathy, paresthesia, hand–foot syndrome

Through the sense of touch we become aware of our physical boundaries and thus of ourselves. Neurotoxic drugs can massively impair this sense under certain circumstances. It is not uncommon for patients to be forced to discontinue chemotherapy due to the severity of the symptoms. Prophylaxis and therapy are very important. The participation of the patient, after appropriate consultation and guidance, is crucial for successful treatment. In general, good skin care should be ensured.

Treatment to accompany the administration of taxanes and vinca alkaloids (with a doctor's prescription)

■ *Stibium metallicum praeparatum D6* (Weleda) 10 ml amp. i.v.	1 amp. parallel to the application of a cytostatic
■ *Stibium metallicum praeparatum D6* (Weleda) trit.	¼ tsp. during the entire therapy period
■ Rhythmical Einreibung of the hands and feet with *Aconite Nerve Oil* (WALA)	2 x daily and as needed

CAUTION: The use of rosemary ointment can increase symptoms of neurotoxicity!

Treatment to accompany the administration of platinum derivatives, 5–FU (with a doctor's prescription)

The element platinum belongs to the group of precious metals and is characterized by its low solubility in water and its tendency to accumulate in the body. Equisetum arvense and Formica rufa (red wood ant) have proven to be effective in adjuvant therapy of cytostatic drugs that contain platinum.

■ *Equisetum cum Sulfure tostum D6 amp. i.v.* (Weleda)	1 amp. parallel to the application of a cytostatic
■ *Equisetum cum Sulfure tostum D3 trit.* (Weleda)	¼ tsp. during the entire therapy period
■ Rhythmical Einreibung of the hands and feet with *Arnica comp./Formica, Oleum* (Weleda)	2 x daily and as needed

I) Care of irradiated skin
Moisturizing skin care, with:

- ■ *Combudoron* (Weleda) external gel, liquid[13]

- ■ *Wund- und Brandgel* (wound and burn gel WALA)

- ■ *Brandessenz* (burn lotion WALA)

Patients experience oncological treatment and its effects on body, soul and spirit very individually. Especially chemotherapy is associated with many negative effects. In accompanying patients, though, we often observe that they revive due to the suppression of the tumor, become interested in their environment again, participate in life anew and open themselves to spiritual thoughts.

8. Anthroposophic nursing in oncology

Anthroposophic nursing care in oncology is concerned with accompanying the patient in his illness and conveying a healing impulse by means of individual therapeutic and nursing actions.

Again and again we observe inner development in people dealing with the illness. At the same time, we can experience maturation in the nurses as individuals and as a group. The shared idea of helping and the will to heal—emerging from a love of the human being—forms the connecting element between the nurses. We gain valuable impulses for coping with demanding oncological nursing tasks through authentic, sincere encounters and conversations in the therapeutic team—these serve as a source of strength.

> *"It is among human beings that one must seek God. The spirit of heaven reveals itself most brightly in human events, human thoughts and human emotions."*
>
> Novalis (1772–1801)

References

1   Steiner, R. *The healing process. Spirit, nature and our bodies.* SteinerBooks, Great Barrington 2011.

2   von Dach, C.; Heine, R., Heiligtag. R. Anthroposophische Pflege von Krebskranken. *Der Merkurstab* 2009; 62 (4), p. 330–342.

3   Steiner, R. From symptom to reality in modern history. Revised ed. Rudolf Steiner Press, London 2015.

4   Steiner, R. *Theosophy. An introduction to the supersensible knowledge of the world and the destination of man.* Rudolf Steiner Press, London 2011.

5   Steiner, R. *The Christ impulse and the development of the ego consciousness.* Rudolf Steiner Press, London 2014.

6   Sommer, M. Zur praktischen Anwendung des Ingwerwickels. *Der Merkurstab* 2006; 59 (6), pp. 538–540.

7   Stüdemann, G. Borago-Umschläge bei Lymphödem. Beobachtungen aus pflegerischer Sicht. *Der Merkurstab* 2011; 64 (4), p. 357–359.

8   Altmaier, M. *Metallfarblichttherapie.* Mayer Verlag, Stuttgart 2010.

9   Steiner, R. translated by Christian von Arnim, in: Glöckler, M; Heine, R. (eds.). *Leadership questions and forms of working.* Verlag am Goetheanum, Dornach 2016, pp. 182.

10 Steiner, R. translated by Dana L. Fleming and Christopher Bamford, in: *Mantric Sayings. Meditations. 1903–1925.* SteinerBooks 2015, p. 124

11 Meyer, U. Die Schlehe–Heilpflanzen für Zeitgenossen. *Der Merkurstab* 2011; 64 (2), pp. 100–114.

12 Heek van Tellingen, C. *Vade mecum. A handbook of anthroposophic medicine.* Mercury Press, Spring Valley 2000.

13 Novak, M. Die Pflege der bestrahlten Hautfläche während der Strahlentherapie. In: Weleda (ed.). *Pflegeforum* 2006, (1), pp. 7–9.

CHAPTER XXI

Geriatric Care as Care for Human Beings

ADA VAN DER STAR · ANNEGRET CAMPS

Nursing care in facilities for people of advanced age is fundamentally different from nursing care in hospitals. This chapter will examine the special nursing needs of the elderly with regard to the significance of old age in their biographies, and will present the value and meaning of this phase of life on the basis of an anthroposophic understanding of the human being. Both activating and maintaining care must be measured against the concrete needs of the elderly person. Respect for human dignity replaces the often predominant deficit model of old age.

→   Learning objectives, see end of chapter

1.   The difference between nursing the sick and nursing the elderly

In both professions, nursing activities are central. At the same time, their common element involves very different professional tasks.

We call a person "sick" who, for whatever reason, is hampered in performing his everyday life tasks. Whether it is that he cannot digest food, can no longer guide his own thoughts, can hardly move or can only express himself with difficulty: he feels deterred from being the way he wants to be and developing as he would like.

Nursing care takes over activities which patients cannot currently carry out themselves. It supports and encourages them to take their life back into their own hands, to connect with their biography, and finally releases them back into society. A change has taken place. In the ideal case, the patient becomes completely healthy and may learn to behave in such a way that she does not fall back into illness in the future. She may have to accept having to resume her life in a reduced state.

Dying continues to be seen mainly as an unfortunate event in medicine, which people would prefer to avoid or at least postpone.

The tradition of professional geriatric care is still relatively young. Vocational training for it developed from nursing care and it is still often regarded today as a part of ordinary nursing. A "hospital style" often characterizes nursing care facilities for the elderly.

We find "nursing wards," "nurses' rooms," a ward manager, doctor's visits, fixed times at which washing, eating and even emptying of the bowel or bladder are allowed or required. However, the situation of an elderly person in a nursing home is fundamentally different from that of a sick person in the hospital.

The person is not there "to visit" for a short time until she is restored to health. She now lives permanently in the home for the elderly. As long as she lives, this home will be her home, and she will leave it only when she dies.

The path to death always leads through surrender. The person begins by saying goodbye to her own home, to her personal social environment, and she continues to be accompanied by losses: loss of autonomy through clouding of the senses, restrictions of movement, speech, etc.

Nevertheless, old age is not to be understood as an illness, just as we would not consider a newborn who is incontinent, speechless and completely uncoordinated in his movements and who can hardly make use of his sensory organs to be ill! The things that a person learns to grasp with joy in childhood and adolescence, he must often painfully do without again in old age. There is even often a situation in which the old person in need of help becomes like a small child. People say that the elderly are "like children." Externally, this is true to a certain extent, with the difference that the old man has gathered a wealth of earthly experience that the child does not yet have. This includes experiences that were processed, others that led to abilities, and some that sank unprocessed into the depths of the person's soul.

This fact places very specific demands on nursing care for the elderly, which, unlike nursing care in general, does not aim to achieve fundamental changes in the person's life situation, but to accompany a phase that is part of life. Body care is also part of this task. It may even make major demands on nursing staff. The peculiarity of care for the elderly lies in creating a situation in which people can live through this stage of their biography with dignity. Of course, we still also treat diseases and carry out prophylaxis. This is the nursing side of geriatric care.

But it is only a part of it. The real task is rather to accompany people in their aging process, to help them without taking too much away from them or disturbing them too much with well-meant "activation" attempts. The geriatric nurse is a guest of the elderly person, she must adapt to him and his needs and help him to lead his life in the manner appropriate to him, until he finally frees himself from it.

In nursing there are possibilities for specialization, e.g., according to age, sex, or type of illness. In nursing care for the elderly, on the other hand, the fundamental task is to create a protected framework in which many other people, be they relatives, therapists, housekeepers, doctors or pastors, contribute their help. If we look at nursing training for the elderly, we find that these disciplines are all represented in the curriculum.

While in medicine we have our own concrete conceptions of illness and health, it remains difficult to answer the question of how it feels to be "old." It is only in the course of life that one's own experiences occasionally convey an idea of what this must be like. But actually, we can hardly imagine being thirty, forty, or even fifty years older! This discrepancy remains.

And how does the geriatric nurse know whether his work was successful after the old man died in dignity? As long as we have no concrete thoughts about life after death, we can hardly hope for an answer to this question. But this profession may provide fulfillment if we see our task also in preparing the person's life after death as well as possible [→ Chapter "The Accompaniment and Care of the Dying and Deceased"].

2. Structuring one's life and geriatric nursing

"Geragogy" has existed as a subject in geriatric nursing training since the early 1980s. It is often understood to be an educational task on behalf of the elderly, closely related to pedagogy. In fact, many cities or institutions offer a more or less rich range of courses for older people, including "universities of the third age." However, these services are aimed at people who are independent and who do not need the help of nursing staff. Concrete geriatric nursing care finds its educational mission in creating an appropriate living environment for the very elderly and/or sick, in creating a cultural atmosphere in which old people can develop in the truest sense of the word (the Greek word *geraios* = old man, dignitary; the Greek word *agoge* = leadership). These very old people, who are at the end of their lives, have very little time left. The activities of daily life cost very much of their remaining strength. It would be a pity if they had to waste the rest of their energy by just passing the time superficially.

Despite all efforts for renewal in the work with people of advanced age, "afternoons for the elderly" are still widespread, which consist mainly in someone—either grinning or with a compassionate, understanding smile—offering some trivial "pleasure" while enjoying coffee and cake. The beneficiaries sway back and forth to music, talk about the good old days, or Santa Claus hands out presents, maybe a washcloth and a bottle of juice or beer, whichever they prefer! The rest of the time the old people sit in the neon-lit hallway or at the foot of their hospital bed. Instead, geragogy for the elderly can become an instrument for shaping the lives of very old people, by actively shaping their environment and the course of their day in such a way that they are offered a humane living space, e.g., by taking into account the laws of nature, the culture of the people, and by offering specific stimuli to their senses. Nature observation sessions relevant to the season can be adapted to the possibilities of the participants—and may include anything from the simple showing and naming of common plants to sophisticated presentations of ecological systems. Likewise, reading literary texts, listening to stories, attending talks on historical or contemporary topics, listening to music together, looking at pictures or watching films can be designed in such a way that the activity corresponds to the emotional and mental capabilities of the inhabitants. Stimulation of the senses through movement, smells, colors, sounds is a further possibility to create a meaningful life together. More complex are individual biographical work and artistic therapies, such as therapeutic painting and anthroposophic speech formation.

Providing welcoming, cozy rooms, paying attention to the habits, likes and dislikes of the elderly help to turn the institution into a home in which people feel at home. Flower arrangements and small things from nature, such as those on a "seasonal table," as well as animals from the surrounding area, give opportunities to consciously experience the course of the year and set accents by celebrating festivals. Especially disoriented elderly people can experience themselves embedded in time and space and thus find security and orientation. Cultural events and creative-artistic work offer impulses for soul and spirit.

Music occupies a special key position. Concerts and entertainment delight old people, as well as the opportunity to sing well-known songs themselves. Some elderly people in need of help, who appear only passive to us during nursing care, unfold their personality in an undreamt-of way when singing. Their humanity comes to manifestation and radiates into everyday encounters.

The same is true when we make it possible for old people to take part in church services. Very observant geriatric nurses report that the elderly person can appear changed in the aftermath of this experience, as if his human dignity had been affirmed.

Such "magical moments" give caregivers hints on how to deal with the elderly, even in the most everyday activities.

Another area of work that is very concretely related to the individual is to occupy oneself with one's biography, an area which can also involve relatives.

What a treasure of the fruits of life is hidden in an old man! Knowing the person's life stories arouses interest in everyone involved, it engenders understanding and respect for the people entrusted to us, who thereby become givers rather than mere receivers, and who then also end up processing the experiences of their lives by accepting their own mistakes and shortcomings.

To meet all these requirements, geriatric nurses need a high degree of general and individual knowledge.

As important as activating opportunities are, one thing must not be forgotten: old people need a considerable amount of time in which they can devote themselves to merely thinking about things. This contemplation can be seen as a kind of processing of life experiences. Rudolf Steiner described how the aging human being, whether he is aware of it or not, experiences forces releasing themselves from his body according to inherent laws, and thus arrives at a certain kind of wisdom.[1]

We must not, therefore, prevent the very elderly from doing this by offering too many opportunities for activity. When the nurse develops an awareness of the value of this "being immersed in oneself," he will no longer be plagued by the idea, oriented to his own needs, that the people in his care are not experiencing enough variety. The satisfaction of geriatric nurses that results from their insight into the actual wishes of the elderly is the prerequisite for creating a peaceful atmosphere in a care group. This, too, is an aspect of geragogy.

So far in this chapter, we have not considered the care of the elderly at home. Essentially the same applies. The only question that arises is how far the domestic environment really does justice to people in old age. However well the person's caregiving network may be organized, it is often ignored that the elderly are frequently left to themselves and to their helplessness for long periods of time.

SPECIALIZATIONS IN NURSING

Left alone, this helplessness can become threatening. The life forces that are becoming free then do not unfold their positive effect. Elderly people need community. And, society needs old people who view this work benevolently, because work wants to be seen.

Nevertheless, the decision to grow old at home or in an institution is a matter for the elderly and their relatives to decide. Even when it is folly that an old person wants to stay at home, this wish should be respected if the people around him want to and are able to support it.

On the other hand, the—painful—separation from one's own four walls can also offer an opportunity to practice dying already in life. The more voluntarily a person consciously lets go of things in old age, the more peaceful the aging process will be. In addition, experiencing and understanding the processes of detachment helps the people around the person to gain a different relationship to their own lives and to include the worlds beyond life on earth to a greater extent.

3. Views of humanity und motivation in geriatric care

Current views on old age—both in the public mind (reflected in the media) and in science (in scientific theories on old age)—go in two directions. People see old age as being naturally connected with a withdrawal from active life, from work, from one's social environment, even from one's family. This corresponds to the inner need of the old person for peace and contentment. The natural process of deterioration is not only seen as biological, it is also transferred to activities of soul and spirit. People think the old person doesn't want to get involved anymore. He is disengaging.

On the other hand, activity theory is increasingly gaining acceptance, which sees the danger that the old person will be labelled too early as inactive, that existing potentials of creativity, learning ability, knowledge and physical performance will be buried unused: "He who rests, rusts." A growing range of activities in different fields is taking this view into account. Political involvement, including founding a new political party, senior sports, university studies, even senior discos are nothing unusual today.

It is not a question here of deciding which of the two theories is the right one. Truth is contained in both, but each proves problematic when conceived one-sidedly: one shows us the old man caught in his processes of deterioration and justifies his being phased out into having no role or task. The other one seems to be saying: "Don't allow yourself to get old" and ignores the fact that with death we finally have to go through a "separation," which is then only experienced as defeat and therefore has to be postponed and repressed for as long as possible. Preparation for death has no room in permanently active "unretirement."

Both theories are ultimately based on a deficit model of aging that is simply accepted in one case and ignored or combated as far as possible in the other. Depending on the underlying opinion, nursing care for the elderly works either as preserving, protecting, relieving, or stimulating and activating in the sense of helping people to help themselves.

Training today places more and more emphasis on activating care, and it appears to be an expression of good quality care when as many people as possible are dressed in a nursing home during the day and can be found up and out of bed. As an instructor, you quickly find yourself in a dilemma: although trainees are motivated and equipped to provide activating care, such care is often difficult to provide in everyday working life and under increasingly difficult conditions. In line with activity theory and for cost reasons society is leaving old people in their domestic environment for as long as possible, which corresponds mostly also to their personal inclination. As a result, caregivers in homes for the elderly are encountering more and more elderly people who are in great need of care, especially those who are disoriented, i.e., the most helpless of the elderly. Inevitably, activating care takes a back seat in this case, because, with such a heavy workload, care that keeps the person passive and dependent can be carried out more easily and quickly. This already paves the way for a guilty conscience and frustration during training, because the aspiration and the reality cannot be reconciled. Some well-known consequences are nurses lacking ideals who do rote work, or who leave the profession. What remains is joyless tiredness on the part of nurses and those being cared for, which makes a significant contribution to the depressing, musty, unpleasant atmosphere in nursing homes and institutions for the elderly.

The disengagement and activity theories do not offer an image of the human being that can serve as a basis for the long-term motivation that is needed in geriatric nursing care. They may serve as guidelines for how to work in one case or another, but they do not answer the question of the meaning of aging.

Anthroposophy assumes that every day and every hour that a person lives on earth—no matter how frail, disoriented or even unconscious—is important not only for himself, but for his environment and even for the whole of humanity. How can this be?

The abilities that lift the human being beyond any animal are an upright gait, speaking and thinking. Just as small children gradually learn these skills in the first years of life, aging people must gradually give up their abilities at the end of their lives. Walking becomes more difficult; movements can only be carried out with difficulty or not at all. On the one hand, disease-related disorders hinder speech, on the other hand one gets the impression that some elderly people have simply lost the need for communication. In relation to thinking, people lament forgetfulness—short-term memory is known to deteriorate, and this complicates orientation in contemporary everyday life.

To equate these natural aging processes with total deterioration on the level of soul and spirit would mean to understand old age as a failure of the person's forces. This is a view which inevitably leads to "salvation" through active euthanasia as a logical consequence. "Mercy killing" shortens the suffering that is perceived to be senseless.

A key to understanding the meaning of old age can be found when we see an opportunity for higher evolving in the development of soul and spirit within the weakening body, with its decline in function. As the body becomes weaker, drier and more fragile, the higher members of the fourfold human being penetrate and seize it less and less: they let go more and more, the spirit becomes free.

> *"Only now the person does not have the possibility to hold on to it, because here he is facing the physical world and wants to express himself through the body. What is becoming more and more independent and self-reliant only becomes fully apparent after death. So, it is not that the spirit and soul become too dull as the person ages, on the contrary: they are becoming ever freer and freer ... "*[2]

As when one prepares for a journey to a foreign country by acquiring knowledge about it beforehand from books and pictures, so also the experience of the gradual detachment from the body can be seen as a learning process for the 'I', which already during life is getting a foretaste of what it will experience as a purely spiritual existence after death.

The theory of disengagement in old age seems to be justified to a certain degree when one has physical development in mind. Activity in old age is primarily to be related to things of soul and spirit. To engage in activity exclusively on a bodily level will lead to defeat in the end.

Addressing the spirit, no matter to what extent it is still expressing itself through the body, gives the old person an opportunity to experience his or her higher self as a reality, i.e., to feel recognized as a human being.

4.　Stimulation for people in care

Irrespective of whether we are providing activating or protective care, we can always try to stimulate this 'being human' by striving ourselves for orderly movement and upright posture, as well as clear speaking and sincere communication, and earnestly pursuing our own spiritual training and personality development [→ Chapter "Nursing as a Path of Development"].

The following example of straightening up will explain what we mean by stimulating 'being human' in more detail. Heroic deeds and spectacular events are usually made famous with big words. We find out about them in many ways. As a rule, only a few people notice what happens in obscurity.

When you work in the nursing profession, you experience again and again what efforts weak people make when struggling to achieve an upright position. With great effort they confront the forces pressing them down and their own fragility in order to stand on their feet for a short time. Something which the healthy can do countless times without difficulty: for the sick or old person, it can be the event of the day. What power helps people to stand up? Already in ancient cultures—and perhaps more than today—people knew of this power and described it:

> *"... when day breaks you are risen upon the horizon,*
> *and you shine as the Aten in the daytime...*
> *the two lands are in festival, alert and standing on their feet, now that you*
> *have raised them up.*
> *Their bodies are clean, and their clothes have been put on;*
> *their arms are (lifted) in praise at your rising..."*

From "The Great Hymn to Aten," in: Simpson W.K. (ed). *The Literature of Ancient Egypt.* 3rd revised and enlarged ed. Yale University Press, New Haven and London 2003.

Elderly people, including those not in need of care, are naturally exposed to forces of hardening. Any effort to counteract this hardening can mobilize positive strength and buoyancy. Day after day, when people raise themselves up, especially when they overcome heaviness and weakness, they awaken in themselves this power that people in former times experienced as divine, as something carrying them from outside, because it affected the whole earth. Today we experience this power from within.

We may call it the power of resurrection, which was put into our inner being by the Christ impulse as a seed. When we recognize the cosmic dimension of raising oneself upright as an expression of the human 'I', then this motivates us to bring people who are constantly lying in bed into a sitting posture, at least for short moments, or to create the experience of standing on their feet once a day, and to help those who are handicapped in walking to take a few steps, even if it is only for a short distance.

But there are also people who lie heavily where they are, who no longer take part in everyday life, who doze with greatly diminished consciousness, and for whom one almost wishes they could finally be redeemed by death. It is also and especially true for them that, as long as there is still a spark of life in their bodies, this divine power dwells within them and the force of gravity, which the body completely succumbs to only at death, must be countered by the force of life, the power to raise oneself upright.

Raising oneself upright on a physical level happens as described, but an upliftment can also take place in the soul, e.g., in overcoming oppressive moods, resignation, depression, or an upliftment in the spirit can happen through prayer, meditation and cognitive effort. On which level the uprightness is found and with which degree of consciousness this is accomplished, is to be determined individually in the changing states of life. What all efforts to raise upright have in common is that they increase the presence of positive forces in the world.

These forces make working in geriatric care worthwhile! Even, and especially, when the demands on us are becoming more and more difficult. Every humane act of nursing care, even the slightest one, gains meaning for both the elderly person and the nurse.

It is precisely the ailments and pressures of old age that offer us the opportunity to develop these positive forces. Let us try to imagine what potential exists in our presently living old people alone!

Attacks on the 'I' are abundant in the world, e.g., through violence, media, drugs, etc. The cultivation of positive forces, no matter how weak they may be, supports and promotes the 'I'. We see it as a counterweight to all destructiveness and complacent laziness. The efforts of weak, sick and elderly people to raise themselves up are special "heroic deeds," albeit of a modest nature that are not reported in the media. But perhaps so-called "great deeds" are only possible because of these positive forces developed by individuals.

Category	Example learning objectives	Recommended learning path
Skills	You actively permit the "stillness" of old age.	A
Your own learning objective		
Relationships	In your everyday nursing work, you are conscious of the immortal essence in elderly people.	B
Your own learning objective		
Knowledge	You know about the power of uprightness in being human.	C
Your own learning objective		

References

1   Steiner, R. *The connection between the living and the dead.* SteinerBooks, Great Barrington 2017.
2   Steiner, R. *The dead are with us.* Rudolf Steiner Press, London 2006.

CHAPTER XXII
Aspects of Caring for Elderly People Who Are Mentally Ill or Confused

CHRISTEL KAUL

The care of mentally ill and confused elderly people is an immense burden. On the one hand we want to preserve their autonomy and dignity, on the other hand we want to ensure their security and that of their fellow human beings. Only from a differentiated understanding of the consciousness of their patients and with knowledge of the causes can nurses master this task. This chapter will look at mental illness and states of confusion as disturbed aging processes. It will explain this time of having to say goodbye to active life, undergoing necessary transformations, and the shining of the spiritual world into the consciousness of old people. This chapter will give numerous practical suggestions for dealing with completely muddled situations, offer perspectives, and encourage nurses to face up to such difficult encounters.

→   Learning objectives, see end of chapter

1.   On the situation of people with dementia and their nurses

Today, more and more people with severe psychological diseases and dementia are living in nursing homes and institutions for the elderly. Often, they are forced into the institution from home by their circumstances, when they are no longer able to provide for themselves or when no one can deal with them anymore. This means that the threshold at which the old person can still gain an understanding of his new situation and actively shape it has often been crossed a long time ago. The change of location, not deliberately chosen, and the new group of people around the person, dramatically reinforce his lack of responsiveness and lack of ability to express himself. The people who move into an institution under such circumstances fall into dullness and refusal or become restless or aggressive to the point of physical aggression. Often psychotropic drugs additionally put a dense cloud around their consciousness. Such people can no longer get their bearings, new situations appear inscrutable, and they may be constantly searching for their lost home. If they are no longer able to express this verbally, they will find themselves in deep inner despair and forlornness.

The care of such people pushes nurses and, above all, the person's relatives, to their physical and psychological limits, despite the wide range of help given. They suffer equally from the situation and from themselves, from feelings of powerlessness, failure and incomprehension. The aggression of residents can, in turn, trigger aggression and doubts in the nurses about their professional self-image.

Resignation or attempts to force the old person to adapt are often expressions of the excessive demands being made on the nurses.

> A young nurse came out of a resident's room angrily crying and said: "I'm not an aggressive person, but I yelled at Mrs. M. terribly. I'm in despair about myself."

People suffering from dementia are nowadays mostly perceived to be disturbing and frightening. People with dementia confuse the image that we like to have of ourselves. They radically make us question the ideal of self-determination. In a social environment that is characterized by rapid technological development and the illusion that everything is doable, nurses hardly find understanding and support in their work. Great strength and self-development are needed to practice distant compassion and not fall into the maelstrom of despair and hopelessness.

2. The transformation of physical decline into mental and spiritual development

All of human life is permeated by upbuilding and degenerating forces in various metamorphoses. In childhood and adolescence, upbuilding forces necessarily have the upper hand. The infant must grow into the world. In the middle of life, the person reaches a climax of inner and outer strength, and upbuilding and degeneration are in balance. Then a slow reversal begins. The upbuilding of the vital forces decreases and processes of degeneration intensify. Less and less vitality and regeneration are available to counter the degeneration caused by physical and intellectual work. To age is to experience a withdrawal of one's upbuilding forces. The old person is growing out of the physical world, he is "de-living." This process can be observed in increasing coolness, drying of the skin, loss of elasticity and weakening of the sensory organs. The body seems ever more "lifeless." Death in old age occurs when the available life forces have been exhausted.

Aging is characterized by physical degeneration. The aging process of soul and spirit, on the other hand, has its own stages of development. This runs opposite to the upbuilding and degenerating forces described. Childhood and adolescence are characterized by assimilating and learning. In the middle of life, we develop what has been absorbed and learned into abilities and apply them. Each person is independent and responsible for himself. After reaching mid-life, people can more deeply recognize, transform and communicate perceived connections. Tried and tested experiences become more and more clearly comprehensible. The question of the meaning of one's own life path acquires a wider horizon. This process does not happen by itself, it evolves through one's own effort of will. It is shaped by the existential question: "Am I as a human being at the mercy of this process of ongoing physical decline or can my inner development remain free of it?" This question determines the significance of aging for the individual.

If the experience of physical degeneration comes to the fore, there is a danger that old age will be perceived or suppressed as a threat to existence. Rigid adherence to habits, the loss of self-esteem and the resulting problems with the environment are also usually the result of an attitude that sees old age as a deficit. When one succeeds in keeping oneself mentally and spiritually mobile, by opposing the physical degeneration with inner mental stature, then the desire often arises to clarify and work through one's life, to order one's life, to develop serenity, farsightedness, peace and love as gifts to the world. On this path, the human being can remain the architect of his life until the end, despite all adversities and physical limitations. "I no longer look at what I can no longer do, I'm happy about what I can still do and I am thankful for every day. I am ready to go."

It is precisely letting go that opens up the chance of finding the pearls of life in old age. This does not happen without pain. It takes courage and humility to pull away the veil of illusion that had obscured the actually important things of the world during life, which in a certain way also gave protection. The omnipresent physical limitations of aging must be transformed into freedom. Becoming free of being externally pushed and pulled gives peace and serenity. In this quietness we can listen and ask more deeply about ourselves.

Age-related illnesses make it painfully obvious that our physical garment is worn out and cannot be renewed. They intensify the conflict between holding on and letting go. They indicate the path that every human being must follow, whether freely or reluctantly—the path to death. Is the human being only part of living nature or is he also a member of a spiritual world? Is death doom or transformation? Is old age a post-processing of one's biography and a preparation for life in the spiritual world? If so, then old age would be a phase of purification and refining for the threshold crossing. Diseases of old age can mean great pain and yet serve to make people aware of their coming departure. Understanding enables transformation, the soul becomes free. Past experiences acquire a different appearance and weight. The meaning of one's unique path in life shimmers through pain, injuries and omissions.

3. The anthroposophic-anthropological understanding of senile dementia

Over the course of a lifetime, body-bound upbuilding forces are largely transformed into forces of consciousness. If this metamorphosis is not completely successful, then unconscious life processes are pushed abnormally into consciousness. They flood thinking and imagining. It is then no longer the world that is reflected in one's consciousness, but one's own life processes.

There are three areas in which human beings interact with the environment:

- Through nutrition we absorb the world materially.
- Through breathing, we connect to it in a finer and more conscious way.
- Through sensory impressions we take the world entirely immaterially into ourselves.

The following section will describe how nutritional, respiratory and sensory life can lead to disturbances in consciousness if bodily processes are not transformed in an age-appropriate way.

3.1 Food intake and its metamorphosis

Physical food is absorbed by the digestive organs, adapted, broken down and transformed into the body's own substance. Unusable material is eliminated. Nutrition enables upbuilding, regeneration and reproduction of the body. It is to nutrition that we owe the maintenance of our body and thus the ability to become active. With our limbs we deliberately shape the world. Healthy people do not perceive their digestion. Only discomfort makes them aware of it. Unconscious will normally prevails in the metabolism.

Metabolism (uptake—transformation—excretion) enables:			
Inwardly	Upbuilding, regeneration, reproduction	Forming the body	Unconscious will
Outwardly	Limb activity	Shaping the world	Conscious will

Chart: The metabolism and its metamorphoses

3.1.1 The pathology of untransformed metabolic processes in old age

Metabolic activity decreases with age. If the transformation of the bodily upbuilding processes into alertness of soul and spirit did not take place sufficiently in the person's biographical development, then the soul and spirit remain as if "chained" to the body's life processes. The unconscious metabolic processes overwhelm the consciousness and the aging person becomes their plaything. The body's dependence on food corresponds to the enjoyable and pleasurable attachment of the soul to metabolic processes. A balance must be found at an early stage, so that the soul in old age, when the bodily need for food and drink subsides, does not remain bound to the body. Only conscious detachment from physicality offers the soul the chance to avoid following the descending path of the body. If this is not already practiced during life, the condition of the physical body will dominate the feeling of life in old age. Obsessions and feelings of loss will arise.

This can be observed in the following typical behaviors: at first, food intake becomes increasingly important for the aging person affected, until he finally only lives from food intake to food intake. As long as he eats, he exists, in between he seems dissatisfied and claims that he is getting too little or that he has not yet had anything to eat. Maybe every ten minutes he'll ask when there is finally going to be something to eat. The dominant topic of conversation for him is food and the physical sensations associated with it. He does not manage to emancipate himself from the life process of nutrition, and since it is decreasing or dying, he is dying along with it mentally. Connectedness with food can become more and more compulsive, even leading to delusions that are not always associated with the subject of food. Compulsive theft as "compensation" for the perceived material lack can be an expression of the soul being too strongly bound to the body-bound aspect of food.

If the processes at work in digestion penetrate the person's consciousness, he may experience images of destruction and dissolution. The people affected feel torn or forced to destroy themselves. Often these images cause terrible conditions, especially at night. Compulsiveness and fears develop when metabolic processes intrude into the person's consciousness.

3.1.2 Therapeutic nursing measures

First of all, it is important to understand the person's words correctly. A statement can be interpreted in different ways.

"My coat has been stolen." I take the patient to her room and show her the coat. She recognizes it and exclaims, "Oh, there it is!" The incident was therefore an expression of forgetfulness. Perhaps she will soon forget the incident and the coat.

The same thing can happen differently, without insight. The elderly person does not react at all to seeing the coat but continues to search restlessly. She thereby signals: "I am losing my earthly mantle; I can't get to my body anymore." Such people therefore often do not want to take off their clothes and they wear several garments on top of each other. Clothes become their skin. The opposite reaction is also possible: patients experience their body as an obstacle and as a scary encasement. They want to get rid of it and therefore take off their clothes again and again. They run around restlessly—fleeing from themselves.

Here, clothing and food are unconsciously used as code for the body and its preservation. This frequent metaphor, which also occurs in dreams, contains an important therapeutic hint. The body wants to be treated as the covering of the soul. Treatment and nursing care therefore deal with the body as a covering that needs care and protection. The aim is to give support, raise upright, strengthen and at the same time make lightness and loosening possible. The following measures support these gestures:

- Rhythmical Einreibung according to Wegman/Hauschka
- Rhythm in the daily routine
- Warm, enveloping clothing (also in summer)
- To fall asleep: a warm footbath, or preheat the bed with hot water bottles, put wool socks on
- Stroke down the patient's legs and then warm the soles of her feet with the palm of your hand.
- Light a candle, say a poem or prayer, sing a song
- When saying goodnight, put your hand on the old man's hand, deliberately say his name and look into his eyes.
- Go for a walk and perhaps sing a hiking song; draw attention to nature, touch things, touch flowers, smell the scent, pluck wool, etc. (i.e., to experience boundaries and encounters through the sense of touch)

3.2 Breathing and its metamorphosis

A second way in which we absorb the world is through breathing. Through breathing we connect intensively with our environment. The air is initially the outside world, but for moments it becomes our inside world, only to be exhaled again after a short time. A part of the air connects with our organism and is transformed (inhaling oxygen, "combustion," exhaling carbon dioxide). Between inhaling and exhaling there is a short pause, a slight standstill. This interruption of the even flow acts in the subconscious as a wake-up process. In comparison with food intake, contact with the environment is partly more intense, partly more volatile. We inhale the same air together with others and exhale our own into it. There is a social exchange in breathing. The breathing process is semi-conscious, dreamy and strongly connected with feeling, which can be observed well in the coupling of mental moods and breathing rhythms. If the person's breathing is organically disturbed, this has a direct effect on how they feel. But also, the soul influences breathing. A big scare will make us breathless. When we are comfortable, we take regular deep breaths. Our breathing reveals our relationship to our surroundings. A sigh shows that we are not in harmony with the world. The soul and spirit connect with the earthly through breathing in constant alternation and then let go again. The incarnation process begins with the first breath at birth, and the soul detaches itself from the physical world again with the last exhalation at death.

3.2.1 Late-life depression and anxiety as lost mental elasticity

Frequently occurring geriatric depression and the lack of drive associated with it, along with associated mental narrowness and fears, are directly related to the respiratory process. Respiratory movement naturally becomes slower and flatter with age. Often an old person holds back his breath too much, and his mental mobility (immobility) unconsciously follows along.

In asthma and pulmonary emphysema, this process has manifested organically. When there is a tendency to "hold the breath back," the lungs expand over time. They gradually lose their elasticity and an ever larger, poorly ventilated space develops in them. A comparable process takes place in the soul in cases of late-life depression. Many feelings are held back in the soul over the course of life and now the person lacks the mental elasticity to exhale mentally. It gets harder to "inhale" new things. The life of the soul is not experiencing any warming and transparency, it is withering away.

The old man increasingly withdraws into himself, becomes lonely and sad, finally becoming embittered. The soul's stiffness is also expressed in the physical. The body cramps to the point of immobility, the facial expressions become impoverished and stony. The person seems motionless on the outside and on the inside. One has the feeling that the essence of this human being is locked in the body. Cold develops both inwardly and outwardly. Even in sleep there is no real relief, the body remains cramped. A tendency towards inner retreat that has already existed during life can intensify in old age.

3.2.2 Therapeutic nursing measures

Physical warmth, rhythm, movement and soul warmth—love—have a harmonizing effect. Quiet, undiminishing attention is important in the accompaniment of such people. All provocative gestures will make them close up even more. Specifically, we can offer the following:

- Rhythmical Einreibung of the whole body, especially intensive treatment of the hands and feet
- Warm clothing
- Raising upright (mentally and physically)
- Short walks
- Full baths with stimulating bath additives (e.g. *Rosemary Invigorating Bath Milk* (Weleda), *Pine Reviving Bath Milk* (Weleda), *Citrus Refreshing Bath Milk* (Weleda) or *Lemon Lemongrass Vitalising Bath Essence* (Dr. Hauschka))
- Reading short fairy tales that contain the gesture of giving (e.g., the Star Money fairy tale)

- As a silent gesture, place your enveloping hand without pressure on the patient's hand or around their shoulders; this has a deeply relaxing and liberating effect.
- Stimulate rhythmic movements with the gestures "give and take," "open up and withdraw," "release and bind," "put a ball into their hands and have them give it back"; the gesture intensifies until the ball can be thrown. A further intensification consists in guiding a rod over the head backwards and forwards. To support this exercise, the following text can be spoken rhythmically:

Sower's verse
Measure your step,
measure your swing!
The earth will keep on being young!
There falls a grain
to die and rest.
Its rest is sweet.
It lies at peace.
Here's one that pierces through the clod.
It finds its goodness. Sweet the light.
And not a grain falls out of this world.
And each falls as it pleases God. Conrad Ferdinand Meyer (1825–1898). Translated by
Matthew Barton, in: Berg P. The moon gardener. *A biodynamic guide to getting the best from your garden.* Temple Lodge, Forest Row 2012.

These measures provide opportunities to talk about stressful experiences. Especially laughter can be freeing; depressed people are known to find this difficult.

An old lady was regularly visited by her son on weekends and was invited to go on excursions into the beautiful surroundings. When she came back and I asked her if it had been nice, she always said: "Yes, but now they're gone!" A very short bright "yes" and then the curtain of the "but." We had a good relationship, so one day I asked her: "May I smile softly every time you say 'yes, but'?" she replied: "Yes, but," and then she smiled herself and said: "I did it again!" She couldn't break the habit anymore but smiled and looked at us very warmly. By doing that she brought herself into balance.

3.3 The metamorphosis of the senses

[→ Chapter "From the Question of Meaning in Cancer to the Cultivation of the Senses"]

Human beings enter into a relationship with the world through their senses. 'I'-consciousness is formed via sensory perceptions. It is through them that the 'I' gains access to the world. Sensory impressions are a kind of subtle nourishment. Just as there are healthy or inferior, digestible or indigestible foods, there are also constructive, life-giving and degrading or damaging sensory impressions. Just as with food, there can be too much or too little. Sensory impressions have a direct effect on a person's physical organization. A frightening stimulus makes the skin turn pale and the breath falter. An inspiring impression warms and reddens the face. Our breathing speeds up. Sensory impressions affect blood circulation, breathing and metabolism. It is well known that a harmoniously designed environment has a healthy effect, while a cold, chaotic one is unhealthy.

If we were not to form the associated concepts by thinking, and relate them to one another, all the contents of perception would exist as incoherent details. The senses allow us to recognize only one side of reality, the other side must be actively added to it. Concepts and ideas that we develop live on within us and become part of our individual world view. In this way, perception and conceptualization continue to affect us, even when the event has long since passed. This content, which has been achieved in the course of life and is often forgotten, enlivens us in old age, especially when our relationship to the world is weakened by the weakness of our senses.

Due to the increasing limitation of sensory perception, the connection with the environment is lost. Life takes place only in one's own imagination. This leads to disorientation and illusion, to numbness and isolation. If the past life of an elderly person was predominantly marked by external, material stimuli and values, then diminished functioning of the senses will become a terrible experience of loss. Only when this loss is countered by a rich spiritual inner life, acquired over the years through interest in the world, does freedom from the physical develop.

> *When seeing is forgotten,*
> *the light becomes infinitely rich!*
> *When hearing is destroyed:*
> *the heart gathers itself*
> *in the eternal depths.*
> *When the senses of perception*
> *are destroyed:*
> *the human being becomes able*
> *to detach himself*
> *from all the stimuli of the world,*
> *pure, open and complete,*
> *in perfect union*
> *with the universe,*
> *wide, boundless*
> *like an invigorating breath of air,*
> *not subject to any divisions*
> *of humanity.*
> Lao Tzu (604–531 BC)

3.3.1 The sense of life transforms into equanimity

Our sense of life conveys perceptions of the state of our own bodily functions. Through it we perceive strength or weakness, vitality or morbidity. When an old person remains fixated on these perceptions, he becomes dependent on the weakness of his metabolism. He is prone to annoyance, bad temper and pessimism. Attention and equanimity towards one's metabolic processes are often the only protection against the withdrawal of one's life forces from one's corporeality.

Helpful nursing measures:
The nurse first tries to use existing resources and gently stimulate the patient's life forces. This is done via:
- Rhythm in the daily routine
- Age-appropriate, easily digestible food
- Sufficient fluid intake
- Rhythmical Einreibung
- Fresh air
- Refreshing baths
- A feeling of security through the creation of a pleasant environment

3.3.2 The sense of one's own movement and the sense of balance

The sense of one's own movement and balance is transformed into freedom and mental balance within. Restrictions in mobility, due to weakness, stiffness, joint pain or paralysis lead to internal immobility if the metamorphosis from external activity into inner soul activity was not accomplished. Inner rigidity is also expressed in egocentric thoughts circling around oneself.

The sense of balance conveys security and orientation in the environment. Uncertainty, fear, holding on to what is familiar and the feeling of being deprived of one's freedom are mental expressions of a lack of reference to the world.

Helpful nursing measures:
Nursing care to promote elementary experiences of the body:
- Straightening oneself up (also while sitting), making good contact with the ground with one's feet
- Movement in any form (e.g., walking, dancing, swimming or passing a ball around a circle: accept with your left hand, give to yourself, pass on with your right hand; left—middle—right: a feeling of balance develops)
- Put your hand quietly on the elderly person's back, between the shoulder blades.
- Rhythmic speaking, singing and music

3.3.3 The sense of touch transforms into reverence

When the sense of touch weakens, the perception of one's own person dwindles. The "I-am feeling" is increasingly lost. This causes great unrest. Those affected must touch themselves constantly, or they cling to their nurses. They feel uncloaked.

Helpful nursing measures:
- Gently touching, stroking, laying on of hands, giving warmth and envelopment
- Handicrafts with warming materials
- Petting animals

3.3.4 The sense of sight transforms into inner comprehension

Age-related visual disturbances lead to misinterpretations and compensatory additions from one's own imagination. Those affected no longer comprehend what they see. They become jumpy and see danger everywhere.

Helpful nursing measures:
- Approach the elderly person quietly, avoid haste, announce your actions verbally
- Describe the surroundings
- Lead by touch and give security
- Suggest that you close your eyes while sitting together and tell each other how you perceive your surroundings.
- Practice color perception

3.3.5 The sense of smell transforms into compassion

In smelling we take the world deep inside us. The smells trigger dislike or pleasure, antipathy or sympathy in us. When our sense of smell weakens, its stimulation of the soul disappears, and we lose its ability to awaken us to what is foreign. This can lead to dullness and carelessness towards the environment.

Helpful nursing measures:
- Flower fragrances or essential oils awaken the person to their environment and invigorate them inwardly.

3.3.6 The sense of taste transforms into tact and politeness

The organ of taste also loses its vitality. As a result, many elderly people complain constantly about eating, or they want to eat the same food every day. One-sidedness may ensue. Often there is even a certain greed. Nagging and exaggerated demands can be an expression of a weakened sense of taste.

Helpful nursing measures:
- Make the meals tasty
- Create a nice atmosphere
- Stimulate the sense of taste by differentiating between sensory qualities (e.g., by comparing the acidity of an apple with that of a lemon)
- Gentle, respectful oral care

3.3.7 The sense of warmth transforms into patience

Organ and soul warmth influence each other. A cooling of the body leads to mental coldness. When a person retains inner soul warmth and enthusiasm, their body also heats up. Old people produce less heat due to their slower metabolisms. That is why we have to keep them warm from the outside and, if necessary, supply them with heat.

Helpful nursing measures:
- Help the person to enjoy small things
- Bring him together with others whom he can warm to (often it is the affection for small children or animals)
- Warm encounters with relatives and caregivers

3.3.8 The sense of hearing transforms into restraint

Hearing loss can lead to distrust: "The others are talking so quietly because they're talking about me." Or: "They want to shut me out." The person suspects hostility towards him. He doesn't feel understood and doesn't understand anymore.

Helpful nursing measures:
- Turn fully to the person when speaking.
- Communicate understanding and warmth through eye contact and touching the person's hand; this can create trust and release the cramped desire to hear (which also improves hearing).
- Rhythmic sounds through instruments warm up and enliven the sense of hearing.

3.3.9 The senses of the speech, thoughts and the 'I' of the other person transform into courage, silence and renunciation.

The willingness to take in new things and enter into new relationships can be greatly reduced by physical weakness or rigid habits: "Everything used to be better!" "How could anyone understand this!" "Young people today have no morals!" All these statements show how difficult it is to adapt to change.

Helpful nursing measures:
- We, the companions, are the help.
- Our inner flexibility, our understanding for other thoughts and viewpoints opens up possibilities for new things.
- Fairy tales, poems, prayers, gospel texts or imaginative thoughts help people to open these senses.

4.　The double

Another phenomenon, which occurs occasionally in many exceptional mental states, affects some people particularly severely and recurrently: the encounter with their double. Due to the loosening of the higher members of the fourfold human being from the physical body, confused or demented people become border crossers between the physical and spiritual worlds. The past, with its shadows and light, pushes itself into the present, while the spiritual world comes from the future. The double is a kind of shadow image of the human personality. It gathers all those qualities which we as human beings would like to have separated from us, but which are inseparably connected with our being. This state is like a premonition of the experiences that the deceased will have immediately after death.
[→ Chapter "The Accompaniment and Care of the Dying and the Deceased"]

A typical manifestation of the double is a sudden change in a person's personality. He suddenly appears with an ugly charisma. His facial expression becomes a grimace, his eyes rigid, his voice quite strange. This can increase to vulgar expressions and violence. It is often difficult, especially for relatives, not to take these outbreaks personally. It is a real exercise to remain calm in encounters with the shadow being, the double that every person carries within him, and not to react with personal disappointment or anger.

A real help can be:
- to address a petition to the guardian angel of the person concerned.
- to look at the person's biography with the question of what task this person has set himself for this life.
- to look at shortcomings with loving understanding and to emphasize the points of light.

- to look at the person with distance and without fear, and to say his full name loudly and clearly in case of physical aggression. That can bring him to his senses.

In the case of an acute physical attack, it is often a lifesaver to refrain from resisting. People in this situation literally have inhuman powers, and resistance whips them up. If one is in the firm grip of a person in a state of mental emergency, it helps to let the tension out of one's body and become quite limp. That makes it almost impossible for the patient to keep holding you. This "trick" should be practiced with colleagues before use.

Example

An old, very distinguished lady (businesswoman) hit everyone with her stick. You couldn't turn your back on her or she clasped your neck. She screamed and scolded and never calmed down. One day she lay on her bed, completely exhausted, shouting her insults.

I sat down on the edge of the bed, not within arm's reach, and she said in Bavarian, "May your husband die, and I'll rip your ears off." I said calmly: "You don't want that." Her face lost its rigor, and she said in her normal voice: "No." But then the curtain closed again. It became clear that speaking was not a way to relieve the situation. I treated her legs with rhythmic strokes. When I reached her knees, she said in a normal voice: "You won't make it." I just kept stroking and I said: "You want to bet?" When I arrived at her feet, she fell asleep, relaxed.

"These shattering encounters can unsettle and frighten us, but they also help us to answer existential questions: Who am I? What did I want to do? Where have I come from? Where am I going? For who can say that he knows who he is without the other helping him?"
Dorothea Rapp

We all need the help of another, a fellow human being, to become human beings.

Category	Example learning objectives	Recommended learning path
Skills	You can empathize with the consciousness of confused people.	A
Your own learning objective		
Relationships	By your behavior you give orientation to confused people.	B
Your own learning objective		
Knowledge	You are familiar with possible causes of confusion.	C
Your own learning objective		

References

1. Der Doppelgänger. *Flensburger Hefte,* vol. 65. Flensburger Hefte Verlag, Flensburg 1999.
2. Glas, N. *Lichtvolles Alter.* Mellinger Verlag, Stuttgart 1992.

CHAPTER XXIII

Caring for People with Dementia in Inpatient Facilities

HEIKE SCHAUMANN

→   Learning objectives, see end of chapter

1.   Introduction

Caring for people with dementia always challenges us to come up with new ideas and ways of acting. At the beginning of our work in home communities we mainly thought about the concrete aspects of daily life, about the occupations and daily routines to be organized. Over the last few years, the work has evolved, and other issues have come to the fore. It is almost always individual changes in people with dementia that give cause for concern or confront us with new questions. This, in turn, influences the everyday life of the entire group in a home community. It is exciting to experience how the dynamics of individual destinies affect and touch the lives of other residents, including the nurses.

Feelings, emotional experiences, and habits from the past shape our lives together. There is little discussion and there are hardly any conversations that allow us to participate in the inner worlds of the people we are caring for. Much takes place without language, or only fragments of language. That changes things. Reflection, and the pursuit of change, happens among staff members and nurses. The dependency of the people living in the facility can be shocking. We strongly feel responsibility for the circumstances of their lives, for their feelings and their concrete possibilities for expression, which we create, or not. This brings with it a sharp confrontation with our own life questions and abilities (such as the ability to feel alive).

The fact that life and death belong together in this disease results from the drama and the irreversibility of the process. No healing, only certain deterioration and, at the end, death, are predetermined. But within this path there are surprisingly many possibilities that need to be made use of. Any development that may still happen depends on the opportunities offered to the people with dementia by the nurses in their new environment.

This chapter will illuminate various aspects of the lives of people with dementia in inpatient settings. The topics will be derived from concrete experiences in a home community.

Digression

In recent years, new forms of living have developed for people of advanced age and especially for people with dementia. These include home communities, which are usually connected to a standard care facility, or which form their own inpatient facility. The home community comprises one or more small groups of residents living together in family-like living spaces. The focus is on everyday life and on living together as normally as possible.

Outpatient assisted living communities take a different approach to home communities in that, operating separately from an inpatient provider, they emphasize the independence of the tenants to a large extent.

2. Moving into an institution: an increasing loss of space for making decisions and acting as one pleases

The lives of people with dementia take a new turn when they become residents of the "foreign world" of a nursing home, outpatient assisted living community or home community.

As a rule, relatives or caregivers decide on the new place of residence. A point has been reached, also in the biography of the family, which makes deciding on a new life situation unavoidable.

The possibilities for all family members to act and make decisions have become so limited that a good outlook on life no longer seems possible. While people with dementia want to hold on to what they are used to—and despite increasing despair—hold on to what they are familiar with, their relatives are in a relationship crisis. The relatives' understanding, tolerance, love and loyalty towards the person affected by dementia have often reached a low point.

Example

Mrs. M. has been married for 50 years. Her husband has been suffering from Alzheimer's dementia for seven years. She looks after him at home and makes use of ambulant services, such as a nursing service and day care.

Mrs. M. always controlled her husband and he usually did what she wanted him to do. As his dementia progresses, his behavior becomes uncontrollable. He does things Mrs. M. can no longer tolerate. Both are feeling worse and worse. It is no longer possible to maintain their accustomed way of living together. In this situation Mrs. M. falls ill herself. She will no longer be able to care for her husband for an indefinite period of time. Mr. M. has to go to a short-term care facility.

During the consultation it becomes clear that peace has been lost in living together. Their long-established patterns no longer carry them. There have been outbreaks of mutual violence. This is not spoken of openly, but the couple's children later confirm our suspicions. In this troubled situation, the entry of Mr. M. into the institution is initially experienced as a relief.

Mr. M. is involved in the decision-making process, but he can no longer express himself clearly. He accepts the decision without complaint, his independence and decision-making ability are already severely reduced.

Mr. M. is settling in and seems to be feeling comfortable. He has a great urge to move, which makes life difficult for the staff of the institution. His wife has other complaints: Mr. M. is not shaved, he doesn't sing along, his trousers are all dirty, etc. Mrs. M. can only gradually grasp the entirety of her husband's situation. The overall impression is too overwhelming, so she clings to little things. With understanding, but also by setting clear limits, the staff team gradually achieves open discussion of the progression of Alzheimer's dementia.

Mrs. M. mourns in her own way, she must first overcome the loss of living together before she can help to constructively shape her husband's new world, and thus also a new phase in her own life.

Mr. M. turns his grief into movement. His desperation becomes clear when he angrily hits his reflection.

The example of the M. family is individual and yet exemplary. From beginning to end, the relatives are companions and essential co-decision-makers. Almost always, making a home for people with dementia in inpatient facilities will fail if it is not possible to gain the trust of the families or if the trust is lost.

Enduring grief and the feeling of loss is an essential step on the way into the new world of living in a "home." If we announce the integration of a new inhabitant too early in the first weeks and months and too self-confidently, the person's sadness and experiences of loss have not been sufficiently appreciated.

A spouse who after one week only hears how well the affected person is doing does not necessarily react with joy. He wonders if everything he has done has been wrong, he doubts his abilities as a partner.

In addition to helping the person to settle in, our work is also about accompanying these processes of detachment and mourning. Children of people with dementia mourn differently than spouses, and daughters usually differently than sons. What they all have in common is that they had to experience more or less up close how the disease changed their family member. They also have to make tough choices. Children who were not very close to their parents often suffer from the fact that they are now forced to make such a far-reaching decision for their parents, even though they never wanted to. Spouses, on the other hand, have the feeling that they are breaking their vows and abandoning their partner.

Essentially, the decision on how to proceed is made at the beginning of the move into the inpatient facility. Cooperation, transparency and respect for the decisions of the family group form the basis for expanding the space for activity and possibilities for development. In this network, people with dementia—in the best case—begin to revive according to their possibilities and can use their remaining abilities.

3. Integrating into and getting used to one's new home—shaping the way people live together

Adapting and integrating oneself into the new environment costs the affected person a lot of effort. Especially people for whom competence and independence were very important are very afraid that others will notice their insecurity and decreasing ability to remember things. The concealment of deficits is becoming increasingly strenuous. The loss of the accustomed environment and the usual routines must be compensated for step by step.

People with dementia are often looking for "home." They must go to work, find their children, are "called by their parents" and so on. As a rule, this does not refer to their previous places of residence. The search for home stands for the safe place that has been lost in the course of dementia. The further back the longing goes, the clearer it becomes. At the end of their lives, people with dementia sometimes call for their mother, because she, like no other person, provided the first security in their lives.

Caregivers have an important task in the phase of adapting to a new home in that they are called upon to constantly spin new threads that the dementia sufferer can use as orientation. The experience of being known, being given a task, hearing one's name, finding a place in the group—all these are outwardly unspectacular but indispensable aids that caregivers take on anew every day. The more seriously this is done, the safer the residents will feel in their new environment. Gradually it becomes clear which activities are particularly important for which person.

3.1 Feeling at home in the community

Example

Mr. T. was a judge. For him there is a clear distance to other people. He is careful with his contacts. His professional task has lifted him out of the group of "normal" people. He always stays at a certain distance. He doesn't attend any events at first. Gradually he comes out of his room more often and likes to sit in the "second row." An armchair at the edge of the group gives him the opportunity to participate in community life from a certain distance. Thus, it is increasingly possible to establish a secure connection with him, which at the same time enables him to maintain a sovereign position in the inpatient facility.

People develop and look for ways to get involved in their new circumstances, to help shape life in their own way. Even in an advanced stage of dementia, residents can still learn; they make contacts, find their place, entrust themselves to a new environment.

Example

Mrs. U. no longer speaks. She hasn't said a word in months. She watches intensively everything that happens in the living area. She perceives much more than one would expect. Mrs. U. frowns, looks at people who turn towards her, and expresses her feelings in this way. She makes different facial expressions when she wants to show whether she is satisfied or rather sad. Her way of participating in life must first be recognized and understood by the staff.

3.2 Habits create security

Example

Mr. F. is very restless at first. The staff are afraid that he will fall because he wanders aimlessly and waveringly through the living area. Little by little his pathways change. He develops a pattern, goes on certain routes and has three armchairs that he approaches again and again. His gait becomes more stable. The staff get to know his routes and keep them open to him. His habitualness brings a certain peace to all, the danger of falling has been reduced.

Especially people who have lived alone before and were increasingly lonely or isolated tend to flourish in a community. Abilities that had disappeared are revived; some activities can be resumed.

On the other hand, their deficits also become clearer. After a good phase, dementia progresses. Speech disorders intensify and physical symptoms, such as movement disorders and incontinence, are added. It is only when these deteriorations are accepted as part of the journey that new and different ways of participating in community life open up.

3.3 Different forms of dementia

It is important to differentiate between the different forms of dementia. Progressive Alzheimer's dementia follows other laws than, for example, dementia associated with Parkinson's disease.

In vascular dementia, many skills are retained, such as recognizing close people or knowing about the past.
Experience shows that it can be very helpful to know the form of dementia involved. In practice, though, there is still the problem that in many cases there is no exact diagnosis at all. From experience with different individual cases and under certain circumstances, nurses may be able to draw conclusions about a particular disease. This influences their understanding and handling of symptoms, such as hallucinations, or problems with speech and movement.

Delirium is an often-unrecognized condition in people with dementia. This life-threatening deterioration is often experienced in practice as "challenging behavior."

3.4   What skills do staff need?

An important balancing task in the integration of people with dementia in inpatient facilities is to keep an eye on both deficits and opportunities for development in equal measure. This also concerns the facility itself. How well can staff cope with the abilities, strengths and weaknesses, as well as losses, of the people who have dementia?

Nurses who want to work with people with dementia usually have a positive attitude towards the sometimes chaotic circumstances that this work entails. Having well-ordered procedures with habits and comprehensible structures is important but must never be allowed to stand above everything else. Spontaneity and enjoyment in finding creative solutions are essential when residents do incomprehensible and seemingly absurd things.

Staff who have a positive attitude towards life, who tend to look at the available resources—even in themselves—find it easier to pursue this work for years on end. Confirmation comes usually not via words, but much more via non-verbal means: gestures, looks or perceiving that someone feels comfortable and safe.

The same applies to institutions and their self-image: they must ensure that staff have the creative leeway they require. Inpatient forms of care can only function as homes if there is a sense of being responsible for the development of the people with dementia, their families and the nurses.

4.   Dealing with life's remaining opportunities—occupations in inpatient facilities

An important step towards integration into an inpatient facility is being able to be active. While the affected person is settling in, the team must already consider the possibilities of inclusion in the institution's processes. Setting the table, folding laundry, cutting vegetables are all activities that occur in any house or apartment-sharing community. The tasks must be adapted again and again to the actual abilities of the residents. This requires creativity. What happens when no resident wants to take over household chores, is there an alternative in place? Often good ideas cannot be implemented promptly, and later it is much more difficult to practice the activities with the resident. Habits that are not supported by the whole team fail because of the normal procedures of the facility. People with dementia usually do not claim the right to continue doing those things, so that they often lose many competences after a short time.

It sounds paradoxical, but in addition to getting used to being active in the new environment, it is also important to realize that less is sometimes more. In recent years, residents of inpatient facilities have often been overwhelmed with things to do. Every day there are activities such as memory training, remembrance rounds, singing and much more. Often in large groups. These are often options that do not suit people with Alzheimer's dementia, for example. Many sit and seem to be taken care of for this time, nothing more. Sitting quietly at the table, being allowed to watch, sitting silently next to a nurse, these are all things that so far have not been considered "occupations" enough. Professionalism in social care means that one can present such unspectacular activities to others in a comprehensible manner and document them in writing.

Example

Mr. V. suffers from Lewy body dementia that shows Parkinson's-like symptoms. Until a few years ago, he managed a large company. In the residential facility he seems very active. He is on the move all day, almost always busy with his work. Everything he encounters, he reinterprets into his old work processes. He sees the staff members of the institution as his employees, scribbles "orders" on small pieces of paper and asks others to do the inventory with him. Mr. V. lives in his own world.

He has little interest in occupations in the classical sense. He leaves when a group activity is going to start or interprets it as happening in his company: then, however, he is also the boss and gives the appropriate speech in front of his employees.

Mr. V. does not need offers of things to do, he needs people who understand the world he lives in and support him in it. He feels comfortable when he can act as "the boss" and is needed.

The experience of Mr. V. shows as an example how little normal occupations mean to many people with Alzheimer's dementia or Lewy body dementia.

Communication with people suffering from dementia is as diverse and exhausting as life itself. The only difference is often the uncertainty we experience. Are we supposed to take what's been said at face value or not? Which statements are to be taken seriously, which are not? Only the presence of the listener helps in the assessment. The meaning of what is said results from the situation, the seriousness of the encounter, the relationship that already exists. Nurses need to learn to trust their experiences in order to assess the importance of what people with dementia say. These are complex processes: listening, assessing and evaluating, the image of the person concerned, his situation, adapting one's own actions, involving others.

Example

Mr. F. usually speaks only incoherently, people find him very difficult to understand. In a situation in front of the elevator a small conversation happens. Mr. F. is asked how he is. He answers with all clarity: "Bad, and my prospects aren't good either." His conversation partner has no doubt about the seriousness of what has been said. At this moment Mr. F. is aware of his situation and is evaluating it. Over the next few weeks, his condition deteriorates rapidly.

Depending on the clinical picture, the affected person is more likely to be hampered by a slowdown in thinking and speaking, such as in Parkinson's dementia, or by a complete loss of speech, particularly common in advanced Alzheimer's or alcohol dementia.

Example

Mr. P. shows mild dementia in advanced Parkinson's disease. His dementia manifests itself in an increasing inability to oversee and control his life and daily structure. Listening to him is difficult because he speaks very quietly and slowly (a common problem of Parkinson's disease). Some things he can no longer realistically assess: which activities are meaningful, what is affordable, whether his daily routine is much too stressful....

Since communication almost always revolves around him and his illness, it is increasingly important for the nurses to overcome inner resistance. This is not because of his Parkinson's disease or mild dementia, but above all because of his self-centeredness, which is expressed in his many wishes. Is it part of the disease or his personality? The question does not seem clearly answerable. In our communication with Mr. F. we try to find out what is really important to him, where we must show him resistance, and which wishes can be fulfilled, even if we consider them to be absurd. This is not an easy task; nurses are not free from mistakes and injustices. Everyone has something to forgive and must ask for forgiveness. Nevertheless, communication succeeds when both sides accept this unstable balance and can endure it when it swings out to one side or the other.

For successful communication in the work with dementia patients, proven methods that support nurses are available. These include validation according to the gerontologist Naomie Feil and integrative validation according to Nicole Richards (1957–2014). However, such methods require regular practice to be effective. They always remain only a part of the communication between nurses and people with dementia.

5. Adaptation and resistance: previous patterns of behavior may change

As they live on with dementia, people change in different ways. The progression of dementia robs them of their abilities: planning and judgement, initiative, coping with intellectual demands, mobility and movement patterns change. Their patterns of behavior change.

Example

Mrs. H. moves into the home community and very much needs confirmation at the beginning. Several times a day she asks if she's doing everything right. She's looking for recognition that she can adapt well. This goes so far that it is almost impossible to conduct a conversation without this introductory monologue. Over two years there is very little change in her behavior. Then her disease progresses: Mrs. H. is more and more often very confused, she hardly knows how to understand procedures.

Since this turning point, her appearance has also changed: she seems to have a negative and disapproving attitude towards the nurses, she is silent when spoken to, crosses her arms and mumbles evil words to herself. Increasingly, she insults other residents sitting near her. The pattern of wanting to be the "dear" Mrs. H., who does everything just as she should, does not disappear completely, but increasingly. She only reacts positively to men. They can still get her to get out of bed or make her participate in a coffee circle.

One experiences her behavioral change as an increasing loss of control. Against this backdrop, her new challenging behavior appears as a call for resistance in search of her personality. This development is easier to accept when one knows her history of over-adaptive behavior.

Such changes also occur in the opposite direction. People who lived more as loners, always made autonomous decisions, perhaps adopting certain behaviors through their social role, now show other sides of their personality.

Example

Mr. D. was very influential in his family and also in his job. He had clear ideas about his position in life. When he moves into the facility, his daughter warns the nurses that her father will certainly not attend any events. He hasn't done that his whole life. She is then amazed and somewhat offended that her father is very committed and enthusiastically involved in all kinds of activities. He's a passionate singer. Has he rediscovered this side of his personality and lived it out for the first time without intellectual control? He has not forgotten the lyrics of the songs that he sang in childhood, which he never sang again until now. He is obviously enjoying his participation in all sociable offers.

His daughter is insecure, she has always experienced her father as strict, now this new side seems uncanny and a little embarrassing to her. Her father jokes with staff, he seems friendly and interested in people. As much as she is happy that he seems to be doing well, the other Mr. D. was more familiar to her, and he also had her respect, despite all the problems. His daughter must get to know her father again.

6. Letting go—Accepting increasing weakness and accompanying the dying process

Accompanying people with dementia in the last phase of their lives is a challenge that demands a whole new approach from relatives and staff in nursing homes for the elderly. The question of whether people who suffer from dementia die differently is discussed again and again. In principle, dying is as individual as people's lives are. From the point of view of relatives, it seems difficult to make decisions in the interest of the person who has dementia.

Especially when dementia has been shaping a family's life together for many years, it is likely that there has not been a conversation about the issues of life and death for a long time. Relatives are unsure: is what we discussed many years ago still valid today? Does the person with dementia feel differently than before? Does he perhaps see his life in its present state as worth living, even though he had thought that impossible before? This uncertainty accompanies relatives latently. Such questions suddenly become very urgent when a deterioration in the person's physical condition occurs, when there are signs of weakening, of waning, as decisions about possible measures must be taken. In this situation the relatives bear an existential responsibility, because their actions can decide between life and death.

Decisions once made are often questioned years later. Was it right to refuse a tube feeding, would an operation have perhaps restored the quality of life after all? The circumstances and the overall situation in which action was taken are often not significant. The uncertainty remains whether one has decided in line with the wishes of the affected person or over his head. It is therefore very important to reflect thoroughly on these issues, exchange views with other stakeholders and, if possible, allow enough time to make decisions.

6.1 The confrontation with dying

Disease crises such as rapid weight loss, a femoral neck fracture or a general weakening can be very worrying. Should the person with dementia be taken to the hospital or remain in a familiar environment? What measures should be taken? Although such events are usually not completely surprising, in many cases they are experienced as such. Often it seems that the question of dying is being asked for the first time in these moments. In a society that is almost exclusively concerned with life, the confrontation with the possible end is frightening. No matter how old people are and no matter what overall situation they find themselves in, most people are not used to assuming such responsibility. Relatives are often shocked when they realize what a single decision can do.

6.1.1 Building trust

It is very helpful in these situations if there is an environment around the person with dementia and his relatives that is willing to support such decisions. A good exchange between the participants is a prerequisite. If the affected person lives in a home, nurses and treating physicians can form this environment, and attendants or therapists can help. It is important that conversations about these questions be sought again and again. Otherwise, there is a risk that any agreements will no longer be up to date at the time of an acute deterioration and that unnecessary misunderstandings will arise between the parties involved. It can be a great help for the relatives to be in close contact with their family doctor, for example, so that he or she can help them to get through the decision that they have to make in the difficult situation. This requires trust, which only develops within a longer discussion process. Relatives must be able to rely on the acceptance of the decisions that they make.

They are the ones who will live on with the consequences of the decision taken; the relatives therefore need the support and feedback of others in order to make their decision and to implement or revoke it at the decisive moment. Nurses in the institution must accept this, even when from their point of view a good solution is not going to be implemented or a worse alternative has been chosen.

Many stories of growing old and dying show: every new situation, every change in the previous state of people who are in the transitional area between life and death must be perceived anew and discussed between the decision-makers and the wider human environment.

6.1.2 Making decisions

Some examples will describe the particular challenges of decision-making in the final phase of life:

Example

Mrs. P. is 89 years old and has lived in the home for four years. Despite the stroke that led to her being placed there, she's quite well. She has a daily routine that suits her, and she enjoys her contact with other people very much. Suddenly her condition worsens, and heart damage causes her to weaken rapidly. She eats less and less but is balanced and peaceful. A relatively short time ago it was agreed with her daughter not to take Mrs. P. to hospital in such a case. When the critical situation actually occurs, her daughter begins to falter. It is of course one thing to discuss the situation abstractly and quite another to have to act in reality. All the questions come flooding back: could Mrs. P. be helped in the hospital, is there a new therapy, would she still have a few good years?

The nurses and the family doctor are called together and form their own opinion. They have the impression that Mrs. P. wants to go her way peacefully. Her daughter is very uncertain and suspects the nurses of seeking a simple solution. She insists on taking her mother to the hospital. Mrs. P. dies there three days later, lovingly cared for by her daughter. Weeks later the daughter comes back to visit the nursing home, she is grateful for her mother's many years of care. In retrospect, she sees her insistence on hospitalization as an overreaction, as an attempt not to have to take responsibility. But she's okay with it, because despite everything, she was able to be with her mother at the end.

It is obvious that the daughter's uncertainty was the reason for this last change of place and environment from home to hospital. Mrs. P. could no longer decide for herself, so her daughter had to try to find a way that did them both justice. The people around them were willing to support the daughter's decisions.

In the end, it is important to have courage and to trust one's own feelings. The question of whether there can be a "good end" to dying must be answered each time anew and differently. From the point of view of the nurses in this case, a different course would have been possible. Mrs. P. could have died peacefully in the nursing home. In this case, however, her daughter would perhaps have spent a long time worrying about how much more time her mother would have had if she had been admitted to the hospital. What Mrs. P. wanted, what she thought and felt about dying, remains the great unknown. In this example, the bereaved are relieved and have no feelings of guilt. They feel confident that they have acted correctly and have done what seemed possible under those circumstances.

It is often only possible to recognize when the last phase of life has begun in retrospect. Therefore, relatives must trust that their thoughts and considerations will help to shape the dying phase well. They often do not know what the person with dementia thinks and feels about this, or they cannot interpret the signs he gives them. Sometimes, however, the people being cared for express their wishes clearly, and if the people around them are willing to take them seriously, they can be given back a piece of lost self-determination.

Example

Mrs. S. moves into a home community when her dementia is already well advanced. She had been living alone in her large apartment for the last few years. She takes little part in the activities of the living group, looks tired and is very introverted. Due to her poor blood values, tumor disease is assumed, but no one wants to impose the strains of intensive diagnostics on her. Mrs. S. is losing weight. One day at the table, she says she doesn't want to eat anymore. The nurses are outraged and want to persuade her to eat. However, some members of staff experience her statement as being clear and distinct; from this point on Ms. S. appears to be more conscious again. She repeats her statement of not wanting to eat any more to her daughter, who has the same impression. Days later the family doctor talks to Mrs. S. and asks her clearly: "You know you will die if you don't eat?" "Yes, I know that," is her answer. Everyone who has heard her talk about this is sure that Mrs. S. is serious. She's sticking to her word: for eight weeks she lives without eating but continues to drink. She stays in her room for the meals, she is offered food again and again, but continues to refuse it. She appears calm and retains clarity. At the end she lies in her bed and dies very peacefully, one year after her move to the home. During the dying phase, the relatives and staff of the nursing home cannot always understand what Mrs. S. is experiencing or why she can suddenly make such a clear decision. Again and again those involved try to make sure that they are acting correctly and that Mrs. S. really wants to die. The result is always the same. The feeling of having done the right thing does not change after Mrs. S. has died. Everyone feels the relief and peace that death has brought her.

This example shows how a person's decisions can be understood and taken seriously despite their dementia. In the end, Mrs. S. regained her personal sovereignty.

The increasing losses that a person experiences are as noticeable for patients with dementia as they are for any other elderly person. When it becomes clear that their strength is running out, people react very differently, but they often show their environment in one way or another what they are going through in the dying phase.

Example

Mrs. M. with her 98 years has been very mobile for a long time. She likes to tell old stories and yet she is ready to carry on every day. Physically, one hardly notices any changes. She perceives the other residents and gets upset about their supposedly improper behavior. From one day to the next her behavior changes. Mrs. M. suddenly cries a lot, which she had never done before. The people around her are concerned and want to comfort her, but the crying does not stop. Mrs. M. is inconsolable. At the same time Mrs. M. begins to call more and more often for her mother. She increasingly stays in her room, in her bed. There she cries too but is more satisfied overall. Her body, which had been upright and apparently unchanged for a long time, is declining and deteriorating. She seems to completely detach herself from the material world. After a few weeks the crying and shouting stops and another two weeks later Mrs. M. dies peacefully.

Mrs. M. has gone through something very comprehensible in her dying phase: she has returned to her time has a child, as an infant, which led to a deep longing to be with her mother again—cared for and protected. Since she could not simply go back to that time and what her mother stood for did not become tangible, she felt a deep sadness. One can also interpret crying as an expression of feeling sad, letting go and saying goodbye.

However one understands the last weeks of Mrs. M., the people around her had the immediate impression that they must not disturb her farewell. At first it was not easy for relatives and nurses to experience her sadness, but the reasons gradually revealed themselves and it became easier for them to join in her leavetaking.

6.1.3 Accepting the new situation

People with dementia are very dependent on the decisions of the people around them at the end of their lives. In the course of the disease, they have increasingly lost their independence and now no longer make even the smallest decisions independently. The people who have taken care of everything during this time come at the beginning of the last phase of life to a point where they should let go of what they have held on to with all their strength so far: they had reminded the person that he had to eat, they gave him food, told him again and again who they were, took him by the hand and sat him on a chair, brought him into the sun and returned him to the house when it rained.

This makes it difficult to let go at the end of life and do things differently, to give less to eat than before, to refrain from doing everything possible, to realize whether sociability and daily activities are still appropriate, or whether the person might prefer to be alone. These are questions that are not easy to answer.

6.2 Nutrition in the last phase of life

6.2.1 Changing needs

The topic of nutrition is often one of the most difficult in the last phase of life. Whether at home or in a nursing home, the question almost always arises in the course of dementia as to whether the person affected is getting enough food and fluids, as he or she begins to eat less and less or refuses to eat at all. Sometimes only their habits or their taste changes, and if this is recognized and considered, the problem can initially be solved. But if all attempts have failed and no offer—be it finger food, a special favorite food, sieved food or high-calorie food—can stop the "eating less and less" any longer, the question of nutrition arises in a new light: is this changed eating behavior a sign of the dying process, is it natural not to want to eat or not to be able to eat at an advanced age, when one increasingly has other disease symptoms of age and dementia? Nurses often find themselves in a dilemma: they are very afraid that the person entrusted to them will suffer from hunger and thirst and may no longer be able to express this, but on the other hand they do not want to force him to eat. Oftentimes nurses had been able to connect with the person concerned by serving him food or bringing him special favorites, and now this connection also breaks off.

In such a situation, our common perception must be focused on how the person with dementia feels.

Example

Mr. L. has been living in a home community for three years. He is increasingly affected by the consequences of his Parkinson's disease. Dementia has also developed over time. His speech is very difficult to understand, he hardly communicates with other people. From the very beginning he felt comfortable in the community and took part in social gatherings with joy. His movement restrictions are now becoming more and more serious and he is increasingly impaired in his ability to eat. It seems his will has no access whatsoever to his body. His eyes do not open, although Mr. L. is awake, his mouth closes as soon as the spoon comes. He is only able to drink relatively well; he succeeds in absorbing liquid by sucking. Attempts to influence the symptoms of Parkinson's disease no longer have any effect. Feeding him sometimes lasts up to an hour and is bringing all those involved more and more to the end of their strength. Mr. L.'s daughters are asking themselves together with the home community staff what the next steps will be. Various questions have come up: how intensively are we trying to serve Mr. L. food, how long can this take, would a stomach tube be a solution? The home community team keeps a close eye on the situation, exchanges information and makes agreements about when Mr. L. will receive his food.

New points of view arise in a conversation with his two daughters: when he was healthy, Mr. L. experienced how a relative was nourished via a stomach tube for several years, and told his daughters that he was energetically opposed to this for himself. In addition, his daughters find the progressive process of Parkinson's disease more and more life-determining. Mr. L.'s family doctor is included in the conversation and supports the daughters' point of view.

It is agreed that Mr. L. shall not receive a stomach tube, the daughters want to discuss this with him in so far as possible. The time spent feeding him is limited somewhat, and more attention is paid to better using the times in which Mr. L. is awake. Everyone tries to meet Mr. L.'s needs as much as possible. Mr. L. is still oriented towards life and he looks forward to the coming day every morning.

Two weeks later, Mr. L. develops pneumonia. New questions must be answered: the hopeless situation seems to be approaching the end, but it will depend on how the people around Mr. L. respond. After considerations and discussions, the daughters decide that their father will not receive antibiotics and—of course with intensive care—no further measures should be taken. Mr. L. dies three days later. The daughters, who have lovingly cared for him for many years, are happy. They do not doubt for a moment that they have made the right decision.

In this example, the problem and complexity of the decisions to be taken becomes very clear. In itself, every suffering of Mr. L. represents a medically treatable disease. In the overview and the overall situation, the picture emerges from which the decisions of the people around him ultimately result.

6.2.2 Easing the feeling of thirst

For relatives, the idea that the affected person could die of thirst is usually very frightening. Today, however, it is known that the sensation of thirst in people changes during the dying process and the feeling of thirst diminishes. If the mouth and throat are well moistened and cared for, there is no reason to fear that the dying person will "agonizingly" die of thirst.

People who don't eat anymore get weaker and weaker. It is different when people no longer consume fluids—then their vital functions decline rapidly. Soon memory and consciousness will also be affected, a form of confusion that is easily confused with dementia may arise. Judging what to do when a person refuses to drink therefore seems particularly difficult, and the time for intervention is shorter. Counter-measures are often taken quickly out of concern that the person's dying will be accelerated without having exhausted all possibilities and without having understood the cause of their refusal to drink. In old people, this usually means that they are supplied with fluid (usually an isotonic saline solution) through infusions (intravenously, often subcutaneously). It is difficult to decide when to stop such fluids.

Example

Mrs. H. still likes to participate in community life despite her 90 years. Lately she appears to be more tired and, it seems to her relatives, also more confused. She drinks little and rejects offered drinks. The family doctor prescribes infusions. Every evening she now gets 500 ml of liquid, she accepts the procedure calmly. After a few days she is feeling noticeably better, she revives and takes a more active part in the daily routine. Everyone is glad. Mrs. H. drinks more again.

A few weeks later, Mrs. H.'s condition deteriorates again. This time the infusions cause almost no change, Ms. H. increasingly resists them. She is becoming weaker and is withdrawing into herself, the people around her see themselves confronted with new questions. After some conversations it becomes clear that Mrs. H. is in a different overall condition than the first time. It seems that this time it is a matter of saying goodbye. In agreement with her relatives and the family doctor, Mrs. H. is no longer supplied with fluid by infusions. She herself drinks and eats less and less, communication with her is hardly possible anymore. Her relatives and the staff of the nursing facility remain open to changes, they exchange information regularly, but the joint decision is not revoked. Until the end Mrs. H. consumes food and liquid in ever smaller portions. After three weeks, she dies.

In the example of Mrs. H. it becomes clear that there can be no explicit affirmation or denial of fluid intake through infusions. The decision often results from the actual attempt, whereby the team observes the success of the measure and evaluates it for future action.

6.3   Expecting the unexpected

People usually don't die unexpectedly. Often death is indicated by various signs, such as increasing weakness, loss of appetite or a sudden physical illness. Nevertheless, many relatives find death surprising. "My mother is very old, I realize that, but I cannot imagine her no longer being here," explains a woman as her mother begins to say goodbye.

One can adjust to nursing care, to what life brings, but what will change after death is much less tangible.

How will the person live on in my memory, will I even think of him, will the family now break apart completely? Will I be the next to die? The relatives have many questions on their minds that they cannot and do not always want to answer. When the expected happens unexpectedly, any careful considerations and decisions previously made are usually forgotten. The same questions that the relatives asked themselves weeks or months ago suddenly appear to be open again and it seems as if they had never been answered. At this moment, the relatives need support.

Example

Mrs. M. has become increasingly weaker at the age of 95. She has been living in an institution for two years, for a very long time she was active and physically fit. Her children are taking care of their mother and have never consciously imagined a life without her. Now her strength is waning and those involved must begin to accept the thought of her dying. The dying process takes a long time and goes through different phases; occasionally Mrs. M. feels better again, then she seems to be almost her old self, other days she has to spend in bed. Altogether Mrs. M. changes only slowly. Since it is not possible to talk to her about her condition, her relatives exchange their assumptions with the nurses about how Mrs. M. sees her situation, what she feels and how she is experiencing her increasing loss of strength. Then follow two weeks that she spends only in bed and in which she is actually "lying on her deathbed." Her children are helpless at first: what should they do? How much time can, and do they want to spend at their mother's bedside? What will happen at their mother's deathbed? Questions which can only be answered individually, and which depend very much on the empathy of the environment. Mrs. M.'s relatives have never been involved in a dying process, they do not know how everything will develop and how long it will take. Even the staff of the facility do not know this with absolute certainty, but they have already accompanied the dying of some residents of the home community and can report on those experiences. Mrs M.'s children are somewhat reassured when the staff explain their assessment. Mrs. M. now lies more and more often in bed, but she does not give the impression that she is suffering. Over a week, a new closeness develops between the children and their mother, a kind of festive atmosphere develops. Brother and sister tell each other many stories from their life with their mother and share their memories of her. At the end of the week, Mrs. M. dies alone at night. The staff of the home groom Mrs. M. and put clothes on her that had been chosen for this moment. Everyone is in a reflective, but also happy mood: the foreseen has come true and there is no cause for regret and no feeling of having missed anything. Despite all the grief, the situation is full of peace.

In the last two weeks of Mrs. M.'s life, it was thoroughly discussed what should happen after her death. How will Mrs. M. be buried, will there be a funeral service? Who is to be notified? Many important questions could be comfortably answered. At the end of this process, the participants created a very differentiated and thus meaningful image of Mrs. M., the image of a person with all of her inconsistencies, with her developments and setbacks. The people who took part in this process were also able to gain certainty for the questions relating to their own lives. To accompany the death of Mrs. M. in this way has given them the certainty that a "good death" is possible.

7. The professionalism of nurses

Designing spaces in which people with dementia can spend a life that both allows for development and meets an increasing need for calm and retreat is a complex task.

What is professionalism in this field of work? Living together in residential groups and home communities with people who have dementia needs the nurses to be close to the people that they are caring for in order to make liveliness possible. At the same time, they need a high degree of knowledge about clinical pictures and methods in dealing with typical behavior patterns. The interaction of knowledge derived from training and knowledge derived from experience is professionally stimulating.

The team of nurses lives from the exchange and from the diversity of views and approaches when people with dementia get into crises or their behavior causes turbulence in the community. An essential aspect of professional action is to use the knowledge gained from these experiences. This includes discussions within the team that look at crises that have been overcome and reflect on the entire process. The team tries to act from the knowledge of the situation of the individual and the community. Working with "small" solutions, sometimes tiny steps in situations that seem overwhelming and almost unsolvable, has proven to be successful.

Professionalism also includes the involvement and partnership of relatives and attendants. Respect for family ties is an important step in promoting the self-determination of people with dementia.

Example

Mr. L. is on the move all day. He can't be stopped, and he goes outside as often as he can. At first, there's always someone with him. Sometimes he is already on his way and has to be searched for with the police.

The family agrees to this arrangement after a few conversations. They understand that Mr. L. experiences any form of restraint as a deprivation of liberty. The situation is not happy. An attempt is made to involve the environment. Neighbors often bring Mr. L. back: they are not always friendly. Mr. L. needs a lot of attention. The team discusses taking turns accompanying him. The situation remains tense for weeks. The other residents are neglected, a change in medication hardly brings any relief, so it is reversed again. Then Mr. L changes. He seems calmer, but also less lively. Over the next few weeks his overall condition changes dramatically. He increasingly refuses food and drink. Attempts to figure out whether he is in pain fail. Again and again the team is looking for a way to positively influence the situation. The family and experts are consulted until all parties understand that Mr. L. is coming to the end in his own way. He dies a few weeks later.

The team remains full of questions, but also feels encouraged. All have tried to contribute one or more solutions. When it became apparent that things could not go on like that for him, staff respected it. His family experienced it in a similar way.

Working with people with dementia requires as much closeness and empathy as it requires distance through case discussion and method work. Achieving liveliness and the "normality" that is so often demanded in care facilities is a lengthy and laborious process.

Adapting this quotation from Karl Valentin, "Art is beautiful, but takes a lot of work," we can say: "Community with people who have dementia is beautiful but takes a lot of work."

What drives nurses is their vision of an everyday, fulfilled life, which despite dementia allows people to experience highlights and normality. This includes the willingness to accept what people with dementia offer their nurses: moments of insight, gratitude and spontaneous devotion. Giving and taking belong together to form a community.

8. People with dementia in the hospital

One of the great fears that relatives and nurses have in nursing homes is that those affected by dementia will have to go to a hospital. Usually there are bad experiences with hospital stays. Time pressure and lack of nursing staff have a very negative effect on people with dementia. The hectic pace of life in many hospitals is difficult to bear, because normally you need a lot of patience and time to adjust to the rhythm of life of people with dementia.

In hospitals there is no time to give food, answer questions, prepare or adequately accompany the patient to examinations. The confusion, resistance and sometimes aggression of those affected are caused and intensified by such circumstances. After a prolonged hospital stay, people with dementia often return in a very disoriented state and with worsened symptoms. Patients are increasingly being discharged from the hospital very quickly, even after major surgical procedures, for example. This has the advantage that the confusion is still reversible, but the disadvantage that healing processes and aftercare after surgery are not complete. Nursing homes must adapt more and more to this, whereby a better cooperation with the hospitals would be helpful, e.g., regarding instructions on wound care, etc. More and more often, rehabilitation measures after surgical interventions are carried out in the elderly care facility in order not to further unsettle people with dementia by changing their environment again by placing them in a rehabilitation facility.

Some clinics have begun to focus on the topic of "dementia in hospitals." Special areas for patients who have orientation and perception disorders are set up. They are characterized by spatial orientation aids such as colored walls and doors, handrails or common rooms. Some clinics set up accompanying services for dementia patients before and after major operations or make it possible to admit someone to accompany them. A special dementia day-care project is offered by Herdecke Community Hospital, where people with a concomitant diagnosis of dementia are cared for during the day by geriatric nurses and voluntary helpers.

9.   People with dementia in outpatient care

New nursing legislation has fundamentally improved outpatient care for people with dementia. Nursing care options have been expanded and can be used in various combinations. Families can make use of care services, day-care facilities and low-threshold treatment services and thus often find support for keeping their loved one at home for a long time.

All this makes sense if the family situation is reasonably stable, and a network connects the offers in such a way that the relatives and the affected person can benefit.

For people with advanced dementia and increasing disorientation, being in their own home gradually loses importance. "Home" is then above all an inner place to which they retreat. Patients who live alone often suffer more from isolation and loneliness than from the loss of their familiar environment as dementia progresses. Especially since they often don't recognize this environment as their home anymore. Spouses have been known to lament that their partners affected by dementia want to "go home" in the evening, even though they have been living there for forty years.

Here it is important to recognize when outpatient care no longer meets the person's basic needs. However, a desire for change will hardly be expressed by the affected people themselves, since precisely this ability—to assess one's own life situation—is already more or less limited. Experience has shown that the act of moving into a nursing home is much less dramatic than family members fear. People with vascular dementia often benefit longer from outpatient care, as their recognition and enjoyment of their familiar home environment tends to persist for longer. But the loneliness of this disease also makes life among people seem meaningful. This can often be ensured for a long time by visiting a day-care facility.

The support and assistance of relatives is important in outpatient care. The relatives need to be able to talk to each other in order to cope with the stress that everyday life brings with it, despite all the possibilities for help. People with dementia are the focus of their family's efforts because of their illness, so that relatives often forget their own needs for a long time and consider them less important. Sudden illnesses and states of exhaustion on the part of the relatives caring for the person are therefore not rare and may cause the entire domestic help system to collapse.

In recent years, more and more caregiving spouses of people with dementia have approached the consulting services of inpatient providers because, despite a wide range of outpatient services and support, they no longer feel able to cope with the emotional and physical strain of caring for the patient. Good counselling can shed light on the situation of dementia sufferers and their relatives alike. Psychosocial aspects are often more decisive for the decision to provide outpatient or inpatient care than the availability or awareness of suitable outpatient services.

Category	Example learning objectives	Recommended learning path
Skills	You can describe a daily routine from the perspective of a resident.	A
Your own learning objective		
Relationships	You find ways of addressing inner resistance against residents, diseases, disabilities, colleagues and of openly approaching solutions.	B
Your own learning objective		
Knowledge	You know the factors that must be taken into account so that a resident can find a good home in a home community.	C
Your own learning objective		

CHAPTER XXIV

Palliative Care

CHRISTOPH VON DACH · SASHA GLOOR

→   Learning objectives, see end of chapter

1.   Introduction

Palliative care has been an important area of anthroposophic nursing care since its inception. Patient histories from 1921, which have survived to this day, show that even then patients were cared for and treated who today would be described as requiring palliative care. The Ita Wegman Archive contains all the files from the early years of the original clinic near Basel, Switzerland (Klinisch Therapeutisches Institut, now called Klinik Arlesheim). There are, for example, cases of patients with tuberculosis and patients with cancer. Anthroposophic nursing can look back on a very long tradition in the field of palliative care. Palliative care was provided long before the term came into being.

Many treatments, such as external applications, have been administered by nurses since then. This means that interprofessional cooperation, which is the aim of palliative care, already has a very long tradition.

This chapter will first look at the model and the extended approach of anthroposophic palliative care, then present specific external applications that can be used. This chapter will not follow classical symptom management as can be found in many palliative care textbooks. Anthroposophic palliative care seeks a salutogenetic and not a mechanistic approach. It is based on a holistic view of the human being and the world. Instead of being symptom orientated, the focus is on life processes and health-promoting aspects right up to the dying phase.

1.1   The origins of palliative care

Palliative care began at St. Christopher's Hospice in London. Dame Cicely Saunders (1918–2005) founded a movement there which was initially called the hospice movement. The first hospice opened in 1967. The idea was to enable terminally ill people—mainly cancer patients at that time—to die with dignity. The Canadian physician Balfour Mount coined the term "palliative care" only later, in 1975.

Over the past decades, the meaning of the term "palliative care" has been constantly changing. Originally it referred to cancer patients who had arrived at the last phase of life and were about to die. Today, palliative care refers to a much longer period in the course of a disease that is highly likely to lead to death. Current research results show that early palliative support, in addition to medical care, helps people to improve their quality of life and reduce pain, and can reduce health-care costs. In addition, one study showed that the survival time of people with cancer is up to 30% higher among patients who receive palliative care early on.[1] The paper highlighted the importance of palliative care, not to shorten life, but to maximize the quality of the remaining lifespan and possibly even prolong it. Professional nursing care plays a decisive role in this. Consequently, palliative care is not only provided for people in the last phase of life, i.e., during dying, but also much earlier, in some cases shortly after the diagnosis.

Palliative care is currently based on definitions of various organizations, such as the World Health Organization (WHO, 2002), the European School of Medical Oncology (ESMO, 2003) and the European Association for Palliative Care (EAPC, 1998). They show that today palliative care is understood and applied much more comprehensively and is no longer or should no longer be exclusively restricted to the care of people with cancer.

The term palliative care is derived from "pallium" and "care." A "pallium" is an enveloping, warming mantle. One could say that it describes the primal nursing care gesture of enveloping, which also underlies Rolf Heine's model of nursing-care gestures [→ Chapter "The Concept of Nursing Gestures as a Model for Nursing Care"] and the effect that we know from *Solum oil* (WALA) or a Rhythmical Einreibung treatment of the whole body. 'Care' is an English term that does not exist in this way in the German language. It is much more comprehensive than the meaning of the German word for nursing (*pflegen*). The term was originally used in the transcultural nursing movement by Madeleine Leininger (1925–2012) to mean care provided by non-professionals, and later by various theorists for the concept of "caring" (Watson, Benner). Caring in this sense is a comprehensive, empathetic way of caring for sick people. It is an approach that consciously distances itself from a mechanistic understanding of nursing care.

In the context of Anthroposophic Medicine, palliative care describes the nurse's inner striving to offer the sick person as much relief from his symptoms as possible and a high quality of life. It is much more about "how" something is done than just "what." This does not mean that we no longer provide treatment or that we give up the will to heal, rather, the inner questions of the practitioner become different [→ Chapter "Illness and Destiny"]. The anthroposophic understanding of palliative care is to care for the seriously ill and dying person in the awareness that their development is possible and should be promoted right up to the last breath and beyond. This presupposes the awareness that life is not finished with physical death and that human beings continue on a spiritual path.

2.   When does dying begin?

Palliative care should start early—parallel to medical treatment. The question is: "When does dying begin?" Many textbooks do not deal with this question because a clear answer cannot be given. Nevertheless, the question is important for our understanding of the dying process.

When the heart stops beating or the brain stops functioning, death occurs. But when does the process of dying begin? Is it when the person's breathing changes and turns into Cheyne-Stokes respiration or agonal breathing? Is it when a person is no longer responsive? Is it when cachexia becomes evident? Is it when the person concerned starts thinking about dying? Is it the diagnosis of an incurable disease? Or the beginning of the aging process? Is it when a child has grown up? Does the dying process begin already at birth?

To understand dying, we must look not only at birth, but at the moment when the soul is still outside the physical body and the first cell clusters, the placenta and the various layers emerge that will surround the fetus. The placenta and the enveloping layers form a very interesting and mysterious structure. Rudolf Steiner spoke about it in different places. It is tissue that prepares new things and without which no baby, no new physical life can emerge. As the infant grows within these enveloping layers, tethered to the placenta, he develops the future characteristics and prerequisites that he will need to live out the possibilities of his destiny (karma). One can imagine that the soul of the unborn child stands beside the growing embryo, bringing with it that which shapes the biographical consequences of the past. This then acts via the placenta and the enveloping layers on the developing baby and prepares the "plan" for the coming life of this newly emerging human being. It is not a fixed plan that simply plays itself out, but an infinite number of possibilities that can be lived in the future. The principle of being human is to have freedom and free will. The embryo develops within these protective layers and is surrounded by the placenta. Almost throughout the entire gestation period, the embryo looks (to the extent that one can already speak of seeing) at the placenta as if at a starry sky, perhaps also seeing possible predispositions in its future life path.[2]

This is the moment, I believe, when dying begins. The placenta becomes sclerotic very quickly and shows clear signs of aging once it has been expelled when the baby is born. The placenta dies as the first part of the newborn to die and not as part of the mother, because the placenta originates from the baby's cells. Wolfgang Schad wrote: "With birth, only the internalized organization remains alive. The enveloping layers that carried and sustained us up to this point now withdraw and die. This makes us more incomplete from birth onwards than we were before. The basic experience that remains existentially with us for the rest of our lives—that we can only be a piecemeal part of ourselves—does not leave us from birth onwards. It is a topos belonging to every Christian self-understanding."[3] Steiner said that the spiritual substance of the placenta and the enveloping layers then accompany the human being invisibly through the whole of life. They are like the carriers of the karmic possibilities that guide the person through life. Therefore, the moment of the embryo being created, and the death of the placenta plays a decisive role in our confrontation with dying and the time of death. This mystery, which takes place at the very beginning of life, influences our entire earthly lifetime and thus also our last breaths.

2.1 Living and dying as a process

"Shouldn't there also be a death over there, the result of which would be earthly birth? When a spirit dies, it becomes a human being. When a human being dies, he becomes a spirit."

Novalis (1772–1801)

Actually, life as a whole can be understood as a process of dying, with the two opposite movements of immersing oneself into physical matter and extracting oneself from the earthly world again. In the first half of life the human being becomes increasingly earthly and incarnates thereby. With this deep incarnation into the physical body, human beings transform their life forces. So, toddlers and children are still very full of life. Adults lose part of this vitality and gain instead the ability to think consciously. Their life forces diminish. So, you could say that human beings are dying in the physical world. When the moment comes in which a human being detaches himself from the body again (and this does not happen only during the dying process) then life forces become free and the human being lives, so to speak, into the spirit or, we could say, into death. Thus, older people can think about things much more intensively, because their life forces are now available for thinking, for involvement with spiritual matters. Birth at the beginning of physical life is also a form of dying, namely from the spirit into physical life, while dying is a birth into the spiritual world.

3. The fourfold human being

The fourfold nature of the human being has already been described in detail in a previous chapter [→ Chapter "The Anthropological Foundations"]. Here we shall examine how it relates to the dying process. The fourfold human being is a dynamic interaction of four different aspects—the physical, the etheric, the soul and the 'I'. These four aspects are intimately connected and interwoven. They are more or less closely connected over the course of the day and night, and their connection also varies over the course of a person's biography. There is an ongoing alternation between loosening and binding. Rudolf Steiner described that during the day, when human beings are awake and conscious, this fourfold nature is closely interwoven, whereas at night, in the phase of deep sleep, the four members are only loosely connected. This release gives the physical body the opportunity to regenerate. The next morning the person feels restored and ready for the beginning day. A very similar releasing process of the fourfold nature occurs in dying. What remains behind is the physical body and the etheric body, while the soul body and 'I' withdraw. The 'I' is then in the spiritual world to develop further there. Only at death does the etheric body also separate from the physical body. During and before the dying process, by observing the physical body, we can discern how the interaction of the four members of the human being changes. Trained observation allows an assessment of the person's current situation. Thus, careful and exact perception of the patient's physical body forms the basis for anthroposophic nursing and palliative care. An example of this is the moment when edema forms in the body and we can observe a general weakening of the etheric forces.

4.   The seven life processes

Physical life always goes hand in hand with life processes, as existence is only possible where life is present. These processes work both at the beginning and at the end of life. Rudolf Steiner described seven definitive processes that are decisive for incarnation and that remain with us until we leave the physical body again. Life processes are thus closely related to dying and to the dying process, because dying is also a part of life.

5.   Pain in anthroposophic palliative care

Palliative situations and the dying phase often confront patients and nurses with pain. Pain is always multidimensional and is experienced individually by each person. Thus, it is not possible to judge from the outside whether another person is experiencing intense or mild pain. Pain is always what the affected person feels and describes.[4] It should be taken seriously and treated. Not treating it would be unethical. Anthroposophic palliative care does not see pain primarily as a "by-product" of a disease. Pain is rather an expression of being human and is thus part of existence. It always affects the whole person. Pain can make development possible, but it can also prevent it by blocking the affected person and restricting his life. For nurses, it is crucial not to hold preconceived opinions. People who suffer from pain and wish to receive treatment must receive the best possible treatment according to current guidelines and with all available analgesics. However, those who do not wish to receive pain therapy, or only reduced pain therapy, must also be respected. The decision lies solely with the patient.

5.1   Palliative sedation

Palliative sedation is increasingly used in many institutions. This means that medication is used to bring patients—usually in the final phase of life—into a comatose state for a defined period or until physical death occurs. The decision for this requires very careful consideration, based on high ethical standards. Ideally, such a decision takes place in discussion with the patient, the relatives, and the entire medical team. Since development is possible up to the moment of death, and even beyond, from the point of view of anthroposophic palliative care, such a decision must be carefully weighed. However, palliative sedation is not excluded in the setting of anthroposophic palliative care. The patient's needs and wishes, as well as his or her autonomy, must guide the decision.

6. Principles for external applications in palliative care

Each external application is preceded by a differentiated assessment of the situation. What should be supported, and which aspects need to be considered? Does the patient need warmth or cold? What can be said about the interaction of the members of his fourfold nature? Only when these questions have been carefully clarified can an external application be chosen.

Basically, the following applies to external applications in palliative care:

- **Less is more**
  One to a maximum of three external applications per day are enough. The question of what the patient needs (support or relief) gives orientation.

- **No irritating substances**
  As a rule, no irritating substances, such as mustard powder or horseradish, are used to accompany the dying.

- **Ask about previous experiences**
  The patient and his relatives must be involved in decisions on external applications. Have there been good or bad experiences with certain substances or applications?

- **Sufficient time**
  The organism must be given sufficient time to react to the application. This applies in particular to the post-treatment rest period.

- **Evaluating the effect**
  After the application, the effect should be checked and evaluated. The patient or relatives can record the effect in a journal.
  It is not enough to simply note that the application "felt good."

- **Individual choice of substances**
  The substances used in the external applications must be individually adapted to the patient. This is especially true for palliative and dying patients.

7. External applications in palliative care

The following are examples of external applications to accompany the last phase of life, as well as the dying process, in a soothing way. They are based on the results of a working group that has collected reports on external applications worldwide.[5] For this chapter, they are arranged according to the seven life processes. Pain, as an overriding phenomenon, will first be discussed independently of this system.

7.1 Pain

External applications show very good effects in the treatment of pain. They address the affected person holistically. It is especially the experience of being attended to so intensively by the nurse that allows the patient to feel that she is being taken seriously in her very difficult situation. External applications do not replace pain medication, they support it. A careful assessment is carried out before treating the pain to determine the intensity and type of pain. Various evaluation instruments are available for this purpose (e.g., the Numerical Rating Scale (NRS), Visual Analog Scale (VAS), Zurich Observation Pain Assessment (ZOPA)). It is often helpful for patients to describe their pain, perhaps by means of a symbol or a picture, while someone listens to them attentively. There are types of pain that respond very well to warmth, such as pain from bone metastases, and others that respond better to cold, such as inflammatory processes. External applications support opiate therapy and often provide additional pain relief.
To accompany the treatment of bone pain:

■ Oil compresses with *Solum oil* (WALA)	2–3 x daily
■ Flax seed poultices (hot) [Instructions → Chapter "Anthroposophic Nursing Care in Oncology"]	2–3 x daily
■ Partial Rhythmical Einreibung with *Solum oil* (WALA)	3–4 x daily
■ Larix/Olibanum beeswax compress (Klinik Arlesheim Pharmacy)	as needed

Neuralgic pain:

■ Warm oil compress with *Aconite Nerve Oil* (WALA) or *Aconitum e tubere W 5%, Oleum (WALA)*	2–3 x daily
■ Partial Rhythmical Einreibung with *Aconite Nerve Oil* (WALA) or *Aconitum e tubere W 5%, Oleum (WALA)*	2–3 x daily

SPECIALIZATIONS IN NURSING

Inflammatory pain:

- Cool farmer's cheese compresses (until the farmer's cheese warms up and dries)   2–3 x daily

- Cold pack application (until the pack warms up)   as needed

- Compresses with *Luvos medicinal clay 2* (Luvos Heilerde 2) and *Arnica Essence* (WALA, Weleda) (until the paste warms up and dries)   as needed

Headache due to brain tumors/metastases:

- Head or forehead compresses with *Arnica Essence* (WALA, Weleda) (cold, possibly dilute with ice water)   3–4 x daily

7.2 Breathing

Breathing has a very central effect on human well-being. On the one hand, it is an expression of a person's emotional state and mood, and, conversely, it also influences their inner state. For example, fear accelerates a person's breathing and makes it superficial, while obstructing their breathing often leads directly to fear. Relaxed, calm breathing is an expression of well-being and relaxation. Breathing exercises (i.e., conscious guidance of breathing) engender of sense of well-being. This is especially true for people in palliative situations or in the dying process.

To treat shortness of breath (not asthmatic):

- Chest compresses with *Lavender 10% oil* (Weleda) or *Lavandula, Oleum aethereum 10%* (WALA)   1–2 x daily

- Chest compresses with with *Thymus, Oleum aethereum 5%* (WALA)[6]   1 x daily

- Rhythmical Einreibung treatment of the thorax with *Lavender 10% oil* (Weleda) or *Lavandula, Oleum aethereum 10%* (WALA)   2–3 x daily

- Rhythmical Einreibung treatment of the feet and/or lower legs with *Lavender 10% oil* (Weleda) or *Lavandula, Oleum aethereum 10%* (WALA)   2–3 x daily

For acute shortness of breath:

- Back strokes with *Eucalyptus, Oleum aethereum 10%* (WALA)   as needed

- Back strokes (over the clothing, without a substance)   as needed

Support in case of fear and agitation:

- A Pentagram Rhythmical Einreibung treatment on three consecutive days with *Gold rose-blossom lavender oil* (Dr. Heberer), then two subsequent treatments, each following a one-week interval

- Rhythmical Einreibung treatment of the feet with *Red Copper Ointment* (WALA)   2 x daily

- Rhythmical Einreibung treatments with *Gold rose-blossom lavender oil* (Dr. Heberer)   1–2 x daily

- Rhythmical Einreibung treatments with *Hypericum, Flos 25% oil* (Weleda) or *Hypericum ex herba 5%, Oleum* (WALA)   1–2 x daily

- Rhythmical Einreibung treatment of the hands with *Rosa e floribus 10%, Oleum* (WALA)   2–3 x daily

- Heart ointment compresses with *Aurum/Lavandula comp. cream* (Weleda)   at night

- Heart compresses with *Arnica Essence* (WALA, Weleda)   as needed

- Wrist compresses with *Arnica Essence* (WALA, Weleda)   as needed

- Solar plexus strokes with *Aurum/Lavandula comp. cream* (Weleda)   1–2 x daily

- Hand or foot baths with *Lavender Relaxing Bath Milk* (Weleda) or *Moor Lavender Calming Bath Essence* (Dr. Hauschka)   1–2 x daily

- A sounding bath with, e.g.,
  Lavender Relaxing Bath Milk (Weleda) or   several times
  Moor Lavender Calming Bath Essence (Dr. Hauschka)   daily

Fear in the night/experiences of shock:

■ Abdominal ointment compress with *Oxalis, Folium 10% ointment* (Weleda)	at night
■ Rhythmical Einreibung treatment of the abdomen with *Oxalis, Folium 10% ointment* (Weleda)	2 x daily
■ Warm wrist compresses with *Lavender 10% oil* (Weleda) or *Lavandula, Oleum aethereum 10%* (WALA) in combination with *Oxalis Essence* (WALA) or *Oxalis, Folium 20% tincture* (Weleda)	2 x daily
■ Abdominal ointment compress with *Oxalis Essence* (WALA) or *Oxalis, Folium 20% tincture* (Weleda)	2 x daily

Pleural effusion:

■ Farmer's cheese thorax compresses, body temperature	1–2 x daily
■ Rhythmical Einreibung treatment of the thorax with *Plantago Bronchialbalsam* (bronchial balm, oil for external use, WALA)	2 x daily
■ Rhythmical Einreibung treatment of the thorax with *Lavender 10% oil* (Weleda) or *Lavandula, Oleum aethereum 10%* (WALA)	2 x daily
■ Rhythmical Einreibung of the thorax with *Thymus, Oleum aethereum 5%* (WALA)	2 x daily
■ Abdominal compress with buckwheat (mix buckwheat flour with a little lukewarm water)	2 x daily
■ Place a *Stannum metal foil patch* (Weleda Switzerland, Apotheke an der Weleda) on the throat (with the fabric side on the body)	1 x daily
■ Compress with *Stannum metallicum 0.4% ointment* (Weleda) (place the stannum-coated side of the cloth on the thorax)	1 x daily

Human life is accompanied by very specific body warmth. Even before the first breath is taken, the organism needs warmth to be able to live. Warmth is an expression of well-being, interest and enthusiasm. A lack of warmth is an expression of anxiety, tension and discomfort. It can also indicate the beginning of the actual dying process, when the extremities become cold and changes occur in the blood circulation of the skin, causing discoloration. A great deal of relief can be achieved for patients by encouraging their warmth organisms, especially in the phases of palliative care and dying. A warm hot-water bottle or a simple foot rub often eases the patient. There are certain disease conditions in which the dying person does not tolerate heat—on the contrary, they may even want cold, such as ice cubes to suck or an open window in winter. We should follow these wishes if possible.

People also experience warmth in the soul. Here it is important to cultivate warmth as a basic attitude in nursing and in conversation. Artistic therapies engender inner soul warmth in patients.

Applications to support the warmth organism:

- Oil dispersion baths with various additives, e.g., *Prunus spinosa e floribus W 5%, Oleum* (WALA)[7] — 1 x daily

- Oil compresses (abdomen, chest, kidneys) with warming oils, e.g., *Solum oil* (WALA) — 1–2 x daily

- Beeswax compresses with various substances

- Rhythmical Einreibung treatments (partial and whole-body treatments) — 1 x daily

- Pentagram Rhythmical Einreibung treatments with *Aurum/ Lavandula comp. cream* (Weleda) — 2–3 x week

- Ginger kidney compresses with ginger powder or fresh ginger — 2–3 x week
  [Instructions → Chapter "From the Question of Meaning in Cancer to the Care of the Senses"]

- Footbaths, with various substances, e.g., *Lavender Relaxing Bath Milk* (Weleda), *Moor Lavender Calming Bath Essence* (Dr. Hauschka), *Rosemary Invigorating Bath Milk* (Weleda), *Citrus Refreshing Bath Milk* (Weleda) or *Lemon Lemongrass Vitalising Bath Essence* (Dr. Hauschka) — 1 x daily

Shortly after birth, infants receive their first food in the form of mother's milk, and from then on, they must feed themselves steadily until their body dies. Nutrition also plays an important role in the palliative care of patients. It is often precisely here that very central and ethically significant questions arise. Should nourishment be administered parenterally? Should fluid be given intravenously? How much fluid should be given? It often helps to discuss this with the patient, the relatives and the entire medical team.

Thorough and regular oral hygiene is very important. A person's feeling of thirst during the dying phase does not only depend on the amount of fluid in the body, it is also determined by the condition of the oral mucosa. Nausea often prevents adequate nutrition.

Support in case of nausea:

■ Ginger tea from fresh ginger	as needed
■ Compresses with *carraway 10% oil* (pharmacy formula) (for gas, 30 minutes to 2 hours)	3 x daily and as needed
■ Compresses with chamomile tea (for stomach cramps, 30 minutes)	3 x daily and as needed

To support liver activity:

■ Yarrow liver compresses [Instructions → Chapter "From the Question of Meaning in Cancer to the Care of the Senses"]	1 x daily
■ Liver compresses with *Stannum metallicum 0.4% ointment* (Weleda)	1 x daily

To support organ activity:

■ Rhythmical Einreibung treatments of the organs, with the appropriate metal ointments	1 x daily
■ Metal foil compresses (Weleda Switzerland, Apotheke an der Weleda)	1 x daily
■ NOURISHING BATHS: Mix 2 tbsp. honey, 100 ml cream, ½ l milk, 1 tbsp. olive oil and the juice of one lemon in a bottle, shake well, and pour into the bath water.	2–3 times a week

Creative mouth refreshment:

- Frozen fruit juice cubes to suck

- Pieces of fruit, e.g., pineapple, to suck

- Mouth rinses with flavors preferred by the patient

7.5   Elimination

Elimination as a life process seems somewhat strange at first. Here it is a matter of digesting ingested food and breaking it down into smaller molecules. The organism absorbs these molecules or eliminates them. Life depends on the processes of absorption and elimination taking place continuously and to the right degree. When the body takes in too much, it becomes unhealthily overweight; when it can no longer absorb enough, cachexia occurs. The question of absorption and elimination arises in an exceptional way in the dying process. What still has to be absorbed? What support does the dying person require? Vomiting and constipation are also linked to this life process. On the level of soul, a central question arises, especially in the dying process: "What belongs to me and what do I want or need to part from?"

To treat congestion/edema:

■ Compresses with *Borage Essence* (WALA)	1–2 x daily
■ Ointment compresses with *Borage 5% ointment* (Apotheke an der Weleda)	1–2 x daily
■ Farmer's cheese compresses (temperate, 45 minutes)	1–2 x daily
■ Cabbage compresses (overnight) [→ Chapter "Compresses in Anthroposophically Extended Nursing"]	1–2 x daily
■ Leg compresses with lemon juice, *Citrus Refreshing Body Oil* (Weleda) or *Lemon Lemongrass Vitalising Bath Oil* (Dr. Hauschka) (45 minutes)	1 x daily
■ Compress with *Luvos Healing Earth 2* (Luvos) and *Arnica Essence* (WALA, Weleda) (make a spreadable paste, duration: until the paste dries out and crumbles)	1–2 x daily

To treat ascites:

■ Abdominal compresses with Equisetum tea[8]		1 x daily
■ Ginger kidney compresses, with ginger powder or fresh ginger		1 x daily
■ Abdominal compresses with lukewarm farmer's cheese		1 x daily
■ Abdominal compresses with buckwheat (mix buckwheat flour with a little lukewarm water)		2 x daily
■ Abdominal ointment compresses, with *Mercurialis ointment* (WALA) or *Mercurialis perennis 10% ointment* (Weleda)		2 x daily
■ Rhythmical Einreibung of the back, with *Solum oil* (WALA)		1–3 x daily

To treat constipation:

■ Rhythmical Einreibung treatment of the thighs or abdomen with *Oxalis, Folium 10% ointment* (Weleda)		1 x daily
■ Abdominal compresses with *Oxalis Essence* (WALA) or *Oxalis, Folium 20% tincture* (Weleda)		1 x daily
■ Abdominal compresses with anise caraway fennel tea		1 x daily
■ Figure-eight Rhythmical Einreibung treatments of the patient's sides with *Chamomilla e floribus W 10%, Oleum* (WALA)		1 x daily

To treat diarrhea:

■ Abdominal compresses with *Chamomilla e floribus W 10%, Oleum* (WALA)		1–2 x daily
■ Abdominal compresses with *carraway 10% oil* (pharmacy formula)		

7.6 Maintenance

Maintenance makes the ingested and broken-down food components available to the organism. This life process ensures that the required substances are integrated into the organism. With regard to palliative care, maintenance means ensuring that the body's remaining functions, such as movement, breathing or intact skin and mucous membrane boundaries, are maintained. That is why prophylaxis is also included. On a soul level, this refers to integrating experiences into one's reality.

Prophylaxis:

SKIN:
- Partial Rhythmical Einreibung treatments, with *Solum oil* (WALA)

PNEUMONIA:
- Rhythmical Einreibung treatment of the thorax, with *Eucalyptus, Oleum aethereum 10%* (WALA)

CONTRACTURES:
- Regular movement and Rhythmical Einreibung treatments of the extremities with *Solum oil* (WALA), *Primula (primrose) Muscle oil* (WALA), *Arnica, Flos H 10%* (Weleda) or *Arnica e floribus W 5%, Oleum* (WALA)

Care of the oral mucosa:

- *Sea buckthorn berry oil* (diluted 1:10, e.g., with avocado oil   several times daily

- *Propolis mother tincture* (diluted in water)   several times daily

- *Mouth balm, liquid* (WALA)   several times daily

For people who are bedridden for a long time:

- Partial Rhythmical Einreibung treatments, with *Citrus Refreshing Body Oil* (Weleda) or *Lemon Lemongrass Vitalising Bath Oil* (Dr. Hauschka)

To maintain the feeling of uprightness while lying down or during dizziness:

- Stroke the soles of the patient's feet, or Rhythmical Einreibung   as needed treatments with *Cuprum metallicum praeparatum 0.4% ointment* (Weleda) or *Copper Ointment* (WALA)

Constant growth is necessary to maintain the human organism. The organism can live for a long time thanks to the renewal of skin, mucous and corneal cells, as well as countless other tissues. Physical life means constant growth. This also applies to palliative care or to the care of the dying. In the dying phase, growth in the figurative sense (apart from the body) plays a very important role. Anthroposophic nursing care accompanies a dying person in the awareness that development and inner growth are possible and meaningful up to the last breath. Growth in this phase of life is understood in the sense of inner development.

To accompany the dying process:

- A Pentagram Rhythmical Einreibung treatment on three consecutive days with *Gold rose-blossom lavender oil* (Dr. Heberer), then two subsequent treatments, each following a one-week interval

- Music therapy

- Biography work

7.8   Reproduction

Reproduction is the ability of the physical organism to reproduce life and create new life, ranging from DNA strands and individual body cells to an entirely new body. In a broader sense it is about the world of thoughts, in which it is possible to rethink things or form new ideas. Regarding palliative care, this may mean, for example, achieving reconciliation in existing situations of conflict or forgiving the mistakes of others. So, right up until the moment of physical death it is possible to develop new insights or new aspects of life.

■ Ginger kidney compresses with ginger powder or fresh ginger	2 times a week
■ Biography work	2 times a week

8.   The dying process—Observations from the daily work of a nurse

When accompanying the dying we perceive more than physical changes. Much more is happening than we can explain through physical phenomena.

In my (Sasha Gloor) many years of work in oncology I have been able to accompany many people and have witnessed numerous moments of death. I repeatedly noticed how individual dying is. It is no less unique than a person's biography, yet typical phases can still be experienced. The dying process carries people through what is happening, without them having to become aware of the overarching composition of their individual path.

It became clear to me that dying is a process, a path, and not an isolated event that marks the end. In nursing, our knowledge of such processes is of great importance for our support of our patients. The model that I describe here refers to people with cancer. But it can also be applied to other palliative situations. In a slightly differentiated form, this model can also be fruitful in nursing care for the elderly and in accompanying the very elderly.

8.1   The dying process as a journey with seven stages

I shall now describe the stages that I believe that we can observe in the journey of oncological disease up to the crossing of the threshold, first from the patient's perspective and then from the nurse's point of view.

The length of the journey and the time spent in each individual stage are individual. Many ill people only travel part of the journey, they then "disembark"—it may seem to outside observers—and return to life. Distant acquaintances or neighbors often describe these people as being healthy again.

Yet it is noteworthy that the cancer patients themselves usually experience this differently. Many are aware of having a more conscious experience of time, finiteness, quality of life, illness and health, in some cases also a different appreciation of life and their fellow human beings. They are in a process from which one cannot simply "disembark" on the level of soul and spirit. With some people these feelings and thoughts remain more diffuse. Their feelings may be expressed, e.g., in fear, agitation or helplessness, while other affected people realign and restructure their whole lives, both internally and externally.

Oncological diseases often reappear years later, then the affected person and the relatives have already proceeded part of the way and at a certain point they are again accompanied by the life processes described.

It is very important to me that you do not read the process steps described below as if they were a train schedule. Figuratively speaking, patients walk at their own pace, and we nurses are allowed to support and sometimes accompany them, but we cannot plan or predict the next train station or the duration of the stop.

Assigning planets to the stages of the illness can help us understand them pictorially. Linking up with these qualities enables a different approach to the process of dying than a purely intellectual one.

8.2 The seven planets as an analogy for the phases of the dying process

Most people today perceive the planets as being very far away. They do not see them as shaping forces in our world. This was not always the case. For example, the names of the weekdays are derived from the seven planets. We still use these terms today without being constantly aware of what they refer to. Monday–Moon, Tuesday (French mardi)–Mars, Wednesday (French mercredi)–Mercury, Thursday (French jeudi)–Jupiter, Friday (French vendredi)–Venus, Saturday–Saturn, Sunday–Sun.

The planetary forces are to be understood as archetypes and not as the physical celestial bodies. In the order of the weekdays they are an expression of developmental processes and evolution.

8.2.1 Self-perception

Self-perception–Moon
- Unclear perception of a change, intuiting, sensing
- Fatigue, exhaustion, night sweats, up to the point of discovering a lump
- The person experiences herself differently than before
- Triggers uncertainty, questions, sometimes also panic

Self-perception is not the same as a diagnosis in the medical sense. It is a diffuse or perhaps a clear perception that something in me or about me feels different than before (days, weeks or months ago).

This could be tiredness, for example. Some patients describe it as a sudden awareness that something is wrong, that they are always tired even though they are not doing more than usual. Or they may have bronchitis that simply doesn't heal, a cough that doesn't improve, and then this feeling that "something is wrong."

Especially in women with breast cancer, self-perception often involves discovering a lump in their breast. The reaction to this perception is quite individual. One patient told me she hadn't touched her breast directly for two weeks. Other women immediately tell someone and/or go to the doctor. In each case, however, self-perception triggers a reaction; whether the person takes a defensive attitude or embraces immediate action.

One patient told me that she had tried not to think about the lump in her breast and had first gone on vacation with her husband without informing him of her suspicions. These were then her best holidays. For other women such an approach would be inconceivable, they describe how they immediately wanted certainty about what was "wrong" with them.

Moon qualities

The Moon reflects sunlight and, when full, stands like a huge mirror in the sky. The Moon quality has to do with becoming visible, displaying an image of something. I perceive only what is reflected on a surface, I do not see what is underneath. Observation, self-perception and reflection are the topics. Moon forces are related to sensing and dreaming, not to rational perception.

8.2.2 Confrontation

Confrontation—Mars

- The person becomes a patient
- Visits to doctors and hospitals
- Diagnosis, being confronted with the facts
- Triggers fear, anger, despair and disbelief

The medical diagnosis is a radical confrontation. The person becomes a patient, goes from being healthy to being sick. Especially with cancer, the people affected suddenly feel themselves to be terminally ill or doomed to die. Most people think of cancer and death as an inseparable symbiosis and they ask: how much more time do I have? How long will I live? What will happen to my children when I die?

As a nurse I have experienced that this is felt less strongly when people are diagnosed with serious heart disease, for example, than when they are diagnosed with cancer.

Most people carry pictures of cancer around with them: I will have to have chemotherapy and then I will lose all my hair, I will die soon, I will have to be admitted to a hospital, I will suffer unspeakable pain. Fear, despair and anger arise.

Patients often wonder: "Why me? I never smoked and now I have bronchial carcinoma." A feeling of injustice, of having been betrayed by life, or a sense of being punished can occur.

Some people go to the doctor with a strong suspicion, others with a rather diffuse uncertainty. When they hear the diagnosis, this is almost always a shock. Oncological diseases in particular are often discovered by chance. People go to a doctor for a "checkup," and then the doctor diagnoses prostate cancer, for example. In this situation I have often experienced that patients cannot believe it at first. One man told me that he had gone to three family doctors, hoping that there had been some confusion with his documents. The unexpected diagnosis catapults the person from a supposedly healthy state into a seriously ill one. I remember some patients who told me that the scariest thing about the disease for them still today is that it developed unnoticed. How could this cancer grow in me without me noticing anything?

Mars qualities

The Mars quality is very powerful and fast. Mars does not have the time to weigh things up for a long time; it gets right down to acting on them. *Confrontations* are inevitable. Mars forces confront themselves and others. The Mars quality is involved in standing up and fighting for a cause.

8.2.3 Deciding

Deciding—Mercury

- Deciding on treatment, enormous time pressure and lack of time, flood of information
- Often not yet processed
- "Mindless" acting out of fear, very active relatives
- Triggers fear, and sometimes hope, too
- Can give security again
- Patients often cannot yet connect inwardly with their decision

As soon as the person concerned has received the diagnosis and has begun to understand what is "wrong" with him, he must already make *decisions*.

Patients are confronted with prognoses and information about the disease. If the person does not come from a medical or related profession, the technical language alone can often be overwhelming. Their intellectual grappling with the diagnosis, their consideration of the choice of therapy and the often different suggestions proposed by the doctors address a completely different part of them than the emotions that arise upon hearing the diagnosis. This is an enormous burden for most patients.

Add to that the fear for their lives, that time is running out.
In addition, there may be external time pressures (e.g., an urgent operation, or the start of chemotherapy as soon as possible). Those affected are hardly able to keep up with this rapid decision-making process.

The fact that virtually all clinical pictures, prognoses, courses of treatment, x-rays, personal presentations, comments and alternative therapy suggestions can be found on the Internet in large quantities today does not make the decision easier for patients.

Follow-up examinations are almost always prescribed, patients must go to the hospital or to specialists and undergo different diagnostic procedures. Each new examination, each consultation highlights different aspects of the disease. Every new finding is accompanied by new fear and hope.

In almost all cases, those affected see themselves forced to act before they can deal with the diagnosis and connect themselves in some way with the subsequent decisions and measures.

I remember a person who, after the diagnosis and the prescribed follow-up examinations and consultations, consciously took a break and withdrew to a monastery for meditation before undergoing surgery and starting chemotherapy.

Most patients describe this time in retrospect as if they had felt overwhelmed by the flood of information and their own emotions. They found themselves forced to make decisions without a clear overview of the multitude of possibilities and details.

Mercury qualities

Information, knowledge and movement: these mediating elements are pure Mercury qualities. The metal that represents it is fluid, hard-to-contain mercury. In Mercury we meet speed; it was only just here—and now it is already gone again. The Mercury quality has the power to collect. There are numerous possibilities open to the Mercury principle. The Mercury quality accompanies the absorption of polar opposite information and different possibilities.

8.2.4 Finding one's own

Finding one's own—Jupiter

- The person is in the middle of treatment, or the first cycle is completed.
- Marked by the treatment
- Hope may be partially or not fulfilled, zero point (what happens next? Where am I? What do I want?)
- Going my own way
- Triggers sadness, hopelessness, doubt, but also the opportunity to grasp life anew, to seek new paths
- Questions about spiritual dimensions and the meaning of life

The entry into an anthroposophic clinic very often represents a part of or the starting point in the process of *finding one's own.*

Most of the patients treated in the Lukas Clinic* did not come to us at the beginning of the disease, they usually came during the course of treatment.

I remember one statement in particular; the patient answered my question about her expectations for her hospital stay: "I want to know where I've gone! All that's left is cancer, disease—but where am I?" Another answer to the same question: "Oh, you know, I need a vacation now, a vacation from this cancer!"

When entering the Lukas Clinic, most people expressed the wish to find out what this disease had to do with them at all and to actively participate in their own recovery or handling of the disease.

The topic of *finding one's own* is about determining an individual path with and in the disease situation, or redefining terms such as health and disease for oneself.

Some patients enter into opposition to the doctor treating them and/or their own family. They accept the incomprehension of their next of kin in order to better understand themselves and their illness.

---

* This facilty is now called Klinik Arlesheim.

Example

A man came to the clinic after an operation. He had started practicing Qigong, had become a vegetarian and was now meditating every evening. His wife told me that she didn't have any problems with her husband's cancer, but she did have a problem with his new "craziness."

The need to find new insights into the illness and one's personal life situation seems to me to be central in this phase. Old things are suddenly discarded, and new things are eagerly absorbed. From the outside this is not always understandable, some relatives experience a kind of alienation towards these new interests. Some patients go to very extreme lengths, such as eating almost nothing but raw garlic.

Jupiter qualities

Jupiter, the father of the gods, wisely takes care of his subjects and does not forget his own needs. This love of life, this joy in life are Jupiter qualities. Jupiter does not lose himself in daily events; he keeps the scepter firmly in hand in crisis situations. The Jupiter quality accompanies the steadfastness to continue on one's way.

8.2.5 Creating order

Creating order—Venus

- The disease becomes a reality, the person with cancer and the people around him are now living with his cancer.
- A time of tidying up and organizing
- Viewing the past
- Biography work
- Preparation of a will and testament, preparation for the time afterwards
- Triggers deep emotions, strong mood swings
- Memories come back
- New questions arise, relatives are often intensely involved

In a figurative sense, the time of creating order has a lot to do with tidying up and sorting. The disease topic is quite different here, it has become a fact. The affected person is living with the disease and his or her environment has adapted to it.

It seems to me that creating order occurs very differently in this phase. Usually, this is followed by an initial *creating of order* after *finding one's own*, in which patients think about all the things that need to be arranged in case they suddenly die, e.g., their will and testament, the signing over of the company while they are still alive, and the like. In this stage of *creating order*, we often experience that couples "suddenly" marry after having been together for decades, for example.

But *creating order* can also happen under great time pressure, e.g., when the person's disease is progressing rapidly. This is where quite intense arguments may occur, which additionally burden the dwindling forces of patients. I remember a mother for whose children an adoptive family was being sought—under great time pressure—as she needed a family to take her children in so that they would not have to go to a home after their mother's death.

The priorities for what has to be brought into order result from the biography and the life situation of the person concerned. The mother from the example above used all her remaining strength to be able to "go in peace."

Some patients are more likely to create order in the personal, private sphere, such as by seeking forgiveness for disputes that have arisen over the course of their lives. In such cases it may be important for a certain person to come to visit them, or for an important conversation to take place.

Some people have a strong need to communicate something that has been kept secret until then. For instance, a long since grown-up child learned who his biological father was without having asked about it.

Family members and friends are often strongly involved in *creating order*, they can be supportive, but sometimes they remain perplexed. People who have gained the certainty for themselves that they will not live much longer often have the courage to address unusual or previously taboo topics.

It is not uncommon for there to be a long period of time between *finding one's own* and the stage of *creating order*, during which the affected person goes back to participating fully in life again. In this case, external things, such as financial arrangements, have already been completed.

Nevertheless, I have never experienced that this sixth step was skipped. Patients usually go through a personal process. It is not uncommon for them to deal again intensively with their own biographies or with individual, particularly pleasant or unpleasant times in their lives. I remember one person reading all her travel journals and reflecting intensely on those journeys.

Depending on the person's life, very strenuous and painful processes may be in progress, or it may be a matter of looking back, finding closure for and reflecting on everything that has been lived through. Emotional fluctuations, fears, anger and despair are always possible when creating order. But so are making peace, forgiving and giving away, as well as clarifying.

Religious topics often come to the fore—they too need time and space. Many patients prepare their funeral, write down their life story for the funeral service or decide on the content of their obituary.

Venus qualities
Relationships, affection, dislike and the establishment of comprehensive harmony are the central themes of Venus. Venus's need for harmony is not superficial, it is essen-

tial. Where there is conflict, no beauty—in the figurative sense—can arise. The quality of Venus accompanies the handling of emotions.

8.2.6 Preparation

Preparation—Saturn
- The time of creating order is over, there is more and more reconciliation with the situation and with what is happening
- The approaching death becomes a reality, the veil to the spiritual world becomes thinner
- Preparing for the new that is coming
- The pain subsides, the nausea lessens, the cough disappears
- Deep peace sets in, which also grips the people around
- The person gives more than he takes
- Peace is in the air, transcendence becomes almost tangible

When preparing, the activities that were still necessary when creating order are no longer in the foreground. All in all, there is much greater peace and serenity. Highly emotional moments occur less often or are completely absent. Many people seem reconciled with what is happening to them—at least over long periods of the day or night.

It is not uncommon for physical symptoms such as pain, coughing or persistent itching to subside. Many patients fall asleep during the day. With this sleep it seems as if patients were "far away" and their sleep seems actually quite peaceful. When you ask people in this state whether they dreamt anything, they often describe pleasant images, often images from childhood or special moments in life. These descriptions and the mood in which people find themselves very often have something conciliatory and calm about them; there is a coherence that is not easy to describe and that sometimes seems surprising to outsiders.
Nevertheless, there are always phases in which the patients linger in this special sleep, but appear restless and tense, perhaps speaking, holding their hands in the air or fiddling around with the blanket. If one addresses them, they are not completely oriented, they are more likely anxious or insecure, and they may describe images from less pleasant dreams. One lady in this situation asked us several times whether she was still alive or already with the angels.

From observing such sleep, we can say that it is special. It is not ordinary sleep: it is easy to interrupt, yet the person sleeping seems more "absent" than during normal sleep. They already seem to be looking a little beyond the threshold, into the spiritual world.

Patients who have lived religiously often find great peace when representatives of their faith perform religious rituals with them. Such patients feel protected and accompanied by their faith.

Saturn qualities

The principles of calmness and internalization are the central aspects of Saturn. There is nothing more that can or must be done quickly anymore, everything has its time and its validity. Activity and mobility are never at the forefront of the Saturn principle, where stability and tranquility prevail. The Saturn quality involves finding peace, concentrating on essentials.

8.2.7 Detaching oneself from this world

Detaching oneself from this world—Sun
- The actual dying process, the shortest phase
- Birth into the spiritual world, leaving the body behind as an empty shell
- For the relatives this is often much more difficult than for the affected person himself—we remain behind

Detaching oneself from this world is the shortest moment of the seven stages in terms of the time it takes. This refers to the person's birth into the spiritual world and to their departure from our world and their physical body. In the medical sense, this is the moment of death.

The dying person follows his own rhythm. The process can neither be stopped nor temporarily interrupted from the outside, it is already being helped along by the spiritual world.

Each person is on their own in this moment. Nurses, relatives and friends remain on the side of life and can do little. Purely practical actions lose their significance and one has to allow the spiritual element instead.

Sun qualities

The metal associated with the Sun is gold and the organ equivalent is the heart. We carry the Sun forces of our heart with us—gold and its shadow—when we stand at the threshold. Everything bright, everything dark that our heart holds, we will transform it on our journey after death, until it is time for a new incarnation.

The quality of the sun accompanies the human 'I' across the threshold.

8.3 How can nurses accompany the dying process?

Now that we have presented the patient's situation, let us look at the associated practical nursing tasks.

8.3.1 Self-perception

- Listen and take time
- Observe the patient's thinking and world view

As a nurse I have no contact with the patient when he is in the stage of *self-awareness*. He tells me about this experience looking back on it. Here I am needed as a listener. The great art is to perceive the patient's need (e.g., his wish to tell the whole story) to take the time and listen, despite the hustle and bustle of everyday life. This allows us, for example, to learn something about our patient's way of thinking and world view: how does the person see this experience in relation to her life? Did she want immediate certainty? Did she get very scared, was she paralyzed and could not act at all? Did she think that she would react like this, or was she surprised by her feelings?

We often accompany patients through medical examinations in which new, different, better or worse findings are obtained. When I already know how a person has dealt with a "suspected" condition, I can treat him more individually than I could a person who is completely unknown to me.

Example

I remember a woman who experienced pain when coughing and immediately thought that it was "the same cancer" that her mother had already died of. Later lung carcinoma was actually diagnosed and before each follow-up examination she gave herself a (very bad) prognosis. It was not possible to encourage her, we had to wait with her for the findings and endure the uncertainty. Only when she was wrong several times did this pattern finally fall apart.

8.3.2 Confrontation

- Shock at the diagnosis
- Support the patient's etheric forces
- Consider the patient's temperament

We nurses are usually not present at the actual diagnosis. We often encounter the patient shortly afterwards or somewhat later in the course of the illness.

From my experience I know that the diagnosis usually represents a mild to severe shock to those affected. From the point of view of anthropology, a shock always has an effect on the person's fourfold constitution. Since this fourfold constitution is not a fixed configuration, it is a mobile and fragile system that needs support and compensation in extreme situations. In oncology it is important never to ignore this. Creating order and supporting the patient's life forces (etheric forces) always plays a role.

Many anthroposophic medications have a stabilizing effect on the four members constituting the human being. We can also give the patient structure and support by administering a Pentagram Rhythmical Einreibung treatment [→ Chapter "Rhythmical Einreibung According to Wegman/Hauschka"]. Every rhythmical pattern supports the patient's etheric forces, be it the daily structure, regular meals, a figure-eight bath (a bath in which the nurse moves the water in a figure-eight pattern) or a Rhythmical Einreibung treatment according to Wegman/Hauschka.

Many patients speak again and again about the moment when they were first informed of the diagnosis. Often, they are given an estimate of their remaining time to live, whether it was because the patient or relatives asked directly, or because the doctor simply volunteered the information. Such numbers are almost indigestible for many people. The information remains in their consciousness like a meteorite that has crashed in. As a nurse, you must be very careful with this and it is often necessary to explain what is meant by an "average survival time." It is necessary to consider the temperament of the patient. For a choleric person it might be good if he can first criticize the doctor who gave the diagnosis before talking about the topic itself.

I have increasingly noticed that when the diagnosis is made by chance, patients blame themselves for not having noticed the disease sooner. In this case it relieves many people to hear that this often happens. Patients often talk about it with each other and thereby overcome the feeling of it being their own fault.

8.3.3 Deciding

- Time constraints, time pressure
- Information
- Creating an interior space

In this phase, the pressure of time—the awareness of being ill now and having to make the right decision immediately—seems to me to be the greatest source of distress.

Some patients do not get as far as asking themselves what they think about possible treatments. Others, in contrast, lose sight of an overview due to their many options. They inform themselves about as many concepts as possible and do not find a decision due to the sheer variety. Some patients seem to have no will at all and hand over the responsibility to the attending physician.

As a nurse, I try to assess the patient's level of information, to find out what the person wants to hear again, what they would like to learn that is new, and what I "cannot" confront them with again.

This is the informative side of this stage. All information forms an exterior space, a perimeter around the patient. Often this is an area that offers little protection and is rather threatening in character.

That is why another aspect seems to be very important for the patient to be able to make a decision at all. Patients often cannot keep up emotionally with what is happening to them externally. When I have the possibility to accompany patients in this phase of decision-making, I create as much peace and equilibrium as possible. I help the person concerned to create an inner space, to find access to himself. Moments of equilibrium can be created with the help of Rhythmical Einreibung according to Wegman/Hauschka, or we can administer compresses. The patients have lost their accustomed protection and are facing a new unknown situation. We work a lot with *Solum oil* (WALA) to support such protection from outside. Solum envelops the patient, it separates the inside from the outside.

8.3.4 Finding one's own

- Searching
- What does this illness have to do with me?
- What else do I want to experience, leave aside or rediscover?

At this stage, as mentioned above, I have gotten to know most patients. On this part of the journey, people are consciously looking for a way to deal with the disease that is right for them. This can be very different for different people. Some simply no longer want to talk about the disease and they return to everyday life with a lot of activity and confidence. Others pause to find out what the meaning of their suffering might be. Patients often change their lives and dare to make a new start: a new partnership, a different job, a new place of residence.

Here it is helpful to pay attention to the biographical phase and seven-year period in which the person finds himself [→ Chapter "Illness and Destiny"]. This may give an indication of which questions are or could become important. Thus, the person's individual situation can also be viewed from the point of view of general laws. As a nurse, I do not have the skills to work with patients on their biographies; a specialist has to be consulted for that. From experience, I know that teams often discuss whether or not a particular patient has become too extreme in restructuring his life, and that biographical considerations can contribute to greater objectivity.

As we move into new territories, we sometimes overshoot the target on our way to finding the middle ground. That is why extreme diets, a rejection of any treatment at all, and forms of self-healing are always an issue in the phase of *finding one's own*. Such approaches do have positive aspects, but they can turn into dangerous one-sidedness. Here it is helpful if the nurses in the team determine one or two nursing gestures for working with this person. This gives support and stability in a phase in which the patient is in a state of upheaval. The nursing gesture model is a structuring concept for both sides (the nurse and patient) [→ Chapter "The Concept of Nursing Gestures as a Model for Nursing Care"].

I have noticed time and again that patients who are seeking answers have approached me not as a caregiver or nursing specialist, but as a person. "What do you personally think?" When I was new to the profession, I used to find such situations difficult. Over time I recognized a very positive aspect to this question, as it gives you new freedom and an opportunity to enter into a more intense relationship with the patient. You always have the freedom to say, "as a nurse, I must urge you to do so... but if I myself were in your situation, I can imagine...." Authenticity seems to be central in the stage of *finding one's own*. People are often very open and interested, looking for spiritual nourishment in the form of books, conversations or art.

Finding one's own way of life, one's personal center, can be very well supported by Rhythmical Einreibung according to Wegman/Hauschka, art therapy, eurythmy therapy and, of course, biography work.

8.3.5 Creating order

- Cleaning up and sorting
- Emotions
- Involving family members

There are different aspects to creating order. As nurses, we often organize very practical things. A religious representative or a notary may arrive, or a former schoolmate from the USA needs to be called. Usually the people around the sick person are important in this phase. This can be very exhausting for patients on all three levels (physical, mental, spiritual). Often the nursing staff must structure the patient's daily routine rhythmically, with times for care, visiting times and the very important rest periods. Often there are strong emotions, because the affected people are beginning to realize that they may be seeing certain people for the last time. Saying farewells and giving voice to things become central elements as soon as patients assume that they are not going to return to everyday life.

Here, strong demands are made on nurses with regard to looking after the people around the patient. Especially distant acquaintances sometimes cannot assess the situation correctly and need support. Patients often comfort their visitors. It may happen that those affected will talk very freely about their situation and about dying, but only with the nurses and not with the family. The family members usually do not dare to mention what is coming, so a nurse may need to mediate.

Some patients prepare everything for the time of death. They determine the clothes that they want to wear and express wishes as to whom one should first notify or which lipstick they want to have applied after their death. It is extremely important to settle and address these things. Again and again, I have seen people arrange their obituaries and the funeral. A patient once said to me: "Well, that's done. Now I can go in peace. My sons would have organized this quite differently and I assume that I will see it from above. It's got to be done the way I want it, right?"

"Fear of the night" increasingly becomes a topic during the phase of creating order. In a sleeping person the 'I' and the soul body are much more detached from the physical and etheric bodies than in an awake person. We also find this natural loosening process in people who are dying. Normally we do not experience this pulling out or loosening as unpleasant. People who are very ill or who are already closer to the threshold of death often experience agitation and fear of falling asleep. They can be startled when they fall asleep and feel that they are falling back onto the bed. Others are afraid to close their eyes because they are already experiencing a sensation of falling backwards. Sensations of this kind have to do with the detachment of the two higher members of the person's fourfold nature ('I' and soul body) and they are very often observed during this period of *creating order*, when patients are physically already greatly impaired. This "fear of the night" can be alleviated by a Rhythmical Einreibung of the feet, with

- *Rosa e floribus 10%, Oleum* (WALA)

- *Lavender 10% oil* (Weleda) or *Lavandula, Oleum aethereum 10%* (WALA)

or by a heart ointment compress, with

- *Aurum/Lavender/Rose cream* (Weleda)

Some people find it helpful when relatives or friends spend the night in the room.

8.3.6 Preparation

- Give the person space
- Relieve them
- Take over tasks for them

The stage of *preparation* is calmer and more relaxed than that of *creating order*. Nurses accompany, monitor and take charge of, e.g., personal hygiene, positioning and excretion processes. It relieves the patient when the nurse takes care of body-related maintenance activities. Patients can do whatever their powers allow, and everything else they leave to the nurse. This giving up of what they used to do for themselves varies in difficulty for different people, since it always means letting go of everyday abilities that they will never win back. This requires a lot of empathy from the nurse, usually it is a process that must be carefully accompanied day by day to optimally care for the patient. It is very helpful to work with nursing gestures in such cases, especially when it is difficult for a patient to let go of being active.

Usually the phases of sleeping become longer, and daytime sleep occurs, as described. Oral hygiene becomes increasingly important. The focus is on caring for the skin, which involves working extensively with oils and other substances. Rose oil is often used, as rose accompanies threshold transitions gently and comfortingly. Solum oil is used to protect the skin and to form an enveloping layer, but lavender oil and mallow oil are also suitable for application and Rhythmical Einreibung.

- *Rosa e floribus 10%, Oleum* (WALA)

- *Solum oil* (WALA)

- *Lavender 10% oil* (Weleda) or *Lavandula, Oleum aethereum 10%* (WALA)

- *Mallow oil* (WALA)

Other relieving applications, such as farmer's cheese compresses for ascites, can be administered as long as the patient experiences them as being effective.

As a rule, we do not administer applications that irritate the skin or strain the circulation, such as brush baths. Measures of this kind have an incarnating effect, make the patients wide awake and generate a strong physical presence. In contrast, this person is occupied with shedding her body to enter the spiritual world.

If agitation ensues that is not caused by pain or sluggish excretory processes, it can help to administer:

- Rhythmical Einreibung treatments with *Lavender 10% oil* (Weleda) or *Lavandula, Oleum aethereum 10%* (WALA)

- Heart compresses with *Aurum/Lavandula comp. cream* (Weleda)

Music therapy and eurythmy therapy can accompany patients very nicely, without them having to become active themselves. Numerous anthroposophic medicinal products are used to gently and effectively treat agitation in the *preparation phase.*

Often relatives are grateful when they can take over small tasks and thus help care for the patient. However, it is equally important to relieve the burden on relatives when necessary and to ensure that they sleep and eat as much as needed. Patients sometimes no longer engage in conversations, so it is important to tell their relatives that patients usually listen, nonetheless.

It is helpful to accompany the patient's relatives very closely, as there are usually interactions between the relatives and the patient in terms of tension and relaxation.

The process of *preparation* requires space—telephone calls or similar should better happen outside the patient's room. Nurses are usually tasked with organizing the surroundings.

8.3.7 Detaching oneself from this world

- Being present in the moment
- Dignity
- Shaping one's surroundings

People die as individually as they have lived. Each moment of death is unique. Some people die when they are alone in the room, others when their loved ones are with them. Many people seem to wait for a certain person before they can go.

The actual threshold crossing can only be accompanied from the moment. The spiritual world is already helping to determine how it will happen. Very often relatives report that it was beautiful—and are themselves amazed at what they have just said.

Dignified treatment of the deceased and the three days after death seem to me to be valuable moments both for the deceased and for the relatives. The deceased needs three days to completely detach himself from his lifeless body and withdraw his etheric body. During this time the person's appearance often changes, many people seem to rejuvenate themselves. During the three days, the relatives have time to say goodbye and to accompany the person spiritually and/or religiously. The setting plays an important role: What does the laying-out room look like? Are there flowers? May there be Christian religious symbols in the room, or should these be temporarily replaced by others?

A description of the soul's journey in the spiritual world after death until the next incarnation would go beyond the scope of this chapter. I would therefore just like to conclude by saying that spiritual accompaniment by the living does not have to end after these three days. From an anthroposophic point of view, the soul after death ascends through the planetary spheres on its way to a new incarnation. Rudolf Steiner described different stages of this journey through the planetary spheres. Knowledge of these phases can support us in accompanying a person who has died.

Category	Example learning objectives	Recommended learning path
Skills	You use external applications to support the seven life processes in dying people.	A
Your own learning objective		
Relationships	You bring empathy to accompanying people who have been diagnosed with a disease that is likely to soon lead to death.	B
Your own learning objective		
Knowledge	You know the inner developmental stages that a person passes through when dying.	C
Your own learning objective		

References

1 Temel, S.; Joseph, A.G., et al. Early palliative care for patients with metastatic non-small-cell lung cancer. *New England Journal of Medicine* 2010; 363 (8), pp. 733–742.

2 Steiner, R. *Physiology and healing. Treatment, therapy and hygiene—spiritual science and medicine.* Rudolf Steiner Press, London 2013.

3 Schad, W. *Die verlorene Hälfte des Menschen—Die Plazenta vor und nach der Geburt in Medizin, Anthroposophie und Ethnologie.* Verlag Freies Geistesleben, Stuttgart 2008, p. 72.

4 Mc Cafferey, M.; Beebe, A.; Latham, J. Schmerz. *Ein Handbuch für die Pflegepraxis.* Ullstein Buchverlage, Berlin 1997.

5 von Dach, C.; Heine, R.; Heiligtag, H. Anthroposophische Pflege von Krebskranken. *Der Merkurstab* 2009; 62 (4), pp. 330–341.

6 Lerch, A.; Meyer, U. Thymianöl—Einsatz in Phytotherapie und anthroposophischer Medizin. *Der Merkurstab 2008*; 61 (2), pp. 163–165.

7 Meyer, U. Die Schlehe—Heilpflanzen für Zeitgenossen. *Der Merkurstab* 2011; 64 (2), pp. 100–114.

8 Meyer, U., et al. "Rechnen Sie auf die Kieselsäure"—Pharmazeutische Gesichtspunkte zu einer möglichen Optimierung der Equisetum-Therapie. *Der Merkurstab* 2012; 65 (2), pp. 112–116.

CHAPTER XXV

The Care and Accompaniment of the Dying and the Deceased

GUDRUN BUCHHOLZ

This chapter will describe the soul's passage out of the body into a new existence after death. The fruitfulness of viewing human existence from an anthroposophic perspective is particularly evident when dealing with death and dying, and modern near-death research has confirmed it. This presentation will be based on fundamental suggestions for how to support people who are dying, suggestions that have been developed over decades of cooperation between doctors, nurses and priests. We shall explain the practice of caring for and laying out the body, as cultivated in anthroposophic hospitals, showing its significance for both the deceased and the bereaved.

→   Learning objectives, see end of chapter

What we call the beginning is often the end
And to make an end is to make a beginning...
We shall not cease from exploration
And the end of all our exploring
Will be to arrive where we started
And know the place for the first time.
                                        T. S. Elliot (1888–1965)

1.   Introduction—An attempt at an approach to death and dying

Some years ago, I had the following deeply memorable experience. The four-year-old son of friends, who had been suffering from an incurable tumor for two years, died. At this news, friends of the family, including me, went to the children's ward to say goodbye and support his parents.

We felt great uncertainty because we did not know how to meet them at such a moment. However, the boy's mother came down the ward corridor towards us with a glowing expression on her face and said: "It was so beautiful." At first, I was stunned by this exclamation and was strangely touched. How can a mother say such a thing immediately after the death of her child? We stepped into the room where the boy was laid out on his little bed. A primeval wisdom emanated towards us from this child. We, who were previously uncertain and troubled, suddenly felt lighter, happier. It was as if a peace-giving veil of light had descended upon us. Someone suddenly remembered that Johannes had always liked to sing. So, we sang his favorite songs for him. The result was a wonderfully cheerful, light atmosphere, and we all left the room feeling strengthened and richly blessed. This experience had a decisive influence on my attitude towards people who have died. It showed me that death does not have to be met exclusively with melancholy and that it can also give us something if we only look at it correctly.

Often, however, we encounter the opposite. When a patient dies in a hospital ward, those present at the moment of death flee the room after a short time, or they don't even enter the room, saying: "We want to remember him the way we've always known him."

In our Western culture we no longer dare to look death in the eye. For us, death usually means the failure of medicine, the failure of the doctor. Yet from the first minute of life, nothing is more certain than death. Every living being is affected by death and dying at some point. Human beings are exceptional only because they must know this consciously. But the thought of death seems to be so unbearable that people keep repressing it and making it taboo. It could be that when we made death a taboo, we also lost the meaning of life. People increasingly suffer from loneliness, existential insecurity and feelings of deep senselessness in their lives. In the past, even into the early 20th century, death used to be seen as a natural part of existence. People felt the approach of death and they prepared themselves for it by arranging for anything that needed to be taken care of, such as sewing a shroud, bringing order into their circumstances and saying goodbye to their relatives.[1]

Today in the West, people usually die lonely—often in a hospital, and there they may be pushed out of the way into a bathroom.

Since we cannot look death in the eye, we have also lost the culture in which ritual actions used to be performed for the deceased and for our own coping with grief.[2]

Confronting ourselves with dying can illuminate the meaning of life in a special way. To acquire an idea of what death means becomes a necessity when we work in a profession that constantly confronts us with it. An anthroposophic-anthropological understanding of death can help.

2.   The anthroposophic view of dying and death

One of the fundamental communications of spiritual science, besides giving insight into the human fourfold constitution (which consists of a physical body, etheric body, soul body and 'I') is the idea of reincarnation. "Human beings are seen as beings of soul and spirit, who appear through physical corporeality at birth. Their origin lies in the spiritual world, to which they return after each life on earth. The core of their being, their individuality, is eternal. The goal of life on earth is to develop further towards freedom and the ability to love, and towards growing spiritualization. For each life on earth, human beings set themselves certain tasks before they are born. Illness often plays an important role in mastering such tasks. In our encounters with other people, we form connections of destiny which continue in repeated lives on earth.

Every human being participates in the overall development of humanity through his or her actions and is part of a larger cosmic context."[3]

Based on this conception of the human being, the anthroposophic approach to nursing care and medicine encompasses the whole human being. Through knowledge of reincarnation and karma, every encounter between people takes on a very special meaning. An endeavor of Anthroposophic Medicine and nursing care is therefore not merely to restore the same state of health as before the disease, but also to address what wants to develop into the person's future.

2.1   What happens to our fourfold nature after death?

Death occurs through a change in the connection between the members of the four-fold constitution.[4] The etheric body (which is responsible for maintaining the form and functions of the physical body) joins the soul body and the 'I' as they detach themselves from the physical body, leaving the physical aspect subject to decay. However, the soul body and etheric body do not separate from each other immediately after death. All the memories of the finished life are recorded in the etheric body as if in a journal. "During the waking state, the many sensory impressions conveyed by the physical body prevent all the memories from being present in our consciousness. They are forgotten. After death, this impediment ceases to exist and the etheric body— freed from its task of upbuilding and regenerating—reveals the entire memory of the soul in a kind of panorama of the person's life. "[5] The soul body connected to the etheric body conjures all the person's memories into one comprehensive, vivid panorama. In contemplating this panorama after death, one does not experience oneself as the main actor, but as an observer.

There are many reports of people who were deemed "clinically dead" and yet returned to life. They almost unanimously report on experiences of looking back on their life, e.g., George Ritchie[6] and Stefan von Jankovich.[7] The American physician Raymond Moody collected several hundred experiences of people who were "clinically dead" and who reported very similar things independently of one another: After being released from their physical body they found themselves in a transparent, weightless, spiritual body, which they described as a kind of force field.[8]

At this stage of death, they did not experience their consciousness as being extinguished. Instead they experienced a wonderfully peaceful clarity in which they looked back on their life.[9] People who have had such an experience are generally no longer afraid of death, and the event changes their further life on earth. About three days after death, the etheric body disperses completely into a general world of formative forces. Elisabeth Kübler-Ross (1926–2004) described this condition as the untethering of the silver cord.[10] At this point, only the soul body and the 'I' are left. We have a similar state in sleep, where the soul body and 'I' come out of the physical body yet remain oriented towards the physical body. However, there is one essential difference to death: during sleep the soul body is filled with the day's experiences from the physical world and the 'I' is occupied with processing these experiences. After death the 'I' is free from this task, so it can now become aware of the much more subtle spiritual experiences that the soul is having in its non-physical surroundings. Nevertheless, in the first period after death the soul still retains a certain connection to the experiences gained through life on earth, which must be processed during a phase of purification.

There are three types of attachment of the soul to the physical body:

- Needs like thirst, hunger and love are determined by the physical body and must be satisfied by the intake of fluids, food and human attention.

- Mental needs, such as to engage in science, art or religion, which can be satisfied only with the help of physical organs.

- The enjoyment of pleasures, drives, desires and passions that go beyond physical needs. The deprivations that the soul now has to endure until it has completely overcome its attachment to the physical body have been described by various religions as purgatory or consuming fire, because this third type of desire must be completely swept out of the soul in 'kamaloka' (the place of desire: *kama* = "desire" in Sanskrit, *loca* = "place").

The time of purification after death is about one third of the foregoing human lifetime. During this time the soul looks back on its life in reverse, beginning with the moment of death and working back to the moment of birth, objectively judging every one of its subjective acts and thoughts during its life on earth. That is, during this review the 'I' must itself experience all the pain and joy that it inflicted on other people. Through such self-evaluation, the 'I' can absorb the necessary moral impulses for making amends and further perfecting itself. After this period of purification and retrospection, part of the soul body disperses, while the part necessary for the continued existence of this individual connects with the 'I' as a "life extract." The 'I' then returns to its spiritual homeland, where further experiences await it.[11]

2.2   The psyche of the dying person

We are interwoven with the world around us with a thousand threads. Our lives, our plans, our goals are directed towards this life, and we need interaction with the world in order to stand within it in a healthy way. Being told that one has been diagnosed with a fatal disease profoundly changes this relationship. Where there used to be active engagement with life, there should now be saying goodbye to it, and not just temporarily for a long journey, but for the last great journey itself. Not everyone is mentally prepared to cope with such a blow, especially not immediately. Why is this? A relatively small amount of soul energy is enough for the fulfillment of our daily duties. The amount of energy required increases when an inner predisposition or a hard blow of fate causes someone to start to think about life in general or his own life in particular. Prayers and/or meditations lead to an increase in the soul's life energy. Living in the face of death is a kind of permanent meditation prescribed by fate. Thus, a person who has been practicing meditation or something similar may succeed better and faster in adjusting to the path from life to death than someone who is hit by the diagnosis entirely in the here and now. We are not referring to the ability to concentrate in general, which is very much in demand in the world today and which happens in the mind with the participation of the will. We mean the middle human being, which can experience the richness of life in joy and sorrow, the weaving beauty of nature, the deepening that can be won through art, and which is not left untouched by the religions and worldviews of humanity. More precisely, we do not mean the middle human being of feeling, we mean the one for whom the light and the clarity of the head have been widened into the heart. And since the head analyses but the heart synthesizes, this middle aspect can see many areas of life in context. It is the spiritual human being capable of thinking with the heart.

This level of developmental maturity is demanded ad hoc of a person when they are unprepared and are suddenly diagnosed with a fatal disease, which is usually enormously overwhelming. This is accompanied by the danger of the person becoming predisposed to a new disease, first psychologically, then psychosomatically. The ill person must first learn to look death in the eye and then gradually transform it into a teacher and friend who can show him what is essential and enduring in his life and who can help him to grow beyond his little earthly ego.

What are the problems and fears that arise at the moment that people hear the doctor's diagnosis?

Especially for a person who has been fully active in the world up to now, it is not just having to say goodbye to his life's task, it is the feeling of no longer being useful to society and the fear of no longer being respected because of this, and of falling into social isolation. There is also the fear of becoming a burden to other people, especially relatives, or of being separated from them by long hospital stays. The idea of having to make the change from a familiar to a foreign environment in a weakened state is also very distressing. Last but not least, it is the fear of becoming dependent on overburdened, indifferent, unknown people.

The disease itself also sometimes triggers massive fear of pain, prolonged infirmity, possible disfigurement and changes in consciousness.

Finally, the ill person will have to live through the next period of time with the already existing and still to come physical suffering in full knowledge of the hopelessness of his condition. He is about to say goodbye to his loved ones and his wider social environment, but also to nature as he currently sees and loves it. In addition, there is the burden of what remains unresolved in his biography, such as unfinished work, unachieved goals, unresolved relationship problems, and mistakes that haven't been made good. In addition, there is a deep-seated elementary fear of death because, with rare exceptions, people lack their own experience with it and have a more or less high degree of uncertainty as to what happens after death.

The dying person is initially faced with enormous psychological burdens before he can develop a more relaxed attitude. He experiences eons of loneliness in which he undergoes developments that even those close to him often cannot understand or relate to.[12]

Elisabeth Kübler-Ross divided the dying process into five stages which people go through in a variety of ways and sequences. Her great concern was to awaken understanding for what a person experiences in the dying process.[13]

3. Birth and death

> *"When a human being is born, a spirit dies, when a human being dies, a spirit is born."* Novalis (1772–1801)

When we look at the two gates of human life, the first as well as the last breath represents a sacred moment, which we accompany with joy on the one hand and sadness on the other.

"What we call birth is nothing but the other side of death, another name for the same process from the opposite point of view, just as we call the same door an entrance or an exit, depending on whether we are looking at it from the outside or the inside. One may rightly wonder why people do not remember their last death, and this is the reason why most people do not believe that they have ever experienced it. But they do not remember their birth either, yet they do not doubt for a moment that they were born. They overlook the fact that active memory (i.e., the memory underlying our conscious will) is only a small part of our normal consciousness, and that our 'subconscious memory' has registered and preserved all the impressions and experiences that have long slipped away from our waking consciousness."[14]

According to the interviews that Helen Warnbach[15] conducted, regarding the recollections of a group of people under hypnosis, the subjects unanimously stated that they had experienced everything—i.e., the time before and during pregnancy, the birth process, including the words that were spoken—fully consciously. Only then did they become an infant, a toddler, and so on, in terms of consciousness. People who have come back from the threshold of death tell of similar spiritual experiences in many variations.

So, according to all these reports, when we stand grieving or reverent beside a person who has died, we are certainly not alone. The person who has died is present with us (and may also need our thoughts as guidance in this new plane of existence). From this we can see that a long period of suffering before death allows a dying person to enter the spiritual world with a more mature consciousness than a sudden quick death. Both variants are in the hands of the powers of destiny and the above makes it very clear that we are by no means entitled to replace the one that is more protracted and painful for us with the one that is more pleasant and comfortable.

If we could empathize before with the fact that a person who is still in the midst of life initially does not want to acknowledge the certainty of death associated with a diagnosis and rebels against it, we can understand on the other hand the keen wish of some severely suffering patients to be released as quickly as possible from their agony. These are very human emotions in the life of soul, so finding meaning in what is happening to oneself is absolutely necessary. Meaning can be found only from the inclusion of life after death. Birth and death are real limits to our power. If I respect them, I will be kindly received and accepted into higher laws.

4. The transformation of the dying person

Dying is a process that takes place in phases and is concluded by death as the end of all life processes.

4.1 Time perspectives

When a person is dying, he is undergoing omnipresent suffering in all time periods—in the past, the present and the future. By our readiness to talk, we or other people close to him can help him as he looks back on and reappraises his life, until his biography has become a readable script to him. Looking at the present, the dying person perceives everything that surrounds him very finely and sensitively through an increased sensitivity of his senses.

The seriously ill and the dying have very clear perceptions of our truthfulness or dishonesty. Masking our true thoughts does not work. Eckhard Wiesenhütter, for example, described his experience of dying. He was able to clearly perceive the thoughts and feelings of the people who came to his bedside.[16]

The sense of taste and the sense of smell become much more pronounced, so that certain food smells or fragrances, barely perceptible to us, can cause nausea. Color sensations also become much more intense. Colors which the healthy can hardly see because of their subtlety can be experienced by the dying as being unbearably intense. Art therapists who have worked with dying people report on this phenomenon. The sense of hearing is also more finely developed. It is the last sense to be lost. The dying person feels excluded when people whisper in his environment.

During the dying process we often observe that the dying person's eyes seem to look into a far distance, as if covered by a veil, perceiving something we cannot see, similar to the gaze of a newborn baby who sees so much, but not yet us.

Thinking of the future of the dying person, the people around him should give him the certainty that they will not immediately forget him. Many people seem to feel the need to continue on in some way, in memory. It is also possible to discuss the person's wishes for the funeral and the form of burial. This spares him from having to experience something quite foreign to him after death. The idea of reincarnation offers further help, since it enables us to know that in the future, we will be able to overcome past failures and take on new tasks. Nevertheless, the idea of reincarnation does not completely console us about having to say farewell to our loved ones as they are this time around. That is unrecoverable in its present richness.

Most people fear death less than pain. So, for many dying and seriously ill people, a pain therapy concept (such as pain therapy according to C. Klaschik and F. Nandl, based on the WHO's step-by-step scheme) can be a great help.[17] Treatment according to this concept makes pain more tolerable and contributes to an improved quality of life. Nevertheless, there are dying and seriously ill patients who cannot be treated according to this concept because, even with regularly administered peripheral analgesics or morphine, it is not always possible to achieve sufficient pain relief. It is also often the case that painkillers are not tolerated, or they cause paradoxical effects.

Some patients who took morphine described that they had thoughts that were not their own, which irritated them. Also, their sense of their own body changed, so that they felt strangely divided into two. From anthroposophic spiritual science it can be seen that opiates intervene deeply in a person's being. We can observe that patients who are lovingly accompanied by relatives, friends and helpers, and who experience pain relief or no pain when taking morphine, hardly experience any impairment of their inner path. However, there are also many ill people who have neither loving relatives, nor friends nor a spiritual background. Under the influence of strong pain medication, they are led further and further away from themselves, instead of to themselves. With these patients, the dying process often takes a long time, and one always has the impression that they are still waiting for something.

4.3   Pain relief

It is important for nurses to know that pain therapy with opiates can facilitate the patient's inner path, but also block it, depending on the external conditions around the patient.

There are many possibilities for relieving pain, e.g., pain therapy with potentized medicinal plants.[18] With the availability of external applications—such as oil dispersion baths, Rhythmical Einreibung and compresses—we nurses have important tools to address the whole person, as well as the person's pain locally where it hurts. By doing something for this person, by preparing myself, by administering a treatment on him and with him, I am giving him very personal attention, which in itself—if done with inner compassion—is healing in addition to the outer action.

In every person, no matter how sick and full of pain he may be, there also lives a healthy side, which asks to be addressed, so that it can develop further. Self-healing forces are part of the whole human being. If they are suppressed by negative influences, they remain ineffective. To stimulate these forces, it is therefore of great importance that we know about the patient's potential for development and that we are able to convey real hope from this. If we succeed in directing the patient's interest more towards the environment and the outside world, be it literature, music, painting or nature, then his perception can move into a mental realm that can become a source of strength for him. The pain does not only call for treatment with chemical substances, it challenges us as individuals and as a therapeutic community to contribute ourselves as human beings and as healing remedies. Pain needs our love to be healed.

We have experienced again and again that hardly any pain killers are needed shortly before death. The higher members of the person's being—the soul body and the 'I'—which feel the pain, slowly detach themselves from the body, making the body less and less perceptible.

4.4   The encounter with the double

Often, shortly before death, we can perceive a clear change in the dying person's nature, which can manifest itself in states of fear, anger and aggression. He may almost look as if he is battling something. His relatives are often distressed and astonished, and even the nurses are strangely touched and may feel attacked. Such a phase of change can last from a few hours to days. Then it passes and the person seems to be transformed. He proceeds towards death with equanimity and inner peace. From anthroposophic anthropology we know that in this phase the dying person is having an encounter with his double. Who is this double? He is described as a real spiritual being who is not perceptible to our normal everyday consciousness. He is made up of our life's thoughts, words and deeds. Just before we cross the threshold of death, we meet him. Usually it is not a very pleasant encounter, because the double is a merciless mirror of ourself. Rudolf Steiner described him as extremely ugly and frightening, while at the same time having great sternness and love.[19] His appearance expresses something like the following: "Here in me you see the sum of your thoughts, words and deeds from your life on earth. It is up to you to make me ever more beautiful and perfect. By your striving, I can transform myself into a radiant being of light."

If the encounter with this guardian of the threshold strikes a person unprepared, it can cause great fear and terror. At the same time, though, a strong impulse can arise in him to contribute more and more to perfecting his humanity in a new life. If we, as nurses, perceive such a change of being knowingly and understandingly, we can help the dying person in our thoughts. Such encounters with the double are also experienced by people who gain access to the world of spirit through spiritual training. You must pass by him if you want to enter the world of spirit. But in order not to perish from it, you need preparation, spiritual training.

When we fall asleep, our 'I' and soul body withdraw from the physical body and visit the world of spirit, where they get nourishment for the next day's work. Here, too, we must pass the guardian of the threshold, but we don't notice him because we are "unconscious." Our lack of consciousness is a protection, because we could not bear the sight and could be driven insane by it, as it is described in Bulwer Lytton's *Zanoni*, for example.[20] Several other works of world literature also describe encounters with the double.[21]

SPECIALIZATIONS IN NURSING

5. Nursing care for people who are dying

Caring for a dying person is a great challenge because we are constantly confronted with our own insecurity. It takes courage to stick with this uncertainty, overcome it and create within ourselves the composure with which we can approach the patient. An important aspect of nursing care is to meet the dying person again and again and find out what inner unspoken question he may be living with. Although there are many possibilities to help the dying, we must not hide the fact that accompanying the dying is not a technique that can be learned, it is a highly personal act that can only be performed out of human compassion. "All our knowledge about dying is lost to the dying person, even precisely chosen words cannot reach him if they do not come from the root of real humanity. To really meet the dying person and thus help him can only be done by someone who strives and works hard to become a loving person. Love requires that we say yes to our own humanity, also saying yes to allowing feelings of fear and helplessness."[22]

To follow, as nurses, a path of practice in the sense of the six "supplementary exercises" as described by Rudolf Steiner can form a foundation for self-knowledge, knowledge of human beings, and a constantly growing capacity for love, through which real encounter becomes possible [→ Chapter "Nursing as a Path of Development"].

The age of a dying person is decisive for nursing care. The younger the patient, the more we deal with the relatives as sufferers and as helpers. In children's wards, mothers are admitted along with their child to give their child enveloping protection. The death of a child or a young person is a destiny that strikes a community, the death of an elderly person is more of an individual fate. The younger person still has, the older person has once again, a stronger relationship to the spiritual world. Middle-aged people fight the hardest to free themselves from the earthly. Accordingly, care of the dying looks different for each age group.

Here are some suggestions to expand upon the usual, generally known nursing care measures available.

WARMTH: Warmth plays an important role in the care of the seriously ill, warmth on all levels. Dying people often lack the strength to produce their own warmth. Their weakened warmth organism must therefore be protected from outside. When a person is surrounded by warmth, she develops trust and feels secure. It can be a blessing for the seriously ill to be offered warm tea sometimes, instead of cold water. It then makes sense to have a thermos flask with tea ready on the bedside table.

In all nursing activities, we must take care to ensure that the patient does not get cold. We can achieve comprehensive warming and at the same time have a very calming effect on a dying person by giving her a warm footbath in bed, or hand and arm baths. The warmth conveys—as already described—a feeling of security, making it easier for the dying person to let go.

WATER: In addition to warmth, the element of water also plays an important role when administering such treatments. In water, people live in their primal element, which was their home during embryonic development. Water conveys lightness, vastness and basic confidence. At the same time, it can relieve pain for a while.

EXCRETIONS: Excretions are important in the care of dying people. Regular digestion is essential. It is difficult for a dying person who has not voided for several days to free himself from his body, because he is oppressed in the truest sense of the word. Rhythmical Einreibung treatments of the patient's abdomen with *carraway oil* (*Oleum aethereum Carvi 10%, extemporaneous pharmacy preparation*) can help.

SWEATING: Lemon water washes can be refreshing when people sweat a lot (cut open an unsprayed lemon under water and squeeze it out). Sage or peppermint tea washes are also pleasant. Plant extracts are also available as washing emulsions (e.g., *Lemon Lemongrass Vitalising Bath Essence* (Dr. Hauschka) or *Citrus Refreshing Bath Milk* (Weleda)).

NUTRITION: In terms of nutrition, care must be taken to ensure that patients receive light, mildly spiced food, so that their organisms are not additionally burdened by hard-to-digest foods. It often happens that patients only have water or highly acidic fruit juices on their bedside table to drink. These juices may taste too intense and burn on the tongue. In that case, as already mentioned, it can be very beneficial for the patient to have a glass of warm tea ready. Fruit juices can also be warmed up. Care should be taken to ensure that enough fresh fruit is always available. Even a small piece of an orange can be very invigorating, sometimes even when you only smell it. Cutting a lemon in the patient's room has proven its worth in promoting salivary secretion. The resulting scent is usually very pleasant and refreshing to patients. Make sure that they consume enough fluids.

ORAL CARE: Caring for the mouth (using mixed teas, e.g., chamomile-sage-lemon-rose-honey tea, in addition to mouth sprays) and keeping the lips moist are a matter of course in the care of such patients and does not need to be explained in more detail here.
We always prepare fresh tea for rinsing the mouth.

INSTRUCTIONS: Pour 200 ml boiling water over three to five chamomile flowers and one sage leaf and allow to steep for 30 seconds, add two to five drops of lemon juice and a half teaspoon of honey. Cover the tea mixture and allow to cool to 30°C (86°F). If the tea herbs are left to steep longer, the tea will acquire a bitter and astringent flavor. Lemon juice has a salivary effect and must be avoided in case of mucous membrane injuries. Rose honey sweetens and nurtures mucous membranes.

ENVIRONMENT: The external environment is also important and should not be underestimated. We can change the patient's room by hanging up pictures that mean something to him. It can become a nightmare to always have to look at the same disliked picture on a wall. Natural objects, such as flowers, beautiful stones or shells, can connect the patient to the outside world.

It goes without saying that order should prevail in the room, because outer order is transferred to inner order.

MUSIC: Music appeals to most people deep in their soul. Ill people experience a sense of security, of being welcomed in, when they hear the tones of a lyre (a small harp-like instrument).[23] The music makes them feel light and lifts them up. Some people will be able to let go, finally cry again, through music, through hearing sounds. This can be very liberating. When we take the time to play something on a lyre or flute for the seriously ill person, or when we encourage the relatives or even the dying person herself to play, we enable her to achieve balance and inner peace.

A music therapist, who works with comatose and ventilated patients in an intensive care unit, reported that music reaches people deep within and that people can be led to a slow awakening with the help of music. Some of the comatose patients confirmed to her afterwards that the sounds had played a decisive role in bringing them back into life.[23]

READING TO THE PATIENT: Another way of accompanying the dying is to read fairy tales, stories and poems to them. Fairy tales are generally read to children up to a certain age. Children seem to drink in fairy tales and live quite naturally with them. Elderly and dying people often find a new connection to fairy tales. The stories awaken memories and longings that may have rested locked up within them for a long time. They feel at home again in the fairy tale images, which often tell of transformations. What is the reason for this? If we look at the fairy tales of different cultures, we notice that all—no matter what culture they come from—have a similar basic motif. They tell of good and evil, pain and suffering, transformation and redemption. The fairy tales show, in pictures, what spiritual reality is. Thus, a language has been found which all people understand, when they listen with their hearts, as well as their ears. Elderly and dying people can find themselves in the images of fairy tales and connect with the spiritual world. Stories and poems which describe the way of the soul after death can also be fundamentally helpful.[24]

PASTORAL CARE: An important aspect in the care of the dying is pastoral care. One can often observe that patients need nothing more urgently than someone who cares for their soul. Nevertheless, when they are asked whether they would like to speak to a priest, they often reject the idea quite firmly. Such strict rejection can, however, diminish over the course of the disease. It is therefore important that we find the courage to ask repeatedly. It is precisely in the last days or hours of life that the need for a pastor or priest arises. Some people can cross the threshold more peacefully when they have spoken, prayed, or received the sacrament of the Anointing of the Sick from a priest. We should be vigilant for the moment when the dying person may call non-verbally or verbally for a pastor.

One challenge for nurses that comes up again and again is the accompaniment of their patients' relatives. This plays a particularly prominent role in the care of dying children. It is often helpful for relatives to be involved in nursing activities. It makes them feel like they can still do something. They can also be encouraged to read something aloud, to play an instrument or even to just be there and hold the hand of the dying person. They need our confirmation that even when they are seemingly just sitting there passively, they can still do a lot for the dying person through their thoughts and feelings.

Helplessness, uncertainty and fear of loss characterize the situation of relatives. This is also felt by the dying person, and it is often difficult for both the dying and their relatives to talk about it. In such cases, a nurse's mediating and open words can open the door, so that the people involved can move towards each other again through honest conversation. How often are the bereaved burdened by unsaid words! A truly open, truthful conversation between the dying person and his or her relatives can become the most intense experience of recent years for everyone, once again connecting them intimately with each other. The nurse is neither in the situation of the dying nor in that of the rather helplessly compassionate relative. He is in the midst of what the dying person is no longer: active and in a profession, strong, healthy. Only great consciousness can bridge this abyss: reverence for death in its larger dimension, respect for the personality and the lived life of the one who is about to cross the threshold.

Here we must look again at the inner training required by nurses, which so far occurs little, or mostly not at all, in nursing training. When we have a dying person in front of us, we have a person who, with greatly weakened physical powers, is at the same time required to make a very great effort of consciousness, and he must be able to find support in us. This happens first of all through insightful compassion for his situation. But feelings tend to become depleted when they are not fed by spiritual sources. Only through the nurse's work on herself can the strength grow to reach across the abyss that separates people.

6.   Death

Day after day the media confronts us with death, yet we push it far away from us. Only when we ourselves are directly confronted with death do we stand there stunned, and it is difficult for us to really look it in the face. We hand all post-mortem care over to the undertaker.

When a person dies in a hospital, he is usually "gotten rid of" quickly and inconspicuously. Pushed along the darkest cellar corridors, he finally ends up in a room that lacks any human dignity. Completely naked, wrapped only in a sheet, he is slid into a refrigerator compartment, where several other corpses above and below him have already been stored just as lovelessly. If relatives express the wish to see their deceased loved one just once more, this is only possible for a very short time in the ward. Otherwise, a visit to the mortuary can be a shock unless an empathetic person has created an appropriate atmosphere for that moment.

6.1 External features that indicate that death is about to occur

As the dying person's etheric body begins to detach, inner pressure on the tissues decreases, their body temperature drops, the sphincters of their eyes and lips begin to fail. The cold that slowly rises from the limbs to the torso gradually takes hold of the body. Typical death characteristics appear. The skin color changes and becomes a marbled bluish grey. The face looks as if it has been chiseled out, the nose appears more pointed, the eyes lie deep in their sockets and no longer close completely. The face is pale. A white triangle forms from the nose to the corners of the mouth. The skin is clammy, the lines of the hands disappear more and more.

6.2 The moment of death

At birth, a new baby is lovingly received, wrapped in a warm cloth and placed in his or her mother's arms. All hectic activity is avoided to make the adjustment to the new situation as beautiful as possible for mother and child.

The moment of death is usually marked by grief, by the pain of those who are left behind. It is perhaps a great loss of earthly closeness for the relatives, yet a threshold crossing for the deceased. Very often this is described as a tunnel, at the end of which a wonderful bright light receives the person. We can imagine this tunnel as a soul reality when we think of how we are connected to earthly existence through the channels of our senses. At the moment of death, we withdraw from our environment and go through a process of turning inside out—from the world of the senses into the world of our soul and its spiritual home. Those left behind do not see anything of this new life. But they can know about it, follow it in thought and celebrate the arrival of death in all its greatness and dignity. They can do so externally by placing flowers and candles as an image of that light, and inwardly by saying a prayer, a poem or engaging in religious worship. We can empathetically give form to the moment of death by acknowledging that we are now letting go of the person instead of receiving him, as is done at a birth, and by lovingly accompanying this fact. Proper letting go is something that is usually very difficult for us in life, whether we are saying goodbye to loved ones, are having to give up a familiar environment, or must give up a habit that we have grown fond of. Already in everyday life we can practice letting go, which always has something to do with overcoming pain. We know from experience that this overcoming ultimately gives us the great strength to openly encounter something new and to develop ourselves further.

7. Care of the deceased in anthroposophic institutions

To enable the soul of the deceased to be undisturbed as he or she detaches from the body, we do not begin any actual external care until about half an hour to one hour after death. If necessary, we wash the deceased and, if possible, dress him in his own clothes, otherwise we dress him in hospital clothes. We dress any wounds with bandages and put in the person's dentures, if possible. After putting fresh sheets on the bed, we comb his hair. We cover the body with a sheet up to under the arms. We close his eyes with warm, moist compresses that should remain on the eyes for only a few minutes! A chin rest made of plastic or a roll of fabric supports the chin, which is not tied up with a bandage, as it used to be, because that disfigures the person very much. We cover the neck of the deceased with a cloth or a scarf so that the chin rest is not visible. The hands now lie on top of each other on the bed sheet. The deceased should be exposed to as little movement as possible while we do all this. Everything superfluous is removed from the room. A candle burns, taking care that no shadow falls on the face.

We do all this together with the relatives, if possible. Often, they report later how important it had been to them to be able to take care of these last acts together, also as a way of dealing with their grief.

It is customary for the deceased to remain in his room for a few hours. This gives relatives, friends, ward staff, nurses, doctors and therapists the opportunity to say goodbye, individually or collectively. They may say a prayer, read a text from the Bible, recite a verse or a poem, and/or sing a song. Singing can loosen up the atmosphere and release people from feeling oppressed. Fellow patients can also be included in this farewell. For them it can be a great help to experience that the previously suffering person appears relaxed and liberated after death. Even when they are initially insecure, they are usually grateful to have been included in this farewell. It creates space for questions that they had not yet thought of or had not yet dared to speak of.

7.1 The laying out of the deceased

When I was a young nurse working in a university hospital, the following experience left a deep impression on me: one day three people died in our ward, whom I had nursed for a long time. I was deeply shocked when the pathology nurse came with a zinc tub and threw in all three people naked on top of each other, as if they had never been human beings. Nowhere was there a room where someone could have visited the deceased again. My displeasure and my massive complaint about it to the appropriate people was only met with pitiful smiles.

All anthroposophic clinics and homes for the elderly have one or more rooms in which the deceased can be laid out with dignity. These rooms are designed with fitting architecture and colors.

After everyone on the ward has said goodbye, the nurses take the deceased, accompanied by relatives if possible, to the laying-out room, where he is laid out on the catafalque, which is covered with a sheet. To the left and right of the catafalque there are candles, which are lit and, as long as the deceased is lying there, burn constantly. The relatives have the possibility of leaving the deceased in this room for three days. They can hold the vigil there and arrange the room in their own way.

7.2 Changes after death

When one observes the deceased during the first three days after death, one can notice amazing changes: quite apart from the fact that wrinkles smooth out, the expression on the face also changes. It often appears to be divided into two, into a serious half and a smiling half.

Something of the life of the deceased is still perceptible in the atmosphere around him. It may be that people feel his loneliness, his having been "torn out of life" or how fulfilled his life was very clearly, without having known him before. If one visits the deceased more often in the room where he is laid out, one can perceive a changing mood there. After two and a half to three and a half days, though, it is over: one notices that only a shell remains lying here, like a cocoon abandoned by a butterfly.

If the deceased is collected by an undertaker, the body is placed in the coffin in the presence of a nurse. She ensures that this takes place with dignity and she accompanies the deceased out of the building.

7.3 The laying-out group

In Herdecke community hospital there is a circle of people who have made it their task to care for the deceased. They visit the deceased at least once a day. They pay attention to changes in the deceased in order to be able to intervene if necessary, e.g., if the process of decay is rapid. Furthermore, this group makes sure that candles and possibly incense are burning constantly. They read a poem, a prayer, a passage from the Gospel of John or other texts, as appropriate. After autopsies, the deceased are washed, dressed and laid out again. A further important task is to assist, with words and deeds, members of staff who have questions about dying and death. The laying-out group consists of volunteers from the nursing staff who have taken over this task free of charge and can be reached at any time by wireless communication. The group also includes a Protestant minister, a Catholic priest and a priest of the Christian Community. The group meets regularly every two weeks to discuss topics and organizational matters. The work of this group has proven to be very meaningful, because time and again there are staff members who are overwhelmed by dealing with death situations, who feel helpless. The work also creates contacts and conversations with relatives.

It is very much to be hoped that more and more hospitals will consider creating a dignified space and framework for the deceased. This will help the bereaved to cope better with their grief. Ultimately, though, it is done for the deceased, who is being born into the spiritual world at the time of death.

Category	Example learning objectives	Recommended learning path
Skills	You provide the dying with relief through body care.	A
Your own learning objective		
Relationships	You answer the dying person's questions regarding the dying process appropriately and honestly or you enlist the help of therapists, colleagues or priests.	B
Your own learning objective		
Knowledge	You are familiar with the path of the dying as it is described by anthroposophic spiritual science.	C
Your own learning objective		

References

1   Ohler, N. *Sterben und Tod im Mittelalter.* Patmos-Verlag, Ostfildern 2003.

2   Canacakis, J. *Ich sehe deine Tränen.* Kreuz-Verlag, Stuttgart 2002.

3   Translated from the mission statement of the short-term care facility Turmalin in Witten, Germany.

4   Steiner, R. *Theosophy. An introduction to the supersensible knowledge of the world and the destination of man.* Rudolf Steiner Press, London 2005.

5   Maurice, M. *Anthroposophy—Was ist das?* Novalis Verlag, Schaffhausen 1987.

6   Ritchie, G.G. *Return from tomorrow.* Reprint Baker Publishing Group, Ada 1995.

7   von Jankovich, S. *Ich war klinisch tot.* Drei Eichen Verlag, Ergolding 2011.

8   Moody, R.A. *Life after life.* 25th anniversary ed. Rider, London 2001.

9   Ritchie, G.G. *Return from tomorrow.* Reprint Baker Publishing Group, Ada 1995.

10   Kübler-Ross, E. *Über den Tod und das Leben danach.* Verlag Silberschnur, Neuwied 1989.

11   Maurice, M. *Anthroposophy—Was ist das?* Novalis Verlag, Schaffhausen 1987.

12   Senft, H. Erfahrungen eines Krebspatienten. Unpublished lecture of November 16, 1989.

13   Kübler-Ross, E. *On death and dying. What the dying have to teach doctors, nurses, clergy and their own families.* Reissue ed. Scribner, New York 2014.

14   Lama, A.G. Die Bedeutung des Tibetanischen Totenbuches für den modernen Menschen. *Deutsche Krankenpflegezeitschrift* 1985; 38 (3).

15   Wambach, H. *Life before life.* Bantam Books, New York 1981.

16   Wiesenhütter, E. *Blick nach drüben.* Gütersloher Verlagshaus, Gütersloh 1991.

17   Klaschik, E. *Medikamentöse Schmerztherapie bei Tumorpatienten.* Mundipharma, Limburg 2008.

18   Simon, L. *Schmerztherapie mit homöopathisch potenzierten Heilpflanzen.* Haug Verlag, Heidelberg 1998.

19   Steiner, R. *How to know higher worlds—a modern path of initiation.* Anthroposophic Press, Great Barrington 2002.

20   Bulwer-Lytton, E. *Zanoni. A Rosicrucian tale.* 2nd ed. SteinerBooks, Hudson 1989.

21   Wilde, O. *The picture of Dorian Gray.* Reprint Dover Publications, Mineola 1993.

22   Juchli, L. *Pflegen, Begleiten, Leben.* Recom Verlag, Basel 1985.

23   Gustorff, D. Die Kunst der Musik in der Therapie. Unpublished lecture of September 28, 1991, held at the conference "Kunst im Krankenhaus" in Münster, Germany.

24   Lagerlöf, S. *Thy soul shall bear witness.* 1921.

Epilogue

The Future of Professional Nursing

"Anthroposophic Medicine is young and just at the beginning of its development. To a large extent it is still engaged in laying its own groundwork... within it lies a comprehensive and profound possibility for humanizing medicine through a differentiated spiritual understanding of the human being. To collaborate on this is the greatest need. Until this has happened to an ever greater extent, there remains a feeling of gratitude and indebtedness towards the results and methods of modern medicine, which has researched so much and has developed aspects that are indispensable for the future."[1]

The author of these lines was Thomas McKeen (1953–1993), an outstanding anthroposophic physician and founder of the Anthroposophic Medical Seminar at the Filderklinik hospital. This book on nursing care is dedicated to him. His words speak of modesty towards the achievements of Anthroposophic Medicine, confidence and trust in its possibilities for development, as well as respect and admiration for the achievements of medical science.

The relationship of anthroposophic nursing care to nursing care in general, to medicine in general and to Anthroposophic Medicine is shaped by a similar attitude. The very small number of anthroposophic nurses worldwide and the marginal degree of academic competence available call for the utmost modesty towards the "big" world of nursing care and medicine.* That is why we look with amazement and admiration at the cures made possible by modern medicine and at our colleagues who give their best for their patients every day all over the world. We are grateful for the opportunity to participate in this medicine and to be part of the nursing profession.

But we nurses are driven by a longing and a certainty: to bring about a real cure, every treatment should appeal more and more to the patient's own will to develop and change. Medications and surgical procedures provide physical relief, silence symp-

---

* Initiatives for anthroposophic nursing care now exist in more than twenty countries, on all continents. Several advanced training courses for professional nurses have been established, especially in connection with the worldwide spread of International Postgraduate Medical Training (IPMT) for physicians. Today, around 2500 professional nurses work in the environment of anthroposophic institutions worldwide. About 1000 nurses are self-employed or employed at medical institutions that do not have an anthroposophic orientation. About 20 percent have completed at least 200 hours of training in anthroposophic nursing. The overwhelming majority of anthroposophic nurses live in Germany. About 2000 nurses have gained qualification there over the last 40 years by completing a three-year, state-recognized anthroposophic training.

toms, and relieve pain. In contrast, the life forces in the depths of the human body that respond to therapeutic interventions, that allow surgically stabilized bones to grow together again, or that cause blood formation after cytostasis, do not require treatment, they require the patient's will to live and develop, and they require nursing care. The art of healing of the future will be successful when patients acquire an inner understanding of how diseases work in them and how only their cooperation and powers of transformation make healing possible. Neither today's medicine nor nursing care take this sufficiently into account. More and more patients are therefore rightly looking for a "hearing" form of medicine—a form of medicine that senses what people require from their desires, needs, worries, and suffering and then lets them retain responsibility for it (or gives back the responsibility and expects the person to take it on). Only with patient responsibility will a medication or treatment heal—"make whole"—in the true sense of the word.

It is the project of Anthroposophic Medicine to uncover the mysterious relationship between the self-responsible human 'I' and the person's life forces, so as to enable these life forces to have a healing effect. Anthroposophic Medicine can only do this if it learns from and with its patients.

What is the task of nursing care in the healing art of the future? More and more, nursing care must transform the living environments of those in need of care (at home, in homes for the elderly, in hospitals) into real healing places. Ideally, nursing care will enable long-term treatment and illness as a path of development, give the person in need of care resonance for his process of change, and create a light-filled, joyful, sometimes concentrated and quiet atmosphere. It will rejoice in recovery and be a source of hope. It is the task of anthroposophic nursing care to delve ever deeper into everyday human life and to explore the mysterious relationship between the external environment and the habits and moods of the person in need of care, and to help influence these. Perhaps that is why (according to oral tradition) Rudolf Steiner recommended that hospitals be run by nurses.

Such a project requires new forms of cooperation between doctors and nurses, which are outlined below. Forms need to be developed in which the resources and questions of the patient or the person in need of care form part of the therapy in a comprehensive sense.

Aspects of collaboration between doctors and nurses[2]

Physicians and nurses do different things for patients, so in each of these two professions some skills are more developed than others. This begins with the more academic education of physicians compared with the more hands-on nursing training. Not least it is individual destiny that predisposes people towards their chosen profession, and each profession therefore has its own constitution. Taking these constitutional differences into account we shall examine various aspects of the way physicians and nurses work together.

Everyone is a caregiver. Things in need of care can be found in all life contexts. The kingdoms of nature "under" us, our social relationships with one another, and our links with the spiritual world require constant attention if they are to remain within the sphere of human culture.[3] If we did not take care of them they would lose the special stamp that we give them and revert to a state of nature.

Elements of caregiving can also be found in the work of physicians. A doctor who, as a general practitioner, cares for a patient for many years, performs a (social) care-giving service that may be more significant than the sum of all acute interventions.

In contrast to the limited duration of a medical intervention, nursing takes place almost unnoticed in a rhythmic timelessness. This unpretentious nature of nursing care resembles the inconspicuous course of healthy physical, psychological, social, and spiritual life. Only when a malfunction occurs in the accustomed rhythmical flow do pain or incapacity make us aware of our life processes. This irruption of awareness brings with it the quest for treatment and, if the incapacity has become severe enough, care of ourselves is replaced with care given by others.

Every therapeutic intervention changes the consciousness of the person being treated.[4] Nursing care, on the other hand, has the task of maintaining "the normal interaction between the individual and the environment."[5] This "normality" has to be determined for the respective condition of the patient and the nursing actions have to be adapted accordingly. For example, the normal way to wash a baby differs from washing a feverish or paralyzed person.

Nursing shapes the patient's day. By sharing and shaping the patient's daily routine the nurse uses powers of consciousness that differ from those of the physician called in a crisis. Symptoms of illness wake up both the patient and the one who is called in to examine and diagnose the disturbance. Everyday routine, on the other hand, tempts us to succumb to the sleepiness of habit. Nursing work trains us to adapt to the life processes and rhythms of the patient. An archetypal image of this is a breastfeeding mother. Her whole body is bound up with her baby. Though nurses do not nourish sick people with their bodies, they do "lend them their hands, their ears, their heart," forming a kind of functional unit with them.

Devotion and compassion are important components of nursing activity. The tendency to lose alertness, brought about by devotion and adaptation to the rhythmic flow of habitual life, can be called a constitutional weakness of the nursing profession.

The doctor, on the other hand, who is active in dealing with the disease, is constantly exposed to impressions that bring about alertness and enhanced awareness. The reasons for his actions do not primarily result from empathy, involvement, and resonance with the patient, but from recognizing the causes of the disease expressed in the symptoms. Symptoms show what has become. History-taking relates to the past, and the diagnosis ascertains what has happened up to the present moment. Recognizing the illness (in the spiritual-scientific sense) brings realization of what will heal it. This culminates in a prescription. The will impulse concentrated in finding the remedy flows over into the work of pharmacists, therapists, and nurses. Physicians rarely carry out the treatment themselves. Constitutionally, it is thinking and ideas that dominate in the physician's awareness.

Two different approaches resulting from the different professional constitutions thus exist in the therapeutic community of nurses and doctors:

Doctor	Nurse
Emphasis on knowledge and will	Emphasis on feeling and will
Observing what has become	Experiencing what is evolving
Past-oriented	Committed to the present
Giving impulses for the future	Providing space for the future
Awakening–emerging	Dreaming–delving in
Light	Warmth

Another difference between physicians and nurses arises from the karmic relationship between the patient and the physician on the one hand and the patient and the nurse on the other. The patient seeks out a specific physician and wants individual treatment. The healing conveyed by the physician makes it possible for changes in destiny to come about and opens the way for the development of new faculties.

Past karma is resolved through treatment and a path to the future opens up. The purpose of some illnesses is not so much to overcome karmic consequences as to acquire future capacities (as, for example, with chronic diseases). In these cases, the physician takes on a role resembling that of a nurse, a role that accompanies the patient with compassion.*

Patients do not seek out a specific individual for a nurse. Trust in the nurse is based more on moral status than on specific expertise. Confidence arises in response to the nurse's moral attitude rather than any particular specialized knowledge. The patient wants to be recognized as a human being by the nurse, and in this sense, nursing supersedes the individual. It is concerned with the universally human aspect, with the human being in the human being.[6]

A brotherly or sisterly relationship quality (in the universal sense, not in the sense of family) is developing through nursing care, one which will only fully determine relationships between people in the future.

---

* Chronic diseases require the patient to actively participate in the healing process. The patient must adjust his life to pain, disability, social exclusion. He "practices" patience, the capacity to endure suffering, perseverance, steadfastness between hope and despair, learns to "live" "his" life despite his complaints and disabilities. In this way, the patient cultivates forces for the future. In contrast, acute diseases mobilize completely unconscious self-healing powers, e.g., in wound healing, fever, vomiting, diarrhea or when receiving external help, such as artificial respiration, the removal of damaged organs, osteosynthesis. The latter requires precise expert action from the physician. In case of chronic illness, one would not want to do without expert action, but empathy is needed above all.

The constitutional one-sidedness of each of these professions has its beneficial counterpart in the other. Working together, specialized and yet complementing one another, they do something that must find a synthesis in every individual. The nurse must lift into the light of consciousness the treasures won from compassion, must wring alertness from the daily routine in order to achieve full possession of his or her nursing skills or reach an inner source of strength. The physician, by diving into the daily routine of the patient and the therapeutic community, will win a wider horizon of knowledge and action, especially where it is a matter of comprehending the illness imaginatively. Collaboration develops from the readiness to awaken through the other for one's own task—and this is no mere addition of abilities, it is an independent, new space of consciousness, which encourages and fires individual achievements in undreamt-of ways.

Collaboration such as this enables nurses to carry the guiding principle of the therapy right into everyday tasks. For the physician, the therapeutic community becomes a vessel in which his healing impulse continues to have an effect. In everyday life, as the space of time and consciousness in which doctors, therapists, nurses and patients meet, it will ultimately become clear whether we as a therapeutic community are in a position to create a healing atmosphere.

Where there is danger, there is also something growing that can save us*

The art of healing as we know it in the prosperous countries of the world is chronically threatened from two sides. On the one hand, it is not self-evident that our societies will maintain the will to ensure access to medical and nursing care for everyone who needs it in the future. Will the next generations honor our aging societies with adequate medical and social care, or will major distribution battles flare up over precious access to health and education?

On the other hand, commercialization and bureaucratization are paralyzing the "will to heal" of those currently active in the healthcare system. The treatment of chronic diseases, which so often follows acute intervention, costs time and patience—as the word 'chronic' indicates. Another old word—"patient"—which describes both the patience and the suffering, has been replaced by the terms "customer" or "client." The paradigm of establishing health by repairing an imperfect body still determines the functional spaces of our clinics and pharmaceutical laboratories. We say "still determines"—because one day the laboratory table must become an altar[7] and the healing of a disease must become a musical resolution (Novalis).[†] Then recovering people will be hopeful people, healthy people will be those endowed with the gift of health,

---

[*]   Friedrich Hölderlin (1770–1843)

[†]   In the words of Novalis: "Every illness is a musical problem; healing comes through musical resolution. The shorter and yet more complete the resolution, the greater the musical talent of the doctor. (Diseases can be resolved in many ways. The choice of the most expedient determines the talent of the doctor)." Translated from: Kamnitzer E. *Novalis. Fragmente*. Jess Verlag, Dresden 1929. Chapter 11.

and health itself will be a miracle. Then even clinics will become so beautiful that they will be admired and cared for centuries later, just like Gothic cathedrals today.

ROLF HEINE
NETWORK FOR ANTHROPOSOPHIC NURSING CARE IN GERMANY
(NETZWERK ANTHROPOSOPHISCHE PFLEGE IN DEUTSCHLAND) /
ACADEMY FOR NURSING PROFESSIONS AT THE FILDERKLINIK
(AKADEMIE FÜR PFLEGEBERUFE AN DER FILDERKLINIK)
JUNE 2017

References

1   McKeen, T. *Anthroposophische Medizin. Einführende Vorträge und Aufsätze.* Salumed Verlag, Berlin 2016, p. 50 and 52.

2   This section first appeared in the Circular Letter of the Medical Section at the Goetheanum, St. John's Tide 1994 (no. 6) under the title: "Physicians and nurses—two occupations with different constitutions. Aspects of professional collaboration."

3   Compare chap. "Nursing as a Path of Development."

4   Cf. Steiner, R. Lecture of September 8, 1924, in *Broken vessels. The spiritual structure of human frailty.* Anthroposophic Press, Great Barrington 2003.

5   Cf. note 4.

6   Cf. the six works of mercy in the Gospel of Matthew: "Inasmuch as you have done it unto one of the least of these my brethren, you have done it unto me." (Matthew 25:40).

7   Steiner, R. Lecture of February 27, 1910, in *The reappearance of Christ in the etheric. Selected lectures.* Revised ed. Rudolf Steiner Press, London 2003.

List of products mentioned with US and European equivalents

USA	Germany (DE) / Switzerland (CH)
Aconite Nerve Oil (Wala) Acontium D3 Oleum (Weleda US) Lavender Quartz Oil (Uriel)	Aconit Schmerzöl (DE) Aconitum/Camphora comp., Oleum (CH)
Aconitum e tubere W 5%, Oleum (WALA) Aconitum 5% oil (Uriel, can make on demand)	Aconitum e tubere W 5%, Oleum (DE)
Aesculus/Prunus comp., essence (WALA) Aesculus Quercus essense (Uriel)	Aesculus/Prunus comp., Essenz (DE)
Amara drops (Weleda US) Chicory Ginger Bitters (similar, Uriel)	Amara Tropfen (DE, CH)
Arnica comp./Formica Oleum (Weleda) Weleda US: Arnica comp. Formica ointment	Arnica comp. / Formica Ölige Einreibung (DE) Arnica comp. / Formica Oleum (CH)
Arnica e floribus W 5%, Oleum (WALA) Arnica 5% Oleum (Uriel, same) Weleda US: Arnica Oleum D1 oil dispersion	Arnica e floribus W 5%, Oleum (DE) Arnica e floribus W 5%, Oleum pro balneo (CH)
Arnica essence (WALA, Weleda US, Uriel))	Arnika Essenz (DE, CH)
Arnica, Flos H 10% (Weleda) see above	Arnica, Flos H 10% (DE)
Aurum Lavender Rose ointment (Weleda US) Aurum Lavender Rose Cream (Uriel)	Aurum / Lavandula comp. Creme (DE) Aurum / Lavandulae aetheroleum / Rosa Unguentum (CH)
Baby Tummy Oil (Weleda US)	Baby-Bäuchleinöl (Weleda) (DE)
Blackthorn Toning Body Oil (Hauschka) Malva Tiliae Body Oil (Uriel)	Schlehenblüten Pflegeöl (DE) Schlehenblüten Pflegeöl (Hauschka-CH)
Borage 5% ointment (Weleda US) Borago/Lavandula Lotion (similar, Uriel)	Borago 5% Salbe (DE)
Borage essence (WALA)	Borago-Essenz (DE) Borago ex herba, Tinctura (CH)
Brandessenz (burn lotion WALA) Combudoron Liquid (external) (Weleda US) Arnica Nettle Gel and Spray (similar, Uriel)	Brandessenz (DE)
Calcea wound cream (WALA) Wound Care (Weleda US)	Calcea Wund- und Heilcreme (DE)
Calendula Baby Cream (Weleda)	Calendula Babycreme (DE) Calendula Pflegecreme (CH)
Calendula D4 eye drops (Weleda) Calendula 3X (Uriel)	Calendula D4 Augentropfen (DE, CH)
Calendula essence (WALA, Weleda US)	Calendula Essenz (DE) Calendula officinalis, Tinctura (CH)
Calendula essence (Weleda US)	Calendula Essenz (DE, CH)
Calendula ex herba D3 amp. (WALA)	Calendula ex herba D3 Amp. (DE)
Calendula Wind & Weather Balm (Weleda US)	Calendula Wind- und Wetterbalsam (DE, CH)

USA	Germany (DE) / Switzerland (CH)
Chamomilla e floribus W 10%, Oleum (WALA, Weleda US) Chamomilla 10% (Uriel)	Chamomilla e floribus W 10%, Oleum (DE) Chamomilla e floribus W 10%, Oleum pro balneo (CH)
Citrus Refreshing Bath Milk (Weleda US)	Citrus Erfrischungsbad (DE, CH)
Citrus Refreshing Body Oil (Weleda US) Citrus 10% Oil (Uriel)	Citrus Erfrischungsöl (DE, CH)
Citrus, Oleum aethereum 10% (Weleda US) Citrus 10% Oil (Uriel)	Citrus, Oleum aethereum 10% (DE) Citri aetheroleum 10%, Oleum pro balneo (CH)
Combudoron external gel (Weleda US) Burn Care liquid (Weleda US) Arnica Nettle Gel and Spray (Uriel)	Combudoron Gel (DE, CH)
Comforting Baby Oil (Calendula) (Weleda US)	Calendula Pflegeöl (DE, CH)
Comforting Body Lotion (Weleda US)	Calendula Pflegemilch (DE, CH)
Comforting Cream Bath (Weleda)	Calendula Bad (DE)
Cuprum metallicum praeparatum 0.1% ointment D3 (Weleda US)	Cuprum metallicum praeparatum 0.1% Salbe (DE)
Cuprum metallicum praeparatum 0.4% ointment (Weleda US)	Cuprum metallicum praeparatum 0.4% Salbe (DE) Cuprum metallicum praeparatum 0.4% Unguentum (CH)
Rose Copper (0.4% cuprum oxyd.) (Uriel)	
Equisetum cum Sulfure tostum D3 trit. (Weleda US) Equisetum with Sulfure Tostum 6X (Uriel)	Equisetum cum Sulfure tostum D3 Trit. (DE) Equisetum cum Sulfure tostum D3 Trituration (Formula magistralis, verschreibungspflichtig) (CH)
Equisetum cum Sulfure tostum D6 amp. i.v. (Weleda US)	Equisetum cum Sulfure tostum D6 Amp. i.v.
Equisetum cum Sulfure tostum D6 trit. (Weleda US)	Equisetum cum Sulfure tostum D6 (DE) Equisetum cum Sulfure tostum D6 Trituration (CH)
Equisetum ex herba W 5%, Oleum (WALA) Equisetum D1 Oleum Equisetum 5% oil (Uriel)	Equisetum ex herba W 5%, Oleum (DE) Equisetum ex herba W 5%, Oleum pro balneo (CH)
Eucalyptus, Oleum aethereum 10% (WALA) Eucalyptus 10% oil (Uriel)	Eucalyptus, Oleum aethereum 10% (DE) Eucalypti aetheroleum 10%, Oleum pro balneo (CH)
Farmer's cheese	Quark (DE, CH)
Gentiana comp. pillules (WALA) Gentiana/Absinthium pellets (Uriel)	Gentiana Magen Globuli velati (DE)
Gold rose-blossom lavender oil (Dr. Heberer) Aurum Lavender Rose Cream and Oil (Uriel)	Gold-Rosenblüten-Lavendel-Öl (DE)
Hypericum ex herba 5%, Oleum (WALA) Hypericum 5% oil (Uriel, Weleda US)	Hypericum ex herba 5%, Oleum (DE) Hypericum perforatum ex herba 5%, Oleum (CH)
Hypericum, Flos 25% oil (Weleda US) Camphor Hypericum oil 15% (Uriel)	Hypericum, Flos 25% Öl (DE) Hypericum, Flos 25% Oleum (CH)

USA	Germany (DE) / Switzerland (CH)
Larix/Olibanum beeswax compress (Klinik Arlesheim Pharmacy)	Larix/Olibanum Bienenwachsauflage (Klinik Arlesheim Pharmacy) (DE, CH)
Lavandula, Oleum aethereum 10% (WALA) Lavender 10% body oil (Uriel)	Lavandula, Oleum aethereum 10% (DE, CH)
Lavender 0.1% oil (pharmacy formula)	Lavendelöl 0.1% (Apothekenrezeptur) (DE)
Lavender 10% oil (Weleda US)	Lavendelöl 10% (DE) Oleum aethereum Lavandulae 10% Oleum (CH)
Lavender Relaxing Bath Milk (Weleda) Lavender Bath (Uriel)	Lavendel Entspannungsbad (DE, CH)
Lemon Lemongrass Vitalising Bath Essence (Hauschka) Lemon Bath (Uriel)	Zitronen Lemongrass Bad (DE, CH)
Lemon Lemongrass Vitalising Bath Oil (WALA) Lemon Bath (Uriel)	Zitronen Lemongrass Pflegeöl (DE, CH)
Luvos Medicinal Clay 2	Luvos Heilerde 2 (DE, CH)
Mallow oil (WALA)	Malvenöl (DE) Malva comp., Oleum (CH)
Melissa ex herba W 5%, Oleum (WALA)	Melissa ex herba W 5%, Oleum (DE)
Melissa oil (WALA) Melissa D1 oleum (Weleda US) Melissa Oil (Uriel) Marjoram Melissa Oil (Uriel)	Melissenöl (DE) Melissa comp., Oleum (CH)
Mercurialis ointment (WALA) Mercurialis D1 ointment (Weleda US) Mercurialis Calendula ointment (Uriel)	Mercurialis Salbe (DE) Allium cepa/Mercurialis comp., Unguentum (CH)
Mercurialis perennis 10% (Weleda)	Mercurialis perennis 10% (DE) Mercurialis perennis 10% Unguentum (CH)
Moor Lavender Calming Bath Essence (Dr. Hauschka)	Moor Lavendel Bad (DE, CH)
Moor lavender oil (WALA) Solum Aesculus oil and cream (Uriel)	Moor Lavendel Pflegeöl (DE, CH)
Mouth Balm, liquid (WALA) Echinacea Quartz - liquid and gel (Uriel)	Mundbalsam flüssig (DE) Antimonit/Rosae aetheroleum comp., Solutio (CH)
Nursing Tea (Weleda US)	Milchbildungstee (DE)
Oleum aethereum Carvi 10% (extemporaneous pharmacy preparation)	Oleum aethereum Carvi 10% (Apothekenrezeptur) (DE)
Oleum aethereum Lavandulae 10% oil (Weleda US)	Lavendelöl 10% (DE) Oleum aethereum Lavandulae 10%(CH)
Oleum aethereum Melissae indicum 10% (Weleda)	Oleum aethereum Melissae indicum 10% (DE)
Oleum aethereum Salviae 10% (extemporaneous pharmacy preparation)	Oleum aethereum Salviae 10% (Apothekenrezeptur) (DE)
Oleum Menthae piperitae 10% (extemporaneous pharmacy preparation)	Oleum Menthae piperitae 10% (Apothekenrezeptur) (DE)

USA	Germany (DE) / Switzerland (CH)
Oxalis e planta tota W 10%, Oleum (WALA), Oxalis D1 ointment (Weleda US) Oxalis Oil 10% (Uriel) Oxalis Gel 10%, 20%, 30% (Uriel)	Oxalis e planta tota W 10%, Oleum (DE) Oxalis e planta tota W 10%, Oleum pro balneo (CH)
Oxalis essence (WALA)	Oxalis-Essenz (DE)
Oxalis, Folium 10% ointment (Weleda US)	Oxalis, Folium 10% Salbe (DE) Folium 10% Unguentum (CH)
Oxalis, Folium 20% tincture (Weleda US)	Oxalis, Folium 20% Tinktur (DE) Oxalis, Folium 20% Externum (CH)
Phytolacca D30 (DHU)	Phytolacca D30 (DHU) (DE)
Pine Reviving Bath Milk (Weleda US) Spruce Bath (Uriel)	Edeltannen Erholungsbad (DE, CH)
Plantago Bronchialbalsam (WALA) Plaintain Beeswax Ointment (Uriel)	Plantago Bronchialbalsam (DE, CH)
Plumbum metallicum praeparatum 0.4% ointment (Weleda US), also D3 ointment (Weleda US)	Plumbum metallicum praeparatum 0.4% Salbe (DE) Plumbum metallicum 0.4% Unguentum (magistral formula, only available by prescription) (CH)
Primula (primrose) muscle oil (WALA)	Primula Muskelnähröl (DE) Primula comp., Oleum (CH)
Propolis mother tincture (Hanosan)	Propolis Urtinktur (DE)
Prunus spinosa e floribus W 5%, Oleum (WALA) D1 Oleum (Weleda US) Prunus 5% Oil (Uriel)	Prunus spinosa e floribus W 5%, Oleum (DE) Prunus spinosa e floribus W 5%, Oleum pro balneo (CH)
Ratanhia comp. Mouthwash (Weleda US)	Ratanhia comp. (DE) Ratanhia comp. Flüssigkeit zur Anwendung in der Mundhöhle (CH)
Red Copper Ointment (WALA) Rose Copper ointment (Uriel)	Kupfer Salbe rot (DE) Cuprum oxydulatum rubrum 0.4%, Unguentum (CH)
Revitalising Leg & Arm Tonic (Hauschka) Venadoron Leg Toner (Weleda US)	Rosmarin Beinlotion (DE, CH)
Rosa e floribus 10%, Oleum (WALA) Rose Oil 10% (Uriel)	Rosa e floribus 10%, Oleum (DE) Rosa e floribus comp., Oleum pro balneo (CH)
Rose Day Cream (Hauschka, WALA, Weleda US)	Rosen Tagescreme (DE, CH)
Rosemary 10% ointment (Weleda US) D1 Oleum (Weleda US)	Rosmarin-Salbe 10% (DE) Oleum aethereum Rosmarini 10% Unguentum (CH)
Rosemary Invigorating Bath Milk (Weleda) Rosemary Bath (Uriel)	Rosmarin Aktivierungsbad (DE, CH)
Rosmarinus 10% ointment (Weleda US)	Rosmarinus 10% Salbe (DE) Oleum aethereum Rosmarini 10%, Ung. (CH)
Rosmarinus, Oleum aethereum 10% (WALA) Rosemary Oil 10% (Uriel)	Rosmarinus, Oleum aethereum 10% (DE)
Silicea D10 trit. D6, D12 (Weleda US) : Quartz 12X pellets (Uriel)	Quarz D10 Trit. (DE, CH)

USA	Germany (DE) / Switzerland (CH)
Solum oil (WALA) Solum Aesculus Oil (Uriel)	Solum Öl (DE) Solum uliginosum comp., Oleum (CH)
Spruce Needle Bath Oil (Wind und Wetter Bad) (Hauschka) Spruce Bath (Uriel)	Wind und Wetter Bad (DE, CH)
Stannum metal foil patch (Weleda US)	Stannum Metallspiegelfolie (DE, CH)
Stannum metallicum 0.4% (Weleda US)	Stannum metallicum 0.4% (DE) Stannum metallicum 0.4% Unguentum (CH)
Stibium metallicum praeparatum D6 10 ml amp. (Weleda US) Stibium D6 ampule (Uriel)	Stibium metallicum praeparatum D6 10 ml Amp. (DE, CH)
Stibium metallicum praeparatum D6 trit. (Weleda US) Stibium D6 trit. pellets and liquid (Uriel)	Stibium metallicum praeparatum D6 Trit. (DE, CH)
Thymus, Oleum aethereum 5% (WALA, Weleda US)	Thymus, Oleum aethereum 5% (DE) Thymi aetheroleum 5%, Oleum pro balneo (CH)
Venadoron (Skin Tone Lotion) (Weleda US)	Venadoron Gel (DE, CH)
Wund- und Brandgel (wound and burn gel) (WALA) Burn Care (Weleda US) Arnica Nettle Gel (Uriel)	Wund- und Brandgel (DE) Argentum/Urtica comp., Gelatum (CH)
Yarrow 5% in olive oil (Dr. Heberer)	Schafgarbe 5% in Olivenöl

About the Authors

Rolf Heine

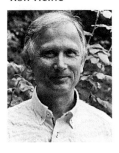

Rolf Heine (born 1960) is a certified nurse and anthroposophic nursing specialist (IFAN). He completed his training at the Filderklinik Independent Nursing School in Filderstadt, near Stuttgart, Germany. From 1986 to 2016 Rolf Heine worked as a nurse at Filderklinik hospital, initially on the ward for internal medicine. This was followed by a teaching position at the Filderklinik Independent Nursing School and work heading a nursing research project on external applications of mustard and ginger. As a member of the nursing management at Filderklinik hospital Rolf Heine was responsible for the gynecology/obstetrics, internal medicine, and oncology wards. He has many years of experience in the areas of quality assurance and nursing development. In 2012 he founded the Academy for Nursing Professions at the Filderklinik hospital and served as director. Today he maintains the Network for Anthroposophic Nursing Care in Germany.

He was a member of the board of the Association for Anthroposophic Nursing for 18 years. He is a member of the German Nursing Council (DPR) and a member of the board of the umbrella organization for Anthroposophic Medicine in Germany (DAMiD). He is also active as the coordinator of the International Forum for Anthroposophic Nursing (IFAN) in the Medical Section of the School for Spiritual Science at the Goetheanum and is a member of the International Coordination of Anthroposophic Medicine (IKAM). He is president of the International Council of Anthroposophic Nursing Associations (ICANA).

He has published numerous contributions on the topic of anthroposophic nursing in books and professional journals. He lectures and teaches seminars in Germany and abroad.

Klaus Adams

- Born in 1961
- Has been a nurse on an open psychiatric ward in the Friedrich-Husemann-Klinik in Buchenbach, near Freiburg/Breisgau, Germany since 1990
- Community service in the field of geriatric care and work with people with disabilities
- 1984–1987 Nursing training at Herdecke Community Hospital (GKH)
- 3 years of experience in the neurology ward at GKH
- 1995–1997 Further training in psychiatric nursing in Freiburg im Breisgau/Emmendingen, Germany
- Anthroposophic nursing specialist (IFAN) since 2009
- Auditor for the International Coordination of Anthroposophic Medicine (IKAM) since 2012

- Many years of teaching experience in training nurses
- Lecturer on soul exercises and other anthroposophic-psychiatric topics

Frances Bay

- Born in 1962
- Independent practice in anthroposophic nursing and as an expert for Assessment and Rehabilitation after severe accidents (e.g., tetraplegia, brain trauma, multiple amputations, and medical errors) for the The National Accident Compensation Corporation (ACC) of New Zealand
- Training as a nurse at the Royal Infirmary of Edinburgh, Scotland, 1983–1986
- Advanced training in nursing in Anthroposophic Medicine at the Ita Wegman Clinic in Arlesheim, near Basel, Switzerland, 1987–1988
- Training as a teaching nurse at the Continuing Education Institute for Nursing and Care for the Elderly in Bad Liebenzell-Unterlengenhardt, Germany in 1989
- 1992 Bachelor of Arts in Nurse Education, Manchester Victoria University, England
- A registered nurse (RN) for the past 28 years
- Intensive Care Unit and Heart Transplant Surgery at Wythenshaw Hospital in Manchester, England, 1990–1991
- Lecturer in nursing at Keele University, England, 1992–1995
- Head of ward and practice development, emergency ward, Russels Hall Hospital in Dudley, England, 1999–2004
- Since 1990: courses in anthroposophic home care for parents and teachers at Waldorf Schools in England and New Zealand
- Co-editor of the second edition of this book

Annegret Camps

- Born in 1951
- Nurse, teacher for nursing professions, KOMED mediator (conflict settlement and mediation)
- Nursing training at Herdecke Community Hospital
- Anthroposophic nursing specialist (IFAN)
- Many years of nursing experience in surgery, accident surgery, internal medicine, geriatrics and geriatric care
- Founded the first anthroposophically oriented training in nursing care for the elderly in Ahrensburg, near Hamburg, Germany, in 1983
- Head of the Seminar for Geriatric Care in Frankfurt/Main, Germany, 1991–2012
- Freelance lecturer since 2012

Bernhard Deckers

- Born in 1957
- Nursing training at Herdecke Community Hospital
- Anthroposophic nursing specialist (IFAN)
- Nurse at the Filderklinik hospital in Filderstadt, near Stuttgart, Germany, since 1986
- Project point for external applications
- Research associate at the ARCIM research institute (Academic Research in Complementary and Integrative Medicine) at Filderklinik hospital

Carola Edelmann

- Born in 1959
- Nurse and pediatric nurse
- Rhythmical massage therapy practitioner
- Anthroposophic nursing specialist (IFAN)
- Olgahospital in Stuttgart, Germany, 1979–1984
- Filderklinik, in Filderstadt, near Stuttgart, Germany, 1985–1989
- Continuing education in anthroposophic parent counseling
- Home pediatric nursing and rhythmical massage therapy with the home care provider Häusliche Kinderkrankenpflege e.V. in Stuttgart, Germany, since 1991
- Parent counseling

Sasha Gloor

- Born in 1968
- Certified physical education teacher
- Nurse HF (higher vocational school)
- Anthroposophic nursing specialist (IFAN)
- Expert in Rhythmical Einreibung according to Wegman/Hauschka (IFAP)
- Nurse HF in the Lukas Clinic in Arlesheim, near Basel, Switzerland for 12 years
- Coordinator and lecturer in the Soleo nursing continuing education course at Klinik Arlesheim, Switzerland, since 2009
- Lecturer in the basic and advanced course for anthroposophic nursing in Nagoya, Japan, since 2010

Christel Kaul

- Born in 1943
- Geriatric nurse
- Waldorf teacher
- Conflict consultant
- Management of the inpatient nursing home Altenwerk Marthashofen, in Grafrath, Germany
- Lecturing activity

Monika Layer

- Born in 1957
- Certified nurse, teacher for nursing professions
- Master of Advanced Studies (MAS) in Public Management at the college Zürcher Fachhochschule (ZFH)
- Anthroposophic nursing specialist (IFAN)
- Expert in Rhythmical Einreibung according to Wegman/Hauschka (IFAP)
- Certified nurse in Germany and Switzerland (including Klinik Öschelbronn in Öschelbronn, Germany, and Lukas Clinic in Arlesheim, Switzerland)
- Teacher for nursing professions and head of the Independent Nursing School at the Filderklinik Hospital
- Training and continuing education of nursing staff, including Head of Further Training and Education at Frauenfeld Cantonal Hospital (Switzerland) and Head of Education at Winterthur Cantonal Hospital (Switzerland)
- Various specialist publications, including publication of the work "Praxishandbuch Rhythmische Einreibungen nach Wegman/Hauschka", 2nd ed. Hans Huber Verlag, Bern 2014. Translated as *Handbook for Rhythmical Einreibungen according to Wegman/Hauschka*, Temple Lodge, Forest Row 2006
- Head of Nursing at the Center for Integrative Medicine at St. Gallen Cantonal Hospital, Switzerland, since 2010
- President of the Swiss Nursing Association (APIS-SAES)
- Member of the Board of the International Forum for Anthroposophic Nursing (IFAP)
- Lecturing activity

Heike Schaumann

- Born in 1962
- Nurse
- Certified social worker/social educator
- Nursing training at Herdecke Community Hospital, 1983–1986
- Social worker in a counseling center for people with dementia and their relatives in Kassel, Germany, since 2004
- Head of a home community for people with dementia in Kassel, Germany, since 2007
- Teaching activity at a nursing school for the elderly
- Advanced training courses on dementia

Jana Schier

- Born in 1976
- Nursing training at the county hospital KKH Grossenhain in Germany
- Two years of experience as a nurse in the surgical ward of KKH Grossenhain
- Nurse in the oncology hospital Helios Klinik Dresden-Wachwitz (formerly Humaine Klinik Dresden) in Dresden, Germany, 1998–2008
- Participation in the Anthroposophic Nursing Seminar in Dresden

- Basic anthroposophic course, advanced training in compresses and Rhythmical Einreibung according to Wegman/Hauschka at Filderklinik hospital in Filderstadt, Germany
- Nurse in the Center for Integrative Oncology at the Filderklinik hospital, with a focus on antitumoral therapy (implementation, patient support, side-effect management) since 2008
- Collaboration in the area of nursing care within the cancer network Onkologischer Schwerpunkt Esslingen
- Lecturing activity

Ada van der Star
- Born in 1949
- Nurse and kinesthetics trainer
- Studied medical education at the Martin Luther University of Halle-Wittenberg
- Studied eurythmy in Vienna, Austria (Bildungsstätte für Eurythmie)
- Anthroposophic nursing specialist (IFAN)
- Many years of nursing experience in internal medicine, neurology, psychiatrics, geriatrics and geriatric care
- Founded the first anthroposophically oriented training in nursing care for the elderly in Ahrensburg, near Hamburg, Germany, in 1983
- Head of the Seminar for Geriatric Care in Frankfurt/Main, Germany, 1991–2012
- Freelance lecturer and biography guide since 2011

Christoph von Dach
- Born in 1966
- Nurse HF (higher vocational school)
- Master of Science (MS) in Palliative Care
- Anthroposophic nursing specialist (IFAN)
- Head of Nursing at the Lukas Clinic in Arlesheim, near Basel, Switzerland, for 15 years
- Clinical Nursing Scientist at the Center for Clinical Nursing Science of the University Hospital Zurich
- Project Manager for Palliative Care at the University Hospital Zurich
- Module manager "Palliative Care" at the Kalaidos University of Applied Sciences in Zurich, Switzerland
- Co-initiator of and lecturer for the foundation courses and continuing education courses in anthroposophic nursing in Fair Oaks, near Sacramento, USA
- Lectures in Germany and abroad

Gabriele Weber
- Born in 1960
- Certified vocational educator (FH)

- Certified nurse
- Anthroposophic nursing specialist (IFAN)
- Several years of experience in internal medicine, including at Herdecke Community Hospital
- Work as a nursing educator in training, further training and continuing education, including for the Association of Anthroposophic Nursing Professions since 1991
- Nursing educator and director of the Dörthe Krause Institute in Herdecke, Germany, focus on further training and continuing education

Index

Onions 302
Open-mindedness 116
Organ Rhythmical Einreibung 263
Osteoarthritis
  Cabbage compress 286
Over-excitedness 301
Overheating 247
  Local 247
Oxalis e planta tota W 10%, Oleum 442,
  453–455
Oxalis Essence 442, 517
Oxalis, Folium 10% 359, 442, 517
Oxalis, Folium 20% 442, 455, 517

P
_____

Pain
  Cancer 446
Painful conditions
  Rhythmical Einreibung 272
Pain relief 549
Palliative Care 508
  Breathing 515
  Dying processes 510
  Elimination 520
  External applications 513
  Growth 523
  Maintenance 521
  Nutrition 519
  Origins 508
  Pain 512
  Reproduction 523
  Sedation 513
Palliative therapy 434
Parental counselling 347–348
Parent-child relationship 375
Paresthesia
  Cancer 457
Partial body Rhythmical Einreibung 263
Passive heat treatment 247
Pastoral care
  Dying people 553
Path of development 78, 95
Patients 52, 242
  social impact 75
  Somnolent 242
Patient review 85
Peat lavender oil 154
Pentagram Rhythmical Einreibung 264
Peppermint 255
Perception 46
Personality 35

Personality disorders 402
  Guidelines 403
Phenomenological-physical perspective 319
Physical body 39, 544
Physiology 39
Phytolacca 358
Pine Reviving Bath Milk 253, 477
Placenta 510
Plantago Bronchialbalsam 246, 449, 517
Plant extracts 292
Platinum derivatives 458
Pleural effusions 250, 449
Plumbum metallicum 0.4% 517, 394, 519
Pneumonia 240, 255, 316
  Pneumonia prophylaxis 245, 255
Point-Circle meditation 106
Polyneuropathy
  Cancer 457
Positivity 91, 116
Post-treatment rest 309
Poultices 277, 289, 303
Prayer 103
Pregnancy 337
Preparation 109
Pressure relief 248
Primal rhythm 203
Primula (primrose) muscle oil 522
Propolis mother tincture 522
Protecting 136
  Child 136
  Dying people 156
Prunus spinosa e floribus W 5%, Oleum 267,
  268, 452, 457, 518
Psychiatrics 384
Psychoanalysis 42
Psychoeducation 379
Psychosis 392
Psychotherapy 42, 394
Psychotropic drugs 383
Puerperium 343, 348
Pulse 101
Purification
  After death 545

Q
_____

Quartz sand 302

R
_____

Randomized Controlled Trial 322
Rathania comp. 457